ANTIBIOTIC RESISTANCE:
CAUSES AND RISK FACTORS,
MECHANISMS AND ALTERNATIVES

PHARMACOLOGY – RESEARCH, SAFETY TESTING AND REGULATION SERIES

Poisons: Physiologically Active Substances
S. B. Zotov and O. I. Tuzhikov
ISBN: 978-1-60741-973-0

Antibiotic Resistance: Causes and Risk Factors, Mechanisms and Alternatives
Adriel R. Bonilla and Kaden P. Muniz (Editors)
2009 ISBN: 978-1-60741-623-4

PHARMACOLOGY – RESEARCH, SAFETY TESTING AND REGULATION SERIES

ANTIBIOTIC RESISTANCE: CAUSES AND RISK FACTORS, MECHANISMS AND ALTERNATIVES

ADRIEL R. BONILLA
AND
KADEN P. MUNIZ
EDITORS

Nova Science Publishers, Inc.
New York

Library of Congress Cataloging-in-Publication Data

Antibiotic resistance : causes and risk factors, mechanisms and alternatives / [edited by] Adriel R. Bonilla and Kaden P. Muniz.
   p. ; cm.
 Includes bibliographical references and index.
 ISBN 978-1-60741-623-4 (hardcover : alk. paper)
 1. Drug resistance in microorganisms. I. Bonilla, Adriel R. II. Muniz, Kaden P.
 [DNLM: 1. Drug Resistance, Bacterial. 2. Anti-Bacterial Agents--therapeutic use. QW 52 A6287 2009]
 QR177.A55 2009
 616.9'041--dc22
                                                                    2009024616

Published by Nova Science Publishers, Inc. ✦ *New York*

Contents

Preface

Antibiotic resistance is the ability of a microorganism to withstand the effects of antibiotics. There are three mechanisms that can cause antibiotic resistance: prevention of interaction of drug with target, decreased uptake due to either an increased efflux or a decreased influx of the antimicrobial agent and enzymatic modification or destruction of the compound. In the past couple years, antibiotic resistance has become an increasing public health concern. Tuberculosis, gonorrhea, malaria and childhood ear infections are just a few of the diseases that have become hard to treat with antibiotic drugs. This book addresses the concern that over the past few years, there has been a major rise in resistance to antibiotics among gram-negative bacteria. New antibacterial drugs with novel modes of actions are urgently required in order to fight against infection. Novel antibiotics such as linezolid, carbapenem ertapenem, daptomycin and gemifloxacin are examined in this book. The genetic approaches used in risk assessment of antibiotic resistance dissemination are looked at as well. Furthermore, this book discusses the present studies on the use of veterinary antibiotics in agriculture, on the occurrence of antibiotic compounds and resistant bacteria in soil and water and clearly demonstrates the need for further studies.

Chapter I- The extraordinary capacity of a number of bacterial organisms to develop resistance to antibiotic compounds remains a hot topic on the minds of doctors, hospital staff, reporters, and the community since several years. It is also heralded as a textbook example of "Darwinian evolution" continuously in action. As a consequence, these multiresistant bacteria are being studied also by "evolutionary" scientists, with the hope that they will reveal secrets or trace a pathway as to how molecules-to-man evolution could have happened.

Chapter II - Probiotics are live microorganisms that could confer health benefits on the host once administered in adequate amounts. One of the main benefits of probiotic organisms is their ability to improve gastrointestinal health, where they act as an important biodefense in preventing colonization and subsequent proliferation of pathogenic bacteria in the intestines. Additionally, they have also been used to treat and/or prevent antibiotic resistance in the host via indirect mechanisms. Various studies have shown that probiotics could modulate the immune system of the host leading to a reduced use of antibiotics, and could suppress the growth of pathogenic bacteria thus limiting their transfer of resistant genes to the host.

A long history of safety has contributed to the acceptance of probiotics as a safe food adjunct. However, recent studies have reported the occurrence of antibiotic resistance in probiotics. Probiotics have also been found to translocate and were isolated from infected lesions such as bacterial endocarditis and blood stream infections. These have led to the need for further assessment of probiotics so that their negative consequences do not outweigh their benefits. Antibiotic resistance and the ability to translocate of probiotics are now emphasized and are suggested to be made as criteria for safety assessment and labeling prior to their use as food supplements.

Much attention has been given to the factors and mechanisms involved on the acquired antibiotic resistance of probiotics. Some studies have found that the species and origins of the strains could affect the acquiring of antibiotic resistance, while others have demonstrated that genes coding for antibiotic resistance are transferable among bacteria of different origins. Recent laboratory advances have provided more details and information on some postulated mechanisms. Probiotics could be antibiotic resistant inherently or acquired via vertical evolution such as inactivation of enzymes, alteration of membrane protein channels and efflux pumps, and/or via horizontal evolution of gene exchange.

Although antibiotic resistance of probiotics is rarely life threatening, it may serve as a marker of more serious underlying diseases. This review will also present some in-vitro and in-vivo evidence of the detections and isolation of antibiotic resistant probiotics, epidemiology of strains found, and their surveillance, monitoring and disposal once detected. There are also efforts to evaluate the need for elimination of antibiotic resistance although few probiotics meant for human consumption are classified as resistant. Past reports have found that a failure to demonstrate in-vitro horizontal gene transfer could not be used as a yardstick to exclude the risk of dissemination of genes. It has been suggested that genetic approaches are needed to eliminate antibiotic resistance, one being selective removal of plasmids coding for antibiotic resistance. However, the issues of phenotypical and genotypical alteration of the strain arise and that the impact of the genetic changes on the probiotic properties remains unknown. The present review will also highlight the genetic approaches used in risk assessment of antibiotic resistance dissemination.

Chapter III - An ever increasing dependence on conventional therapeutics coupled with an alarming escalation in antibiotic resistance has facilitated the emergence of a new faction of bacterial adversaries, the antibiotic resistant 'superbugs', the aetiological agents of nosocomial infections. Against this backdrop scientists and clinicians are now struggling to find viable therapeutic alternatives to antibiotics. One such alternative involves the use of probiotics; live microorganisms, which when consumed in adequate amounts, confer a health benefit to the host. Furthermore, a new generation of probiotics termed 'designer probiotics' have been engineered to target and neutralise specific bacterial pathogens, viruses and toxins while at the same time persisting for longer periods in foods and other delivery vehicles prior to ingestion and subsequently within the gastrointestinal tract.

Chapter IV - Antibiotics are among the most beneficial drugs ever introduced but their utility has been compromised by the emergence and spread of antibiotic resistant bacteria. Currently useful antibiotics impose enormous selective pressure on bacterial populations and the use and overuse of these agents has led to the evolution, in a relatively short timeframe, of multidrug-resistant pathogens capable of rapid and efficient horizontal transmission of genes encoding resistance determinants. New antibacterial drugs with novel modes of action are urgently required in order to continue the fight against infection: unfortunately, the upturn in the incidence of resistance has coincided with a marked reduction by the pharmaceutical industry in efforts to develop new agents. Even "professional" pathogens such as *Staphylococcus aureus*, a bacterium equipped with an impressive array of virulence effectors for damaging the host, require a reduction in the host's defenses in order to colonize, enter tissue and cause infection. Correction of this imbalance between host and pathogen may provide a novel approach to the therapy of severe bacterial infections, by either shoring up immune defenses or modifying the bacteria at the site of infection to render them less able to survive in the host. Thus, pathogens may survive, multiply and cause infection because they are virulent or resistant to antibiotics; therapeutic agents that modify these properties *in vivo* may resolve infections, either alone or in combination with conventional antibiotic chemotherapy, in a way that may not readily lead to drug resistant bacterial survivors. Examples of such modifiers of the bacterial phenotype, together with other emerging approaches to the treatment of bacterial infections, are described.

Chapter V - *Staphylococcus aureus*, *Streptococcus agalactiae* and *Enterococcus* spp. are bacteria with a high capacity for acquiring determinants of resistance to antibiotics, giving rise to multi-resistance problems. It is assumed that this is related to consumption of antibiotics. The study objectives were to determine the antibiotic susceptibility of these three species in two Spanish hospitals and establish the relationship between consumption of antibiotics and their activity. The activity of antibiotics was evaluated against 1000 clinical isolates of *S. aureus*, *Enterococcus* spp. and *S. agalactiae* identified in the Microbiology Services of San Cecilio Hospital in Granada and Valme Hospital in Seville, determining the relationship between the consumption of antibiotics and susceptibility findings. Glycopeptides and linezolid were the only antibiotics active against 100% of clinical isolates of *S. aureus*, with cotrimoxazole and rifampicin also showing excellent activity. All isolates of *S. agalactiae* were susceptible to ampicillin, cefotaxime, vancomycin and linezolid, with an excellent activity for levofloxacin. All enterococci were susceptible to ampicillin, glycopeptides and linezolid. Finally, a statistically significant inverse relationship was found for the whole set of antibiotics between their consumption and the susceptibility to them of *S. aureus*. The three species retained susceptibility to glycopeptides and linezolid. A good susceptibility was also shown by *S. aureus* to cotrimoxazole and rifampicin and by enterococci and *S. agalactiae* to ampicillin. There was a significant association between antibiotic consumption and rates of resistance to *S. aureus*.

Chapter VI - The past few years have seen a major rise in resistance to antibiotics among Gram-negative bacteria (beta-lactamase [ESBL]-producing enterobacteria, carbapenem-resistant *P. aeruginosa* and *A. baumannii* ...) and, especially, among Gram-positive bacteria (methicillin-resistant *S. aureus* [MRSA], glycopeptide-intermediate [GISA] or resistant *S. aureus* [GRSA], vancomycin-resistant enterococci [VRE], multi-drug resistant *S. pneumoniae* [MDRSP]). This trend has considerably reduced therapeutic options and brought about a need for novel antibiotics, which have been approved by the Food and Drugs Administration (FDA) since 2000.

The first of these was linezolid, an oxazolidinone for the treatment of nosocomial and community-acquired pneumonias and skin and soft tissue infections caused by Gram-positive bacteria, including MRSA, GRSA, VRE, and MDRSP. The cephalosporin cefditoren pivoxil was approved to treat community-acquired respiratory infections (upper and lower airways) and uncomplicated infections of skin and soft tissues produced by Gram-positive or -negative bacteria that are not resistant to this group of antibiotics.

The carbapenem ertapenem is indicated for the treatment of intra-abdominal, skin and soft tissue infections, and community acquired pneumonia caused by Gram-positive or-negative microorganisms and is especially indicated for infections produced by ESBL-producing enterobacteria. Doripenem is a new carbapenem that can be used against intra-abdominal and urinary infections due to Gram-negative or -positive microorganisms at a lower dose than required for other antibiotics in this group.

Daptomycin is a useful antibiotic for monotherapy of bacteremia and skin and soft tissue infections caused by Gram-positive multiresistant bacteria (MRSA, GISA, GRSA).

Gemifloxacin is a new quinolone for treating respiratory infections (e.g., community pneumonia or bronchitis) caused by Gram-positive and –negative bacteria, including MDRSP. Telithromycin offers an alternative treatment for community-acquired pneumonia due to Gram-positive and –negative microorganisms, including MDRSP.

Tigecycline was approved for intra-abdominal, skin, and soft tissue infections caused by Gram-positive and–negative bacteria, including multi-resistant bacteria (ESBL, MRSA).

Retapamulin is used topically for impetigo produced by Gram-positive microorganisms.The objective of our study will be to review the *in vitro* antibiotic activity, action mechanisms, and resistance (if reported) of the above antibiotics and to describe their pharmacokinetic and pharmacodynamic properties.

Chapter VII - Bacteriophages (phages) and bacterial cell wall hydrolases (BCWHs) have been recognized as promising alternative antibacterials. Phages are bacterial virsuses that kill bacteria by causing bacteriolysis. It is estimated that there are about 10^{31} phages on earth and approximately 5,100 have been identified and reported towards the end of last century, providing a vast pool of candidates for applications such as phage therapy. Phages are highly effective and specific to target bacteria. They have been generally accepted as effective antibacterials that could potentially provide safe and cost effective means for the treatment and prophylaxis of bacterial infections. BCWHs are lytic enzymes that cause bacteriolysis by hydrolyzing the peptidoglycan of bacterial cell wall. BCWHs are also called enzybiotics because they are enzymes that have antibiotic-like antibacterial activities. They are produced by amost all cellular organisms including microorganisms, plants, and animals. Virolysins (also called lysins, endolysins) are a special group of BCWHs encoded by phages but produced naturally by bacteria infected by lytic phages. They are probably the most promising enzybiotics.

Chapter VIII - Antibiotic resistance can occur via three mechanisms: prevention of interaction of the drug with target; decreased uptake due to either an increased efflux or a decreased influx of the antimicrobial agent and enzymatic modification or destruction of the compound. Herein we review the results from computational studies on said mechanisms. For the first mechanism, the bacteria produce mutant versions of antibiotic targets. This process has been studied using several levels of theory, from costly quantum mechanics calculations to classical molecular dynamics calculations. For the decreased uptake mechanisms, since the atomic structure of several influx pores and efflux pumps were resolved recently, homology modelling studies and large molecular dynamics simulations allow us to understand this resistance mechanism at the molecular level. Computational studies with antibiotic molecules (mainly *β*-lactam compounds) studying the resistance mechanism in which the antibiotic compound is transformed will be also summarized. *β*-lactamases are bacterial enzymes responsible for most of the resistance against *β*-lactam antibiotics. These defensive enzymes, prevalent in nearly every pathogenic bacterial strain, hydrolyze the *β*-lactam ring and release the cleaved, inactive antibiotics. Computational studies on this reaction provided us with knowledge on the molecular mechanism of action of these enzymes. The results may prove valuable in the design of new antibiotic derivatives with improved activity in resistant strains. Finally, a case study on the mechanism of resistance of fluoroquinolones is explained in detail. Extensive use and misuse of fluoroquinolones in human and veterinary medicine has led to the emergence and spread of resistant clones. These have appeared mainly through mutations in the structural genes that encode their intracellular targets (DNA gyrase and topoisomerase IV) as well as via modifications in membrane permeability (e.g. decreased influx and/or increased efflux). We analyzed bacterial resistance to fluoroquinolones that arises from mutations in the DNA gyrase target protein. We studied the binding mode of ciprofloxacin, levofloxacin, and moxifloxacin to DNA gyrase by docking calculations. The binding model obtained enabled us to study, at the atomic level, the resistance mechanism associated with the most common gyrA mutations in *E. coli* fluoroquinolone-resistant strains.

Chapter IX - Multidrug efflux pumps are important in microbial resistance to antibiotics. The energetics of some systems has been characterised in vitro but the impact on whole cell energetics is less studied. In this chapter, after the rapid presentation of the different MDR efflux families, the energetics of some MDR transporters will be described. The impact of these transporters on cell energetics is discussed and the difficulties in studying MDR efflux energetics in whole cell systems will be presented with a description of available techniques. The importance of this field of investigation will be demonstrated with an example of a microbial global strategy to resist to a cationic compound.

Chapter X - The activity of 12 antibiotics in Mueller-Hinton (MH) broth and Nutrient-Broth (NB) was assessed by microdilution in 50 clinical isolates of *Escherichia coli* producers of extended-spectrum beta-lactamases (ESBLs). In addition, the expression pattern of OmpC and OmpF porins was analyzed after culture of isolates in the two media. Three porin expression patterns were obtained: 13 isolates expressed both porins in both media, 8 expressed one porin in both media, and 29 expressed both porins in NB and one in MH. Analysis of the relationship between modification of porin expression and MIC values of the different antibiotics tested was unable to demonstrate, using this methodology, that porin loss was responsible for clinically relevant changes in the MIC of these clinical isolates.

Chapter XI - China has become the largest mariculture country of the world. The extensive and intense use of antibiotics in mariculture for the prevention and treatment of microbial infections of the farmed marine animals exerts a selective pressure on environmental bacteria. The mariculture environment may have become a reservoir and dissemination source of antibiotic resistance. The prevalence of antibiotic resistance may undermine the effectiveness of various antibiotics, alter the natural microbiota, disturb the ecological equilibria, and create a potential threat to human health and welfare. The emergence of antibiotic resistant bacteria in mariculture and related environments has become a great concern of environmental and human health. There is an urgent need to develop a monitoring platform to investigate the antibiotic resistant bacteria and their resistance mechanisms in mariculture environments, for effective prevention and control of the spread and evolution of harmful antibiotic resistant bacteria and their resistance determinants. Certain research effort has been made to evaluate the abundance and diversity of the antibiotic-resistant microbes and their resistance genes in China mariculture environments. A preliminary review on this issue is provided in this paper. As the biggest mariculture country, China will take the responsibility and resolution for the control and elimination of antibiotic resistance in mariculture environment.

Chapter XII - Understanding the origin of fecal pollution is essential in assessing potential health risks as well as for determining the actions necessary to remediate the problem of waters contaminated by fecal matter. As a result, microbial source tracking (MST) methods aimed at determining sources of fecal pollution have evolved over the past decade. Antibiotic resistance analysis (ARA) has emerged as one MST tool that has proven useful for determining the sources of fecal pollution in environmental waters.

Antibiotic resistance analysis is a simple, rapid, and inexpensive method for performing MST. It is a published method that has been independently validated by a variety of tests designed to improve library-based methods, and is currently being used in laboratories across the United States as well as internationally.

The ARA method is based on the rationale that antibiotics exert selective pressure on the fecal flora of the animals that ingest antibiotics. Different types of animals receive differential exposure to antibiotics and as a result, different animals will have bacteria with at least reasonably source-specific patterns of antibiotic resistance. The ARA procedure involves the isolation and culturing of a target organism, (usually *Escherichia coli* or *Enterococcus sp.*), then replica plating the isolates on media containing various antibiotics at pre-selected concentrations. After the plates are incubated, the organisms are scored according to their resistance to the antibiotics to generate an antibiotic resistance profile (phenotypic fingerprint). These fingerprints are then evaluated by a multivariate statistical method such as discriminate analysis (DA).

Discriminant analysis classifies the bacteria based on shared patterns of antibiotic resistance, and the results are pooled to form a "known source database" (or library) of antibiotic resistance patterns from different fecal sources. The known source database is summarized in the form of a classification table. The average rate of correct classification is the average rate that known source isolates are correctly classified, and is used to measure the reliability of the library. Additional method performance criteria to ensure the reliability of the database are also used, including library decloning, construction of larger libraries representing more diverse host populations, and realistic tests of method accuracy, such as incorporating independently collected proficiency isolates and samples. Isolates recovered from water samples are compared to the known source database to identify an isolate as being either human or animal derived.

Antibiotic resistance analysis is an MST tool that is most appropriate for small, relatively simple rural watersheds. The application of ARA to large-scale complex systems is more problematic as the wider genetic variability present in target organism populations impacts the phenotypic expression of antibiotic resistance. The potential of this genetic diversity occurring in many different host sources leads to the concern of not being able to fully capture that diversity in a known source library, with subsequent reductions in classification accuracy of water isolates (unknown sources). This is particularly relevant when multiple sources of pollution are contributing to watershed contamination at comparatively similar levels. However, the method performance issues that must be addressed with ARA (and are described in this chapter) are identical for any library-based approach and can also be modified to evaluate library-independent MST methods as well.

This chapter describes the advantages and disadvantages of ARA, presents case studies where the method has been used in a variety of different environmental situations, responds to criticisms of ARA, and details six method performance criteria that should be applied to every MST method. Such evaluations are long overdue in the rapidly developing field of MST.

Chapter XIII - The response of bacteria to a given antibiotic or other toxic agent that does not immediately kill them results in an adaptive response that secures their survival. This response may involve a number of distinct mechanisms, among which is the activation of genes that promote the appearance of transporters that extrude the agent prior to its reaching its target. These transporters extrude a large variety of chemically unrelated compounds and hence they bestow on the bacterium a multi-drug resistant (MDR) phenotype. The appearance of this MDR phenotype during therapy makes therapy problematic. Understanding the genetic and physiological properties of MDR efflux pumps is an absolute requirement if MDR bacterial infections are to be successfully managed. There is much to learn and methods that afford the needed understanding will eventually pave the way for the successful management of an MDR bacterial infection. Therefore, the application of recently developed methods that assess the MDR bacterium at its genetic and physiological levels is the focus of this chapter. The material presented in this chapter is only the beginning for the evaluation and assessment of MDR efflux pumps.

Chapter XIV - The reemergence of Mycobacterium tuberculosis with increasing numbers of multi-drug resistant (MDR) strains has increased the need for rapid diagnostic methods.

Molecular bases of drug resistance have been identified for all of the main antituberculous drugs, and drug resistance results from changes in several target genes, some of which are still undefined. Drug resistance in M. tuberculosis is due to the acquisition of mutations in chromosomally encoded genes and the generation of multidrug resistance is a consequence of serial accumulation of mutations primarily due to inadequate therapy. Several studies have shown that resistance to isoniazid (INTI) is due to mutaions in kat G gene. The rpo B gene, which encodes the subunit of RNA polymerase, harbors a mutation in an 81 bp region in about 95% of rifampicin (RIF) reistant M. tuberculosis strains recovered globally. Streptomycin (STR) resistance is due to mutations in rrs and rpsl genes which encodes 16S SrRNA and ribosomal protein S12 respectively. Approximately 65% of clinical isolates resistant to ethambutol have a mutation in the embB gene.

Several susceptibility phenotypes methods have been developed. Among them were radiometric systems such as the BACTEC460 TB system reduces the test time considerably, but they still labor intensive, expensive and require manipulation of radioactive substances.

Rapid promising approach to determine drug resistant strains especially for rifampicin (RIF) is the use of mycobacteriophage. A number of low-cost colorimetric AST assays, such as the 3-(4,5-dimethylthiazol- 2-yl)-2,5-diphenyl tetrazolium bromide (MTT) assay, the Alamar blue assay, and an assay based on microscopic detection of cord-like growth by *M.*

tuberculosis, have been described. However, these tests have limitations; mycobacteria other than *M. tuberculosis* can produce cord factor, and INH can interfere with the formazan production in the MTT assay and give rise to false resistant results. Moreover, the use of a liquid medium in a microtiter plate format in these tests may be disadvantageous not only as a biohazard but also due to possible Contamination between wells.

The goal of the present study is to characterize 100 drug-resistant Mycobacterium tuberculosis (MTB) isolates with respect to their drug susceptibility phenotypes to four common anti-tuberculosis drugs (rifampicin, ethambutol, isoniazid andstreptomycin) and the relationship between such phenotypes and the patterns of genetic mutations in the corresponding resistance genes (rpoB, embB, katG, Rpsl) METHODS: The MIC values of the aforementioned anti-tuberculosis drugs were determined for each of the 100 drug-resistant MTB clinical isolates by the absolute concentration method and by BACTEC460). Genetic mutations in the corresponding resistance genes in these MTB isolates were identified by PCR-single-stranded conformation polymorphism/multiplex PCR amplimer conformation analysis (SSCP/MPAC).

Phenotypic resistance was found in all isolates. All isolates were resistant to ethambutol, 70% isolates were resistant to isoniazid, 50% isolates were resistant to streptomycin and 20% of the isolates were resistant to rifampicin. Genotypic mutations in the studied resistance to rifampicin, isoniazid, streptomycin and ethambutol were 20%, 70%, 80%, and 100% respectively.

These findings expand the spectrum of potential resistance-related mutations in MTB clinical isolates and help consolidate the framework for the development of molecular methods for delineating the drug susceptibility profiles of MTB isolates in clinical laboratories.

Chapter XV - In the last decades, osteoporosis has become a major subject in the field of drug discovery and design. One of the proteins recently considered relevant to use as a drug target is the membrane-bound enzyme H^+-V_O-ATPase. This proton pump is located in the osteoclast cells, which are positioned at the bone surface. In these cells the enzyme controls the proton flux to the bone and consequently bone resorption. One major task on drug design is the knowledge of the secondary and tertiary structure of the enzyme involved. The topology of the V-ATPase protein complex has been largely established, however, the three-dimensional structure is only known for some individual subunits. This chapter reviews our recently published work on the secondary and tertiary structure of the proton translocation channel located in subunit *a* of the V-ATPase complex. For this purpose, we designed two peptides consisting of 25 and 37 amino acid residues, representing the seventh transmembrane segment of subunit *a*, which encompass the proton translocation channel as well as the region of interest for interaction with possible inhibitors. Using a combination of NMR (nuclear magnetic resonance) and CD (circular dichroism) spectroscopy the structure of these V-ATPase peptides was studied in different membrane-mimicking environments. The results indicate that a primordial transmembrane segment of this protein region adopts an □-helical conformation and is longer than proposed by topological studies. Moreover, this segment exhibits a hinge region located near the cytoplasmic end of the channel. It is proposed that the presence of this hinge allows the opening and closing of the proton translocation channel and provides flexibility for the channel to act as a binding pocket for inhibitors. These findings can be used as tools in the design of new drugs that can control the activity of V-ATPase in osteoclast cells, helping in this way the fight against osteoporosis.

Chapter XVI - The emergence of antimicrobial-resistant microorganisms in both humans and livestock is a growing concern. In recent years, increased focus has been given to food as a carrier of antibiotic resistance (AR) genes. However, there have been few systematic studies to investigate acquired AR in lactic acid bacteria (LAB), which constitute common components of the microbial community of food and play a relevant role in food fermentation. In Europe, the Food Safety Agency (EFSA) received a request to assess the safety of microorganisms throughout the food chain and proposed the Qualified Presumption of Safety (QPS) approach. In the QPS approach, safety assessment will depend upon the body of knowledge available for a given microorganism. Apparently, there are no specific concerns regarding most of the food-associated LAB species, which have a long history of safe use in the food chain, provided that the lack of acquired AR is systematically demonstrated. Consequently, increased efforts have been devoted in recent years to gain more insight into the diffusion of AR phenotypes within food-associated LAB, with particular emphasis on those applied as starter cultures or probiotics. Presently available literature data support the view that, in antibiotic-challenged habitats, LAB (especially enterococci) like other bacteria are involved in the transfer of resistance traits over species and genus borders, with important safety implications. The prevalence of such bacteria with acquired genetically-exchangeable resistances is high in animals and humans that are regularly treated with antibiotics. This led to the European ban of the antibiotics used as growth promoters in animal feed. Such measures should, however, be complemented by a more prudent use of antibiotics in both human and animal clinical therapy.

Chapter XVII - Lactic acid bacteria (LAB) consist of the genera *Lactobacillus, Carnobacterium, Lactococcus, Enterococcus, Streptococcus, Leuconostoc, Pediococcus, Desemzia, Isobacilum, Paralactobacillus, Tetragenococcus, Trichococcus, Weissella, Oenococcus* and *Melissococcus* and are present in many different habitats, including food and the human and animal intestinal tract. The long history of LAB with fermented foods have bestowed on them GRAS (generally regarded as safe) status. Intestinal strains play an important role in ensuring a healthy microbial balance. Their presence may lead to increased cytokine production and they may even play a role in preventing the growth of carcinogenic cells. A few rare cases of excessive immune stimulation, systemic infections, arthritis and the formation of hepatobiliary lesions have been reported for some strains of LAB. Such symptoms are usually associated with strains penetrating the mucus layer and epithelial cells. Lactic acid bacteria in food and the gastro-intestinal (GI) tract could act as a potential reservoir of antibiotic resistance genes and may participate in the exchange of genes with strains present in same environment to produce multidrug resistant strains. *Lactobacillus, Pediococcus* and *Leuconostoc* spp. have a high natural resistance to vancomycin. Some *Lactobacillus* spp. are by nature resistant to bacitracin, cefoxitin, ciprofloxacin, fusidic acid, kanamycin, gentamycin, metronidazole, nitrofurantoin, norfloxacin, streptomycin, sulphadiazine, teicoplanin, trimethoprim/sulphamethoxazole, and vancomycin. A few cases of *Enterococcus* infection have been associated with abnormal physiological conditions, underlying disease and immunosuppression. *Enterococcus faecalis* is the most dominant species in general GI infections, whereas *Enterococcus faecium* may cause enterococcal bacteremia. Enterococci have intrinsic resistance to cephalosporins, beta-lactams, sulphonamides and low levels of clindamycin and aminoglycosides. Resistance to chloramphenicol, erythromycin, high levels of clindamycin, aminoglycosides, tetracycline, β-lactams (β-lactamase or penicillinase), fluoroquinolones and glycopeptides is usually acquired. Vancomycin-resistant enterococci (VRE) with *van*A, *van*B, *van*C1, *van*C2, *van*C3, *van*D and *van*E genes have led to a number of nosocomial infections. VanA-type strains confer high level inducible resistance to vancomycin and teicoplanin, whereas VanB-type strains display variable levels of inducible resistance. VRE are highly resistant to most antibiotics and successful treatment is a major problem. The aim of this review is to discuss antibiotic resistance amongst LAB and highlight the genetic determinants involved in horizontal and vertical transfer of resistance genes.

Chapter XVIII - One of the major medical advances of the 20th century has been the development of effective antibiotics which have had a profound impact on the quality of human life. The ability to treat and cure deadly infections and bacterial diseases has forever changed our medical profession and way of life, providing unprecedented relief from pain, suffering, and death due to microbial infection. However, consistent overuse and misuse of powerful broad-spectrum antibiotics over several decades has added to and indeed accelerated the spread of microbial drug resistance. Resistance mechanisms have been found for every class of antibiotic agent used clinically. A major global healthcare problem relates to serious infections caused by bacteria having resistance to commonly used antibiotics. Not only are such infections typically more severe than those of antibiotic-responsive ones, they also require more aggressive interventive measures and are thus significantly more difficult and expensive to treat. Consequently, as we enter the 21st century, a pressing need exists for novel approaches to effectively deal with drug-resistant microbes and the health problems they pose. Nature may provide answers to help guide us, in the form of viral warriors known as bacteriophages, as a means to control and subdue pathogenic bacteria in their natural habitat. Like phages, which emerged presumably through a long evolutionary process, researchers now are acquiring the capabilities to target and neutralize deadly bacteria with *nano*particle-based anti*biotics*, or *nanobiotics*. This chapter discusses the different types of nanobiotics being investigated for delivering and improving therapeutic efficacy of a wide assortment of anti-infectives. The emphasis will be on nanoparticle containers or vehicles to overcome bacterial drug resistance that in essence protect and deliver various classes of antibiotic drugs, including □-lactams, fluoroquinolones, gentamycin, and vancomycin. A brief synopsis is provided on the role nanobiotics could play in drug discovery and development.

Chapter XIX - In this chapter, recent studies on the fate of antibiotics, and especially antibiotics used in animal husbandry, are evaluated under the aspect of potential risks for human health. Because the assumed quantity of antibiotics excreted by animal husbandry adds up to thousands of tons per year, major concerns about their degradation in the environment have risen during the last decades. One main problem with regard to the excessive use of antibiotics in livestock production is the potential promotion of resistance and the resulting disadvantages in the therapeutic use of antimicrobials. Since the beginning of antibiotic therapy, more and more resistant bacterial strains have been isolated from environmental sources showing one or multiple resistance. After administration, the medicines, their metabolites or degradation products reach the terrestrial and aquatic environment indirectly by the application of manure or slurry to areas used agriculturally or directly by pasture-reared animals excreting directly on the land.

After surface run-off, driftage or leaching in deeper layers of the earth, their fate and the impact on environmental bacteria remains rather unknown. Especially against the background of increasing antibiotic resistance, the scientific interest in antimicrobially active compounds in the environment and the possible occurrence of resistant bacteria has increased permanently. On the one side, scientific interest has focused on the behaviour of antibiotics and their fate in the environment, on the other hand, their impact on environmental and other bacteria has become an issue of research. With the advances of modern analytical methods, studies using these new techniques provide accurate data on concentrations of antimicrobial compounds and their residues in different organic matters. Some antibiotics seem to persist a long time in the environment, especially in soil, while others degrade very fast. Not only are the fate of these pharmaceuticals, but also their origin and their possible association with resistant bacteria objects of scientific interest.

This chapter presents an overview of the present studies on the use of veterinary antibiotics in agriculture, on the occurrence of antibiotic compounds and resistant bacteria in soil and water and clearly demonstrates the need for further studies.

In: Antibiotic Resistance: Causes and Risk Factors
Editors: A. R. Bonilla and K. P. Muniz

ISBN 978-1-60741-623-4
© 2009 Nova Science Publishers, Inc.

Chapter I

The Phenomenon of Antibiotic Resistance in an Evolutionary Perspective

*Roberto Manfredi**

Department of Internal Medicine, Aging, and Nephrologic Diseases,
Division of Infectious Diseases, "
Alma Mater Studiorum" University of Bologna,
S. Orsola-Malpighi Hospital, Bologna, Italy

Conflict of interest, sponsorship, fundings, acknowledgments: none.

Keywords: Antimicrobial resistance, spread, evolutionary perspective.

The extraordinary capacity of a number of bacterial organisms to develop resistance to antibiotic compounds remains a hot topic on the minds of doctors, hospital staff, reporters, and the community since several years. It is also heralded as a textbook example of "Darwinian evolution" continuously in action [1, 2]. As a consequence, these multiresistant bacteria are being studied also by "evolutionary" scientists, with the hope that they will reveal secrets or trace a pathway as to how molecules-to-man evolution could have happened [2, 3].

Basically, antibiotics are natural substances secreted by bacteria and fungi in order to kill other bacteria that are competing for limited nutrients; in fact, the majority of present antibiotics are synthetic derivatives of these natural products. Scientists are dismayed to discover that some bacteria have become resistant to antibiotics, mostly through various genomic (chromosomal-, plasmid-, or transposon-carried) mutations.

* Correspondence: Roberto Manfredi, MD. Associate Professor of Infectious Diseases, University of Bologna. c/o Infectious Diseases, S. Orsola Hospital. Via Massarenti 11. I-40138 Bologna, Italy. Telephone: +39-051-6363355. Telefax: +39-051-343500. E-mail: Roberto.manfredi@unibo.it

Changes in natural echosystems, including the release of large amounts of antimicrobial agents in the environment as happened in the last decades, might act on the population dynanmics of microorganisms too, including the selection of resistance determinants, with the visible consequences for human health, in terms of spread of multiresistant organisms in the commumity and especially in hospital facilities [3].

Hospitals have become a breeding ground for antibiotic resistant bacteria, and all microorganisms as whole. In these settings, bacteria proliferate in an "artificial" environment filled with sick people who have some underlying cause of immunodeficiency and concurrent diseases, and where antibiotics have eliminated competing bacteria that are not resistant to used compounds [3].

However, the history learns that bacteria which became resistant to modern antibiotics have even been found in the frozen bodies of people who died long before those antibiotics were discovered or synthesized [4].

As known, antibiotics were first discovered through a providential experiment conducted by Dr. Fleming in late 1920s. His work eventually led to the large-scale production of penicillin from the mold *Penicillium notatum* in the 1940s. Almost concurrently, as early as the late 1940s, resistant strains of penicillin-resistant bacteria began to appear [5]. Currently, it is estimated that over 70% of the different species of bacteria that cause hospital-acquired infections prove resistant to at least one of the antibiotics currently used to treat them [6].

Antibiotic resistance continues to expand for a very broad spectrum of reasons, including over-prescription of antibiotics by physicians, non-completion of prescribed antibiotic treatments by patients, self-prescription of antibiotics by patients themselves, use of antibiotics in animals as growth enhancers, increased international travel, and poor hospital hygiene [5].

In extreme synthesis, bacteria are known to develop antimicrobial resistance through two primary ways:

- By gene mutation, and
- By using a built-in design feature to swap DNA (called horizontal gene transfer); by this last way, bacteria have the possibility to transfer resistance genes among different species which share the same environment.

An antibiotic kills a bacterial cell by simply disrupting an essential structure, or by blocking a critical metabolic function [2]. Antibiotic resistance of bacteria also encompasses a loss of structural and/or functional systems. Anyway, on a general basis the evolutionary mechanisms require a gain of functional systems for bacteria, to evolve into more adaptive organism. For instance, an antibiotic may bind to a specific bacterial protein, so that this last protein cannot function properly. The normal protein is usually involved in copying the DNA, making proteins, or building the bacterial cell wall, all necessary mechanisms for bacteria, to grow and reproduce themselves. If the bacteria have a mutation in the DNA which encodes for one of those proteins, the compound cannot bind to the altered protein; as a direct consequence, the mutant bacteria survive and multiplicate. In the presence of antibiotics, the process of natural selection will occur, favoring the survival and reproduction of the mutant bacteria [2, 3]. Obviously, the mutant bacteria are better able to survive in the presence of the stated antibiotic(s), and will continue to cause illness in the patient, and to increase morbidity and mortality rates.

Although the mutant bacteria can survive well in the hospital environment, from an evolutionary point of view every change occurs at some cost. Actually, i.e. the altered protein is less efficient in performing its normal function, making the bacteria less fit in an specific environment, without the inducing antibiotics [2, 3]. Typically, the non-mutant bacteria are better able to compete for resources and reproduce faster than the mutant form. However, also adaptive mechanisms are activated by resistant microorganisms: the inhibition of some penicillin-binding proteins has been shown to elicit compensative responses in surviving colonies of *Pseudomonas aeruginosa* [7].

Bacteria can also become antibiotic-resistant by gaining mutated DNA from other bacteria. But this still is not an example of evolution in action. No new DNA is generated (a requirement for molecules-to-organism evolution), it is just DNA sequences moving around. However, this mechanism of exchanging DNA is necessary for bacteria to survive in extreme or rapidly changing environments like hospitals or nursing home facilities, or in experimental conditions [2, 8].

The mechanisms of bacterial mutations and natural selection aid microorganism populations in becoming resistant to antibiotics. However, mutation and natural selection also result in bacteria with defective proteins that have lost their normal functions. In general, the evolution process requires a gain of functional systems for bacteria to evolve [2, 3]. Mutation and natural selection, thought to be the driving forces of evolution, only lead to a loss of functional systems. Therefore, antibiotic resistance of bacteria is not an example of "evolution in action", but rather variation within a bacterial kind. It is also a testimony to the wonderful design "the destiny" gave to bacteria, master adapters and survivors in a sin-cursed world [2, 3].

Actually, evolutionary medicine is relevant also to family practice and family physician training, in a wide spectrum of perspectives [9]. Its incorporation into medical training and practice is underway, since its potential scientific burden may be supported by the generation of testable hypotheses and practical applications in relation to both disease pathogenesis, prevention, and treatment [1, 9].

References

[1]   Alpert JS. In Medicine, signs of evolution are ever-present. *Am. J. Med.* 2006; 119:291.

[2]   Gilmore MS. The molecular basis of antibiotic resistance: where Newton meets Darwin. *Int. J. Med. Microbiol.* 2002; 292:65.

[3]   Martínez JL. Antibiotics and antibiotic resistance genes in natural environments. *Science* 2008; 321:365-7.

[4]   Bacterial antibiotic resistance: proof of evolution? www.apologeticspress.org/articles/439

[5]   Antibiotic resistance: How did we get to this? flemingforum.org.uk/slides/antibiotic_resistance.pdf.

[6]   The problem of antimicrobial resistance, National Institute of Allergy and Infectious
       Diseases. www.niaid.nih.gov/factsheets/antimicro.htm/.
[7]   Blázquez J, Gómez- Gómez JM, Oliver A, Juan C, Kapur V, Martín S. PBP3 inhibition
       elicits adaptive responses in *Pseudomonas aeruginosa*. *Mol. Microbiol.* 2006; 62:84-9.
[8]   Is natural selection the same thing as evolution? In *"The New Answers Book"*, Ken
       Ham Ed., Master Books, Green Forest, Arkansas, 2006.
[9]   Naugler CT. Evolutionary medicine: update on the relevance to family practice. *Can.
       Fam. Physician* 2008; 54:1265-9.

In: Antibiotic Resistance: Causes and Risk Factors
Editors: A. R. Bonilla and K. P. Muniz

ISBN 978-1-60741-623-4
© 2009 Nova Science Publishers, Inc.

Chapter II

Antibiotic Resistance and Probiotics: Roles, Mechanisms and Evidence

Min-Tze Liong, Siok-Koon Yeo, Chiu-Yin Kuan,
Wai-Yee Fung and Joo-Ann Ewe*
School of Industrial Technology, Food Technology Division,
Universiti Sains Malaysia, 11800 Penang, Malaysia

Abstract

Probiotics are live microorganisms that could confer health benefits on the host once administered in adequate amounts. One of the main benefits of probiotic organisms is their ability to improve gastrointestinal health, where they act as an important biodefense in preventing colonization and subsequent proliferation of pathogenic bacteria in the intestines. Additionally, they have also been used to treat and/or prevent antibiotic resistance in the host via indirect mechanisms. Various studies have shown that probiotics could modulate the immune system of the host leading to a reduced use of antibiotics, and could suppress the growth of pathogenic bacteria thus limiting their transfer of resistant genes to the host.

A long history of safety has contributed to the acceptance of probiotics as a safe food adjunct. However, recent studies have reported the occurrence of antibiotic resistance in probiotics. Probiotics have also been found to translocate and were isolated from infected lesions such as bacterial endocarditis and blood stream infections. These have led to the need for further assessment of probiotics so that their negative consequences do not outweigh their benefits. Antibiotic resistance and the ability to translocate of probiotics are now emphasized and are suggested to be made as criteria for safety assessment and labeling prior to their use as food supplements.

Much attention has been given to the factors and mechanisms involved on the acquired antibiotic resistance of probiotics. Some studies have found that the species and origins of the strains could affect the acquiring of antibiotic resistance, while others have demonstrated that genes coding for antibiotic resistance are transferable among bacteria

---

* Corresponding author: Dr Min-Tze Liong. Phone: +604 653 2114 ; Fax: +604 657 3678. Email: mintze.liong@usm.my

of different origins. Recent laboratory advances have provided more details and information on some postulated mechanisms. Probiotics could be antibiotic resistant inherently or acquired via vertical evolution such as inactivation of enzymes, alteration of membrane protein channels and efflux pumps, and/or via horizontal evolution of gene exchange.

Although antibiotic resistance of probiotics is rarely life threatening, it may serve as a marker of more serious underlying diseases. This review will also present some in-vitro and in-vivo evidence of the detections and isolation of antibiotic resistant probiotics, epidemiology of strains found, and their surveillance, monitoring and disposal once detected. There are also efforts to evaluate the need for elimination of antibiotic resistance although few probiotics meant for human consumption are classified as resistant. Past reports have found that a failure to demonstrate in-vitro horizontal gene transfer could not be used as a yardstick to exclude the risk of dissemination of genes. It has been suggested that genetic approaches are needed to eliminate antibiotic resistance, one being selective removal of plasmids coding for antibiotic resistance. However, the issues of phenotypical and genotypical alteration of the strain arise and that the impact of the genetic changes on the probiotic properties remains unknown. The present review will also highlight the genetic approaches used in risk assessment of antibiotic resistance dissemination.

Introduction

Probiotics are live microorganisms that could exert health benefits on the host when consumed in adequate amounts. Strains of lactic acid bacteria (LAB) from animal, human, plants and the environment have been isolated and adopted as probiotics. Some of the genera include *Enterococcus, Lactobacillus, Lactococcus, Bifidobacterium*, and yeasts such as *Saccharomyces* and *Candida*. The beneficial effects of probiotics were first reported nearly two decades ago from studies on the Maasai tribes that often consume liters of fermented milk daily. The initial health benefits mainly focused on the improvement of gastrointestinal health, and many studies have been conducted on the effects of probiotics on gastrointestinal disorders, including travelers' and rotavirus diarrhea, constipation, Crohn's disease, irritable bowel syndrome, lactose intolerance and allergy-related intestinal discomfort. The scope of research has since widened and recent research has focused other beneficial effects that involve the utilization of probiotics to improve general health and as an alternative to the administration of drugs to treat a number of diseases. Clinical evidence has suggested a role for probiotics in the treatment of hypertension, the improvement of blood lipid profiles, the alleviation of post-menopausal disorders, the prevention of colonic, prostate and ovarian cancers, the enhancement of the immune system and the improvement of nutrient bioavailability.

New and emerging infectious diseases caused by the rapid evolution of antibiotic-resistant bacteria have led to the need for new antimicrobial compounds. This has subsequently further increased the emergence of antibiotic resistance among bacteria. This resistance is obtained via two distinct mechanisms: intrinsic and acquired. Intrinsic resistance is an inherent chromosomal characteristic that is often not transferable and naturally present in bacterial strains of a similar species. However, acquired resistance is present only in some strains of bacteria within a specific genus or species. It can be obtained either from mutations in endogenous bacterial genes or through the acquisition of exogenous genes from another bacterium that codes for an antibiotic resistance. The latter gene transfer route is transferable and can spread among different bacterial populations (Courvalin, 2006).

The probability of gene transfer depends on the nature of the genetic material to be transferred (e.g., plasmids or transposons), on the nature of the donor and recipient strains, on the population concentrations, and on the presence of antibiotics. Many strains of probiotics have resistance to antibiotics either naturally or acquired through mutation or genetic modification. This resistance can be hazardous when antibiotic resistance genes are transferred to pathogenic bacteria or infections with antibiotic-resistant probiotics occur (Marteau and Shanahan, 2003).

Although probiotics have been found to prevent and/or treat antibiotic resistance indirectly, a key requirement for safe probiotic strains is that they should not carry transmissible antibiotic resistant genes. The safety of probiotics is of utmost importance because most probiotics are marketed for human consumption. Probiotics from fermented products may act as a pool of antibiotic resistance genes that could be transferred to pathogens (Mathur and Singh, 2005). The mechanisms of antibiotic resistance gene transfer have been widely studied. Although clinical evidence has shown that antibiotic-resistant probiotics can be isolated from immunocompromised hosts, little information is available on the proper documentation for their detection, regulation and elimination. A proper risk assessment on antibiotic resistance dissemination in probiotics is needed prior to their consumption.

Roles of Probiotics in Preventing and Treating Antibiotic Resistance

Prevalence of Probiotics in Preventing Antibiotics Resistance

Antibiotic resistance has become an emerging issue and the number of new antibiotic-resistant bacterial strains that have been isolated from patients has increased tremendously throughout the years. The emerging problem of antibiotic resistance has been mainly attributed to two vital factors: the misuse of antibiotics in treating disease and the resistance genes acquired by potential pathogens. In recent years, the development of novel antibiotics to treat infection has slowed down and is unlikely to keep pace with the emergence of new antibiotic resistance strains. Therefore, new therapies are needed to limit the propagation of this problem. Given the beneficial effects of probiotics, using probiotics to prevent antibiotic resistance is possible. Probiotic-mediated prevention of antibiotic resistance can be achieved by two mechanisms: a reduced use of antibiotics and disrupting the transfer of resistance genes among pathogens.

Previous in vitro and in vivo studies have demonstrated that extensive and/or misuse of antibiotics could be a risk factor for the acquisition of resistant bacteria. The antibiotic used would clearly act as a driving force in the dissemination of antibiotic resistance. Under normal physiological conditions, resistant bacteria are suppressed by the dominant commensal microflora. However, extensive use of antibiotics could alter the microbial ecology by eliminating the normal gastrointestinal flora, which would make it easier for resistant bacteria to establish colonization (Roghmann and McGrail, 2006). Probiotics are often used as supplements to replenish the population of beneficial bacteria and in the regularization of the endogenous microflora. As the number of probiotics increases, the number of harmful bacteria decreases. As a result, probiotics could prevent infection by pathogens and even when an infection occurs, it could be treated effectively and successfully as the gastrointestinal tract is predominated by drug-susceptible beneficial bacteria. Therefore, the use of antibiotics could be prevented or reduced. In fact, Hataka et al. (2001) has demonstrated that consumption of milk containing *Lactobacillus rhamnosus* GG (LGG) for seven months by 571 healthy children, aged 1–6, reduced both the incidence of respiratory infections and the need for antibiotic treatment of respiratory infections. The children were given milk containing either no probiotic or $5–10 \times 10^5$ CFU/ml of LGG. The authors reported a 19% relative reduction in the use of antibiotics to treat respiratory infections in the group given milk containing probiotics.

Reducing the use of antibiotics is important in preventing the establishment of antibiotic resistance among bacteria. Probiotics are seen as an alternative to antibiotic treatment due to their ability to improve immune system. It has been widely reported that immunocompromised patients are more susceptible to nosocomial infections. However, colonization with beneficial microflora such as probiotics could lead to an improved immune system.

The consumption of probiotics is capable of stimulating the immune system due to the ability of probiotics to enhance both cytokine and secretory immunoglobulin A (sIgA) production. Cytokines play a significant role in stimulating the immune response to pathogens by activating immune cells once a pathogen is encountered. The chief function of sIgA is the prevention of the binding of foreign bacteria to epithelial cells and the penetration of harmful microorganisms (Erickson and Hubbard, 2000). Thus, probiotics could protect the gastrointestinal tract from the invasion of pathogens and opportunistic bacteria, which would subsequently reduce the risk of infection. In such cases, the use of antibiotics to treat illnesses would be reduced thereby inhibiting the development of antibiotic resistance. Gorbach (1996) demonstrated that *Lactobacillus* GG fed to adults was effective in treating gastrointestinal illnesses without the need for antibiotics. The preventative potential of probiotics in patients suffering from infectious diarrhea and upper respiratory tract infections has led to the suggestion that they could be used as an alternative to antibiotic treatment, thus lowering the occurrence of antibiotic resistance.

Generally, the digestive tract is colonized by a complex microflora content. Therefore, the digestive tract could act as a gene pool for the transmission of antibiotic resistance genes among the gut microflora, which can subsequently lead to the evolution of multidrug-resistant bacteria. Another important factor contributing to the dissemination of antibiotic resistance is the ability of the specific bacteria to acquire the antibiotic resistance gene. The acquired resistance genes could be transferred from one bacterium to another leading to the accelerated emergence of antibiotic resistance. Various mechanisms could contribute to the dissemination of resistance genes but conjugation is thought to be the main mode of antibiotic resistance gene transfer. Therefore, interfering with this stage could lead to the prevention of antibiotic resistance. Probiotics could be useful in disrupting the transfer of antibiotic resistance genes.

This has been illustrated by Moubareck et al. (2007) who conducted a study to evaluate the role of the potentially probiotic bifidobacteria on the transfer of resistance genes between enterobacteria. The transfer of *bla* genes encoding extended-spectrum β-lactamases (SHV-5 and CTX-M-15) were studied in the absence or presence of bifidobacteria. The authors reported that *B. longum, B. bifidum*, and *B. pseudocatenulatum* could decrease the transfer frequency of genes mediating resistance to β-lactams, kanamycin and tetracycline among enterobacteria. Their results suggest that the inhibition of antibiotic resistance gene transfer was due the production of thermostable metabolites by bifidobacteria that subsequently affected the conjugation process.

The conjugation process generally involves intimate physical contact between the two bacteria that exposes the sex pilus of the donor to the recipient cell surface. Thus, any modification of the conjugation process would lead to the alteration of the cell surface of the recipient cells or the tip of the donor pili and to a decreased efficiency of gene transfer. Although strain-specific, probiotics have the potential to serve as an effective method to limit the spreading of antibiotic resistance genes.

To date, however, there have been limited studies examining the effectiveness of probiotics to limit antibiotic resistance. Past studies on the prevention of antibiotic resistance by probiotics have shown conflicting results. Sullivan et al. (2004) demonstrated that there are limited effects of *Lactobacillus* sp. strain F19 in preventing the establishment of resistant bacteria in the gastrointestinal tract of 36 patients who received either placebo or active probiotic products in conjunction with antibiotic treatment. The subjects were chosen on the basis that they had been admitted and would be receiving antibiotic treatment but had not been treated with antibiotics in the three months prior the study. No appreciable differences between the probiotic- and placebo-supplemented groups were observed and both groups showed an increase in quinolone resistance during quinolone treatment.

On the other hand, Moubareck et al. (2007) reported that probiotics could limit the emergence of antibiotic resistance. The authors evaluated the inhibitory effects of different Bifidobacteria strains on the transfer of resistance genes among Enterobacteriacea in a gnotobiotic mouse. Three of the five selected bifidobacteria strains could successfully inhibit the transfer of antibiotic resistance genes and subsequently decrease the development of antibiotic-resistant Enterobacteriacea in digestive tract. Similarly, Zoppi et al. (2001) reported that *Bifidobacterium* and *Lactobacillus* could be used to prevent antibiotic resistance.

These probiotics are able to decrease the production of beta-lactamase in the fecal flora after treatment with a β-lactam antibiotic. This is an important finding that demonstrates that probiotics could prevent the establishment of antibiotic resistance among intestinal microflora because β-lactamase is an enzyme that breaks the β-lactam ring structure subsequently leading to the deactivation of the β-lactam antibiotic. Production of this enzyme often leads to an increase in the bacterial resistance to β-lactam-based antibiotics.

Prevalence of Probiotics in Treating Antibiotic-Resistant Infections and Reducing Pathogens with Antibiotic Resistance

Preventing acquisition of antibiotic resistance is clearly a challenge. Therefore, under conditions when prevention is impossible, treatment is obviously the best alternative to eliminate or reduce antibiotic-resistant strains. Most antibiotic-resistant strains are opportunistic pathogens that could adhere and colonize the mucosal surfaces. This could lead to multidrug-resistant infections when there is a rupture in the colonized area. Once this resistance has been developed and amplified, it is sometimes difficult and even impossible to treat successfully. Given the increased frequency of antibiotic-resistant infections, there is a need to discover a better alternative to curb this problem. The use of probiotics is seen as an alternative to treat antibiotic-resistant infections and to reduced the number of antibiotic-resistant pathogens in the gut.

In fact, past studies have demonstrated that probiotics could treat antibiotic-resistant infections. Manley et al. (2007) monitored the effects of *Lactobacillus rhamnosus* GG (LGG) in vancomycin-resistant *Enterococcus* (VRE)-positive patients and found that patients treated with yogurt containing LGG could clear fecal VRE colonization. A total of 23 VRE-positive patients were randomly assigned to two groups, the treatment group received 100 g daily of yogurt containing LGG, while the control group received yogurt containing no probiotics. All 11 patients in the treatment group cleared the VRE, while only 1 of the 12 patients in control group cleared the VRE after three weeks of treatment. Therefore, live *Lactobacillus rhamnosus* GG could be administered to treat VRE. Likewise, another study reported that probiotic *Bacillus coagulans* could reduce the density of some VRE strains (Donskey et al., 2001). A total of 71 mice were colonized with different VRE strains and were fed either with 0.5 ml of *B. coagulans* culture, bacitracin antibiotic or 0.5 ml of saline. Treatment with *B. coagulans* significantly reduced the colonization of VRE compared to the saline-treated group. While a reduction in the colony density was observed in the antibiotic-treated group, the effect of antibiotic was only transient as the colonization of antibiotic-treated group subsequently rebounded to a level higher than the saline-treated mice at later stages of the study. The colonization density of the antibiotic-treated group was approximately three logs higher than the saline-treated group on the eleventh day of treatment. Therefore, given the transient effect of antibiotics, treatment with probiotics could be a better alternative.

Various mechanisms have been proposed to explain the ability of probiotics to reduce the number of antibiotic-resistant bacteria and to treat infections by antibiotic-resistant strains. One of the proposed mechanisms is competitive colonization. In order for antibiotic-resistant bacteria to cause infection, these bacteria must colonize the site of the infection. Colonization subsequently progresses to infection when there is a break in the skin or mucous membrane which enables the opportunistic pathogen to evade the host defense. Therefore, the ideal approach to treat antibiotic-resistant infections is by competitive colonization of the infected site with susceptible strains. Probiotics provide a new line of potential therapy because they could effectively decolonize the antibiotic-resistant strains without increasing the risk of future resistance. By encouraging the regrowth and repopulation of probiotic strains, the resistance level could be controlled by out-competing the potentially pathogenic antibiotic-resistant strains.

Colonization with probiotics could possibly counteract the colonization of antibiotic-resistant strains, given the ability of probiotics to bind to the enteric epithelium and inhibit the adhesion of pathogenic strains. Competitive colonization is possible due to the relatively higher adhesion ability of probiotics compared to the antibiotic-resistant strains at the target site. Vesterlund et al. (2006) demonstrated that *L. rhamnosus* GG and *Lactococcus lactis* subsp. *lactis* were able to reduce the binding of *Staphylococcus aureus* to human colonic mucosa by 39–44% due to their higher adhesion ability compared to the pathogenic strains. Therefore, probiotics are often chosen for their ability to adhere to epithelial cells. Adherent probiotics could reduce the viability of pathogenic bacteria.

Manley et al. (2007) has proposed that competition for nutrients by probiotics could be a potential mechanism to clear intestinal infections. Under normal physiology, the gastrointestinal tract is such a rich source of nutrients that it may seem unfeasible that such mechanism could influence the composition of the gut microflora. Nevertheless, it only requires the absence of one limiting essential nutrient to trigger this mechanism. Under limited nutrient conditions, probiotics could compete more efficiently for the essential nutrient than the antibiotic-resistant strains. This mechanism could have been partly responsible for the effectiveness of probiotics to eliminate or reduce antibiotic-resistant strains in the gut. *L. rhamnosus* GG has been suggested to compete with VRE for consumption of essential nutrients (e.g., monosaccharides), leading to slower VRE growth (Manley et al., 2007).

In addition to competitive colonization, probiotics could exert antimicrobial activity against various antibiotic-resistant strains. This antagonistic action is due to the production of antimicrobial substances such as bacteriocin and hydrogen peroxide. The use of bacteriocins is often preferred against the administration of antibiotics, as they are perceived to be more natural due to their long history of safe use in foods. Lacticin, the two-peptide (LtnA1 and LtnA2) lantibiotic produced by *Lactococcus lactis* subsp. *lactis* was reported to act against various Gram-positive pathogens, including methicillin-resistant *Staphylococcus aureus* (MRSA), vancomycin-resistant *Enterococcus faecalis* (VRE) and penicillin-resistant *Pneumococcus* (PRP) (Galvin et al., 1999). The possible mode of action for lacticin towards Gram-positive pathogens involves a lipid II binding step by the LtnA1 peptide, followed by insertion of LtnA2 peptide into the membrane. This leads to pore formation and ultimately cell death (Morgan et al., 2005). Therefore, bacteriocin and other antimicrobial peptides produced by probiotics could be promising therapeutic agents to treat antibiotic-resistant infections.

In fact, bacteriocin-producing probiotics could also be used to prevent the growth of antibiotic-resistant strains. The production of these antimicrobial factors in the gut would have an antagonistic effect on the resistant strains, which would confer a competitive advantage to the bacteriocin-producing bacteria in the microenvironment. The competitive exclusion of other microorganisms from this niche would affect the overall composition of the microbiota (Millette et al., 2008). Therefore, it is expected that bacteriocin-producing probiotics could reduce the colonization by antibiotic-resistant strains.

Past studies have demonstrated that strains of *L. lactis* and *Pediococcus acidilactici* that produce nisin or pediocin can substantially reduce the intestinal colonization of VRE following infection (Millette et al., 2008). The bacteriocin and other antimicrobial peptides produced by the probiotic strains are inserted into the cytoplasmic membrane of pathogenic strains and trigger the activity of bacterial murein hydrolases. This eventually leads to the damage or degradation of the peptidoglycan and lysis of the cell (Giacometti et al., 2000). In another in vitro study, *Enterococcus faecalis* demonstrated antimicrobial activity against MRSA in liquid culture (Ohhira et al., 1996). The authors postulated that the active component responsible for the antimicrobial property was a low molecular weight substance produced by the probiotic strain. This substance can inhibit the growth of MRSA. In addition, the production of metabolites (e.g., short-chain fatty acids) could decrease the density of the pathogenic strains. Acetic acid and lactic acids could lower the colonic pH and favor the growth of less pathogenic organisms.

The exact mechanisms by which probiotics limit the spread of antibiotic resistance are diverse and often strain-dependent. Although in vitro studies have demonstrated that probiotics could prevent and treat antibiotic resistance, more studies must be performed to determine the efficacy of probiotics in vivo. However, in vivo trials can be variable due to the variation and complexity of the intestinal microbiota between different mammals. Other probiotic selection criteria that must be taken into consideration include the survival and persistence in the host, safety and technological suitability. Figure 1 illustrates some of the factors that contribute to the dissemination of antibiotic resistance and the roles of probiotics in preventing and treating the infection.

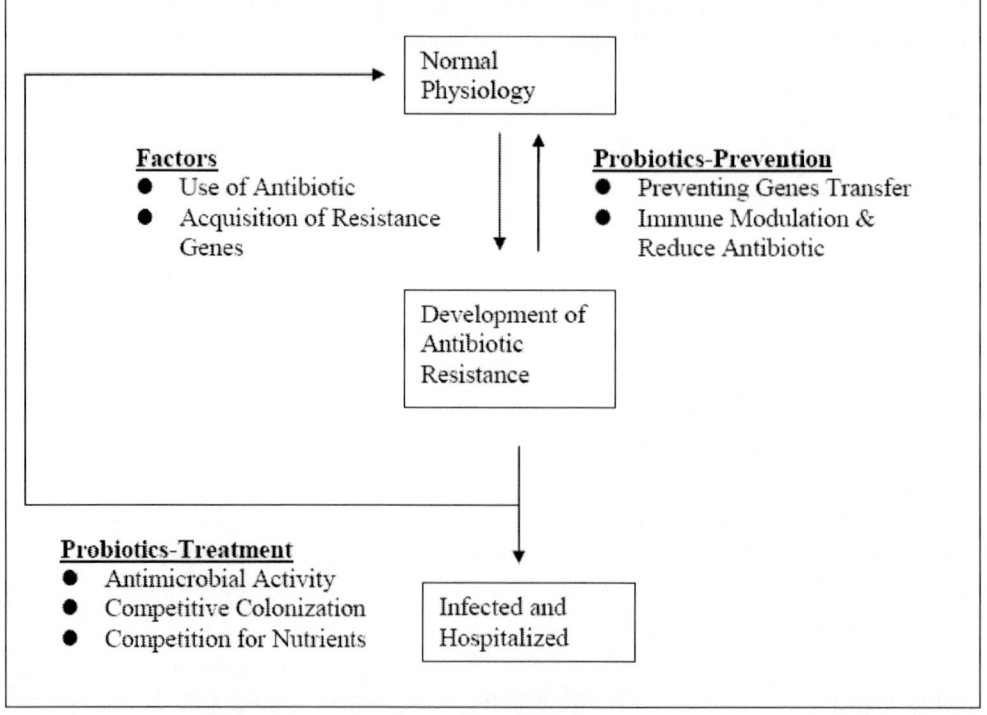

Figure 1. Factors contributing to the development of antibiotic resistance and the roles of probiotics in the prevention and treatment of antibiotic resistance.

Non-Antibiotic Resistance as a Criterion for Probiotics

Although most probiotics are known as "Generally Regarded As Safe" (GRAS) due to their long history of safe use, their potential negative side effects are not zero (Mathur and Singh, 2005). The presence of potentially transferable antibiotic resistance is a concern in the safety of probiotics. Therefore, it is important to assess the safety of food products containing probiotics before they are marketed so that the risks do not outweigh its benefits. This is of utmost importance for new strains of probiotics, because it cannot be assumed that these newly identified probiotics share the same historical safety of traditional strains (Salminen et al., 1998).

Recently, many researchers have speculated that the commensal bacteria may act as carriers of antibiotic resistance genes and transfer these genes to pathogenic or opportunistic bacteria (Mathur and Singh, 2005). Probiotics that have been long considered to be non-infective have been isolated from lesions in patients with bacterial endocarditis and systemic infections (Ishibashi and Shoji, 2001). Therefore, probiotics that possess transmissible antibiotic resistance genes and the ability to translocate need further assessment prior to their use in food supplements.

Importance of Non-Antibiotic Resistance as a Criterion for Probiotics

The susceptibility of probiotics to antibiotics varies with the strain and its final application. Some probiotics are naturally sensitive to the majority of antibiotics but others are naturally antibiotic-resistant. For example *Leuconostoc* is naturally vancomycin-resistant, as are certain lactobacilli (Mathur and Singh, 2005).

Probiotics can also be rendered multi-antibiotic-resistant by mutation or genetic modification. This is important for the pharmaceutical industry so that these probiotics can survive oral antibiotic treatment. This probiotic antibiotic-resistance would help the prevention of gastrointestinal side effects during antibiotic treatment (Courvalin, 2006). However, there is a drawback in this application: a higher risk of horizontal antibiotic resistance genes transfer from these multi-antibiotic-resistant probiotics to other gut pathogenic bacteria. This is because antibiotic resistance genes acquired by the exogenous genes has a greater possibility of gene transfer than the intrinsic chromosome-encoded genes or the resistance acquired through mutations, both of which are not transferable (Ammor et al., 2007).

As suggested by Marteau and Shanahan (2003), probiotics with antibiotic resistance are not necessarily a hazard unless the antibiotic resistance genes could be transferred to potential pathogens. This transfer would result in negative therapeutic consequences, including the emergence of more virulent pathogenic bacteria that cannot be treated by a previous successful antibiotic regimen. The more virulent bacteria would require an increased antibiotic dosage or the use of more powerful antibiotics, which will incur higher treatment cost, in order to clear the infection.

It is not uncommon that antibiotic resistance genes are transferred among microorganisms in the same habitat. There have been many studies demonstrating the in vivo and in vitro transfer of vancomycin resistance genes from enterococci probiotic strains to food-borne pathogenic bacteria such as *Staphylococcus aureus* and *Listeria*. Despite the possible transfer of antibiotic resistance genes, multi-antibiotic-resistant probiotics themselves can become pathogens in clinical infections and render these cases untreatable. Although there are rare occurrences of probiotic infections, a zero-risk infection does not exist, especially in immunocompromised patients (Marteau, 2001). Some of the common infections among immunocompromised patients caused by antibiotic-resistant probiotics are infections caused by strains of *Enterococcus faecalis*, *E. faecium* and certain LAB (Teuber et al., 1999).

It is difficult to assess the transfer of antibiotic resistance genes in vivo and in vitro and it is even more difficult to state what level of gene transfer is acceptable (Marteau, 2001; Marteau and Shanahan, 2003). Therefore, the implementation of non-antibiotic resistance as a criterion for probiotic selection needs thorough evaluation and assessment to determine its feasibility in ensuring the safety of the hosts.

Legislation and Recommendation on Antibiotic Resistant Probiotics

The presence of acquired antibiotic resistance is highly undesirable, more so in Europe than in the United States of America. In the USA, the safety of most probiotics that have been given GRAS status is the responsibility of the manufacturer and these GRAS products are exempted from the statutory premarket approval requirements (Mathur and Singh, 2005). However, the European countries have more stringent point of view on the safety of bacterial products.

The Scientific Committee on Animal Nutrition (SCAN) in European countries proposed the criteria to assess the safety of microorganisms resistant to antibiotics and probiotics used in animals. In its 2001 opinion that was later revised in 2002, the minimum inhibitory concentration (MIC) thresholds (mg/L) that categorize probiotics bacteria such as *Lactococcus lactis*, *Streptococcus thermophilus*, *Enterococcus*, *Pediococcus*, *Propionibacterium, Leuconostoc, Lactobacillus, Bifidobacterium* and *Bacillus* species as antibiotic resistant or antibiotic susceptible have been evaluated (SCAN, 2003). These thresholds are set by studying the distribution of the MICs of the chosen antibiotics in the specific species of probiotic. Ten types of antibiotics that belong to different groups of antibacterial compounds that have human clinical and veterinary importance were chosen for this determination of the MIC: ampicillin, vancomycin, gentamycin, kanamycin, streptomycin, erythromycin, clindamycin, quinupristin/dalfopristin, tetracycline and chloramphenicol (FEEDAP, 2008).

FEEDAP (2008) suggested several quantitative methods for the MIC determination. First, serial two-fold dilutions in agar or broth with the relevant quality control strains should be used during the assessment of the antibiotic resistance of the bacterial strains. All of the test procedures should be performed using specific internationally recognized standards such as those recommend by the Clinical and Laboratory Standard Institute (Mathur and Singh,

2005; FEEDAP, 2008). New technologies using quantitative nucleic acid methods such as PCR, Southern blot and conjugation are recognized and could also be used.

Selection of growth media, dilution method and incubation conditions must be based on existing scientific information related to the specific bacterial strains in order to avoid the possible occurrence of media and growth interference during incubation. All indirect qualitative or semi-qualitative determinations of the MIC value (e.g., the diffusion method) are generally not acceptable. Quantitative methods in antibiotics resistance determination must be used for bacterial genera such as *Lactobacillus* spp., *Propionibacterium*, *Bifidobacterium* and *Leuconostoc* that have no well-standardized procedures or quality control strains unless properly justified (FEEDAP, 2008).

The final conclusion is that live organisms that will be used in animals must demonstrate the absence of transmissible antibiotic resistance determinants against antibiotics that are important in human or veterinary medicine (SCAN, 2003). However, probiotics with inherent antibiotic resistance or antibiotic resistance acquired by mutation of chromosomal genes would generally be acceptable. This is because they have a decreased risk of horizontal antibiotic resistance gene dissemination (FEEDAP, 2008)

The European Food Safety Authority has taken over the tasks of SCAN and proposed a framework for the safety evaluation of microorganisms in the food chain (Courvalin, 2006). The EU-funded project ''Biosafety Evaluation of Probiotic Lactic Acid Bacteria used for Human Consumption'' was carried out from January 2002 to June 2006. The overall objective of this project was to propose recommendations for an evidence-based safety assessment of probiotics for human use. Antibiotic susceptibility and the possibility of horizontal antibiotic resistance gene transmission were studied to determine the safety of probiotics. Results from this study suggested that strains possessing one or more acquired resistance mechanisms should not be developed as a human or animal food adjunct without proper risk assessment (Vankerckhoven et al., 2008).

The Food and Agriculture Organization (FAO) and World Health Organization (WHO) have been collaborating to establish standard procedures for the evaluation and labeling of probiotics in foods. "Guidelines for the Evaluation of Probiotics in Food" has been generated by joint working group of FAO and WHO. This report outlined the recommended criteria and methodology for the evaluation of probiotics and the identification of the data required to substantiate the health claims for food containing probiotics. The minimum requirements needed for probiotic status are the study of the strain identity, the in vitro functional characterization to screen for the probiotic strain, the assessment of probiotic safety and an in vivo study for efficacy (Pineiro and Stanton, 2007).

The determination of the pattern of antibiotic resistance of the probiotics strain, epidemiological post-marketing surveillance and an assessment of the infectivity of the probiotic strain in immunocompromised animals are also recommended in safety assessment of probiotics (Pineiro and Stanton, 2007). After the safety assessment, strains that demonstrate an absence of transferable antibiotic resistance and are non-infectious will be subjected to an efficacy study using randomized, double blind, placebo-controlled animal and human studies that will be carried out at more than one center to confirm the results. Any adverse effects in these clinical trials will be monitored and published in order to demonstrate the efficacy of a particular probiotic strain (FAO/WHO, 2002)

In the case of antibiotic-resistant probiotics the related infections, identification and characterization of isolates should be performed in at least one taxonomic expert lab or an appropriate national reference center that is equipped with specialized detection technology, sufficient reference material and trained personnel for the reliable molecular identification (Borriello et al., 2003; Vankerckhoven et al., 2008).

All clinical isolates should be deposited in international culture collections center under conditions of restricted distribution. Descriptive and fingerprinting data related to the isolates should also be stored in a database that could be made accessible to the authorized medical association and personnel from different countries (FAO/WHO, 2002; Pineiro and Stanton, 2007; Vankerckhoven et al., 2008). It is important for diagnostic and epidemiological purposes to have a definitive identification and characterization to the species level (Borriello et al., 2003) of probiotic strains. The existing documentation are merely recommendations and reports regarding the safety issue of probiotics in foods that have been published by various regulatory bodies from different countries. More global efforts are needed in order to generate an international consensus on a standardized analytical method to assess the safety of potentially new probiotic strains (Borriello et al., 2003).

Translocation of Antibiotic-Resistant Probiotics

Translocation of antibiotic-resistant probiotics is defined as the passage of viable antibiotic-resistant probiotic cells from their endogenous habitat in the gastrointestinal tract to extra-intestinal sites where they are not normally found (e.g., the mesenteric lymph nodes, liver, spleen and bloodstream). Traditionally, translocation can be detected by the culture of viable cells from mesenteric lymph nodes. However, a recent detection method using the polymerase chain reaction to detect bacterial DNA has been described (Quigley and Quera, 2006).

In healthy adults, the translocation of antibiotic-resistant probiotics, along with other endogenous bacteria, across the mucosal epithelium is continuously occurring at a low level. The translocated bacteria and associated by-products will then be rapidly eliminated in the lymphoid organs and have no negative effects on the host (Marteau and Shanahan, 2003). Therefore the risk of antibiotic-resistant probiotic infection in healthy subjects is extremely low. However, infections caused by the translocation of antibiotic-resistant probiotics could be more damaging to immunocompromised hosts that have a weakened immune system. The host could be overwhelmed by the high concentration of antibiotic-resistant probiotics present in their gastrointestinal tract and the translocation of the probiotics may occur when the intestine is diseased or anatomically altered due to a previous illness (Quigley and Quera, 2006).

Rare cases of local or systemic infections (e.g., septicemia or endocarditis) caused by the translocation of antibiotic-resistant probiotic bacteria after the ingestion of a probiotic product has been reported. Probiotic strains that normally associated with these infections are *Lactobacillus, Leuconostoc, Pediococcus, Enterococcus* and *Bifidobacterium.* Cannon et al. (2005) reported localized infections including abdominal abscesses, pneumonia, other pulmonary infections and peritonitis that were caused by β-lactam- and vancomycin-resistant

Lactobacillus species. Salminen et al. (2004) also detected vancomycin-resistant lactobacilli isolates from cases of *Lactobacillus* bacteremia. Ofloxacin-resistant lactobacilli also have been isolated from clinical infections (Ishibashi and Shoji, 2001). *Enterococcus* isolates that responsible for most of the probiotic-associated nosocomial infections have showed an increasing resistance to vancomycin (Marteau and Shanahan, 2003).

Carbapenem-resistant *Leuconostoc lactis* strains have also been isolated from a human ventriculitis infection (Deye et al., 2003; Ammor et. al., 2007). Gollrdge et al. (1990) isolated vancomycin-resistant *Pediococcus acidilactici, Enterococcus faecium, Leuconostoc mesenteroides*, and *E. rhusiopathiae* from multiple blood cultures taken from a leukemic patient with septicemia. Additionally, the isolation of vancomycin-resistant lactobacilli probiotics, specifically *L. rhamnosus, L. fermentum* and *L. acidophilus* have been reported from three neutropenic patients with pneumonia after consuming probiotic products containing lactobacilli (Sriskandan et al., 1993; Land et al., 2005).

It is well-known that bacterial translocation results in various negative clinical infections to the host. However, antibiotic-resistant probiotic translocation is even more detrimental to the health of the patient than the translocation of endogenous bacteria. The transfer of live antibiotic-resistant probiotics from the gastrointestinal tract to other organ via the circulation may potentially cause systemic infections such as bacteremia, septicemia and multiple organ failure (Liong, 2008).

Metabolites produced by either live or non-viable translocated antibiotic-resistant probiotics have also been reported to produce negative side effects in the host. For example, large quantities of lactic acid metabolites produced by translocated lactobacilli in the circulation reduced the sensitivity of host towards certain antibiotics and aminoglycosides antibiotics lost activity due to decrease in pH (Slover and Danziger, 2008). This phenomenon results in inefficient antibiotic treatment. A higher dose of antibiotics, or multiple antibiotic treatments, is required for the complete eradication of infections caused by antibiotic-resistant probiotics that have translocated. Consequently, an increase in the length of the hospital stay, hospitalization costs and a rate of mortality and morbidity are often observed in these antibiotic-resistant infections compared to drug-susceptible illnesses.

Additionally, the resistance genes that located on transmissible genetic elements of antibiotic-resistant probiotics, particularly *Enterococcus* probiotic strains, (Borriello et al., 2003; Marteau, 2001) may be horizontally transferred to other pathogenic microorganisms present in the infected region. This results in other more virulent infections in the hosts. Figure 2 illustrates a schematic diagram showing the route of antibiotic-resistant probiotics translocation and the associated negative effects.

The ability to translocate is a highly recommended indicator for the assessment of probiotic safety globally (Marteau and Salminen, 1997). The inability to translocate in antibiotic-resistant probiotics serves as a safety indicator for the particular probiotic strains used in food products or animal feeds. Therefore, there is a detailed understanding of the host and microbial factors that affect antibiotic-resistant probiotic infections, including the mechanisms underlying translocation, the survival of the probiotic cells and the infectivity of the probiotic cells, is necessary. Isolates of antibiotic-resistant probiotic infections should be sent to reference centers for molecular characterization and confirmation. The report of any incidences of antibiotic-resistant probiotic infection should be made mandatory. All of the records accompanied by isolate preservation and characterization and the number of infections involved should be maintained at the culture collection centers for future reference (Borriello et al., 2003).

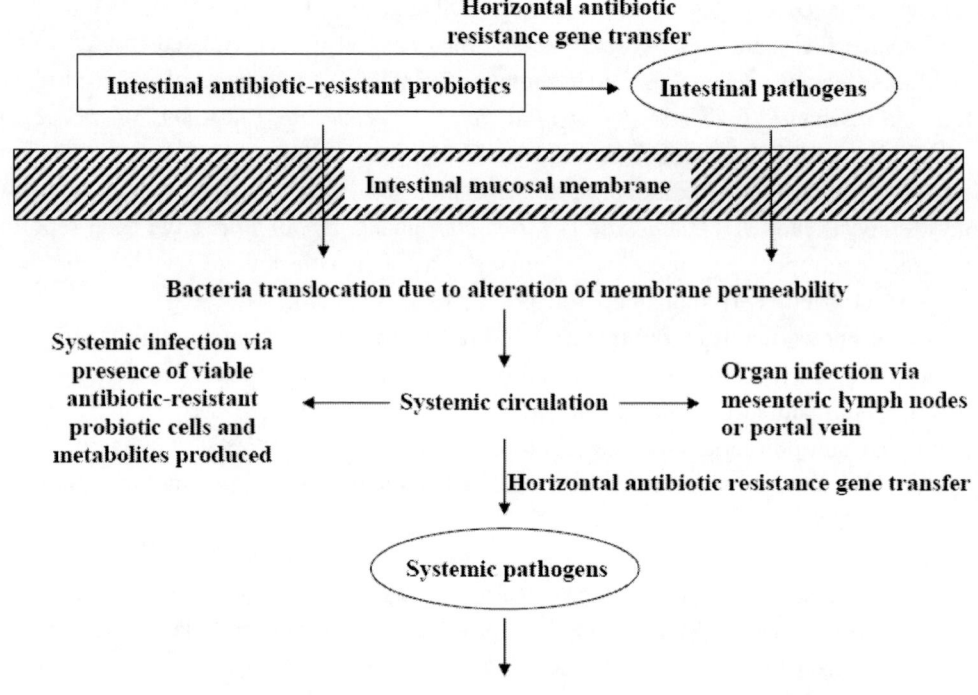

Figure 2. Route of antibiotic-resistant probiotic translocation and associated negative effects.

Mechanism of Acquiring Antibiotic Resistance in Probiotics

Although the use of probiotics in food and food supplements has increased considerably because of their health benefits, antibiotic-resistant probiotics are also co-administered with antibiotics to counter antibiotic-induced dysbiosis and diarrhea. Concerns have been raised over the spread of antibiotic resistance among bacteria and probiotics. Despite known susceptibilities to the majority of antibiotics, in addition to possessing intrinsic resistance, probiotics have displayed the ability to acquire antibiotic resistance from gut commensal bacteria or co-existing microbiota in the food matrix. This forces scientists to reconsider the imminent consequence of losing clinical control over the administered probiotics, which may overweigh the intended beneficial effects. Concerns were heightened following the report of a probiotic, *Enterococcus faecium* that was found to be a possible recipient of the glycopeptide resistance *vanA* gene (Lund and Edlund, 2001). This concern towards increasingly resistant probiotics is justified as the transfer of resistance to pathogenic microorganisms may create new super-bugs. Additionally, the containment of translocated resistant probiotics in the human system results in adverse clinical effects. Thus, transferable and acquired antibiotic resistance has become one of the most emphasized safety criteria for the selection of potential probiotics.

Actions of Antibiotics and Antibiotic Resistance

Generally, probiotic strains of the genera *Lactobacillus, Pediococcus, Leuconostoc* and *Streptococcus* are rather susceptible to clinically relevant antibiotics such as penicillin G, ampicillin, tetracycline, erythromycin and chloramphenicol (Hummel et al., 2007). Additionally, bifidobacteria has been shown to be more susceptible to these antibiotics than lactobacilli (Moubareck et al., 2005).

Antibiotics, natural and synthetic, exert anti-microbial effects via several mechanisms: interference with the synthesis of physiologically important components (e.g., the cell wall, proteins and nucleic acids), the inhibition of metabolic pathways and the disruption of membrane structures. The major mechanism underlying antibiotic resistance evolved on a common principle of inhibiting the antibiotic—target interaction (Courvalin, 2008).

β-lactam drugs (e.g., penicillin, cephalosporin and carbapenem) inhibit cell wall synthesis by interfering with the enzymes required for the synthesis of the peptidoglycan layer. This inhibition leads to cell lysis and death (Biswas et al., 2008). β-lactams also interfere with the permeability of the cell wall envelope, thus increasing the susceptibility of microorganisms to antimicrobial agents like aminoglycosides. Another postulated antimicrobial effect is the disruption of the membrane structure resulting in increased membrane permeability, which leads to the leakage of the bacterial contents, as exerted by polymyxins (Storm et al., 1977).

A resistance mechanism used to counteract such drugs is the production of drug detoxification enzymes (e.g., β-lactamase and aminoglucoside phosphoryltransferase). These enzymes efficiently breakdown the drugs before they can exert their antimicrobial properties against the targeted microorganism. A chromosome-encoded ß-lactamase, *BCL-1*, with a hydrolytic profile encompassing penicillins, narrow-spectrum cephalosporins and cefpirome, has been characterized in probiotic *Bacillus clausii* (Girlich et al., 2007).

Macrolides, aminoglycosides, tetracyclines and chloramphenicol inhibit bacterial growth by selectively binding to the 30S and 50S subunit of the ribosome and inhibiting protein synthesis (Tenover, 2006). Resistance by modification of the target leads to a reduced affinity and binding capacity of the antimicrobial agent to its targeted site (e.g., methylation of 23S rRNA, mutation of amino acid sequences of topoisomerase and other post-transcriptional or post-translational modifications) (Davies, 1997). The resistance of *Bacillus clausii* to macrolides and rifampicin is associated with chromosomally triggered target modifications (Courvalin, 2006).

Fluoroquinolones and rifampicin interrupt nucleic acid synthesis and cause lethal breaks in DNA by inhibiting the bacterial topoisomerase enzymes involved in DNA metabolism and inhibit the DNA-dependent RNA polymerase, respectively. Metronidazole, a drug active against virtually all obligate anaerobes, initiates the preferential reduction of the parent compound by the bacterial ferredoxin system, which generates an intermediate product responsible for breaks in double-stranded DNA (Miller-Catchpole, 1989). Intracellular accumulation of these compounds can be prevented by several mechanisms including the development of impermeability (e.g., through the reduction of the number of pores in the external membrane) in Gram-negative bacteria and the active efflux of antibiotics (Teuber et al., 1999, Courvalin, 2008). *L. lactis* subsp. *lactis* MG1363 has been found to possess multiple drug efflux proteins which are associated with ethidium bromide resistance (Marthur and Singh, 2005).

Since antibiotics are classified according to chemical structure, antibiotics within the same class, sharing the similar structures and possibly target sites, are subjected to cross-resistance by target alteration and drug detoxification (Courvalin, 2008). Thus, it not surprising that studies of antibiotic resistance over the years have yielded inconsistent results. This can be attributed to the different methods used, the lack of a standard procedure for the MIC determination and the different criteria used to interpret the susceptibility tests (Salminen et al., 2006). However, many studies have demonstrated the dependence of antibiotic resistance on the genus, species, strain and phase of logarithmic growth (Bernardeau et al., 2008).

Intergenera and interspecies differences and the species-dependency of *Lactobacillus* spp. antibiotic resistance have been well-documented. Species of the *Lactobacillus* group (*L. acidophilus, L. gasseri, L. crispatus, L. johnsonii, L. delbrueckii* and *L. amylovorus*) were relatively more susceptible to penicillins than other lactic acid bacteria (LAB) species (Klare et al., 2007). The vancomycin resistance appeared to be strain-specific, in which the MIC for *L. rhamnosus, L. plantarum* and *L. paracasei* was more than 256 μg/ml, while it was less than 2 μg/ml for *L. acidophilus* (Danielsen and Wind, 2003). The development of vancomycin resistance is concerning since it is one of the last broad-spectrum antibiotics used to treat clinical infections caused by multidrug-resistant pathogens (Zhou et al., 2005).

Types of Resistance

Antibiotic resistance may be inherent to the probiotics or acquired via two processes: vertical gene transfer (mutation and selection) and horizontal gene transfer (exchange of genes between strains and species) (Biswas et al., 2008). Antimicrobial resistance patterns of various species and sources of lactic acid bacteria would have to be compared to distinguish between intrinsic and acquired resistance (Flórez et al., 2005; Teuber et al., 1999). *E. faecium* isolated from food or patients have highly variable resistance profiles, even though many are acquired traits (Mathur and Singh, 2005).

Enterococcus and *Lactobacillus* have been implicated in the transfer of antibiotic resistance genes and mobile genetic elements, to and from lactic acid bacteria (Moubareck et al., 2005). The extensive and imprudent prescription of antibiotics has resulted in a selective pressure for point mutations and the acquisition of genetic elements encoding resistance. This has led to the dissemination of a variety of antibiotic resistance determinants (Teuber et al., 1999; Ouoba et al., 2008).

Under natural conditions, the dissemination of resistance genes occurs at three superimposable levels: bacterial epidemics (resistant bacteria transferred among mammals), plasmid epidemics (resistance gene located in a conjugative plasmid) and genetic epidemics (resistance genes that are part of a transposable element). Due to DNA replication, the dissemination of resistance genes is often exponential. In the second and third level of dissemination, the genetic information can be inherited vertically or horizontally, with the integration of the resistance elements into host chromosomes or into a conjugative plasmid (Courvalin, 2006). Resistance genes located on mobile genetic elements (e.g., plasmids or transposons) have also been characterized in lactobacilli and enterococci isolated from foods (Flórez et al., 2005).

Natural or Intrinsic Resistance

Intrinsic resistance, sometimes designated as insensitivity, is present in all strains of a given genus or species to protect themselves against suicide by the products of their secondary metabolism (Courvalin, 2008). Intrinsic resistance genes are chromosome-encoded and non-transmissible to other bacteria (Zhou et al., 2005).

Lactobacilli possess prominent intrinsic resistance to bacitracin, cefoxitin, ciprofloxacin, fusidic acid, kanamycin, gentamicin, metronidazole, nitrofurantoin, norfloxacin, streptomycin, sulphadiazine, teicoplanin, trimethoprim/sulphamethoxazole and vancomycin (Danielsen and Wind, 2003). Lactobacilli also appear to have intrinsic resistance to aminoglycosides, quinolones and glycopeptides (Moubareck et al., 2005). Strains of *Lactobacillus delbrueckii* subsp. *bulgaricus* that are widely used as a yogurt culture have been repeatedly found to possess intrinsic resistance against mycostatin, nalidixic acid, neomycin, polymyxin B, trimethoprim, colimycin, sufamethoxazol and sulphonamides (Mathur and Singh, 2005).

Previous studies have demonstrated that *Lactobacillus, Pediococcus* and *Leuconostoc* species possess intrinsic and non-transferable vancomycin resistance (Zhou et al., 2005; Mathur and Singh, 2005). Enterococci are intrinsically resistant to cephalosporins (Teuber et al., 1999) and bifidobacteria are known to be resistant to vancomycin, gentamicin, kanamycin, streptomycin, fusidic acid, trimethoprim, norfloxacin, nalidixic acid, metronidazol, polymyxin B and colistin (Teuber et al., 1999). Some of the resistance of bifidobacteria is likely to be intrinsic.

Although intrinsic resistance is recognized and presents predictable resistance upon administration to humans, the chances of the resistance being transferred to other microorganisms in unspecified circumstances are not non-zero. Transfer of chromosomal resistance genes has been documented between *Lactobacillus* and *E. faecalis,* causing concerns for the possible dissemination of the intrinsic resistance of probiotics among microorganisms (Mathur and Singh, 2005).

Acquired Resistance

This type of resistance, which is only present in certain bacteria belonging to specific genera or species (Courvalin, 2006) that are living in environments constantly challenged with antibiotics (Teuber et al., 1999), involves an initially susceptible population of bacteria becoming resistant to an antibiotic and proliferating under the selective pressure of that agent (Tenover, 2006). The presence of accessory genetic elements such as transposons and plasmids, in addition to chromosomes in the bacteria genome, greatly increases the potential for the spread of the resistance gene. This is especially true if the gene is carried by a mobile genetic element or is itself a self-transferable plasmid or transposon (Courvalin, 2006). Genes conferring acquired resistance are often located on conjugative or transferable plasmids and transposons (Teuber et al., 1999).

Vancomycin resistance in enterococci such as *E. faecium* is plasmid-mediated and results from the acquisition of various operons (e.g., the glycopeptide resistance determinants, vanA- and vanB) (Arthur et al., 1996). Additionally, enterococci have been known to possess a high level of antibiotic resistance that is attributed to the possession of broad host range and extremely mobile genetic elements, such as pAMβ1, a conjugative plasmid carrying constitutive MLS (macrolide, lincosamided and streptogramin B) resistance or Tn916, a conjugative transposon carrying tetracycline resistance (Teuber et al., 1999). Certain species of lactobacilli naturally produce a peptidoglycan insensitive to the action of vancomycin (Courvalin, 2006). Despite its extensive intrinsic resistance, some antibiotic resistance genes in lactobacilli may be plasmid-encoded.

Acquired resistance manifests in two distinct mechanisms: vertical evolution (mutations in endogenous genes resulting in non-transferable resistance) and horizontal evolution (acquisition of an exogenous resistance determinant from other bacteria resulting in transferable resistance) (Courvalin, 2006).

Vertical Evolution – Spontaneous Mutation and Selection Process

Vertical evolution is the endogenous resistance arising from structural or regulatory chromosomal gene mutations that is generally not transferable (Courvalin, 2008). In the presence of antibiotics, the selection process leads to the survival and proliferation of newly resistant strains, which pass the resistant genes to its progeny (Tenover, 2006).

Resistance acquired via this spontaneous mutation functions through several mechanisms: the alteration of the target protein by modifying or eliminating the antibiotic binding site, the inhibition of the accumulation of the antibiotic by modifying the outer membrane protein channels required for cell entry and the up-regulation of efflux pumps to expel drug and, the up-regulation of enzymes that inactivate the antibiotic (Tenover, 2006).

Spontaneous mutations occur at a high frequency in lactobacilli and have resulted in acquired resistance to nitrofurazone, kanamycin and streptomycin (Curragh and Collins, 1992). Non-transferable resistance due to mutations is often the case for rifampicin (Danielsen and Wind, 2003). The discovery of a plasmid encoding a new erythromycin determinant, *erm(LF)*, in erythromycin-resistant *Lb. fermentum* strains also suggests the occurrence of this evolution (Mathur and Singh, 2005).

Although natural and vertically evolved resistance has a low risk of horizontal transmission, low-level chromosomal resistance enhances the evolution of high-level resistance by horizontal gene transfer (Baquero et al., 1997). A *tet(M)* gene conferring ribosomal protection against tetracycline in *Lactobacillus* strains, which has homology to the *tet(M)* gene from the *E. faecalis* transposon Tn916, was not plasmid-encoded in *Lactobacillus* (Mathur and Singh, 2005). This suggests a chromosomal location and indicates a possible occurrence of horizontal gene transfer that was then enhanced by vertical evolution. The presence of antibiotics can induce and enhance gene transfer by providing a selective pressure for resistant bacteria to maintain and disseminate resistance genes (Courvalin, 2008).

Horizontal Evolution – Gene Exchange

Acquired resistance via horizontal evolution involves the development of resistance by the acquisition of new genetic material from other resistant organisms (Tenover, 2006). This gives rise to exogenous resistance, which is highly transferable (Courvalin, 2008). Lactic acid bacteria, like all other bacteria, are dependent upon horizontal evolution or gene exchange to survive and adapt in antibiotic-containing environments (Teuber et al., 1999). The transfer of resistance elements can be promoted by several factors. Launay et al. (2006) postulated that the high density and promiscuity between enterococci and human commensal anaerobes in the intestinal environment, combined with the presence of glycopeptide, created favorable conditions for transfer of the glycopeptide resistance determinant, *vanB*. Another factor which promotes the transfer of resistance determinants is the presence of antibiotics. The enterococcal transposon Tn917 demonstrated enhanced transposition and intercellular dissemination of macrolide resistance following exposure to erythromycin (Courvalin, 2008). This demonstrated the stimulating role of antibiotics in mobility of resistance transposons.

Intergenera and interspecies transfer of resistance genes has been well-documented in probiotics. The *tet(W)* gene, which confers tetracycline resistance by mediating ribosomal protection (Kastner et al., 2006), was suggested to have transferred between anaerobic bacteria genera, ultimately conferring tetracycline resistance in *B. pseudocatenulatum* and *B. bifidum* (Scott et al 2000). The gene was previously found in *B. longum* and in three genera of rumen obligate anaerobes (Moubareck et al, 2005).

The transferability of resistance genes under controlled conditions was studied by Ouoba et al. (2008) in a filter mating experiment. This was achieved by filtering a mixture of resistance gene donor and recipient cell suspensions through a membrane filter to trap the cells in the membrane (Sasaki et al., 1988). The cell-packed filter was incubated in the optimal growth conditions of recipient strain and agar plating was performed to determine the presence of trans-conjugant cells. Upon intimate cell-to-cell contact, the authors observed interspecies horizontal transfer of the macrolide resistance gene *erm(B)* from *Lb. reuteri* L4: 12002 to *E. faecalis* (Ouoba et al., 2008).

In another instance of interspecies gene transfer, linA and linA', which are two variants of the antibiotic resistance gene *lnu(A)*, which was originally, and almost exclusively, detected in staphylococci, was recently detected in lincomycin- and clindamycin-resistant *Lactobacillus* strains (Kastner et al., 2006).

Transduction by bacteriophages or conjugation has been identified as the main mechanism of horizontal gene transfer in natural environments. Mobile genetic elements, such as plasmids and transposons, play a pivotal role in the dissemination of antibiotic resistance genes.

These accessory genetic elements aid in the passive and active communication between susceptible lactic acid bacteria and resistant bacteria, a prerequisite for the acquisition of antibiotic resistance genes (Teuber et al, 1999). This has been observed in *Lb. fermentum* isolated from pig feces, which was found to carry a 5.7 kb plasmid expressing an *erm* gene that conferred a high level of erythromycin resistance. This gene was 98.2% identical to the resistance gene found in the enterococcal conjugative transposon Tn1545 (Fons et al., 1997).

Conjugative transposons are exceedingly important in bacterial evolution due to their broad host range (Launay et al., 2006). Transposons, which has been described in enterococci, lactococci and streptococci, facilitate the transfer and incorporation of resistance genes (Tenover, 2006) by inducing the excision of itself and, after conjugative transfer, incorporation into the new host genome (Teuber, 1999).

Transposons, of various sizes between 16 and 70 kb, may be inserted a single copy, or multiple copies, into plasmids or chromosomes and can mobilize plasmids or chromosomal genes (Marthur and Singh, 2005). Conjugative transposons determine resistance to tetracycline (*tet(M)*), erythromycin (*ermAM, erm*), chloramphenicol (*cat*) and kanamycin (*aphA-3*) and have been reported in strains of enterococci and streptococci (Teuber et al, 1999). In filter mating experiments, the Tn916-type transposon TnFO1 was found to aid the transfer of the tetracycline resistance gene *tet(M)* (99.8% identical to gene of transposon Tn916 at the nucleotide level) from *E. faecalis* FO1 to *Lactococcus lactis* Bu2-60 (Mathur and Singh, 2005).

Conjugative plasmids of various size, function and distribution are common elements in enterococci, lactococci, leuconostocs, pediococci and certain strains of lactobacilli and bifidobacteria (Marthur and Singh, 2005). They are also found in Gram-positive bacteria like *Staphylococcus aureus*, *Enterococcus* and *Streptococcus* species (Teuber et al., 1999). Enteric lactobacilli have been shown to participate in promiscuous gene transfer with the aid of conjugative antibiotic resistance plasmids such as pAMβ1, pAMh1 and PIP501, which are capable of both mobilization and intergenera conjugation (Teuber et al., 1999; Tannock, 1987).

Enterococci have been extensively shown to have prevalent antibiotic resistance genes, including erythromycin, vancomycin, tetracycline, chloramphenicol and gentamicin resistance genes, on transferable genetic elements both on plasmids and transposons (Marthur and Singh, 2005). The pAMβ1 plasmid isolated from *E. faecalis*, which carries constitutive MLS resistance, can move from *E. faecalis* into the plasmid-free strain Bu2-60 of *L. lactis* subsp. *lactis* and from *Lactococcus* and *Enterococcus* into *Lb. reuteri* and back again (Teuber et al., 1999; Tannock, 1987).

In Vitro and *In Vivo* Evidence

For several decades, studies on the selection and dissemination of antibiotic resistance have focused mainly on clinically relevant species. However, the spread of antibiotic resistance has recently become a concern after several types of antibiotic resistance were detected and characterized in some starter cultures and probiotic microorganisms that are commonly used in food products.

Emergence of Antibiotic Resistance among Starter Cultures and Probiotic Strains

There is a growing concern regarding the emergence and dissemination of antibiotic-resistant bacteria worldwide. The increased prevalence of antibiotic resistance is an outcome of evolution under the selective pressure imposed by antibiotics and is the result of numerous complex interactions among antibiotics, microorganisms and the surrounding environments (White and McDermott, 2001). Several factors that cause the emergence of resistance are the increased use and misuse of antimicrobial agents, the decline of infection control practices leading to the increase transmission of resistant organisms and the growth of susceptible hosts.

LABs have had a long history of safe use as starter culture bacteria that has contributed to their acceptance as probiotics. However, the presence of antibiotic residues in milk that resulted in failures in milk acidification has drawn attention to the antibiotic sensitivity and resistance of dairy starter cultures. Since then several studies detailing the safety of starter culture bacteria have been performed from the end of 1950 through 1980 (Salminen et al., 1998). The main threat associated with these bacteria is that they can transfer resistance genes to pathogenic bacteria and vice versa (Marthur and Singh, 2005). Additional studies have investigated the antibiotic resistance profiles of these strains. In the earlier studies, most of the antibiotic-resistant lactobacilli strains were isolated from pork and beef and especially from human and animal gastrointestinal tracts. Of the 43 strains of *L. fermentum* that were isolated from human feces, most showed a low-level penicillin resistance with MICs of 0.03-0.44 U/ml. However, two isolates had MICs of 17 and 13 U/ml (Yokokura and Mutai, 1976).

In the 1980s, several animal isolates of *L. acidophilus* and *L. reuteri* were tested for antibiotic resistance by Sarra et al. (1982). All 16 isolates of *L. reuteri* were vancomycin- and polymycin B-resistant but only 4 out of 30 *L. acidophilus* strains were vancomycin-resistant. The inherent resistance of bifidobacteria to neomycin, nalixidic acid and polymycin B was reported by Miller and Finegold in 1976. This was further proven by Lim et al. (1993) when they assayed 37 natural bifidobacteria isolates against 18 different antibiotics. In another study, a total of 26 strains of *Streptococcus cemoris* and 12 strains of *Streptococcus lactis* were challenged with 18 antibiotics was performed by Orberg and Sandine in 1985. The authors found that all strains were resistant to trimethoprim and almost all strains were resistant to sulfathiazole, while resistance to other antibiotics were species-dependent.

According to Tannock (1987), the conjugative plasmid pAM_1 can translocate from *Lactococcus* and *Enterococcus* into *L. reuteri* and back again. Hence, it is not surprising that lactobacilli (e.g., *L. plantarum*, *L. acidophlus*, *L. brevis*, *L. casei*) isolated from 'home-made' Spanish cheese (Serena, Gamonedo, Cabrales) were resistant to penicillin G, cloxacillin, streptomycin, gentamicin, tetracycline, erythromycin and chloramphenicol (Herrero et al. 1996). Additionally, antibiotic-resistant lactococci and leuconostocs were isolated from the same material.

Increased studies on the safety of probiotic strains have gained attention since antibiotic-resistant pathogens have been disseminating. Recently, a study by Zhou et al. (2005) described the antibiotic susceptibilities of four new probiotic lactic bacteria. All of the newly identified *L. rhamnosus* strains (HN001, HN067) were resistant to vancomycin, while two out of three newly identified lactobacilli strains (*L. rhamnosus* HN067 and *L. acidophilus* HN017) were resistant to cloxacillin. Moreover, the latter two strains were also resistant to Gram-negative spectrum antibiotics (e.g., fusidic acid, nalixidic acid and polymyxin-B) and aminoglycosides (e.g., gentamicin, kanamycin, neomycin and streptomycin).

Tang et al. (2007) had performed a study on the antibiotic susceptibility of strains in Chinese medical probiotic products. They reported that the probiotics tested in their study were multidrug resistant. Resistance to vancomycin was seen in three strains of *L. acidophilus* LAP, *L. bulgaricus* LBJ and *Streptococcus thermophilus* STJ. Furthermore, more than half of the tested strains showed slight resistance to tetracycline.

Recently, several antibiotic-resistant probiotic and starters culture strains have also been isolated from dairy and pharmaceutical products by D'Aimmo et al. (2007). Among the 34 strains of *Lactobacillus* and *Bifidobacterium*, and 21 strains of starter culture bacteria, all tested strains were resistant to aztreonam, cycloserin, kanamycin, nalidixic acid, polymyxin B and spectinomycin with $MIC_{90}s$ (lowest antibiotic concentration that inhibited 90% of the tested strains) ranging from 64 to >1000 µg/ml. However, the antibiotic susceptibility levels to the various antimicrobials were species-dependent.

One of the largest studies investigating the antibiotic susceptibility patterns of starter cultures and probiotic bacteria used in food products was conducted by Kastner et al. (2006) and involved 200 isolates. The authors found that 27 isolates exhibited resistances that were not an intrinsic feature of the respective genera. Despite this, the study detected the presence of the tetracycline resistance gene, *tet*(W) in the probiotic cultures of *Bifidobacterium lactis* DSM 10140 and *Lactobacillus reuteri* SD 2112. For the first time, the later strain was found to contain the *Inu*(A) gene, which previously detected only in staphylococci and is known as *linA*. The gene was responsible for lincomycin and clindamycin resistance.

In another study by Klare et al. (2007) evaluating the antimicrobial susceptibility of 473 isolates encompassein 24 species of *Lactobacillus, Pediococcus* and *Lactococcus* isolated from human samples or cultures intended for probiotic or nutritional use, they found that LAB exhibited broad species-dependent MIC profiles of trimetoprim, trimethoprim/sulfamethoxazole, vancomycin, teicoplanin and fusidic acid. Of the 473 probiotic LAB strains tested, 3 *Lactobacillus* strains (*L. rhamnosus* L-015, L-455 and *L. paracasei* L-005) were highly resistant to streptomycin with MICs of ≥2048 mg/L. Intrinsic high-level resistance to glycopeptides was also detected in pediococci and in several *Lactobacillus* species, including *L. rhamnosus, L. paracasei, L. plantarum, L. reuteri* and *L. fermentum*.

Different techniques were used by different groups to evaluate the antibiotic sensitivity. Therefore, the comparison of the data is quite difficult and any definitive conclusions are hard to draw (Salminen et al., 2006). Data from various studies demonstrated that the resistance profiles of probiotics were of different between the genera and species and species-dependent (Bernardeau et al., 2008). This may be because there is no appropriate standard procedure to determine the susceptibility of the isolates to antibiotics. Since transferability studies are not systematic, the incidences may be underestimated since a minority of starter and probiotic strains may show transferable antibiotic resistance (Bernardeau et al., 2008). Several recommendations were made by 60 academic and industrial scientists during a recent EU-PROSAFE workshop. The participants suggested that the MIC distributions of LAB and other relevant species should be assessed according to the PROSAFE reference method or other comparable and standardized methods. Additionally, a central public database encompassing antibiotic susceptibility data on LAB, as well as other relevant species, has been collected for comparison from several EU-funded projects (Vankerckhoven et al., 2008).

The Global Epidemiology of Antibiotic-Resistant Probiotic Strains

The epidemiology of antibiotic resistance is complex and dynamic. However, there have been very few outbreaks caused by LAB and hence less emphasis has been given to systematic studies that investigate the acquired antibiotic resistance in LAB. Most data exist on opportunistic pathogenic enterococci, while the number of reports on other probiotic strains is limited.

Strains of lactobacilli can be resistant to vancomycin (intrinsic), cefazolin, penicillin, tetracycline, trimethoprim-sulfamethoxazole and ciprofloxacin. These strains have been occasionally identified in cases of human *Lactobacillus*-mediated bacteremia (Antony et al., 1992). Cannon et al. (2005) conducted a study on the effects of probiotic infection that encompassed over 200 cases over a period of 53 years. As reported in their study, antibiotics such as penicillin or cephalosporin were used to treat infections caused by *Lactobacillus* spp. as monotherapy, or penicillin combined with an aminoglycoside for a synergistic effect. Patients with *Lactobacillus* bacteremia had a decreases sensitivity to antibiotics such as vancomycin, cefazolin and ciprofloxacin. Another study demonstrated that a vancomycin-resistant strain of *L. casei subsp rhamnosus* caused a case of endocarditis in a 29-year-old man with a mitral valve prolapse. Due to poor response to antimicrobial therapy with penicillin and gentamicin, the patient ultimately required a valve replacement (Monterisi et al., 1996).

Additionally, Majcher-Peszynska et al. (1999) reported a case of bacteremia due to *L. casei* subsp. *rhamnosus* in a 14-year-old girl suffering from acute myeloid leukemia. The patient also suffered from enterocolitis, *E. coli*-septicemia, pancreatitis and pneumonia. Eighteen blood cultures were detectable with lactobacilli in the course of continued cytostatic and antibiotic treatment. Up to 10^9 colony forming units per gram of feces was detected. The *Lactobacillus*-bacteremia disappeared only after 13 months when the cytostatic therapy was terminated.

Salminen et al., (2006) conducted a study on patients who received antimicrobial therapy during the two weeks prior to the onset of *Lactobacillus* bacteremia. In these cases, 23% of patients were given cephalosporins, 33% of patients received β-lactam agents and 11% of patients were given vancomycin. The infections showed a wide variability in the susceptibility to cephalosporins. This suggested that *Lactobacillus* bacteremia may not be effectively treated with cephalosporins.

A case of a 63-year-old woman who developed mitral valve endocarditis secondary to infection with *L. acidophilus* was reported by Makaryus et al. (2005). The patient had a medical history of ovarian cancer and had received chemotherapy treatment. The infection displayed resistance against azithromycin, ceftriaxone and imipenem. Her condition deteriorated and she was placed in the intensive care unit. Her blood cultures showed growth of *L. acidophilus.* Antibiotic treatment was immediately changed to ampicillin and vancomycin and the infection was cleared. This demonstrated that *L. acidophilus* translocated into the blood and the strain was azithromycin, ceftriaxone and imipenem resistant.

Saarela et al. (2007) conducted the first study investigating the effects of antibiotic therapy on the antibiotic susceptibility of simultaneously ingested probiotic strains. The authors investigated the effects of oral therapy with tetracycline-based antibiotics on the probiotic strains *L. acidophilus* LaCH-5 and *B. animalis* subsp. *lactis* Bb-12. A higher proportion of tetracycline-resistant anaerobic bacteria and bifidobacteria was detected in the subjects taking antibiotics than the control group subjects. In addition, several subjects taking antibiotics had fecal *B. animalis* subsp. *lactis* Bb-12-like isolates that showed reduced tertracycline susceptibility. This study suggests a safety risk in the possible emergence of antibiotic-resistant probiotic *B. animalis* subsp. *lactis* Bb-12 and *L. acidophilus* LaCH-5 when an antibiotic was ingested simultaneously. Even though lactobacilli-mediated endocarditis may lead to infection or death, other antibiotic-resistant probiotic strains have also been associated with infections. A well-documented instance of *Leuconostoc*-associated infection was reported by Buu-Hoi et al. (1985). Two strains of *Leuconostoc* spp. that were highly resistant to vancomycin were isolated from immunocompromised patients with bacteremia. In another case, Coovadia et al. (1987) reported the isolation of a *Leuconostoc* strain from a 16-year-old girl with purulent meningitis.

Detection and Elimination of Antibiotic Resistance in Probiotics

The type of resistance of a probiotic (i.e., whether it belongs to the natural (intrinsic or inherent) type or the acquired type) is useful when detecting antimicrobial resistance for the probiotic strains (Vankerckhoven, et al., 2008). The EU has set stringent guidelines for microorganisms that are used as feed additives. These microorganisms are required to be evaluated on a 90-day toxicity study that includes the detection of naturally occurring antibiotic resistance markers. The presence of antibiotic resistance markers does not automatically exclude the microorganism from authorization, as the risk assessment is based on the genetic basis of the antibiotic resistance (acquired or intrinsic) and the type of antibiotic for which resistance is expressed (Feord, 2002).

Natural antibiotic resistance is non-transferable and is a specific characteristic of a given taxonomic group. In contrast, bacterial strains with acquired antibiotic resistances are characterized by MICs. The MIC value will be higher than the normal MIC range of the original population of a given taxonomic group. Acquired resistance may transfer foreign DNA from and back to the bacterial cell. From previous studies, the transfer of acquired resistance genes may occur under proper experimental procedures but the failure to demonstrate in vitro gene transfer does not exclude the possibility of the transfer of genes. In addition, it has been shown that transfer of resistance genes occurs more frequently in vivo than in vitro (Vankerckhoven et al., 2008). This often complicates the detection processes even though detection methods using various genetic approaches have been developed.

The development of new molecular techniques such as PCR, molecular beacons and DNA chips enhances the efficacy of detecting and monitoring resistance. However, molecular assays have a number of limitations including underestimating new resistance mechanisms, cost and improper quality control that may lead to questionable results. Presently, the common nucleic acid-based assays used for the detection of resistance still offer advantages over the conventional phenotypic assays (Fluit et al., 2001). For example, a high-level of glycopeptide resistance could be detected via phenotypic methods but low-level resistance and the differentiation between different *Van* types are often underestimated via phenotypic techniques (Chen et al., 1998).

One of the largest studies on the detection of glycopeptide-resistant enterococci was conducted by Biavasco et al. (2007). This study detected the VanA phenotype, which expresses inducible, high-level vancomycin and teicoplanin resistance. The study involved glycopeptide-resistant enterococci of different origins (human, $n = 69$; animal, $n = 49$; food, $n = 36$) and from different geographic areas to gain a better understanding of the involvement of the different reservoirs and transmission routes. *Enterococcus* was studied due to their wide use as starter cultures and probiotics for the production of cheese, fermented sausages and animal feeds, as well as their isolation from the bloodstream, urinary tract and surgical sites of patients with nosocomial infections. The number of isolates that are resistant to all previously effective antibiotics is increasing due to the increased emergence of resistance against multiple antibiotics, including high-level resistance to glycopeptides. The authors reported that in 98% of the strains tested, *vanA* was located on plasmids, which may be involved in the intestinal colonization of animals and humans. Additionally, these plasmids were conjugative and may contribute to horizontal transfer processes. The authors also reported that human colonization by food and animal glycopeptide-resistant enterococci is possible although vertical transmission between reservoirs is infrequent. One of the most important findings of this research was the detection of the same *vanA* and virulence determinants in enterococci of different species and origins. This indicates a lack of host-specific markers and suggests that all glycopeptide-resistant enterococci, irrespective of their origins and species, may be regarded as potential reservoirs of resistance determinants and virulence traits that are transferable to human-adapted clusters.

The detection and characterization of antibiotic resistance traits in probiotics is a great concern, especially when they are detected in readily prepared food products. The use of PCR is well-known and this technique has become broadly used after the introduction of a thermostable DNA polymerase and the development of automated oligonucleotide synthesis and thermocyclers. New emerging developments in labeling technology have also expanded the applicability of PCR (Fluit et al., 2001). Gevers et al. (2003) were one of the pioneers in using the (GTG)₅-PCR DNA fingerprinting technique to demonstrate the taxonomic and genotypic potential of diverse *Lactobacillus* strains isolated from different types of fermented meat products as hosts for plasmid-borne tetracycline resistance. The authors detected 94 tetracycline-resistant lactic acid bacteria from nine different types of fermented dry sausage and subsequently characterized the host organisms and the tetracycline resistance genes that they carry. LAB isolates were identified as *Lactobacillus plantarum*, *L. sakei* subsp. *carnosus*, *L. sakei* subsp. *sakei*, *L. curvatus* and *L. alimentarius*. Tetracycline resistance genes determined by means of PCR indicated high sequence similarities (>99.6%) with those reported in the pathogenic *Staphylococcus aureus* MRSA. Southern blots demonstrated that the isolates contained tetracycline-resistant carrying plasmids, while analysis by PCR revealed that the genes were not located on transposons.

With new emerging antibiotic resistance that is acquired at a fast pace, simple and rapid detection methods are desired. A disposable microarray that could detect up to 90 antibiotic resistance genes in Gram-positive bacteria by hybridization was developed by Perreten et al. (2005). A total of 137 oligonucleotides (26 to 33 nucleotides in length with similar physicochemical parameters) were spotted onto the microarray. The microarrays were hybridized with 36 strains carrying specific antibiotic resistance genes that allowed for the testing of the sensitivity and specificity of 125 oligonucleotides. Among the probiotics tested were well-characterized multidrug-resistant strains of *Enterococcus faecalis*, *Enterococcus faecium*, and *Lactococcus lactis*. The technology developed could complement the standard MIC determination for pathogenic and commensal bacteria, detect silent antibiotic resistance genes and could be used for rapid tracking of newly emerging resistance genes. Such a tool was based on DNA arrays and the principle of hybridization, which allow the mass screening of sequences. A large collection of probes are used and are bound to a solid surface. The target DNA is generally tagged with a fluorescent label and hybridization is detected by using an epifluorescence microscope. The fragment probes are applied to the solid surface after they are generated, whereas oligonucleotides are either applied after synthesis or synthesized in situ. On DNA arrays, cDNAs or PCR products are attached to a solid surface and used for large-scale assessment of gene expression by measuring mRNA levels (Fluit et al., 2001).

The microarray technology is also beneficial for the detection of different resistance mechanisms that may coexist in a particular strain. Ammor et al. (2008) isolated a *Lactobacillus sakei* strain from Italian sola cheese made from raw milk and characterized the functionality of ribosomal protection- and efflux pump-encoding genes (*tet*(M) and *tet*(L)) that are responsible for tetracycline resistance. The DNA microarrays that were used contained 327 oligonucleotides (50 to 60 base pairs long), which included control probes and oligonucleotides specific for 250 antibiotic resistance genes, including 28 *tet* genes. The results obtained were interesting as two different mechanisms conferring resistance to tetracycline were detected in the same strain of a LAB for the first time. The authors found that the tetracycline resistance in the strain was mediated by a transposon-associated *tet*(M) gene coding for a ribosomal protection protein and a plasmid-carried *tet*(L) gene coding for a tetracycline efflux pump.

Once detected, the elimination of an antibiotic resistant trait from a particular strain is desired but the process is often complicated, time consuming and, up to now, there has been no documented guideline. Several approaches have been suggested by scientists for elimination of antibiotic resistance, including the selective removal or curing of plasmids coding for antibiotic resistance. However, it has been heavily emphasized that the cured strains would no longer be similar to their parent cells genotypically and phenotypically and may arise as a new strain since they have been genetically modified (Vankerckhoven et al., 2008).

This approach has been adopted by Huys et al. (2006) who detected the plasmid-encoded tetracycline-(S) gene in *Lactobacillus plantarum* CCUG 43738. The authors demonstrated that lactobacilli from food, feed or fecal origin can harbor acquired antibiotic resistance, which is not considered a desirable and safe trait for potentially probiotic strains. However, plasmid curing with novobiocin produced multiple tetracycline-susceptible derivatives of strain CCUG 43738 that showed significantly reduced MICs for tetracycline. A reduction in MIC for tetracycline from 512 to 16 μg/ml was observed and this was in the range for tetracycline-susceptible *L. plantarum* strains. Upon further molecular characterization of these derivatives, the authors found that the 14-kb plasmid was eliminated, which resulted in the loss of the tetracycline-(S) gene. Further evaluation of the conjugal transfer of the tetracycline-(S) plasmid from strain CCUG 43738 to the *E. faecalis* recipient JH2-2 by filter mating showed that it was not possible. Although this may seem as an alternative to the immediate removal of a resistance trait, this study could not exclude the possibility that this plasmid is transferable to other phylogenetically-related recipients and that the parent and daughter strains may differ in probiotic attributes. In another study, Rosander et al. (2008) evaluated the resistance of *Lactobacillus reuteri* ATCC 55730 against several antibiotics and found that the strain harbored two plasmids carrying *tet*(W) tetracycline and *lnu*(A) lincosamide resistance. Upon removal of the two plasmids, a new daughter strain was derived and was shown to have lost the resistances associated with them. Other than the elimination of resistance traits, a direct comparison of the parent and daughter strains for a series of in vitro properties and in a human clinical trial confirmed that the probiotic properties of the parent strain were retained and not modified.

Although feasible, plasmid curing may not be solution that is suitable for all cases of antibiotic resistance elimination. Chin et al. (2005) isolated strains of lactobacilli from the gastrointestinal tracts of chicken and assessed their susceptibility to antibiotics such as chloramphenicol, erythromycin and tetracycline. All of the strains exhibited varying degrees of resistance to all the antibiotics studied. Seven of the twelve *Lactobacillus* strains that exhibited resistance to at least 50 μg/ml of chloramphenicol or erythromycin and five strains that exhibited resistance to at least 50 μg/ml of tetracycline were subsequently subjected to plasmid curing using novobiocin, acriflavin, SDS and ethidium bromide. The results obtained showed that only five derivatives of *Lactobacillus* were cured of their resistance towards erythromycin while the remaining strains were incurable.

Conclusion

Although probiotics are more documented for their gastrointestinal benefits, they could also be used for the modulation of other health aspects such as the treatment and/or prevention antibiotic resistance in hosts. However, with new evidence showing that they could also harbor antibiotic resistance genes, more emphasis are given to the need for further assessment prior to consumption. It is now suggested that non-antibiotic resistance is set as a criterion for safety assessment of probiotic strains meant for food applications. With better knowledge of the mechanisms involved, the dissemination of antibiotic resistance in probiotic strains could also be better controlled. Although antibiotic resistant probiotics have been isolated from infection sites, they are rarely life-threatening. With new emerging genomic technologies, it is hoped that the detection and elimination of probiotics with antibiotic resistance traits could be made more affordable, rapid and accurate.

Acknowledgment

The authors would like to acknowledge the USM RU grant (1001/ PTEKIND/ 811089), USM fellowship and the eScienceFund Grant (305/PTEKIND/613218) for financial assistance.

References

Ammor, M. S., Flo´ Rez, A. B. N. and Mayo, B. (2007). Antibiotic resistance in non-enterococcal lactic acid bacteria and bifidobacteria. *Food Microbiology, 24*, 559-570.

Ammor, M. S., Gueimonde, M, Danielsen, M., Zagorec, M., van Hoek, A. H. A. M., de los Reyes-Gavilán, C. G., Mayo, B. and Margolles, A. (2008). Two different tetracycline resistance mechanisms, plasmid-carried *tet*(L) and chromosomally located transposon-associated *tet*(M), coexist in *Lactobacillus sakei* Rits. *Applied and Environmental Microbiology, 74*, 1394 - 1401.

Arthur, M., Reynolds, P. and Courvalin P. (1996). Glycopeptide resistance in enterococci. *Trends of Microbiology, 4*, 401-407.

Baquero, F., Negir, M. C., Morosini, M. I. and Blazquez J. (1997). The antibiotic selection process: concentration-specific amplification of low-level resistant populations. In Chadwick. D. J., and Goode, J. (Eds.), Antibiotic Resistance. Origins, evolution, selection and spread (pp. 87-105). Chichester, West Sussex: John Wiley and Sons.

Bernardeau, M., Vernoux, J. P., Henri-Dubernet, S. and Guéguen, M. (2008). Safety assessment of dairy microorganisms: The *Lactobacillus* genus. *International Journal of Food Microbiology, 126*, 278-285.

Biavasco F., Foglia, G., Paoletti, C., Zandri, G., Magi, G., Guaglianone, E., Sundsfjord, A., Pruzzo, C., Donelli, G. and Facinelli, B. (2007). VanA-Type Enterococci from humans, animals, and food: species distribution, population structure, Tn*1546* typing and location, and virulence determinants. *Applied and Environmental Microbiology, 73*, 3307–3319.

Biswas, S., Raoult, D. and Rolain J. M. (2008). A bioinformatic approach to understanding antibiotic resistance in intracellular bacteria through whole genome analysis. *International Journal of Antimicrobial Agents, 32*, 207-220.

Borriello, S. P., Hammes, W. P., Holzapfel, W., Marteau, P., Schrezenmeir, J., Vaara, M. and Valtonen, V. (2003). Safety of probiotics that contain lactobacilli or bifidobacteria. *Clinical Infectious Diseases, 36*, 775-780.

Buu-Hoi, A., Branger, C. and Acar, J.F. (1985). Vancomycin resistant streptococci or *Leuconostoc* sp. *Antimicrobial Agents and Chemotherapy, 28*, 458-460.

Cannon, J. P., Lee, T. A., Bolanos, J. T. and Danziger, L. H. (2005). Pathogenic relevance of *Lactobacillus*: a retrospective review of over 200 cases. *European Journal of Clinical Microbiology and Infectious Diseases, 24*, 31-40.

Chen, Y. S., Marshall, S. A., Winokur, P. L., Coffman, S. L., Wilke, W. W., Murray, P. R., Spiegel, C. A., Pfaller, M. A., Doern, G. V. and Jones, R. N. (1998). Use of molecular and reference susceptibility testing methods in a multicenter evaluation of MicroScan dried overnight gram-positive MIC panels for detection of vancomycin and high-level aminoglycoside resistances in enterococci. *Journal of Clinical Microbiology*, 36, 2996-3001.

Chin, S. C., Abdullah, N., Siang, T. W. and Wan, H. Y. (2005). Plasmid profiling and curing of *Lactobacillus* strains isolated from the gastrointestinal tract of chicken. *Journal of Microbiology, 43*, 251-256.

Coovadia, Y. M., Solwa, Z. and Van de Ende, J. (1987). Meningitis caused by vancomycin-resistant *Leuconostoc* sp. *Journal of Clinical Microbiology, 25*, 1784-1785.

Courvalin, P. (2006). Antibiotic resistance: the pros and cons of probiotics. *Journal of Digestive and Liver Disease, 38*, S261-S265.

Courvalin, P. (2008). Predictable and unpredictable evolution of antibiotic resistance. *Journal of Internal Medicine, 264*, 4-16.

Curragh, H. J. and Collins, M. A. (1992). High-levels of spontaneous drug-resistance in *Lactobacillus. Journal of Applied Bacteriology, 73*, 31-36.

D'Aimmo, M. R., Modesto, M. and Biavati, B. (2007). Antibiotic resistance of lactic acid bacteria and *Bifidobacterium* spp. isolated from dairy and pharmaceutical products. *International Journal of Food Microbiology, 115*, 35–42.

Danielsen, M. and Wind, A. (2003). Susceptibility of *Lactobacillus* spp. to antimicrobial agents. *International Journal of Food Microbiology, 82*, 1-11.

Davies, J. E. (1997). Origins, acquisition and dissemination of antibiotic resistance determinants. In Chadwick, D. J. and Goode, J. (Eds.) Antibiotic Resistance. Origins, evolution, selection and spread (pp. 15–27). Chichester, West Sussex: John Wiley and Sons.

Deye, G., Lewis, J., Patterson, J. and Jorgensen, J. (2003). A case of Leuconostoc ventriculitis with resistance to carbapenem antibiotics. *Clinical Infectious Disease, 37*, 869-870.

Donskey, C. J., Hoyen, C. K., Das, S. M., Farmer, S., Dery, M. and Bonomo, R.A. (2001). Effect of oral *Bacillus coagulans* administration on the density of vancomycin-resistant enterococci in the stool of colonized mice. *Letters in Applied Microbiology, 33*, 84-88.

Erickson, K. L. and Hubbard, N. E. (2000). Probiotic immunomodulation in health and disease. *Journal of Nutrition*, 130, 403S-409S.

FAO/WHO (2002). Report of a joint FAO/WHO working group on drafting guidelines for the evaluation of probiotics in food. 2008 September 27. Available from: ftp://ftp.fao.org/es/esn/food/wgreport2.pdf.

FEEDAP Panel (Scientific Panel on Additives and Products or Substances used in Animal Feed) (2008). Technical guidance - update of the criteria used in the assessment of bacterial resistance to antibiotics of human or veterinary importance. EFSA Journal, 732, 1-15.

Feord, J. (2002). Lactic acid bacteria in a changing legislative environment. *Antonie van Leeuwenhoek, 82*, 353-360.

Flórez, A. B., Delgado, S. and Mayo, B. (2005). Antimicrobial susceptibility of lactic acid bacteria isolated from a cheese environment. *Canadian Journal of Microbiology, 51*, 51-58.

Fluit, A. C., Visser, M. R. and Schmitz, F. J. (2001). Molecular detection of antimicrobial resistance. *Clinical Microbiology Reviews, 14*, 836-871.

Fons, M., Hege, T., Ladire, M., Raibaud, P., Ducluzeau, R. and Maguin, E. (1997) Isolation and characterization of a plasmid from *Lactobacillus fermentum* conferring erythromycin resistance. *Plasmid, 37*, 199-203.

Galvin, Hill, M., C. and Ross. R. P. (1999). Lacticin 3147 displays activity in buffer against gram-positive bacterial pathogens which appear insensitive in standard plate assays. *Letter in Applied Microbiology, 28*, 355-358.

Gevers D., Danielsen, M., Huys, G. and Swings, J. (2003). Molecular characterization of *tet*(M) genes in *Lactobacillus* isolates from different types of fermented dry sausage. *Applied and Environmental Microbiology, 69*, 1270-1275.

Giacometti, A., Cirioni, O., Barchiesi, F. and Scalise, G. (2000). In-vitro activity and killing effect of polycationic peptides on methicillin-resistant *Staphylococcus aureus* and interactions with clinically used antibiotics. *Diagnostic Microbiology and Infectious Disease, 38*, 115-118.

Girlich, D., Leclercq, R., Naas, T. and Nordmann, P. (2007). Molecular and biochemical characterization of the chromosome-encoded class A ß-lactamase BCL-1 from *Bacillus clausii. Antimicrobial Agents and Chemotherapy, 51*, 4009-4014.

Gollrdge, C. L., Stingemore, N., Aravena, M. and Joske, D. (1990). Septicemia caused by vancomycin-resistant *Pediococcus acidilactici. Journal of Clinical Microbiology, 28*, 1678-1679.

Gorbach, S. L. (1996). Efficacy of *Lactobacillus* in treatment of acute diarrhea. *Nutrition Today, 31*, 19S–23S.

Hatakka, K., Savilahti, E., Ponka, A., Meurman, J.H., Poussa, T., Näse, L., Saxelin, M. and Korpela, R. (2001). Effect of long term consumption of probiotic milk on infections in children attending day care centres: double blind, randomised trial. *British Medical Journal, 322*, 1327–1329.

Herrero, M., Mayo, B., González, B. and Suárez, J.E. (1996). Evaluation of technologically important traits in lactic acid bacteria isolated from spontaneous fermentations. *Journal of Applied Bacteriology, 81*, 565-570.

Hummel A. S., Hertel C., Holzapfel W. H. and Franz C. M. A. P. (2007). Antibiotic resistances of starter and probiotic strains of lactic acid bacteria. *Applied and Environmental Microbiology, 73*, 730-739.

Huys, G., D'Haene, K. and Swings, J. (2006). Genetic basis of tetracycline and minocycline resistance in potentially probiotic *Lactobacillus plantarum* strain CCUG 43738. *Antimicrobial Agents and Chemotherapy, 50*, 1550 - 1551.

Ishibashi, N. and Shoji, Y. (2001). Probiotics and safety. *American Journal of Clinical Nutrition, 73*, 465S–470S.

Kastner, S., Perreten, V., Bleuler, H., Hugenschmidt, G., Lacroix, C. and Meile, L. (2006). Antibiotic susceptibility patterns and resistance genes of starter cultures and probiotic bacteria used in food. *Systematic and Applied Microbiology, 29*, 145-155.

Klare, I., Konstabell, C., Werner, G., Huys, G., Vankerckhoven, V., Kahlmeter, G., Hildebrandt, B., Müller-Bertling, S., Witte, W. and Goossens, H. (2007). Antimicrobial susceptibilities of *Lactobacillus, Pediococcus* and *Lactococcus* human isolates and cultures intended for probiotic or nutritional use. *Journal of Antimicrobial Chemotherapy, 59*, 900-912.

Land, M. H., Rouster-Stevens, K., Woods, C. R., Cannon, M. L., Cnota, J. and Shetty, A. K. (2005). *Lactobacillus* sepsis associated with probiotic therapy. *Pediatrics, 115*, 178-181.

Launay, A., Ballard, S. A., Johnson, P. D. R., Grayson, M. L. and Lambert T. (2006) Transfer of vancomycin resistance transposon Tn1549 from *Clostridium symbiosum* to *Enterococcus spp.* in the gut of gnotobiotic mice. *Antimicrobial Agents and Chemotherapy, 50*, 1054-1062.

Lim, K. S., Huh, C. S. and Baek, Y. J. (1993). Antimicrobial susceptibility of bifidobacteria. *Journal of Dairy Science, 76*, 2168-2174.

Liong, M. T. (2008). Safety of probiotics: translocation and infection. *Nutrition Reviews, 66*, 192-202.

Lund, B. and Edlund, C. (2001) Probiotic *Enterococcus faecium* strain is a possible recipient of the vanA gene cluster. *Clinical Infectious Diseases, 32*, 1384–1385.

Majcher-Peszynska, J., Heine, W., Richter, I., Eggers, G. and Mohr, C. (1999). Persistant *Lactobacillus casei* subspecies *rhamnosus* bacteremia in a 14-year-old girl with acute myloid leukemia. A case report. *Clinical Pediatrics, 211*, 53-56.

Makaryus, A. N., Yang, R., Hahn, R.T. and Kort, S. (2005). A rare case of *Lactobacillus acidophilus* presenting as mitral valve bacterial endocarditis. *Echocardiography, 22*, 421-425.

Manley, K. J., Fraenkel, M. B., Mayall, B. C. and Power, D. A. (2007). Probiotic treatment of vancomycin-resistant enterococci: a randomised controlled trial. *The Medical Journal of Australia, 186*, 454-457.

Marteau, P. and Salminen, S. (1997). Demonstration of safety of probiotics. *Demonstration of Nutritional Functionality of Probiotic Foods Newsletter, 2*, 3-8.

Marteau, P. and Shanahan, F. (2003). Basic aspects and pharmacology of probiotics: an overview of pharmacokinetics, mechanisms of action and side-effects. *Best Practice and Research Clinical Gastroenterology, 17*, 725-740.

Marteau, P. (2001) Safety aspects of probiotic products. *Journal of Nutrition, 45*, 22-24.

Mathur, S. and Singh, R. (2005). Antibiotic resistance in food lactic acid bacteria-a review. *International Journal of Food Microbiology, 105*, 281-295.

Miller, L. G. and Finegold, S. M. (1967). Antibacterial sensitivity of *Bifidobacterium (Lactobacillus bifidus). Journal of Bacteriology 93*, 125–130.

Miller-Catchpole, R. (1989). Bifidobacteria in clinical microbiology and medicine. In Bezkorovainy, A. and Miller-Catchpole, R. (Eds), Biochemistry and Physiology of Bifidobacteria, (pp. 177-200). Boca Raton, California: CRC Press.

Millette, M., Cornut, G., Dupont, C., Shareck, F., Archambault, D. and Lacroix, M. (2008). Capacity of human nisin- and pediocin-producing lactic acid bacteria to reduce intestinal colonization by vancomycin-resistant enterococci. *Applied and Environmental Microbiology, 74*, 1997-2003.

Monterisi, A., Dain, A. A., Suárez de Basnec, M. C., Roca, G., Trucchia, R. and Bantar, C. (1996). Native-valve endocarditis produced by *Lactobacillus casei* sub. *rhamnosus* refractory to antimicrobial therapy. *Medicina, 56*, 284-286.

Morgan, S. M., O'Connor, P. M., Cotter, P. D., Ross, R. P. and Hill, C. (2005). Sequential actions of the two component peptides of the lantibiotic lacticin 3147 explain its antimicrobial activity at nanomolar concentrations. *Antimicrobial Agents and Chemotherapy, 49*, 2606-2611.

Moubareck, C., Gavini, F., Vaugien, L., Butel, M. J. and Doucet-Populaire, F. (2005). Antimicrobial susceptibility of bifidobacteria. *Journal of Antimicrobial Chemotherapy, 55*, 38-44.

Moubareck, C., Lecso, M., Pinloche, E., Butel, M. J. and Doucet-Populaire, F. (2007). Inhibitory impact of bifidobacteria on the transfer of ß-lactam resistance among *Enterobacteriaceae* in the gnotobiotic mouse digestive tract. *Applied and Environmental Microbiology, 73*, 855-860.

Ohhira, I., Tamura, T., Fujii, N., Inagaki, K. and Tanaka, H. (1996). Antimicrobial activity against methicillin-resistant *Staphylococcus aureus* in the culture broth of *Enterococcus Faecalis* Th 10, an isolate from Malaysian fermentation food-tempeh. *Japanese Journal of Dairy and Food Sciences, 45*, 4-7.

Orberg, P.K., and Sandine, W.E. (1985). Survey of antimicrobial resistance in lactic streptococci. *Applied and Environmental Microbiology, 49*, 538-542.

Ouoba, L. I. I., Lei, V. and Jensen, L. B. (2008). Resistance of potential probiotic lactic acid bacteria and bifidobacteria of African and European origin to antimicrobials: Determination and transferability of the resistance genes to other bacteria. *International Journal of Food Microbiology, 121*, 217-224.

Perreten, V., Vorlet-Fawer, L., Slickers, P., Ehricht, R., Kuhnert, P. and Frey, J. (2005). Microarray-based detection of 90 antibiotic resistance genes of gram-positive bacteria. *Journal of Clinical Microbiology, 43*, 2291 - 2302.

Pineiro, M. and Stanton, C. (2007). Probiotic bacteria: legislative framework—requirements to evidence basis. *Journal of Nutrition, 137*, 850S–853S.

Quigley, E. M. M. and Quera, R. (2006). Small intestinal bacterial overgrowth: roles of antibiotics, prebiotics, and probiotics. *Gastroenterology, 130*, S78–S90.

Roghmann M. C and McGrail L. (2006). Novel ways of preventing antibiotic-resistant infections: What might the future hold? *American Journal of Infection Control, 34*, 469-475.

Rosander, A., Connolly, E. and Roos, S. (2008). Removal of antibiotic resistance gene-carrying plasmids from *Lactobacillus reuteri* ATCC 55730 and characterization of the resulting daughter strain, *L. reuteri* DSM 17938. *Applied and Environmental Microbiology, 74*, 6032 - 6040.

Saarela, M., Maukonen, J., Wright, A. V., Vilpponen-Salmela, T., Patterson, A. J., Scott, K. P., Hämynen, H. and Mättö, J. (2007). Tetracycline susceptibility of the ingested *Lactobacillus acidophilus* LaCH-5 and *Bifidobacterium animalis* subsp. *lactis* Bb-12 strains during antibiotic/probiotic intervention. *International Journal of Antimicrobial Agents, 29*, 271-280.

Salminen, M. K., Rautelin, H., Tynkkynen, S., Poussa, T., Saxelin, M., Valtonen, V. and Jarvinen, A. (2004). *Lactobacillus* bacteremia, clinical significance, and patient outcome, with special focus on probiotic *L. rhamnosus* GG. *Clinical Infection, 38*, 62-69.

Salminen, M. K., Rautelin, H., Tynkkynen, S., Poussa, T., Saxelin, M., Valtonen, V. and Jarvinen, A. (2006) *Lactobacillus* bacteremia, species identification, and antimicrobial susceptibility of 85 blood isolates. *Clinical Infectious Disease, 42*, 35-44.

Salminen, S., Wright, A. V., Morelli, L., Marteau, P., Brassarte, D., De Vosf, W. M., Fonde'Ng, R., Saxelinh, M., Collinsi, K., Mogensenj, G., Birkelandk, S. and Mattila-Sandholmb, T., (1998). Demonstration of safety of probiotics — a review. *International Journal of Food Microbiology, 44*, 93-106.

Sarra, P. G., Vescovo, M., Morelli, L. and Cabras, M. (1982). Antibiotic resistance in *L. acidophilus* and *L. reuteri* from animal gut. *Annals of Microbiology and Enzymology, 32*, 71-76.

Sasaki, Y., Taketomo, N. and Sasaki, T. (1988). Factors affecting transfer frequency of pAMb1 from *Streptococcus faecalis* to *Lactobacillus plantarum. Journal of Bacteriology, 170*, 5939-5942.

SCAN (Scientific Committee on Animal Nutrition), (2003). Opinion of the scientific coomittee on animal nutrition on the criteria for assessing the safety of micro-organisms resistant to antibiotics of human clinical and veterinary importance, European Commission Health and Consumer Protection Directorate-General. 2008 September 27. Available from: http://ec.europa.eu/food/fs/sc/scan/out64_en.pdf.

Scott, K. P., Melville, C. M., Barbosa, T. M. and Flint, H. J. (2000). Occurrence of the new tetracycline resistance gene tet(W) in bacteria from the human gut. *Antimicrobial Agents and Chemotherapy, 44*, 775-777.

Slover, C. M. and Danziger, L. (2008). *Lactobacillus*: a review. *Clinical Microbiology Newsletter, 30*, 23-27.

Sriskandan, S., Lacey, S. and Fischer, L. (1993). Isolation of vancomycin-resistant lactobacilli from three neutropenic patients with pneumonia. *European Journal of Clinical Microbiology Infection Distribution, 12*, 649-650.

Storm, D. R., Rosenthal K. S. and Swanson, P. E. (1977). Polymyxin and related peptide antibiotics. *Annual Review of Biochemistry, 46*, 723-763.

Sullivan, A., Johansson, A., Svenungsson, B. and Nord, C.E. (2004). Effect of *Lactobacillus* F19 on the emergence of antibiotic-resistant microorganisms in the intestinal microflora. *Journal of Antimicrobial Chemotherapy, 54*, 791-797.

Tang, H., Yuan, J., Xie, C. H. and Wei, H. (2007). Antibiotic susceptibility of strains in Chinese medical probiotic products. *Journal of Medical Colleges of PLA, 22*, 149-152.

Tannock, G. W. (1987). Conjugal transfer of plasmid pAMβ1 in *Lactobacillus reuteri* and between lactobacilli and *Enterococcus faecalis*. *Applied Environmental Microbiology, 53*, 2693-2695.

Tenover F. C. (2006). Mechanisms of antimicrobial resistance in bacteria. *American Journal of Infection Control, 34*, S3-S10.

Teuber, M., Meile L. and Schwarz, F. (1999). Acquired antibiotic resistance in lactic acid bacteria from food. *Antonie van Leeuwenhoek, 76*, 115-137.

Vankerckhoven, V., Huys, G., Vancanneyt, M., Vael, C., Klare, I., Romond, M., Entenze, J., Moreillon, P., D Wind, R., Knol, J., Wiertz, E., Pot, B., Vaughan, E. E., Kahlmeter, G. and Goossens, H. (2008). Biosafety assessment of probiotics used for human consumption: recommendations from the EU-PROSAFE project. *Trends in Food Science and Technology, 19*, 102-114.

Vesterlund, S., Karp, M., Salminen, S. and Ouwehand, A.C. (2006). *Staphylococcus aureus* adheres to human intestinal mucus but can be displaced by certain lactic acid bacteria. *Microbiology, 152*, 1819-1826.

White, D. G. and McDermott, P. F. (2001). Emergence and Transfer of antibacterial resistance. *Journal of Dairy Science, 84*, E151-E155.

Yokokura, T., and Mutai, M. (1976). Penicillin resistance and its elimination by treatment with acriflavine in *Lactobacillus fermentum. Japanese Journal of Microbiology, 20*, 241-242.

Zhou, J. S., Pillidge, C. J., Gopalc, P. K. and Gilla, H. S. (2005). Antibiotic susceptibility profiles of new probiotic *Lactobacillus* and *Bifidobacterium* strains. *International Journal of Food Microbiology, 98*, 211-217.

Zoppi, G., Cinquetti, M., Benini, A., Bonamini, E. and Minelli, E.B. (2001). Modulation of the intestinal ecosystem by probiotics and lactulose in children during treatment with ceftriaxone. *Current Therapeutic Research, 62*, 418–29.

In: Antibiotic Resistance: Causes and Risk Factors
Editors: A. R. Bonilla and K. P. Muniz

ISBN 978-1-60741-623-4
© 2009 Nova Science Publishers, Inc.

Chapter III

When Good Bugs Fight Bad – Designing Probiotics to Control Antibiotic Resistant "Superbugs"

*Roy D. Sleator**
Department of Biological Sciences,
Cork Institute of Technology,
Bishopstown, Cork, Ireland

Abstract

An ever increasing dependence on conventional therapeutics coupled with an alarming escalation in antibiotic resistance has facilitated the emergence of a new faction of bacterial adversaries, the antibiotic resistant 'superbugs', the aetiological agents of nosocomial infections. Against this backdrop scientists and clinicians are now struggling to find viable therapeutic alternatives to antibiotics. One such alternative involves the use of probiotics; live microorganisms, which when consumed in adequate amounts, confer a health benefit to the host. Furthermore, a new generation of probiotics termed 'designer probiotics' have been engineered to target and neutralise specific bacterial pathogens, viruses and toxins while at the same time persisting for longer periods in foods and other delivery vehicles prior to ingestion and subsequently within the gastrointestinal tract.

Expert Commentary

As we reach the 80th anniversary of Fleming's discovery of penicillin; the *wonder drug* which heralded a new era in the fight against infection, the medical establishment is now faced with a new challenge in the form of antibiotic resistance – the bugs are fighting back!

---

* Corresponding author mailing address: Dr Roy D. Sleator, Department of Biological Sciences, Cork Institute of Technology, Rossa Avenue, Bishopstown, Cork, Ireland. Email: roy.sleator@cit.ie Phone 00 353 21 4326885, Fax 00 353 21 4545343.

Moreover, the superbugs, such as MRSA (meticillin resistant *Staphylococcus aureus*) and *Clostridium difficile* appear to be winning.

With life-cycles measured in minutes as opposed to years, bacteria have an extraordinary ability to evolve and adapt rapidly to changes in their environment. Thus, in a world where only the fittest survive those bacteria which have developed resistance to antibiotics will predominate. This is particularly apparent in hospital environments where bacteria are constantly exposed to different antibiotics; such repeated exposure has facilitated the development of multiple antibiotic resistance and what we now refer to as hospital acquired or nosocomial infections.

Faced with an emerging pandemic of antibiotic resistance clinicians and scientists alike are now struggling to find viable therapeutic alternatives to our failing antibiotic wonder drugs. One such alternative may be the bacteria themselves; this *"fighting fire with fire"* approach involves probiotic therapy – the application of so called "good bugs" for therapeutic effect. While the exact mechanisms by which probiotic bacteria inhibit pathogens are as yet poorly understood, some advances have nevertheless been made in our understanding of probiotic function. Recent work, for example, revealed that the therapeutic potential of the probiotic strain *Lactobacillus salivarius* is due, at least in part, to its ability to produce a potent two-peptide bacteriocin; Abp118 [Corr et al., 2007]. Furthermore, Rea et al. [2007] recently showed significant anti-*C. difficile* potential for yet another bacteriocin; the two-component lantibiotic lacticin 3147, produced by *Lactococcus lactis*. Significantly, and in contrast to conventional broad spectrum antibiotics, lacticin 3147 completely eliminates 10^6 c.f.u *C. difficile* ml^{-1} within 30 min (at concentrations as low as 18 µg ml^{-1}).

Many pathogens exploit oligosaccharides displayed on the surface of host cells as receptors for toxins and/or adhesins, enabling colonization of the host and entry of the pathogen or secreted toxins into the host cell. Blocking this adherence prevents infection, while toxin neutralization ameliorates symptoms until the pathogen is eventually overcome by the immune system. 'Designer probiotics' have been engineered to express receptor-mimic structures on their surface which fool the pathogen into thinking that the administered probiotic is in fact their target host cell [Sleator and Hill, 2008a]. When administered orally, these engineered probiotics bind to and neutralize toxins in the gut lumen and interfere with pathogen adherence to the intestinal epithelium – thus essentially "mopping up" the infection (Figure 1). Recently Paton et al. [2006] described the construction of probiotic strains with receptor blocking potential against enterotoxigenic *Escherichia coli* (ETEC) toxin LT and cholera toxin (Ctx). *E. coli* strains have also been described which express a chimeric lipopolysaccharide (LPS) terminating in a shiga toxin (Stx) receptor; 1 mg dry weight of which can neutralize >100 µg of Stx1 and Stx2 [Paton et al, 2000].

In addition to infection control probiotics are also being engineered to function as novel vaccine delivery vehicles which can stimulate both innate and acquired immunity but lack the possibility of toxicity that exists with more conventional vaccines which rely on live attenuated pathogens [Sleator and Hill, 2008b]. Probiotic vaccine carriers administered by the mucosal route mimic the immune response elicited by natural infection and can lead to long lasting protective mucosal and systemic responses. Mucosal vaccine delivery (those administered orally or by nasal spray) also offers significant technological and commercial advantages over traditional formulations including: reduced pain and the possibility of cross contamination associated with intramuscular injection, as well as the lack of a requirement for medically trained personnel to administer the vaccine – important considerations for large scale vaccination protocols in less well developed countries [Sleator and Hill, 2008c].

Gut Lumen

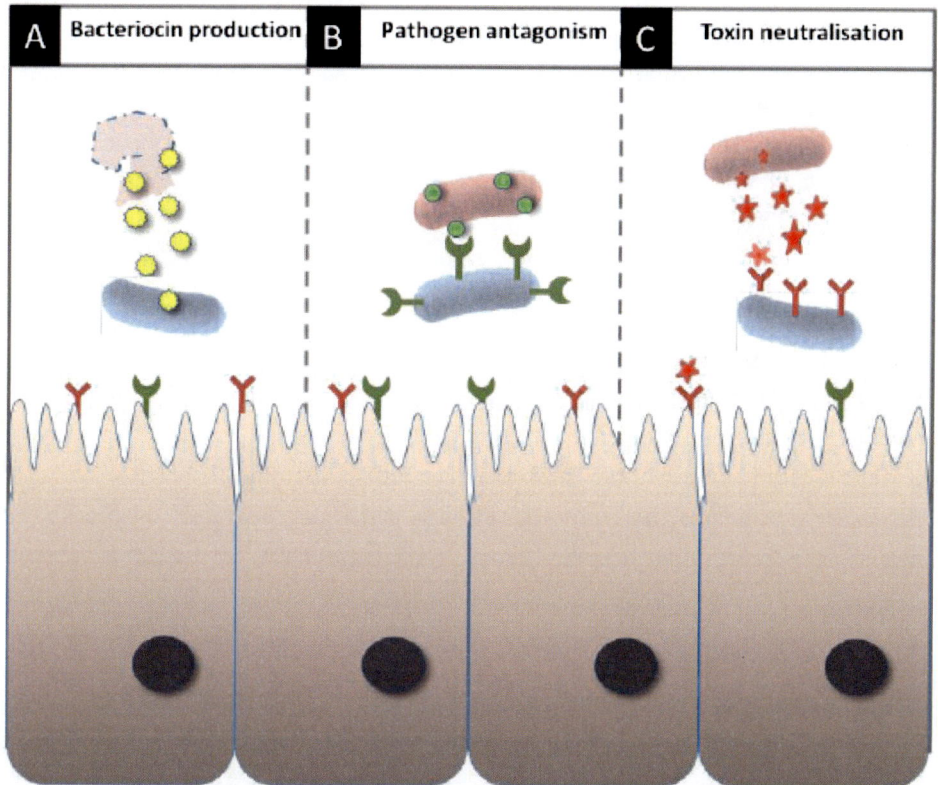

Figure 1. Overview of the anti-infective potential of designer probiotics. Bacteriocin produced by the probiotic (blue) can lyse invading *C. difficile* cells (red) (A) while heterologously expressed receptor mimics on the surface of probiotic cells can antagonise pathogen adherence to the host (B) and neutralise toxin production (C). Reproduced, with permission, from Sleator and Hill, 2008a.

Thus, in the words of The Verve "*Now the drugs don't work, they just make you worse*" - perhaps our only hope of winning the war against the antibiotic resistant "super bugs" will be achieved by recruiting engineered "good bugs" as our allies [Sleator and Hill, 2008d].

Acknowledgments

Dr Roy Sleator is a Health Research Board (HRB) and Alimentary Pharmabiotic Centre (APC) principal investigator.

References

Corr SC; Li Y, Riedel CU; O'Toole PW; Hill C and Gahan CG. Bacteriocin production as a mechanism for the antiinfective activity of Lactobacillus salivarius UCC118. *Proc. Natl. Acad. Sci. USA.* 2007; 104(18):7617-7621.

Paton AW; Morona R and Paton JC. A new biological agent for treatment of Shiga toxigenic Escherichia coli infections and dysentery in humans. *Nat. Med.* 2000; 6(3):265-270.

Paton AW; Morona R and Paton JC. Treatment and Prevention of Enteric Infections With Toxin-binding Probiotics. *Discov. Med.* 2006; 6(31):35-39.

Rea MC; Clayton E; O'Connor PM; Shanahan F; Kiely B; Ross RP and Hill C. Antimicrobial activity of lacticin 3,147 against clinical Clostridium difficile strains. *J. Med. Microbiol.* 2007; 56(Pt 7):940-946.

Sleator RD and Hill C. Designer probiotics: a potential therapeutic for Clostridium difficile? *J. Med. Microbiol.* 2008a; 57(Pt 6):793-794.

Sleator RD and Hill C. Engineered pharmabiotics with improved therapeutic potential. *Hum. Vaccin.* 2008b; 4(4):271-274.

Sleator RD and Hill C. Probiotics as therapeutics for the developing world. 2008c. *J. Infect Developing Countries* 2007; 1(1):7-12.

Sleator RD and Hill C. Battle of the Bugs. *Science.* 2008d. 321(5894):1294-1295.

In: Antibiotic Resistance: Causes and Risk Factors
Editors: A. R. Bonilla and K. P. Muniz

ISBN 978-1-60741-623-4
© 2009 Nova Science Publishers, Inc.

Chapter IV

Modification of the Bacterial Phenotype as an Approach to Counter the Emergence of Multidrug-Resistant Pathogens

Peter W. Taylor, Patricia Bernal and Andrea Zelmer
School of Pharmacy, 29-39 Brunswick Square,
London WC1N 1AX, UK

Abstract

Antibiotics are among the most beneficial drugs ever introduced but their utility has been compromised by the emergence and spread of antibiotic resistant bacteria. Currently useful antibiotics impose enormous selective pressure on bacterial populations and the use and overuse of these agents has led to the evolution, in a relatively short timeframe, of multidrug-resistant pathogens capable of rapid and efficient horizontal transmission of genes encoding resistance determinants. New antibacterial drugs with novel modes of action are urgently required in order to continue the fight against infection: unfortunately, the upturn in the incidence of resistance has coincided with a marked reduction by the pharmaceutical industry in efforts to develop new agents. Even "professional" pathogens such as *Staphylococcus aureus*, a bacterium equipped with an impressive array of virulence effectors for damaging the host, require a reduction in the host's defenses in order to colonize, enter tissue and cause infection. Correction of this imbalance between host and pathogen may provide a novel approach to the therapy of severe bacterial infections, by either shoring up immune defenses or modifying the bacteria at the site of infection to render them less able to survive in the host. Thus, pathogens may survive, multiply and cause infection because they are virulent or resistant to antibiotics; therapeutic agents that modify these properties *in vivo* may resolve infections, either alone or in combination with conventional antibiotic chemotherapy, in a way that may not readily lead to drug resistant bacterial survivors. Examples of such modifiers of the bacterial phenotype, together with other emerging approaches to the treatment of bacterial infections, are described.

Introduction

As we look back eighty years to the discovery of penicillin and contemplate the enormous impact that the introduction of potent antibiotics has had on the wellbeing of societies in industrially developed countries, it is difficult to comprehend the ravages caused by common bacterial infections in the pre-antibiotic era. Potential killer diseases such as puerperal fever, pneumonia, staphylococcal sepsis, scarlet fever, and even tuberculosis were swiftly brought under control for those lucky enough to have access to the new "miracle drugs". Although improving social conditions, access to clean drinking water, better sewage disposal, mass vaccination programs and improved nutrition played key roles, the beginning of a rapid decline in mortality from infectious diseases during the mid-twentieth century coincided with the introduction of the first clinically effective antimicrobial drugs. For example, mortality from infections in the United States fell from 797 to 36 deaths per 100,000 over the period 1900-1980 with a particularly rapid decline from 1938 to 1950 [1]. Comparable steep reductions in infectious disease mortality were also seen in other industrialized countries [2]. In the first decade of the 21st century, the majority of nosocomial and community-acquired bacterial infections can be effectively treated with one or a few of the 150 or so antibacterial agents available for clinical use, even though there are increasingly frequent reports in the medical and scientific literature of infections due to multi-drug and pan-resistant bacteria that will eventually erode the utility of our current antibacterial armamentarium.

Early optimism that vaccines, insecticides, improved surveillance and antibacterial chemotherapeutic agents would provide the tools to suppress permanently the scourge of infectious disease has proven to be wide of the mark. Globally, bacterial infections remain a leading cause of mortality and morbidity and four of the ten leading causes of death are of microbial origin [3]. Infections remain a substantial and entrenched problem in developed countries: each year in the United States alone, nearly two million will acquire bacterial infections during a hospital stay and around 90,000 will die [4]. This contrasts with approximately 10,000 deaths resulting from HIV/AIDS, a figure now surpassed by the number of deaths from methicillin-resistant *Staphylococcus aureus* (MRSA) infections [5]. The reasons for the failure to defeat the threat from infection are complex and encompass socio-cultural change, political and economic upheavals and environmental damage: rural–to–urban migration leading to the creation of high-density slums, increasing long-distance mobility and trade, the social disruption of war and conflict, human-induced environmental damage, climate change and misuse and overuse of antibiotics all provide new opportunities for the spread of infection [6]. "New" infectious agents with the capacity to cause novel diseases seem to emerge with depressing regularity and therapeutic advances have resulted in new groups of individuals, such as transplant patients, susceptible to microbes that do not normally cause disease.

A major threat is posed by the emergence on a global scale of bacteria refractory to currently useful antibiotics: the evolution of acquired antibacterial drug resistance has resulted in significant increases in mortality of hospitalized patients, increased the length of hospital stays and dramatically increased the costs of treatment. Patterns of resistance once found exclusively in bacteria causing hospital-acquired infections are now being found with increasing frequency in the community [7]. Although doom-laden prophesies of "superbugs" and "the post-antibiotic era" are an exaggerated response to the problems we face (for a lively and informed discussion of this topic, see the recent tract from Greenwood [8]), the increasing incidence of antibiotic resistance has contributed in part to the fall from use in countries such as the United Kingdom of heretofore frontline agents such as chloramphenicol, sulfonamides and streptomycin [9]. In addition, the therapeutic utility of currently effective antimicrobials such as the fluoroquinolones, vancomycin and the carbapenems is being eroded by increased frequency of resistance [10]. There is, therefore, an urgent need for new antibacterial drugs effective against today's intractable pathogens and stealthy opportunists but, unfortunately, the traditional suppliers of new antimicrobials, the major pharmaceutical companies, are no longer fully committed to antibiotic drug discovery and development.

The most recent publically accessible comprehensive survey of the status of antimicrobial drug development in the pharmaceutical industry [11] highlights the growing disconnection between medical need in this area and the potential for the introduction of novel anti-infective agents. Of 506 drugs disclosed in 2002 as being in the development pipeline, only six were antimicrobial agents. Pipeline anti-infective agents were outnumbered by "lifestyle medicines" such as drugs for baldness, obesity and impotence that have little or no medical benefit but match more readily the industry's profile of profitable medicines. In the year of the survey, 89 new medicines were introduced, none of which were antibiotics. The situation appears to have declined further in recent years, with reports of only one antibiotic active against multi-drug-resistant Gram-negative bacteria undergoing clinical evaluation [7]. The reasons for the gradual withdrawal of the major pharmaceutical companies from antibiotic discovery and development are well documented [12-14]. Antibiotics are prescribed for short periods of time – usually one to two weeks and rarely more than six weeks; inherent obsolescence due to the inevitability of emergence of resistance; a shift from natural product research to high throughput *in vitro* screens combined with the use of combinatorial chemistry libraries; a regulatory environment that until recently did not take into account issues associated uniquely with antibiotic chemotherapy; pressure on prescribers to restrict the use of new agents; poor return on investment owing to the increasing cost of drug development, combined with consolidation in the industry through mergers and acquisitions. In spite of this climate, there are powerful voices within the industry arguing for continued investment in antibacterial drug discovery [15] and the regulatory, economic and political landscape does appear to be changing for the better [16]. It should also not be forgotten that the market in antimicrobial chemotherapeutic agents is valued at around $35 billion *per annum* and by all rational criteria constitutes an attractive area for the discovery, development and marketing of new drugs.

Although the majority of new antibacterial agents introduced over the last fifteen years are based on established chemical structures, with only two belonging to novel classes and therefore displaying little or no capacity for cross-resistance with established antibiotics, there is a growing feeling that we have come to the end of the road with respect to the advantageous modification of tried and tested classes such as the β-lactams. The hope that the exploitation of genomics and target-based high throughput screening would yield a new generation of novel drugs addressing new molecular targets has not been realized in spite of massive investment [17]; furthermore, a recent molecular analysis of protein expression in experimental infection raises the possibility that we may have already exploited most of the broad-spectrum targets essential for bacterial survival *in vivo* [18]. To a limited extent, smaller biotechnology companies are filling the gap left by the withdrawal of their larger counterparts and, lacking the financial resources of the majors, are either in-licensing part-developed antibiotics or searching for niche products. This new development paradigm may fortuitously present prescribers with what they want – drugs with a narrow spectrum of activity against specific pathogens and the potential for consequent reduction of resistance. As academia and government agencies are being urged to become more involved in the process of antibiotic development [19], the time may be right to begin to exploit some of the more unconventional approaches to the eradication of infection that form the basis of this contribution.

Evolution of Resistance
to Conventional Antibiotics

The emergence and horizontal spread of antibiotic resistance genes in bacteria provide a dramatic demonstration of Darwin's theories of evolution through natural selection. The degree of selective pressure applied by antibiotic use is enormous in comparison to the incremental accumulation of traits that account for more gradual change in higher organisms. The emergence of resistance to bactericidal or bacteriostatic antibiotics is almost certainly inevitable. Sometimes resistance may arise in pathogenic bacteria by a single point mutation, often during the course of an infection, as occurs with AmpC-derepressed *Enterobacter* spp and ciprofloxacin-resistant MRSA [20]. However, some resistance determinants have a longer evolutionary history: in the soil, non-antibiotic-producing bacteria have co-existed with antibiotic producers and evolved a diversified antibiotic resistance gene pool long before the dawn of the "antibiotic era". There is good evidence for extensive lateral gene exchange and recombination processes between microorganisms that occupy seemingly distant microbial ecosystems and it is clear that antibiotic resistance genes harbored within bacterial communities in the soil and other environments have found their way into pathogenic bacteria occupying human and animal ecological niches [21]. Therefore, although resistance may arise by mutation and positive selection of mutants, many resistance traits are acquired by pathogens through lateral transfer of antibiotic resistance genes from ecologically and taxonomically distant bacteria and their clonal selection is realized through intensive antibiotic use and, possibly, other factors.

The major selective pressure driving deleterious changes in the frequency of infections due to antibiotic resistant bacteria is clearly the use, overuse and misuse of antibiotics but the relationship between the volume of antibiotic consumption and frequency of resistance is complex and difficult to quantify due to the lack of a sufficient number of longitudinal studies measuring resistance and drug use patterns. Models based on population genetics and epidemiological observations indicate that a critical level of drug consumption is required to trigger significant and rapidly acquired levels of resistance in community cohorts, followed by a much slower decline in resistance if use of a particular antibiotic is suspended [22]. Such retention of resistance genes in the absence of selection is a well established clinical reality. For example, although sulfonamides and streptomycin are no longer used to any extent in the United Kingdom, levels of resistance to these agents in *Escherichia coli* clinical isolates have not decreased; in fact, the incidence of resistance appears to have increased marginally over the period 1991-2004 [9]. Thus, while acquisition of drug resistance may, in the short term, impose a fitness burden in the absence of selection, compensatory mutations may quickly abrogate any disadvantage and even increase fitness, aiding emergence and dissemination on a global scale of clonally derived pathogens [23]. Thus strategies aiming to preserve clinical utility by the scheduled rotation of therapeutic agents may have limited value, even if a sufficient number of antibiotics were available for use in settings, such as intensive care units, where resistance is most evident [24].

The emergence of antibiotic resistant mutants during the course of chemotherapy should be easier to suppress in comparison to the measures necessary to effect a reduction in the incidence of acquired resistance in populations of bacterial pathogens. Typically, frequencies of mutation to resistance are of the order of 10^{-6} to 10^{-9}; populations of bacteria may reach 10^{10} during the course of severe systemic infection but are unlikely to exceed the size at which an individual bacterial cell contains mutations conferring resistance to two or more antibiotics. Combinations of two or more drugs to which the bacterial population as a whole is susceptible should theoretically prevent therapeutic failure and is the basis of much successful antituberculous chemotherapy, where drugs must be administered for extended periods of time to prevent treatment failure due to emergence of resistance. Quantitative pharmacokinetic and pharmacodynamic models of bacterial population dynamics for single and multiple drug treatments suggest that treatment failure as a result of mutation to antibiotic resistance can be avoided or at least reduced if pharmacokinetic parameters such as frequency of dosing, drug dose, duration of treatment and area under the curve are understood and optimized for a particular drug or drug combination and patient non-compliance is eliminated [25, 26]. For example, the emergence of ciprofloxacin resistance in *Pseudomonas aeruginosa* causing respiratory infections in hospitalized patients could be markedly reduced by maintaining blood levels at an area under the 24 h inhibitory concentration curve (AUC_{24} >110μg/ml) compatible with prevention of bacterial growth [27]. Recently, an elegant approach for the prevention of induction of mutations to drug resistance in *E. coli* has been proposed [28], as a means of combating the evolution of drug resistance by point mutation to quinolone and rifamycin agents. Interrupting LexA cleavage prevents derepression of SOS-regulated proteases that collaborate to induce resistance-conferring mutations, so pharmacological intervention to inhibit LexA during chemotherapy with agents known to give rise to resistant variants may represent an effective means of restraining the emergence of resistance.

It is more difficult to conceive of strategies to suppress dissemination of antibiotic resistance in those, predominantly, opportunistic pathogens that have acquired one or a number of genes conferring resistance from other bacterial communities. With such organisms, antibiotic usage in some patients may increase the risk of colonization or infection with resistant bacteria such as MRSA, vancomycin-resistant enterococci (VRE) and penicillin-resistant *Streptococcus pneumoniae* in individuals who have not received antibiotics [29]. Thus, antibiotics alter the proportion of susceptible to resistant bacteria within populations and increase the likelihood that "third party" individuals will encounter and acquire drug-resistant variants, a concept supported by both epidemiological studies [30] and mathematical models [31, 32]. Prevention of dissemination of resistant commensals and pathogens to susceptible hospital patients by barrier nursing may be one of the few options available in such situations.

Alternatives to Antibiotic Chemotherapy

Although antibiotics have saved more lives than any other group of drugs in the history of humankind, their success has been tempered by the rapid evolution of multi-drug-resistant bacteria. Most antibiotics work by disrupting biosynthetic pathways or inhibiting cellular processes such as key steps in protein biosynthesis; these discrete modes of action present the bacteria with an opportunity to bypass the susceptible metabolic step, to prevent the antibiotic reaching its target or to produce an enzyme which breaks down the antibiotic before it can inhibit cellular processes, and many such mechanisms have evolved through selective pressure. Alternative strategies for treating bacterial infections have been investigated more or less continuously since the "pre-antibiotic era" but have until recently been consigned to the backwaters of therapeutic research. It may now be time to intensify the investigation of some of these approaches: they include the use of photoactive dyes, bacteriophage therapy, phage components such as lysins, compounds that stimulate cellular immune functions and agents that advantageously modify the antibiotic resistance and virulence of bacterial pathogens. As this diverse collection of therapeutic alternatives relies on physical means of cell disruption, on modulation of the host rather than the pathogen or on a diminution in bacterial properties essential for survival *in vivo* but not *in vitro*, they may not so readily select mutants better equipped to evade their antibacterial *modus operandi*.

It has been known for around one hundred years that many microorganisms, including bacteria, selectively accumulate photosensitive dyes and are killed if the dye is activated by light of a specific wavelength. In particular, tetrapyrroles such as porphyrins, phthalocyaninies and bacteriochlorins accumulate in and are selectively retained by a wide variety of abnormal and hyperproliferative cells and tissues. Photoactivation of accumulated molecules by light from the visible part of the spectrum leads, in the presence of oxygen, to the selective destruction of the target tissue due to singlet oxygen-mediated peroxidative damage; free radicals may also be generated and contribute, albeit less effectively, to cell killing. Until recently, photodynamic therapy (PDT) was considered predominantly as a modality for the ablation of solid tumors, but there is growing interest in its potential for the treatment of a variety of non-oncological indications, including infections [33]. Gram-positive bacteria are susceptible to photo-inactivation with a wide variety of dyes and "second generation" cationic photosensitizers have been developed that are able to overcome the barrier function of the outer membrane and efficiently sensitize Gram-negative bacteria [34]. It seems unlikely that resistance to PDT will develop as singlet oxygen and free radicals will cause damage to a wide range of cellular components, including proteins, nucleic acids and lipids [35], although there have been reports that a non-tetrapyrrole photosensitizing agent is a substrate for multidrug efflux pumps in Gram-positive and Gram-negative bacteria

[36]. Indeed, PDT is equally effective against antibiotic susceptible and antibiotic resistant microorganisms and repeated photosensitization has not led to selection of resistant mutants [37]. PDT is particularly effective at disrupting biofilms, killing the component bacteria, and as such is undergoing preclinical investigation for the treatment of oral conditions such as periodontal disease [38]. Other potential clinical applications include localized conditions such as wound infections, burns, soft tissue infections and abscesses, and surface infections of the cornea and skin [35].

Phage therapy, like PDT, is based on physical disruption of target bacteria and has received a great deal of attention in recent years as a therapeutic modality with the potential to resolve infections due to antibiotic resistant bacteria. However, unlike PDT, phage therapy is highly selective due to the nature of the interaction between the phage and its specific host and it therefore could be used eradicate an infection without disturbing the host microbiota. In some states of the former Soviet Union, phage medicines have been used to treat infections in humans since the early 1930s, although they have not been evaluated in clinical trials of a standard acceptable to Western regulatory authorities. This area has been extensively reviewed in recent years [39-41] and its advantages and disadvantages appraised. There is little doubt that phages are effective in eradicating a broad range of non-systemic infections in experimental models and that rapid progress is being made towards the clinical development of medicines based on these self-replicating entities. Regulatory conundrums have in the past proven to be a barrier to the commercial exploitation of phage therapy but the regulatory climate is changing: recent clinical studies have been expedited in Europe under national Medical Ethical Committee guidelines [42]. Non-systemic administration of phage preparations is considered safe [43] and the FDA have recently (April 2006) approved the use of phage cocktails against *Listeria monocytogenes* in ready-to-eat meat and poultry [44].

Resistance to phage is readily acquired by a range of mechanisms and there have been few attempts to minimize the emergence of phage-resistant bacteria either during the course of an infection or in the longer term: like antibiotics, phage therapeutics have the potential to alter the gene compliment of the bacterial components of ecological niches as bacterial host and phage parasite co-evolve [45]. Both *in vitro* and *in vivo*, resistance to phage may develop through genetic changes in bacteria, including mutation, recombination and horizontal transfer of genetic material containing resistance genes, by activation of existing restriction-modification or abortive infection systems and by stationary or other phases of growth that confer temporary resistance to phages [46]. The capacity to generate phage-resistant bacterial mutants during therapy could be minimized by incorporating features of the molecular interactions between host and parasite into the selection and/or design of therapeutic phages [47]. For example, the pathogenesis of neuroinvasive *E. coli* strains carrying the K1 capsule is dependent on the expression of this polysialic acid structure at the bacterial surface [48]: we have noted (P.W. Taylor, unpublished data) that the large majority of laboratory-generated mutants resistant to K1-specific phages are non-capsular and therefore unlikely to survive during neonatal systemic infections caused by the parental bacteria. Thus, phages that target essential virulence determinants at the bacterial surface may be unlikely to select variants that can evade phage therapeutics and still participate in the progression of the infection. The emergence of resistance could also be minimized by consideration of pharmacokinetic and pharmacodynamic parameters for phage therapy. By analogy with antibiotic therapies, Cairns and Payne [46] have used kinetic models to determine the dosing levels of phage that would suppress single-step resistant mutants. Their models show that active therapies, that rely on phage amplification in the host bacterium to generate sufficient progeny through relatively low doses of phage (the "living medicine" approach), are unlikely to avoid problems of resistance if only a single phage is used. Combinations of phage may suppress resistance if they are closely matched with regard to the rate at which they generate progeny. The issue of resistance could be circumvented by passive phage therapy, where doses are sufficiently large to prevent net bacterial growth. In this mode, the phage is used in a fashion analogous to an antibiotic and it may not always be possible to deliver to the site of infection the large doses required. The authors show that combination passive therapy will close the window through which resistant mutants will be selected provided that the concentration of each component phage is greater than the concentration needed to counter bacterial growth. Since the phages are not required to undergo replication in the target bacterial host, restriction-modification, abortive infection mechanisms and interference between phages in multiply infected cells should not come into play, reducing the capacity for resistance to emerge. Whether or not it is practical for such recommendations to be included in the design of phage therapy studies remains to be determined. If not, the use of stand-alone phage therapy may be restricted by the rapid emergence of resistant bacteria during the course of infection.

Alternative ways to exploit phage infection of bacterial pathogens by utilizing phage components rather than intact, infectious phage particles have been gaining ground in recent years. The use of phage-encoded capsule depolymerases to reduce the virulence of encapsulated pathogens will be addressed in a later section. Another group of enzymes attracting a great deal of interest for their perceived therapeutic utility are phage-encoded endolysins [49]. These enzymes facilitate release of mature phage particles from the host bacterium by effecting "lysis-from-within". During the infection cycle phage-directed holins perforate the cytoplasmic membrane of infected bacteria and allow endolysins access to their peptidoglycan substrate; individual endolysins (peptidoglycan hydrolases) can attack a variety of covalent bonds within host peptidoglycan, including those within stem peptides, cross-bridges and the glycan backbone [49]. Thus, the catalytic domains of endolysins display, in the main, amidase or muramidase activity. Extremely rapid lysis of susceptible Gram-positive bacteria can be readily observed *in vitro* after addition of the enzyme to non-infected bacteria [50, 51] and has raised the possibility that such affects also manifest *in vivo*. The enzymes have a narrow spectrum of lytic activity against intact cells and stringent substrate specificity against purified peptidoglycan, due to the capacity of their cell wall-binding domains to recognize subtle differences in peptidoglycan structure. Therefore, the substrate specificities and activities of endolysins can be altered by constructing chimeric proteins combining the catalytic domain of one enzyme with the cell wall-binding domain of another [52]. The utility of endolysins may be restricted due the relatively large amounts of enzyme required to produce "lysis-from-without" but very small quantities of PlyC, an endolysin derived from a streptococcal phage, can effectively sterilize suspensions of group A streptococci within seconds. Single applications of PlyC can protect mucosal oral surfaces in mice against colonization by Group A streptococci and can eliminate heavy streptococcal colonization of the oral cavity [53]. These and other reports of efficacy in experimental models of infection have led to speculation that *in vivo* development of endolysin resistance is unlikely to arise because the enzymes target unique motifs in the cell wall that are essential for viability [54]. However, the mechanism of resistance to vancomycin, involving small changes in peptidoglycan structure, should serve a warning that most bacteria will find a way to circumvent the action of molecules that have the capacity to alter the composition of target bacterial populations.

Traditionally, we look at infection as invasion of the host by pathogens that overwhelm the body's defenses, but this is a simplistic view. Even "professional" pathogens such as *Staphylococcus aureus*, a bacterium equipped with an impressive array of virulence effectors for damaging the host [55], requires a reduction in the host's defenses in order to colonize, enter tissue and cause infection. From an ecological viewpoint, infection is a natural phenomenon resulting from perturbation of the complex relationship between host and parasite, a view that has now gained acceptance many years after it was first mooted by scientific iconoclasts Theobald Smith [56] and René Dubos [57]. From this perspective, the physiological and immunological status of the host is as important as the properties of the parasite in determining whether an infection occurs and the nature of the outcome. It also implies that redressing the balance between host and parasite, either by shoring up the host's defenses or by "disarming" the pathogen, may lead to resolution of the infection without exerting the kind of selective pressure on microbial populations that is inherent in conventional chemotherapy. The idea of limiting infections due to intracellular microorganisms using immune stimulation dates back many years; renewed interest in this approach within the pharmaceutical industry appeared with the realization that resistance was beginning to compromise therapy [58] but has since waned due to changing business priorities. There is evidence that some traditional medicines used by native populations, particularly in Africa and the Far East, may be efficacious in infections due to their capacity to nonspecifically stimulate the immune system; in Europe, at least one over-the-counter formulation based on this principle has been successfully marketed for the treatment of bacterial and viral respiratory infections [59]. A naturally occurring immunomodulating drug, bestatin, reduced the burden of *Salmonella typhimurium* in a murine model of infection [60] and components of native medicines have been shown to stimulate the intracellular killing by macrophages of a number of intracellular parasites, including *Mycobacterium tuberculosis* [61, 62]. Administration of granulocyte-macrophage-colony-stimulating factor (GM-CSF) to forty neutropenic patients with bacterial sepsis resulted in clinical and microbiological improvement or cure but no difference in mortality [63]. These and other studies indicate that immune stimulators may provide useful additions to our palette of anti-infective agents and it is difficult to see how resistance to such agents could develop.

An alternative and perhaps less risky way to enable the host to eliminate virulent or drug resistant pathogens encompasses reduction in the expression by the microbe of determinants that under normal circumstances enable it to gain the upper hand. Thus, "disarming" the pathogen by abrogating antibiotic resistance mechanisms or reducing the expression of virulence effectors at some stage of the infection may tip the balance in favor of the patient in a way that applies less selective pressure than conventional chemotherapy. These ideas form the basis of the remainder of this contribution.

Compromising Bacterial Drug Resistance

The notion that pharmacological intervention can restore the utility of antibiotics made less potent by the evolution of resistance has given rise to one of the most clinically and commercially successful antibacterial drug combinations that have been developed by the pharmaceutical industry. Scientists at Beecham Research Laboratories at Brockham Park, United Kingdom responded to the evolution of β-lactamases in Gram-negative bacteria active against second generation broad spectrum β-lactam agents by discovering and developing the potent β-lactamase inhibitor clavulanic acid [64]. The inhibitor is a β-lactam compound with very modest antibacterial activity but the capacity to bind irreversibly to bacterial β-lactamases. The β-lactamase-inhibiting properties of clavulanic acid were combined with the good oral bioavailability and potent broad-spectrum antibacterial activity of amoxicillin and launched as Augmentin in the United Kingdom in 1981, and subsequently throughout the world [65]. Thus, the clavulanate component restored the activity of amoxicillin against β-lactamase-producing pathogens. The key to its success almost certainly lies in the complimentary pharmacokinetic profiles of the two components: they are well absorbed from the gastrointestinal tract, have similar AUCs and elimination profiles and combining the two does not affect their individual pharmacokinetic properties [65]. *In vitro*, amoxicillin/clavulanate has a very low propensity to select for resistance in comparison to other antibiotics [66]. Resistance in clinical isolates to the combination has been low [67] even though it has been one of the most frequently used antibacterial agents over the last quarter-century; it is however now increasing [68]. It is tempting to speculate that the β-lactam-resistance modulator clavulanic acid exerts reduced selective pressure on target bacterial populations, even though the molecule belongs to the same chemical class as its partner amoxicillin. Subsequent to the introduction of Augmentin, other β-lactam/β-lactamase-inhibitor combinations with clinical utility have been developed [69].

Efflux pumps make a significant contribution to intrinsic and acquired antibiotic resistance of a wide range of clinically relevant bacteria and there have been consolidated efforts in both the academic and commercial fields to find clinically acceptable pump inhibitors. Efflux pumps, such as tetracycline-specific Tet-pumps that are frequently found in a wide range of Gram-positive and Gram-negative bacteria [70], can selectively extrude specific antibiotics or they can expel a variety of structurally diverse compounds with differing antibacterial modes of action. The latter, multidrug efflux pumps, may confer resistance to antibiotics such as the fluoroquinolones, dyes (for example, ethidium bromide), detergents and disinfectants [71]. Clearly, inhibitors of multidrug efflux mechanisms, used in combination with antibiotics whose action is compromised by efflux pumps, would be welcome additions to our chemotherapeutic arsenal, even though the development of combination therapies is notoriously difficult. A number of pump inhibitors have been discovered using high-throughput antibiotic potentiation assays [72, 73] and one class of broad spectrum inhibitor has been extensively characterized [74]. One representative of this class, a competitive inhibitor of resistance-nodulation-cell division pumps, entered Phase I clinical trials in cystic fibrosis patients but the drug was not well tolerated and the trial is currently suspended [73]. This work does, however, indicate a significant potential for the development of small molecule inhibitors and efforts continue in the commercial biotechnology field to develop clinically useful agents of this type [74]. These efforts should be tempered by a recent report that pump inhibitors may select multidrug-resistant mutants, at least in the laboratory [75].

Further opportunities may arise from antibacterial effects associated with Japanese green tea (*Camellia sinensis*). Green tea consumption is linked to a low incidence of various pathological conditions, including cardiovascular disease, diabetes, obesity and cancer. The most abundant polyphenolic component of green tea, (-)-epigallocatechin gallate (EGCg) induces apoptotic cell death and cell cycle arrest in tumor cells but not in their normal counterparts; it also favorably affects several signal transduction pathways and is efficacious in animal models of tumor induction [76]. On the strength of such studies, EGCg has successfully undergone Phase I (human safety) trials [77] and patients with asymptomatic Rai stage 0-II chronic lymphocytic leukemia are currently participating in a Phase I/II trial of EGCg conducted by the U.S. National Cancer Institute. These activities are creating a precedent for therapeutic interventions with natural polyphenols or their synthetic structural analogues. Extracts of green tea have an extremely weak capacity to inhibit bacterial growth but are able to reverse methicillin resistance in MRSA isolates at relatively low concentrations [78-80]. Examination of a range of individual components of tea indicated that this activity was attributable to the catechin gallates, with (-)-epicatechin gallate (ECg) showing greater potency than either EGCg or (-)-catechin gallate (Cg) [81]. Catechins lacking the gallate moiety had no capacity to reverse methicillin resistance [82]. The effect was evident with all β-lactam agents examined (methicillin, oxacillin, flucloxacillin, cefotaxime, cefepime, imipenem, meropenem) and against all forty strains from an international collection of MRSA clinical isolates [82]. Thus, moderate concentrations (3 mg/L or greater) of ECg, EGCg and Cg are able to reduce the MICs of β-lactams for MRSA strains from full resistance (usually >256 mg/L) to below the antibiotic breakpoint (ca. 1-2 mg/L) [78, 82], raising the possibility that such molecules could be used in combination with suitable β-lactam agents to treat MRSA infections.

The galloyl group (D-ring; Figure 1) is essential for β-lactam-resistance modifying activity and epi (*cis*)-configured catechin gallates, such as ECg, are more active than their *trans* counterparts, such as Cg (Figure 1), indicating that the stereochemistry of the C-ring partly governs bioactivity. The relative activities of catechin gallates suggest that reduction in hydroxylation of the B-ring increases resistance-modifying capacity: for example, EGCg is less active than ECg although it differs from this molecule only by the presence of an additional hydroxyl group on the B-ring. Naturally occurring catechin gallates are variably absorbed from the intestinal tract and are rapidly metabolized to inactive products in this compartment due in part to the presence of ester bonds that are susceptible to hydrolysis by bacterial esterases [83]. We have considered these features in order to design, synthesize and evaluate ECg derivatives with a more appropriate pharmacological profile for administration to man. We synthesized the corresponding galloyl amide that, unlike the natural product, is refractory to esterase degradation; it maintains the epi (*cis*) stereochemistry of ECg and is as active as the parent molecule in β-lactam modulation assays [84]. In addition, B-ring-modified derivatives of ECg, such as monohydroxyl compounds and a 3,5-dihydroxy B-ring catechin gallate, have been synthesized and are at least as bioactive as ECg [85].

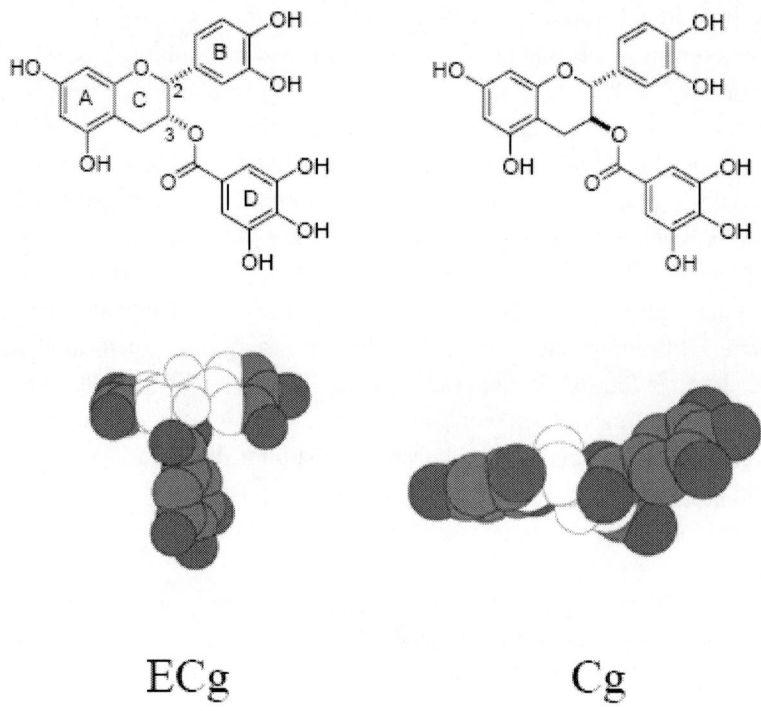

Figure 1. Structures and space filling models of catechin gallates. The colorless regions are hydrophobic domains and the darker regions are hydrophilic domains. Ring nomenclature assignment is shown for ECg.

There is good evidence that natural catechins exert at least some of their biological effects through intercalation into lipid bilayers [86-88] and this goes some way to explaining the structural requirements for β-lactam resistance modification. Catechin gallates bind more avidly than (-)-epicatechin (EC) or (-)-epigallocatechin (EGC) - the non-galloyl counterparts to ECg and EGCg - to small unilamellar vesicles produced from phosphatidyl choline (PC) and ECg has a greater affinity for the bilayer than EGCg [89]. The relative affinity of catechins for membranes reflects their partition coefficients in *n*-octanol-saline [89] and their capacity to modulate β-lactam resistance [82]. We found that these relationships were maintained when catechin binding to staphylococcal cells was examined; we also determined that the binding of ECg is enhanced in the presence of EC [90]. Catechins with epi (*cis*) stereochemistry partitioned into PC liposomes more readily than their non-epi (*trans*) configured counterparts [87]; with epicatechins such as ECg the hydrophobic domain in the region of the ester bond and C-ring (Figure 1; white area) is relatively exposed and therefore liable to perturb the bilayer. Reducing or modifying B-ring hydroxylation increases the dimensions of this hydrophobic domain and in all likelihood increases the capacity to partition into the phospholipid palisade. The rather complex staphylococcal phenotype [91-93] resulting from exposure to ECg and other catechin gallates is likely, therefore, to a be consequence of the intercalation of these molecules into the cytoplasmic membrane of the target cells.

How does ECg compromise resistance to second generation β-lactams such as methicillin and oxacillin? Penicillin binding proteins (PBPs), associated with the external surface of the

CM and the cell wall, constitute the transglycosylases and transpeptidases that catalyse the insertion and crosslinking of newly synthesized peptidoglycan precursors in to the wall; they are the targets for β-lactam antibiotics [94]. Methicillin resistance is associated with an additional PBP, PBP2a, which has a lower affinity for β-lactams and maintains poor transpeptidase activity in the presence of β-lactam concentrations that saturate other PBPs. Synthesis of the pentaglycine cross-bridge, used by PBPs to cross-link glycan chains in peptidoglycan, is catalysed by FmhB, FemA and FemB using tRNA$_{gly}$ as glycine donor [94]; these enzymes are probably on the inner surface of the CM, as their substrates are physically linked to the membrane [94, 95]. Loss of FemA and/or FemB activity results in cells that are hypersusceptible to β-lactams, as PBP2a cannot accept the resulting tri- or mono-glycine interpeptides as substrates [95]. A study by Hamilton-Miller and co-workers [78] suggested that green tea extracts, containing unfractionated catechins in addition to other components, reduced the expression of PBPs in MRSA, including PBP2a. We could not confirm that ECg had a significant effect on the expression of PBP2a. Growth in the presence of ECg did not affect *mecA* gene transcription (Figure 2A), the gene coding for PBP2a, and the gene product was expressed as evidenced by latex/antibody agglutination and quantitative determination of PBP2a in cytoplasmic membrane fractions using an anti-PBP2a antibody (Figure 2B). An alternative hypothesis put forward by Zhao et al., that direct binding of the catechin to peptidoglycan interfered with PBP2a activity with consequent loss or reduction of β-lactam resistance [96], was also investigated: it was found that exogenous peptidoglycan had no significant effect on the capacities of ECg or EGCg to reduce oxacillin resistance in our isolates. This data indicates, therefore, a more complex basis for resistance modification than suggested by these earlier studies, which also fail to explain other elements of the ECg-derived phenotype described immediately below.

Growth in the presence of ECg alters the appearance of *S. aureus* strains when viewed by light and electron microscopy [92, 97]. ECg, but not EC, induced thickened cell walls and pseudomulticellular aggregates, indicating poor separation of daughter cells following division. The clumps of partially divided cocci appeared larger and displayed a rougher surface than control cells (Figure 3). Both ECg [92] and EGCg [91] inhibit the formation of staphylococcal biofilms; formation of these complex surface-associated communities is frequently a prerequisite for colonization and invasion during the course of infections due to *S. aureus*.

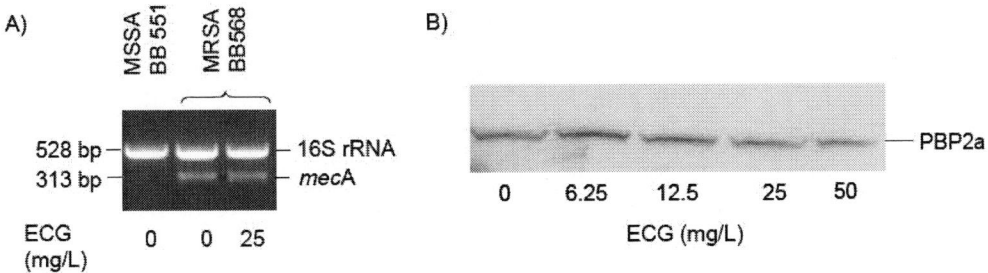

Figure 2. (A). Reverse transcriptase PCR analysis of *mecA* gene transcription. (B). Membrane-associated proteins of MRSA BB568 probed with an anti-PBP2a antibody.

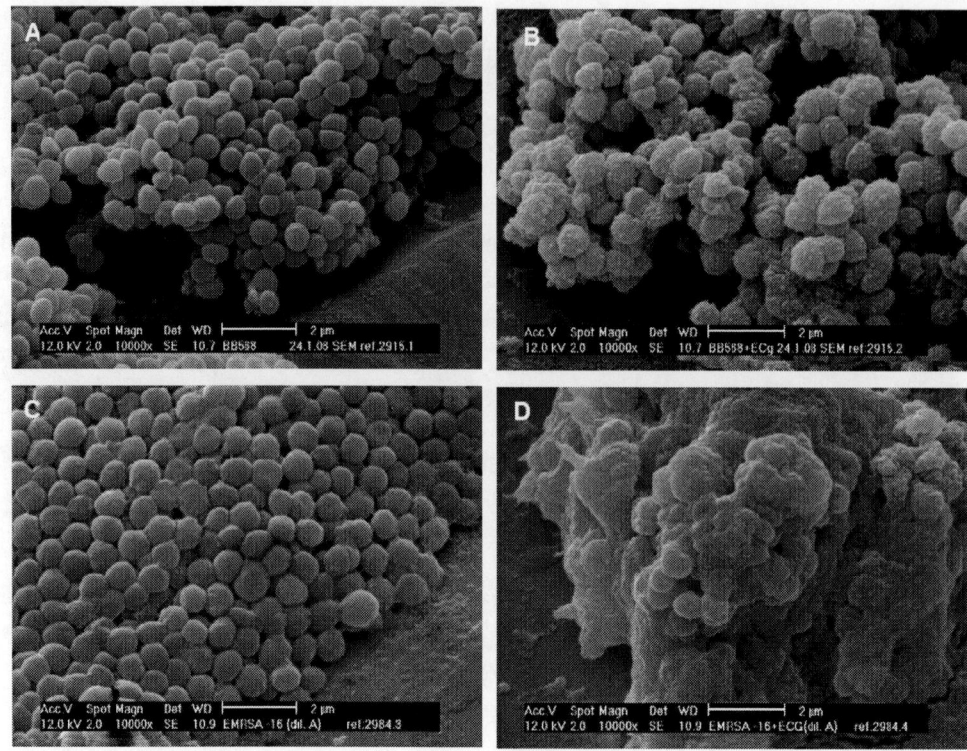

Figure 3. Scanning electron micrographs of *S. aureus* BB568 grown in non-supplemented Müller-Hinton broth (MHB; A), in MHB containing 12.5 mg/L ECg (B). BB568 cells were incubated with cationized ferritin after growth in non-supplemented (C) and ECg-supplemented (D) MHB.

The initial steps of biofilm formation require a balance in the distribution of positive and negative charges at the bacterial surface [98]; an increased negative surface charge leads to electrostatic repulsion and inhibition of biofilm formation. Growth in the presence of ECg appears to increase the net negative charge on the surface of MRSA strains, as ECg-grown cells bind more cationized ferritin than control cells (Figures 3 and 4). ECg markedly suppresses the secretion of the key virulence effectors α-toxin and coagulase by MRSA [93]; indeed, analysis of the extracellular proteome of ECg-treated EMRSA-16 has revealed reductions in secretion of a large number of proteins (Figure 5), suggesting that ECg may abrogate virulence as well as β-lactam resistance in staphylococcal strains. *S. aureus* is remarkably halotolerant, growing in the presence of salt concentrations up to 3.5 M [99]; ECg suppressed the capacity of MRSA strains to grow in medium containing 2% NaCl, KCl and LiCl and it has been suggested that catechin gallates interfere with Na^+-specific antiporter systems operating across the cytoplasmic membrane [100]. The interrelatedness of the components of the ECg-induced phenotype is emphasized by the capacity of NaCl to prevent biofilm formation in much the same way as ECg (Figure 6). Any hypothesis purporting to account for the β-lactam-resistance modifying capacity of catechin gallates must take these effects into account.

The activity of autolysins (peptidoglycan hydrolases), enzymes involved in the orderly cell division, cell wall turnover and cell separation of Gram-positive bacteria, is known to be partly dependent on the charge characteristics of the cell wall [98]; the secretion of autolysins during the cell division cycle is a prerequisite for cell separation [101]. ECg-grown cells retained autolysins within the thickened cell wall, with greatly reduced amounts released into the growth medium [92], and this is likely to account for the observed reduction in cell separation [92, 97].

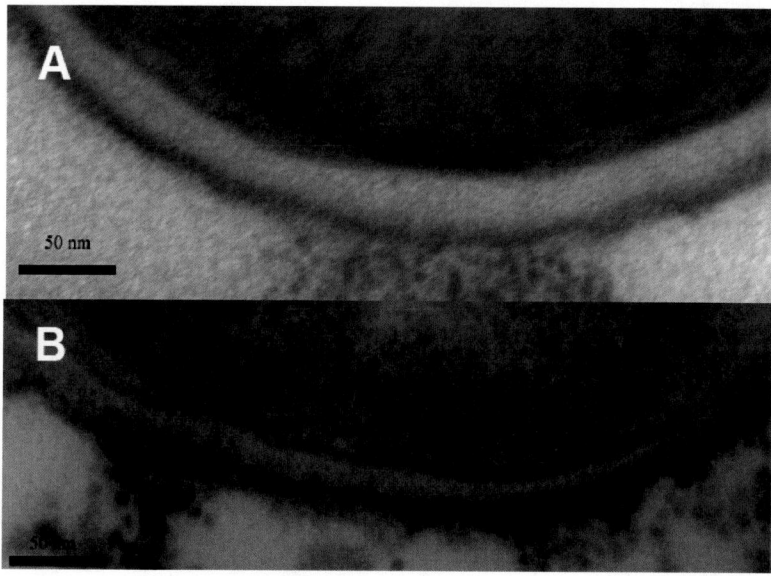

Figure 4. Transmission electron micrographs of ultrathin sections of *S. aureus* BB568 incubated with cationized ferritin (16.6 mg/L final concentration) in the absence (A) or presence (B) of 12.5 mg/L ECg.

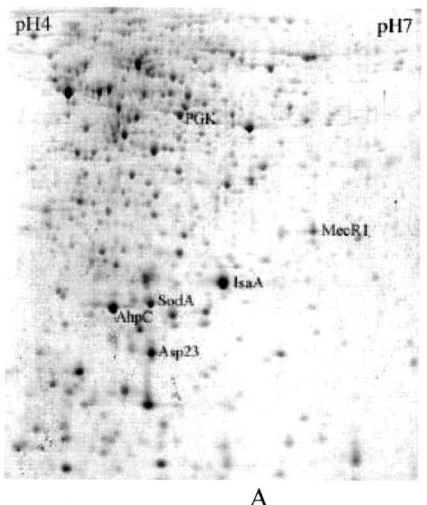
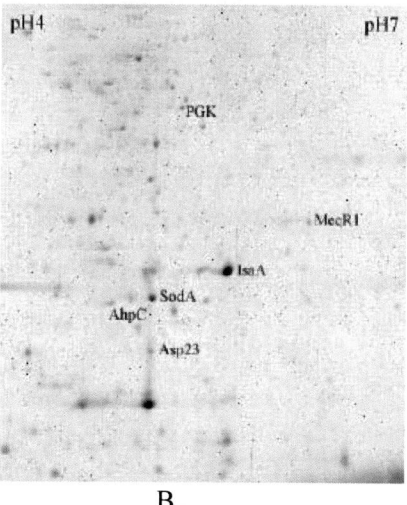

Figure 5. 2-D gel electrophoresis of secreted proteins by *S. aureus* EMRSA-16 in the absence (A) and presence (B) of 12.5 mg/L ECg. Gels were loaded with proteins recovered from the culture medium and standardized on the basis of bacterial cell mass. Cultures were in the stationary phase and bacteria removed by centrifugation. Excised proteins were digested and peptides identified by MALDI-TOF-MS and comparison with established databases.

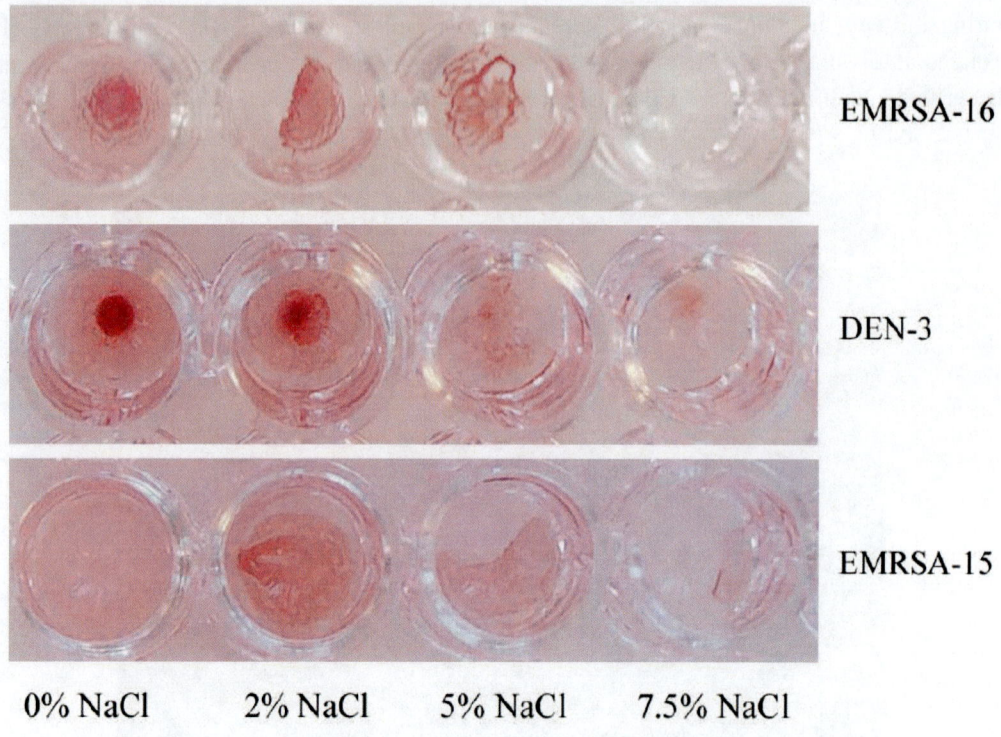

0% NaCl   2% NaCl   5% NaCl   7.5% NaCl

Figure 6. Biofilm formation in plastic wells formed by *S. aureus* clinical isolates EMRSA-15, EMRSA-16 and DEN-3 in the presence of NaCl. The biofilm-forming capacity of these strains varies as follows: DEN-3>EMRSA-16>EMRSA-15.

The processing or enzymatic activity of the autolysins in the cell wall may be compromised, perhaps through binding to charged components [98], as ECg induced a large reduction in Triton-X-100-induced autolysis [92]. Therefore, the abnormal wall thickness of ECg-grown cells is probably related to lower rates of cell wall degradation rather than increased rates of cell wall biosynthesis. Peptidoglycan prepared from cells grown in ECg was more susceptible to hydrolysis by M1 muramidase, an enzyme that breaks glycosidic bonds between the disaccharide units in the peptidoglycan [102], than control cells, indicating that growth in ECg reduces the degree of peptidoglycan cross-linking. This was confirmed by HPLC analysis of the products obtained by mutanolysin hydrolysis of peptidoglycan: ECg reduced the degree of peptidoglycan cross-linking by 5-10%, an amount insufficient to compromise cell wall integrity and likely to be due to relatively modest changes in the levels of PBPs 1 and 3 in the staphylococcal membrane [92]. The pentaglycine cross-bridges, reduced in number, remained chemically unchanged. Surprisingly, growth in ECg markedly decreased susceptibility to lysostaphin [92, 103], a peptidoglycan hydrolase that cleaves pentaglycine cross-bridges between the glycan strands within peptidoglycan. Peptidoglycan-wall teichoic acid (WTA) complexes extracted from ECg-grown cells were less susceptible to lysostaphin hydrolysis than complexes from bacteria grown in non-supplemented medium but after removal of WTA rates of peptidoglycan hydrolysis were identical, regardless of the source of the substrate [92, 103]. This data most strongly suggests that ECg induces alterations in the composition, structure or conformation of WTA. These poly-D-ribitol-phosphate wall components are known to have a significant effect on many of the properties of the Gram-positive cell wall, including modulation of autolysin activity, cation homeostasis, biofilm formation, acid tolerance, expression of virulence determinants and susceptibility to β-lactam and other antibiotics [98].

We determined that growth in ECg alters the structure of WTA in a way that accounts for some aspects of the ECg-induced phenotype. This wall polymer is variably substituted with D-alanine (D-ala) residues that contribute positive charges to the ionic continuum within the staphylococcal cell wall [98]. Growth in ECg led to reductions of up to 50% in the degree of D-alanylation of WTA: in strains BB568 and EMRSA-16, the ratio of N-acetyl glucosamine (a component of the invariant WTA backbone) to D-ala was reduced from 0.6 and 0.49 respectively to 0.3 and 0.28 [103]. Molecular simulations indicated that this resulted in an increase in the net positive charge of the cell wall, which probably accounts for the increased binding of cationized ferritin (Figure 4), and an increase in WTA chain flexibility to a random coil conformation that is likely to provide the molecular basis for changes in lysostaphin susceptibility. Thus, lysostaphin is prevented from binding to the pentaglycine cross-bridge substrate (unaltered by ECg) due to steric hindrance provided by the altered conformation of WTA with reduced D-ala content. *S. aureus dlt* mutants, lacking the capacity to synthesize or attach D-ala to teichoic acids, lose the ability to produce biofilms due to electrostatic repulsion resulting from increased negative surface charge [104] and as such provide parallels with the ECg-induced phenotype. Similarly, anionic sites are necessary for retention of autolysins within the cell wall and are likely to modulate their enzymatic activity [98]. Reduced D-alanylation of teichoic acids correlates with increased susceptibility to cationic antibacterial peptides [105] and glycopeptides antibiotics such as vancomycin [106], and *dlt* mutants may be more susceptible to methicillin [107], suggesting that positive charges within the wall tend to exclude molecules that are anionic at neutral pH. Our data also supports the contention that increased net negative charge in the cell wall leads to increases in antibiotic, and, particularly, β-lactam, susceptibility but we tend to support the view that the very large reductions in methicillin resistance induced by ECg result predominantly from interruption of *mecA*-mediated resistance.

PBP2 is normally located at the division septum in *S. aureus* [108], the primary locus of cell wall synthesis, and is recruited to the division site by externalized peptidoglycan precursor substrate molecules [109]. In β-lactam susceptible *S. aureus*, oxacillin prevents the recruitment of PBP2 and the protein is dispersed over the entire surface of the viable cell [109]. In MRSA strains, PBP2, although fully acylated, is recruited to the septum due to its interaction with oxacillin-refractory PBP2a, which also binds to externalized peptidoglycan precursors [109]. If ECg disrupted the PBP2/PBP2a complex, either by binding to one of the partner proteins or by preventing recruitment and interaction of PBPs through changes in the biophysical properties of the CM, the cell would become phenotypically β-lactam susceptible. We are currently examining this hypothesis, that catechin gallates affect septum formation as the primary mode of action concerned with β-lactam resistance modulation. Intercalation of catechin gallates into the cytoplasmic membrane of MRSA, a process that can be enhanced by the presence of non-galloylated catechins, would alter the biophysical properties and architecture of the bilayer and could account for much of the ECg-derived phenotype. The efficiency of enzymes involved in peptidoglycan synthesis may be reduced, accounting for the small observed reduction in cross-linking, although enzymes involved in synthesis of the pentaglycine cross-bridge are probably unaffected; autolysins are trapped and their hydrolytic activity reduced in a thickening cell wall due to an increased net negative charge conferred on the wall by displacement from the membrane [92] of lipoteichoic acid, the membrane-bound form of teichoic acid that donates D-ala residues to WTA; changes to the charge profile of the ionic matrix in the cell wall affects biofilm formation, salt tolerance and possibly plays a role in increased susceptibility to β-lactam antibiotics; the transport of proteins across the altered membrane are compromised, leading to a less virulent state. For these reasons, we continue to study the interaction of catechin gallates with the membrane bilayer.

The phenotype generated by growth of MRSA strains in ECg is strikingly similar to that noted for vancomycin-intermediate resistant *S. aureus* clinical isolates, so-called VISA strains. These also produce abnormally thick cell walls, separate poorly when grown in antibiotic-free medium and show decreased cross-linkage of the peptidoglycan and altered teichoic acid content compared to vancomycin-susceptible progenitors [110]. Interestingly, VISA isolates also have an increased susceptibility to β-lactam agents. There may be common features to the mechanisms involved in these processes that will provide insights into the relationship between the capacity of opportunistic pathogens to survive in an antibiotic-rich environment and the extent to which their biological fitness is compromised.

Compromising Bacterial Virulence

Directly interfering with the expression of the determinants of bacterial pathogenesis is at first sight an attractive alternative approach to antibacterial therapy. Directed suppression of virulence would not kill the bacterial targets but allow host defenses to overwhelm the compromised invader, providing, at least theoretically, a strategy that would not directly select for resistance to the virulence modifying agent. However, some have argued cogently that any agent which challenges the ability of a bacterium to successfully colonize and disseminate within a host will represent a selective pressure and give rise to pathogens resistant to the agent [111]; this critical issue requires examination both experimentally and from the perspective of evolutionary theory. Gram-positive bacteria, in particular, produce an exceptionally wide array of secreted proteins that contribute, often in concert, to colonization of the host, to bacterial invasion and spread, and to host tissue damage. *S. aureus*, for example, produces virulence effectors that encompass hemolysins, enterotoxins, toxic shock syndrome toxin, adhesins and invasins, as well as superantigens and molecules such as protein A that compromise the humoral response [112]. Compromising individual virulence determinants requires a thorough understanding of the role each factor plays in pathogenesis and in cooperative damage to the host, as removing a single determinant from the complex interaction with the host may not affect outcome. For example, Panton-Valentine leukocidin (PVL) was long thought to contribute significantly to the severity of infections due to community-associated MRSA, but recent evidence suggests that it is primarily a "clonal passenger" [113]. In such situations, agents that affect the expression of the secretome in a relatively non-selective way (such as ECg, above) or interfere with signal transduction leading to the production of whole classes of secreted toxins [114] may be more effective than agents targeting expression of a single virulence effector. That such an approach will have the capacity to provide a favorable therapeutic outcome is highlighted by a recent elegant study demonstrating that LED209, a non-toxic, selective inhibitor of the conserved membrane histidine sensor kinase QseC, associated with Gram-negative pathogens, can prevent death in mice infected with *S. typhimurium* and *Francisella tularensis* [115]. A similar strategy should have an equal or greater effect on the outcome of Gram-positive infections.

Although it is probably unrealistic to consider virulence targeting as anything other than a therapeutic strategy, it does in theory provide the option of intervening at most, if not all, stages of the infection cycle of both intracellular [116] and extracellular [117] pathogens. Many bacteria express virulence determinants in a temporal fashion, with factors associated with colonization appearing early in the process and the synthesis of proteins damaging to the host evident only after the pathogen has become established, a stage often flagged by quorum sensing (QS) systems and global gene regulators [55, 118]. There has been recent progress in the development of QS inhibitors; QS is a cell-to-cell signaling process for promoting collective behavior within a bacterial population, enabling gene expression when the cell density reaches a threshold level. It is involved in the development of tolerance to antimicrobial therapy and to immune modulation, and it up-regulates virulence genes at key stages of infection. Several distinct families of QS molecules have been investigated in both Gram-positive and Gram-negative bacteria and a number of competitive inhibitors of these small molecule extracellular autoinducers developed [119-121], with some *in vivo* efficacy.

Is there any evidence that selective removal of a major virulence determinant from a bacterial pathogen can alter the course of infection? Between the two World Wars, Dubos, Avery and colleagues at the Rockefeller Institute for Medical Research used an enzyme preparation from cultures of a peat soil bacterium to selectively remove the polysaccharide capsule from the surface of type III pneumococci; the capsule represents the pathogen's principle means of defense against immune attack. The enzyme, termed S III, specifically degraded the capsule [122, 123]. Intraperitoneal administration of the enzyme extracts to mice prior to challenge with type III pneumococci gave rise to type III-specific protection [124] and intravenous administration to rabbits with type III dermal infections resulted in early termination of the normally fatal infection [125]. We have used a similar principle to investigate the capacity of a "capsule-stripping" enzyme to alter the course of *E. coli* K1 neonatal systemic infection.

E. coli accounts for 29-53% of isolates from cases of neonatal bacterial meningitis (NBM) [126], an infection usually accompanied by sepsis and with a high case fatality rate. The large majority (80-85%) of these express the K1 capsule [127], a homopolymer of α-2,8-linked polysialic acid (polySia) that mimics the molecular structure of the polySia modulator of neuronal plasticity in the human host. K1 strains colonize neonatal mucosal surfaces, including the intestinal epithelium, and gain access to the bloodstream prior to invasion of the meninges [128]. Following hematogenous spread, the bacteria are thought to enter the central nervous system (CNS) following translocation across the blood-brain barrier at the cerebral microvascular endothelium of the arachnoid membrane [129] or the blood-CSF barrier at the choroid plexus epithelium [130]. Only a limited number of bacterial pathogens are able to invade the brain, due to the protective effect of the physiological barriers between the bloodstream and the CNS, and the overwhelming majority of NBM isolates elaborate a polysaccharide capsule that affords protection against humoral and cellular host defenses [129]. Although K1 strains are found as causative agents of extraintestinal infections such as sepsis and NBM, they exist in the main as components of the commensular gastrointestinal microflora: the factors that underpin the transformation of K1 from commensal to pathogen are poorly understood. The rate of gastrointestinal carriage of K1 in individuals of all ages has been found to be in the range 20-30% [131]. K1 strains are found in the feces of approximately 20% of infants and in the stools of up to 44% of healthy mothers and there is strong evidence of vertical transmission of K1 from mother to infant [131]. The prevalence of K1 in vaginal swabs was found, at 44%, to be higher than that associated with stool samples (21%) [132] and indicates a progressive accumulation of *E. coli* K1 along the fecal-vaginal-neonatal course of transmission.

The antimicrobial properties of amniotic fluid ensure that the intrauterine environment is sterile but, once the membranes rupture or the amniotic fluid is contaminated with meconium, the neonate is exposed to microbes from the maternal genital tract [133]. Contamination of the neonate *in utero* or at birth with *E. coli* K1 [132] or other potential neuropathogens such as group B streptococci [133] increases the risk of development of NBM. The newborn infant displays lower humoral and cellular responsiveness compared to the adult [133, 134] and this is likely to impact on the degree of susceptibility to NBM. In addition, it is highly probable that the capacity of potential neuropathogens to colonize the neonatal gastrointestinal (GI) tract in numbers sufficient to permit their translocation to the blood compartment during the first few days of life also represents a key determinant of outcome, although very little experimental or epidemiological data is available to assess the relative importance of early intestinal colonization. The development of 16S ribosomal DNA arrays for complex microbial populations has facilitated metagenomic analysis of the intestinal microflora [135]; use of this methodology has indicated that incidental environmental exposure to bacteria shortly after birth plays a major role in determining the distinctive characteristics of the evolving microbial community in the GI tract [136].

In order to determine if K1 capsule removal would impact on the progression of this infection, we identified and characterized [137], cloned and sequenced [138], and expressed in high yield [139] an enzyme, endosialidase E (endoE), carried by an *E. coli* K1-specific phage, that rapidly and selectively degrades polySia. The 76kDa enzyme is entirely specific for the α-2,8-sialyl linkages found in polySia and fails to hydrolyse the α-2,3-, α-2,6-, or α-2,9-linkages found in various other human and microbial glycoproteins and polysaccharides. Exposure of a virulent *E. coli* K1 strain to endoE increased its susceptibility to both complement attack [140] and uptake and killing by peritoneal macrophages [141]; the K1 capsule is known to protect against these effectors of the host's immune system [142].

In order to evaluate the therapeutic potential of endoE for the control of neonatal bacteraemia, sepsis and meningitis, we adapted a model of *E. coli* K1 infection in neonatal rat pups developed by Glode and coworkers [143]. The model mimics key features of the human infection: these include non-invasive establishment of infection following colonization of the GI tract, a strong age dependency, temporal development along the gut-blood-brain transit, colonization and penetration of the meninges after invasion of the cerebral spinal compartment and induction of a local inflammatory immune response. We screened a number of *E. coli* K1 strains for their capacity to colonize the GI tract and to produce bacteremia after feeding bacteria to two-day-old (P2) rats [140, 141]. We enhanced the virulence of an isolate from a case of neonatal septicemia (A192) [144], which colonized the GI tract with high efficiency 24 h after oral administration and produced an incidence of bacteraemia of 23%, by serial passage through neonatal rats and designated the enhanced strain A192PP. All pups in each infected litter were colonized within 24 h and translocation to the bloodstream began at P3-P4. By P7 the overwhelming majority of pups (90-100%) were blood culture-positive for *E. coli* K1; without intervention, all bacteremic animals died by P9 (Figure 7). Colonization of the GI tract by A192PP was evident throughout the experiments.

Thus, endoE had no impact on GI colonization by fed K1, suggesting that although *E. coli* K1 expresses polySia in the GI tract [145], the capsule is not required for the maintenance of the K1 gut population. The frequency of bacteremia, but not GI colonization, was strongly age dependent [141]: infected five-day-old (P5) pups showed a much lower incidence of bacteremia and death than younger animals and by P9 pups were refractory to invasion of the bloodstream by GI K1 bacteria. Aerobic culture of flushed luminal intestinal contents at P2 indicated that these pups had not developed an extensive GI microbiota; either no bacteria could be cultured or a light growth of staphylococci, micrococci and *Proteus* spp was found. With K1-fed P2 animals, *E. coli* K1 predominated in P3 luminal samples and was usually the only aerobe or facultative anaerobe detected. In contrast, a more complex luminal microbiota was recovered at P5 and, especially, at P9, raising the possibility that fed K1 cells were unable to compete effectively for sites within the GI tract that would enable them to achieve numbers sufficient to facilitate translocation into the bloodstream.

Intraperitoneal administration of single daily doses (0.25-20μg) of endoE at P3, one day after infection by the oral route, reduced the incidence of bacteremia and death by 80-100%. A similar, but not greater, degree of protection against lethal bacteremia was afforded by five daily 20μg doses administered over P3-P7 [140]. Single doses given at P4 were less effective [141]. Figure 7 shows the outcome of a single intraperitoneal dose of endoE administered at P3 to pups fed *E. coli* K1 at P2. Bacteremia is scored as being present or absent as judged by daily blood sampling; in the treated animals bacteremia was almost always transient in contrast to the very high and persistent blood counts found in untreated animals [146]. The treated animals remained healthy in spite of the transient bacteremia. As the enzyme has no effect on the viability or growth rate of *E. coli* K1 strains, we surmise the therapeutic effect to be due to removal of the protective capsule during the early stages of the infection, allowing the innate defenses of the immature pup to counter the pathogenic mechanisms of the invader. This work clearly demonstrates that abrogation of even one bacterial virulence determinant may compromise the pathogen and supports the view [147] that the polySia capsule is essential for establishment of systemic disease.

In P2-infected pups, *E. coli* K1 cells gain access to the blood compartment at P4-P5, probably via the mesenteric lymph glands [144], where they express the non-*O*-acetylated form of the polySia capsule [146]. Like many O18:K1 isolates, A192PP is lysogenized by prophage CUS-3 [148], which carries the *neuO* gene encoding an *O*-acetyltransferase responsible for non-stoichiometeric *O*-acetylation of sialyl residues at positions C-7 and C-9 of polySia.

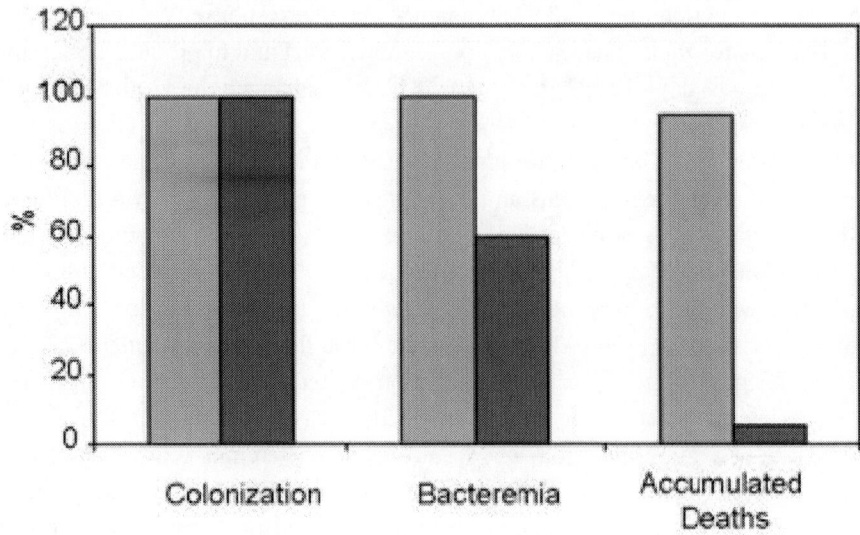

Figure 7. Outcome of feeding *E. coli* K1 strain A192PP to two-day-old (P2) rats. Animals were left untreated (■) or 20 μg endoE was administered at P3 (■); n=22 and n=21 respectively. Colonization was determined daily over P3-P9, although *E. coli* expressing K1 were detected in perianal swabs from almost all animals at P3. Pups were scored as bacteremic if one or more daily blood samples yielded K1 positive colonies. Deaths were recorded over the period represented by P3-P9.

The bacteria transit to the central nervous system and can be recovered in significant numbers from homogenized brain preparations. We determined that the most likely point of entry into the CNS is *via* the choroid plexus, where they can be visualized by immunofluorescence microscopy using surface-antigen-specific reagents [146]. The bacteria colonize the meninges and, interestingly, we could find no evidence that A192PP cells express either the *O*-acetylated or non-*O*-acetylated form of the K1 capsule at this site, even though bacteria recovered from brain tissue retain the capacity to synthesize polySia [146]. Figure 8 shows that the neurons within the cerebral tissue adjoining the meninges contain relatively large quantities of polySia but the meninges contain no detectable polySia, facilitating visualization of the neuroinvasive pathogen with anti-O18 antibody but not with a reagent specific for polySia. The process of invasion and dissemination to the brain is interrupted by endoE; after administration of the enzyme no bacteria can be visualized in blood smears, the choroid plexus, the ventricles or the brain. EndoE is most effective during the early stages of the infection, indicating that down-regulation of capsule expression, which occurs in the meninges and to a lesser extent in the choroid plexus [146], limits the extent to which capsule depolymerization has the capacity to resolve the infection.

Profiling of gene expression using a cDNA microarray comprising over 28,000 genes indicated that meningeal invasion at P5 was accompanied by a highly selective up-regulation of genes characteristic of a local inflammatory response. There was a greater than threefold up-regulation of 416 genes in pooled brain tissue from three infected pups and the expression pattern indicated a complex transcriptional response involving cytokines (in particular IL-1, TNF-α, IL-6), CXC chemokines, complement components associated with the alternative pathway of activation, lipocalins (associated with regulation of the inflammatory response to LPS-mediated endotoxemia [150]) and matrix metalloproteinases, balanced by genes with potential anti-inflammatory effects, such as IL-1 receptor antagonists, xanthine dehydrogenase, xanthine oxidase and superoxide dismutase.

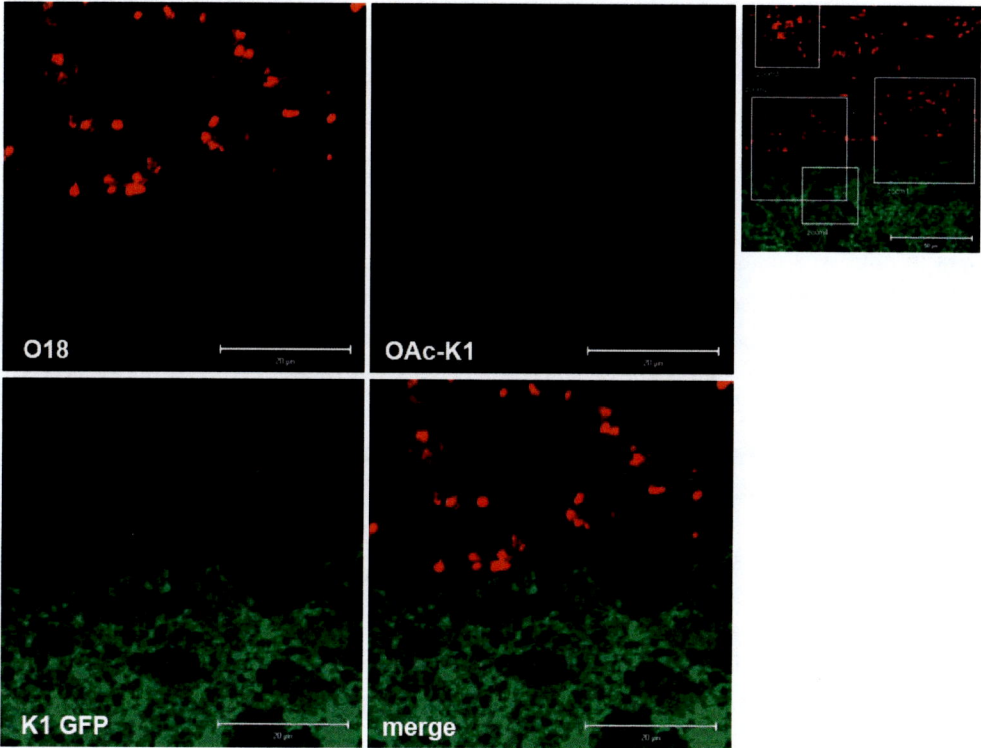

Figure 8. *E. coli* K1 at the meninges-cerebrum interface: non-enhanced confocal images of brain sections from a K1-infected rat pup sacrificed at P5 after feeding of bacteria at P2. Sections were stained with O18 and *O*-acetyl antibodies and K1-GFP reagent [149]. Optical slice of 1 μm; bar = 20 μm in main images and 50 μm in the low power image.

Some key genes were up-regulated up to 3,000-fold. The response could be almost completely prevented by prompt intraperitoneal administration of a single 20 μg dose of endoE. Fundamentally different patterns of gene expression were found in other organs, such as liver and spleen. Many of the products of the up-regulated cytokine and chemokine genes have been found to be associated with neonatal meningitis in the human infant [128]. We conclude that this well-characterized non-invasive model provides an excellent platform for evaluation of the development of neonatal bacteremia and meningitis and for the evaluation of therapies, old and new.

E. coli K1 is an important cause of NBM and sepsis but other encapsulated bacteria also cause these infections. An ideal target for enzyme-mediated capsule depolymerization would be an infection caused by a single bacterial species of which all pathogenic strains produce one structurally unique polymeric capsule that contributes essential features to the pathogenesis of the bacterium. We would consider "capsule-stripping" to be an even more attractive approach if current therapies for any such infection were inadequate and amenable to novel therapeutic paradigms. In our view inhalation anthrax ticks all these boxes. Naturally occurring anthrax is acquired following contact with infected animals or animal products contaminated with the encapsulated, spore-forming Gram-positive rod *Bacillus anthracis* and it usually presents as cutaneous, inhalation or gastrointestinal anthrax [151]. Cutaneous anthrax is the most common and death due to this form of the disease is rare if properly managed. Inhalation anthrax is usually fatal. Natural infections are only rarely encountered in the developed world, but the potential for aerosol-mediated spread of *B. anthracis* spores by rogue states and terrorists is of growing concern. Countermeasures to this threat include vaccination, quarantine and chemotherapy and to this end a limited number of antibiotics have been identified for prophylaxis and treatment [152, 153]. As there have been no clinical studies of the treatment of anthrax in humans, recommended antibiotic regimens are based on empirical treatments for sepsis [153]. Most naturally occurring anthrax strains are sensitive to penicillin, which is approved by the FDA for this indication, as is doxycycline. Likewise, ciprofloxacin has been identified as a suitable alternative due to its efficacy in animal models of anthrax but has not been studied in humans [153]. Resistance to these front-line antibiotics could be engineered into strains of *B. anthracis* and the complete genome sequence of the organism is in the public domain [154].

B. anthracis causes lethal infection due to the elaboration by the vegetative form of a protein exotoxin complex and a capsule composed of a homopolymer of D-glutamic acid linked via the γ amide (PDGA) [151, 155]. These virulence factors are plasmid associated: pXO1 (182 kb) harbours the toxin structural genes *cya*, *pagA* and *lef* encoding edema factor, protective antigen and lethal factor, respectively, whereas pXO2 (96 kb) carries the capsule biosynthetic operon *capBCAD* and the capsule gene regulators acpA and acpB. The products of *capB*, *capC* and *capA* mediate biosynthesis, transport and attachment of large (>100 kDa) capsule polymers to the cell wall [155]; the *capD* gene product is a γ-glutamyltranspeptidase with the primary function of attachment of PDGA to peptidoglycan [156]. It also functions as a depolymerase, effecting the release of diffusible PDGA fragments (<14 kDa) from the surface [156] that may act to inhibit cellular host defenses [157]. *B. anthracis* strains that lack either pXO1 or pXO2 show reduced virulence in animal models of infection in comparison to wild type strains [158, 159]. The key role of the Cap$^+$ phenotype has recently been unambiguously established: strains carrying both plasmids but deleted specifically for *capBCAD* were highly attenuated in a murine inhalation model [160]. Recently, Scorpio and colleagues [161, 162] showed that CapD degraded purified PDGA capsule and removed the capsule from the surface of anthrax bacilli. Exposure to the enzyme enabled murine macrophages and human neutrophils to engulf and kill these otherwise insusceptible bacteria. In addition, parenteral administration of CapD protected mice from challenge with both spores and vegetative *B. anthracis*. Although CapD is a labile enzyme and may not be suited to development as a therapeutic for use in humans, these studies lead the way in defining a novel approach to the treatment of a disease for which there are limited therapeutic options.

Concluding Remarks

It is often pointed out that resistance to antimicrobial chemotherapy is inevitable and will happen sooner rather than later. This is certainly true of conventional agents that eliminate susceptible bacteria from the patient in the short term, from the immediate environment in the medium term and from more extensive bacterial population pools in the long term. Thus, antibiotics alter incrementally the makeup of the microbial world, in particular that part of it that impacts on patients. Some of the new, and so new, therapeutic approaches highlighted in this contribution will do the same. Phages and bacteria have co-evolved for longer than any other components of an interdependent biological association; phages have played a major role in shaping and reshaping the architecture of the bacterial genome and have contributed enormously to the capacity of pathogens to adapt to new hosts and to the emergence of new pathogens or epidemic clones. Any phage used therapeutically will continue this process and phage therapies will need to adapt to the evolution of bacterial targets, as a consequence of phage selection, to remain viable long term options for therapy. For reasons that are less clear, early experiences with efflux pump inhibitors have raised the specter of rapid development of resistance to such molecules.

We have posed the question: is resistance inevitable? Many think that it is, regardless of the nature and degree of the selective pressure applied to the bacterial population in question: but we are not so sure. Even though we are not proposing that endoE be developed for the treatment of *E. coli* K1 infections in the newborn, it is difficult to see how resistance can emerge to an agent that strips away the outer coat essential for survival of the pathogen in the host. Capsule-deprived forms will not survive the attentions of the host's immune system, the bacterium cannot make an alternative protective capsule, decoration of the polySia polymer does not fool the enzyme (at least with regard to *O*acetylation, which seems not to be expressed *in vivo*) and the enzyme will not, as far as we can surmise, be excreted in a form in which it can interact with K1 strains in the environment. The idea that modification of the pathogen, to produce a form less able to survive in patients, is in our view a good place to start a search for a therapeutic paradigm that does not readily produce resistance.

Acknowledgments

Work from the authors' laboratory has been supported by Medical Research Council grants G0000996, G0400268 and G06000064 and British Society for Antimicrobial Chemotherapy grants GA230 and GA382.

References

[1] Armstrong, G.L., Conn, L.A., and Pinner, R.W. (1999). Trends in infectious disease mortality in the United States during the 20th century. *J. Amer. Med. Assoc. 281*, 61-66.

[2] Nelson, K.E., Williams, C.M., and Graham, N.M.H. (2005). *Infectious Disease Epidemiology: Theory and Practice.* Sudbury MA: Jones and Bartlett Publishers.

[3] Mathers, C.D., and Loncar, D. (2006). Projections of global mortality and burden of disease from 2002 to 2030. *PLoS Med. 3*, 2011-2030.

[4] IDSA Report. (2004). *Bad bugs, no drugs.* Alexandria VA: Infectious Disease Society of America.

[5] Klevens, R.M., Morrison, M.A., Nadle, J., Petit, S., Gershman, K., Ray, S., Harrison, L.H., Lyfield, R., Dumyati, G., Townes, J.M., Craig, A.S., Zell, E.R., Fosheim, G.E., McDougal, L.K., Carey, R.B., and Fridkin, S.K. (2007). Invasive methicillin-resistant *Staphylococcus aureus* infections in the United States. *J. Amer. Med. Assoc. 298*, 1763-1771.

[6] Weiss, R.A., and McMichael, A.J. (2004). Social and environmental risk factors in the emergence of infectious diseases. *Nature Med. 10*, 570-576.

[7] Taubes, G. (2008). The bacteria fight back. *Science 321*, 356-361.

[8] Greenwood, D. (2008). *Antimicrobial Drugs: Chronicle of a Twentieth Century Medical Triumph*. Oxford UK: Oxford University Press.

[9] Bean, D.C., Livermore, D.M., Papa, I., and Hall, L.M. (2005). Resistance among *Escherichia coli* to sulphonamides and other antimicrobials now little used in man. *J. Antimicrob. Chemother. 56*, 962-964.

[10] Levy, S.B., and Marshall, B. (2004). Antibacterial resistance worldwide: causes, challenges and responses. *Nature Med. 10*, S122-S129.

[11] Spellberg, B., Powers, J.H., Brass, E.P., Miller, L.G., and Edwards, J.E. (2004). Trends in antimicrobial drug development: implications for the future. *Clin. Infect. Dis. 38*, 1279-1286.

[12] Projan, S.J., and Shlaes, D.M. (2004). Antibacterial drug discovery: is it all downhill from here? *Clin. Microbiol. Infect. 10 (Suppl. 4)*, 18-22.

[13] Norrby, S.R., Nord, C.E., and Finch, R. (2005). Lack of development of new antimicrobial drugs: a potential serious threat to public health. *Lancet Infect. 5*, 115-119.

[14] Overbye, K.M., and Barrett, J.F. (2005). Antibiotics: where did we go wrong? *Drug Disc. Today 10*, 45-51.

[15] Bush, K. (2004). Why it is important to continue antibacterial drug discovery. *ASM News 6*, 282-287.

[16] Nathan, C., and Goldberg, F.M. (2005). The profit problem in antibiotic RandD. *Nature Rev. Drug Disc. 4*, 887-891.

[17] Payne, D.J., Gwynn, M.N., Holmes, D.J., and Pompliano, D.L. (2007). Drugs for bad bugs: confronting the challenges of antibacterial drug discovery. *Nature Rev. Drug Disc. 6*, 29-40.

[18] Becker, D., Selbach, M., Rollenhagen, C., Ballmaier, M., Meyer, T.F., Mann, M., and Burmann, D. (2006). Robust *Salmonella* metabolism limits possibilities for new antimicrobials. *Nature 440*, 303-307.

[19] Royal Society Policy Document. (2008). Innovative mechanisms for tackling antibacterial resistance. http://royalsociety.org/downloaddoc.=5545.

[20] Livermore, D.M. (2000). Epidemiology of antibiotic resistance. *Intensive Care Med. 26*, S14-S21.

[21] Aminov, R.I., and Mackie, R.I. (2007). Evolution and ecology of antibiotic resistance genes. *FEMS Microbiol. Lett. 271*, 147-161.

[22] Austin, D.J., Kristinsonn, K.G., and Anderson, R.M. (1999). The relationship between the volume of antimicrobial consumption in human communities and the frequency of resistance. *Proc. Natl. Acad. Sci. U.S.A. 96*, 1152-1156.

[23] Enne, V.I., Bennett, P.M., Livermore, D.M., and Hall, L.M. (2004). Enhancement of host fitness by the sul2-coding plasmid p9123 in the absence of selective pressure. *J. Antimicrob. Chemother. 53*, 958-963.

[24] Kollef, M.H. (2006). Is antibiotic cycling the answer to preventing the emergence of bacterial resistance in the intensive care unit? *Clin. Infect. Dis. 43 (Suppl. 2)*, 582-588.

[25] Lipsitch, M., and Levine, B.R. (1997). The population dynamics of antimicrobial chemotherapy. *Antimicrob. Agents Chemother. 41*, 363-373.

[26] Austin, D.J., White, N.J., and Anderson, R.M. (1998). The dynamics of drug action on the within-host population growth of infectious agents: melding pharmacokinetics with pathogen population dynamics. *J. Theor. Biol. 194*, 313-339.

[27] Hyatt, J.M., and Schentag, J.J. (2000). Pharmacodynamic modelling of risk factors for ciprofloxacin resistance in *Pseudomoas aeruginosa. Infect. Control Hosp. Epidemiol. 21*, S9-S11.

[28] Cirz, R.T., Chin, J.K., Andes, D.R., de Crécy-Lagard, V., Craig, W.A., and Romesberg, F.E. (2005). Inhibition of mutation and combating the evolution of antibiotic resistance. *PLoS Biol. 6*, 1024-1033.

[29] Lipsitch, M., and Samore, M.H. (2002). Antimicrobial use and antimicrobial resistance: a population perspective. *Emerg. Infect. Dis. 8*, 347-354.

[30] Garber, A.M. (1989). A discrete-time model of the acquisition of antibiotic-resistant infections in hospitalized patients. *Biometrics 45*, 797-816.

[31] Austin, D.J., Kakehashi, M., and Anderson, R.M.. (1997). The transmission dynamics of antibiotic-resistant bacteria: the relationship between resistance in commensal organisms and antibiotic consumption. *Proc. Royal Soc. Lond. B: Biol. Sci. 264*, 1629-1638.

[32] Bonhoeffer, S., Lipsitch, M., and Levine, B.R. (1997). Evaluating treatment protocols to prevent antibiotic resistance. *Proc. Natl. Acad. Sci. USA. 94*, 12106-12111.

[33] Moan, J., and Peng, Q. (2003). An outline of the hundred-year history of PDT. *Anticancer Res. 23*, 3591-3600.

[34] Caminos, D.A., Spesia, M.B., and Durantini, E.N. (2006). Photodynamic inactivation of *Escherichia coli* by novel *meso*-substituted porphyrins by 4-(3-*N,N,N*-trimethylammoniumpropoxy)phenyl and 4-(trifluoro)phenyl groups. *Photochem. Photobiol. Sci. 5*, 56-65.

[35] Hambin, M.R., and Hasan, T. (2004). Photodynamic therapy: a new antimicrobial approach to infectious disease? *Photochem. Photobiol. Sci. 3*, 436-450.

[36] Tegos, G.P., and Hambin, M.R. (2006). Phenothiazinium antimicrobial photosensitizers are substrates of bacterial multidrug resistance pumps. *Antimicrob. Agents Chemother. 50*, 196-203.

[37] Wainwright, M., and Crossley, K.B. (2004). Photosensitizing agents – circumventing resistance and breaking down biofilms: a review. *Int. Biodeterior. Biodegrad. 53*, 119-126.

[38] Konopka, K., and Goslinski, T. (2007). Photodynamic therapy in dentistry. *J. Dent. Res. 86*, 694707.

[39] Alisky, J., Iczkowski, K., Rapoport, A., and Toitsky, (1998). Bacteriophages show promise as antimicrobial agents. *J. Infect. 36*, 5-15.

[40] Levin, B.R., and Bull, J.J. (2004). Population and evolutionary dynamics of phage therapy. *Nature Rev. Microbiol. 2*, 166-173.

[41] Hanlon, G.W. (2007). Bacteriophages: an appraisal of their role in the treatment of bacterial infections. *Int. J. Antimicrob. Agents 30*, 118-128.

[42] Verbeken G, De Vos D, Vaneechoutte M, Merabishvili M, Zizi M and Pirnay J-P (2007). European regulatory conundrum of phage therapy. *Fut. Microbiol. 2*, 485-491.

[43] Bruttin A and Brüssow H (2005). Human volunteers receiving *Escherichia coli* phage T4 orally: a safety test of phage therapy. *Antimicrob. Agents Chemother. 49*, 2874-2878.

[44] Food and Drug Administration. (2006). Food additives permitted for direct addition to food for human consumption: bacteriophage preparation. *Fed. Regist. 71*, 47729-47732.

[45] Lopez-Pascua, L.C., and Buckling, A. (2008). Increasing productivity accelerates host-parasite coevolution. *J. Evol. Biol. 21*, 853-860.

[46] Cairns, B.J., and Payne, R.J.H. (2008). Bacteriophage therapy and the mutant selection window. *Antimicrob. Agents Chemother. 52*, 4344-4350.

[47] Stummeyer, K., Schwarzer, D., Claus, H., Vogel, U., Gerardy-Schahn, R., and Mühlenhoff, M. (2006). Evolution of bacteriophages infecting encapsulated bacteria: lessons from *Escherichia coli* K1-specific phages. *Molec. Microbiol. 60*, 1123-1135.

[48] Schiffer, M.S., Oliviera, E., Glode, M.P., McCracken, G.H., Sarff, L.M., and Robbins, J.B. (1976). A review: relation between invasiveness and the K1 capsular polysaccharide of *Escherichia coli. Pediatr. Res. 10*, 82-87.

[49] Loessner, M. (2005). Bacteriophage endolysins – current state of research and applications. *Curr. Opin. Microbiol. 8*, 480-487.

[50] Krause, R.M. (1957). Studies on bacteriophages of hemolytic streptococci. I. Factors influencing the interaction of phage and susceptible host cell. *J. Exp. Med. 106*, 365-384.

[51] Loeffler, J.M., Nelson, D., and Fischetti, V.A. (2001). Rapid killing of *Streptococcus pneumoniae* with a bacteriophage cell wall hydrolase. *Science 294*, 2170-2172.

[52] Nelson, D., Schuch, R., Chahales, P., Zhu, S., and Fischetti, V.A. (2006). PlyC: a multimeric bacteriophage lysine. *Proc. Natl. Acad. Sci. U.S.A. 103*, 10765-10770.

[53] Nelson, D., Loomis, I., and Fischetti, V.A. (2001). Prevention and elimination of upper respiratory colonization of mice by group A streptococci by using a bacteriophage lytic enzyme. *Proc. Natl. Acad. Sci. U.S.A. 98*, 4107-4112.

[54] Borysowski, J., Weber-Dabrowska, B., and Górski, A. (2006). Bacteriophage endolysins as a novel class of antibacterial agents. *Exp. Biol. Med. 231*, 366-377.

[55] Novick, R.P. (2003). Autoinduction and signal transduction in the regulation of staphylococcal virulence. *Molec. Microbiol. 48*, 1429-1449.

[56] Smith, T. (1934). *Parasitism and Disease*. Princeton NJ: Princeton University Press.

[57] Dubos, R. (1945). *The Bacterial Cell in Relation to Problems of Virulence, Immunity and Chemotherapy*. Cambridge MA: Harvard University Press.

[58] Drews, J. (1980). A role for immune stimulation in the treatment of microbial infections? *Infection 8*, 2-4.

[59] Kolodziej, H., and Kiderlen, A.F. (2007). In vitro evaluation of antibacterial and immunomodulatory activities of *Pelargonium reniforme*, *Pelargonium sidoides* and the related herbal drug preparation EPs® 7630. *Phytomed. 14(Suppl 4)*, 18-26.

[60] Dickneite, G., Kaspereit, F., and Sedlacek, H.H. (1984). Stimulation of cell-mediated immunity by bestatin correlates with reduction of bacterial persistence in experimental chronic *Salmonella typhimurium* infection. *Infect. Immun. 44*, 168-174.

[61] Kolodziej, H. (2000). Traditionally used *Pelargonium* species: chemistry and biological activity of umckaloabo extracts and their constituents. *Curr. Top. Phytochem. 3*,77-93.

[62] Kim, C.E., Griffiths, W.J., and Taylor, P.W. (2009). Components derived from the roots of *Pelargonium* spp stimulate killing of *Mycobacterium tuberculosis* by murine macrophages. *J. Appl. Microbiol. 106*, 1184-1193.

[63] Rosenbloom, A.J., Linden, P.K., Dorrance, A., Penkosky, N., Cohen-Melamed, M.H., and Pinsky, M.R. (2005). Effect of granulocyte-monocyte colony-stimulating factor therapy on leukocyte function and clearance of serious infection in nonneutropenic patients. *Chest 127*, 2139-2150.

[64] Brown, A.G., Butterworth, D., Cole, M., Hanscomb, G., Hood, J.D., Reading, C., and Rolinson, G.N. (1976). Naturally-occurring β-lactamase inhibitors with antibacterial activity. *J. Antibiot. (Tokyo) 29*, 668-669.

[65] White, A.R., Kaye, C., Poupard, J., Pypstra, R., Woodnutt, G., and Wynne, B. (2004). Augmentin® (amoxicillin/clavulanate) in the treatment of community-acquired respiratory tract infection: a review of the continuing development of an innovative antimicrobial agent. *J. Antimicrob. Chemother. 53*, i3-i20.

[66] Davies, T.A., Pankuch, G.A., Dewasse, B.E., Jacobs, M.R., and Appelbaum, P.C. (1999). In vitro development of resistance to five quinolones and amoxicillin-clavulanate in *Streptococcus pneumoniae*. *Antimicrob. Agents Chemother. 43*, 1177-1182.

[67] Leflon-Guibout, V., Speldooren, V., Heym, B., and Nicolas-Chenoine, M.-H. (2000). Epidemiological survey of amoxicillin-clavulanate resistance and corresponding molecular mechanisms in *Escherichia coli* isolates in France: new genetic features of bla(TEM) genes. *Antimicrob. Agents Chemother. 44*, 2709-2714.

[68] Oteo, J., Campos, J., Lázaro, E., Cuevas, Ó., Garcia-Cobos, S., Pérez-Vázquez, M., and de Abajo, F.J. (2008). Increased amoxicillin-clavulanic acid resistance in *Escherichia coli* blood isolates, Spain. *Emerg. Infect. Dis. 14*, 1259-1262.

[69] Coleman, K., Athalye, M., Clancey, A., Davison, M., Payne, D.J., Perry, C.R., and Chopra, I. (1994). Bacterial resistance mechanisms as therapeutic targets. *J. Antimicrob. Chemother. 33*, 1091-1116.

[70] Roberts, M.C. (1994). Epidemiology of tetracycline-resistance determinants. *Trends Microbiol. 2*, 353-357.

[71] Piddock, L.J. (2006). Multidrug-resistance efflux pumps: not just for resistance. *Nature Rev. Microbiol. 4*, 629-636.

[72] Wright, G.D. (2000). Resisting resistance: new chemical strategies for battling superbugs. *Chem. Biol. 7*, R127-R132.

[73] Lomovskaya, O., Zgurskaya, H.I., Totrov, M., and Watkins, W.J. (2007). Waltzing transporters and 'the dance macabre' between humans and bacteria. *Nature Rev. Drug Disc. 6*, 56-65.

[74] Lomovskaya, O., and Bostian, K.A. (2006). Practical applications and feasibility of efflux pump inhibitors in the clinic - a vision for applied use. *Biochem. Pharmacol. 71*, 910-918.

[75] Garvey, M.I., and Piddock, L.J.V. (2008). The efflux pump inhibitor reserpine selects multidrug-resistant *Streptococcus pneumoniae* strains that overexpress the ABC transporters PatA and PatB. *Antimicrob. Agents Chemother. 52*, 1677-1685.

[76] Chen, D., Daniel, K.G., Kuhn, D.J., Kazi, A., Bhuiyan, M., Li, L., Wang, Z., Wan, S.B., Lam, W.H., Chan, T.H., and Dou, Q.P. (2004). Green tea and tea polyphenols in cancer prevention. *Front. Biosci. 9*, 2618-2631.

[77] Chow, S.H.-H., Cai, Y., Hakim, I.A., Crowell, J.A., Shahi, F., Brooks, C.A., Dorr, R.T., Hara, Y., and Alberts, D.S. (2003). Pharmacokinetics and safety of green tea polyphenols after multiple-dose administration of epigallocatechin gallate and Polyphenon E in healthy individuals. *Clin. Cancer Res. 9*, 3312-3319.

[78] Yam, T.S., Hamilton-Miller, J.M.T., and Shah, S. (1998). The effect of a component of tea (*Camellia sinensis*) on methicillin resistance, PBP2' synthesis, and β-lactamase production in *Staphylococcus aureus*. *J. Antimicrob. Chemother. 42*, 211-216.

[79] Zhao, W.-H., Hu, Z.-Q., Okubo, S., Hara, Y., and Shimamura, T. (2001). Mechanism of synergy between epigallocatechin gallate and β-lactams against methicillin-resistant *Staphylococcus aureus*. *Antimicrob. Agents Chemother. 45*, 1737-1742.

[80] Taylor, P.W., Hamilton-Miller, J.M.T., and Stapleton, P.D. (2005). Antimicrobial properties of green tea catechins. *Food Sci. Technol. Bull. 2*, 71-81.

[81] Hamilton-Miller, J.M.T., and Shah S. (2000). Activity of the tea component epicatechin gallate and analogues against methicillin-resistant *Staphylococcus aureus*. *J. Antimicrob. Chemother. 46*, 852-853.

[82] Stapleton, P.D., Shah, S., Anderson, J.C., Hara, Y., Hamilton-Miller, J.M.T., and Taylor, P.W. (2004). Modulation of β-lactam resistance in *Staphylococcus aureus* by catechins and gallates. *Int. J. Antimicrob. Agents 23*, 462-467.

[83] Kohri, T., Matsumoto, N., Yamakawa, M., Suzuki, M., Nanjo, F., Hara, Y., and Oku, N. (2001). Metabolic fate of (-)-[4-^{3}H]epigallocatechin gallate in rats after oral administration. *J. Agric. Food Chem. 49*, 4102-4112.

[84] Anderson, J.C., Headley, C., Stapleton, P.D., and Taylor, P.W. (2005). Synthesis and antibacterial activity of a hydrolytically stable (-)-epicatechin gallate analogue for the modulation of β-lactam resistance in *Staphylococcus aureus*. *Bioorg. Med. Chem. Lett. 15*, 2633-2635.

[85] Anderson, J.C., Headley, C., Stapleton, P.D., and Taylor, P.W. (2005). Asymmetric total synthesis of B-ring modified (-)-epicatechin gallate analogues and their modulation of β-lactam resistance in *Staphylococcus aureus*. *Tetrahedron 61*, 7703-7711.

[86] Caturla, N., Vera-Samper, E., Villalain, J., Reyes Mateo, C., and Micol, V. (2003). The relationship between the antioxidant and antibacterial properties of galloylated catechins and the structure of phospholipid model membranes. *Free Radical Biol. Med. 34*, 648-662.

[87] Kajiya, K., Kumazawa, S., and Nakayama, T. (2001). Steric effects on the interaction of tea catechins with lipid bilayers. *Biosci. Biotechnol. Biochem. 65*, 2638-2643.

[88] Kajiya, K., Kumazawa, S., and Nakayama, T. (2002). Effects of external factors on the interaction of tea catechins with lipid bilayers. *Biosci. Biotechnol. Biochem. 66*, 2330-2335.

[89] Hashimoto, T., Kumazawa, S., Nanjo, F., Hara, Y., and Nakayama, T. (1999). Interaction of tea catechins with lipid bilayers investigated with liposome systems. *Biosci. Biotechnol. Biochem. 63*, 2252-2255.

[90] Stapleton, P.D., Shah, S., Hara, Y., and Taylor, P.W. (2006). Potentiation of catechin gallate-mediated sensitization of *Staphylococcus aureus* to oxacillin by nongalloylated catechins. *Antimicrob. Agents Chemother. 50*, 752-755.

[91] Blanco, A.R., Sudano-Roccaro, A., Spoto, G.C., Nostro, A., and Rusciano, D. (2005). Epigallocatechin gallate inhibits biofilm formation by ocular staphylococcal isolates. *Antimicrob. Agents Chemother. 49*, 4339-4343.

[92] Stapleton, P.D., Shah, S., Ehlert, K., Hara, Y., and Taylor, P.W. (2007). The β- lactam-resistance modifier (-)-epicatechin gallate alters the architecture of the cell wall of *Staphylococcus aureus*. *Microbiology 153*, 2093-2103.

[93] Shah, S., Stapleton, P.D., and Taylor, P.W. (2008). The polyphenol (-)-epicatechin gallate disrupts the secretion of virulence-related proteins by *Staphylococcus aureus*. *Lett. Appl. Microbiol. 46*, 181-185.

[94] Ehlert, K. (1999). Methicillin-resistance in *Staphylococcus aureus* – molecular basis, novel targets and antibiotic therapy. *Curr. Pharm. Des. 5*, 45-55.

[95] Berger-Bächi, B., and Tschierske, M. (1998). Role of Fem factors in methicillin resistance. *Drug. Res. Upd. 1*, 325-335.

[96] Zhao, W.-H., Hu, Z.-Q., Okubo, S., Hara, Y., and Shimamura, T. (2001). Mechanism of synergy between epigallocatechin gallate and β-lactams against methicillin-resistant *Staphylococcus aureus*. *Antimicrob. Agents Chemother. 45*, 1737-42.

[97] Hamilton-Miller, J.M.T., and Shah, S. (1999). Disorganization of cell division of methicillin-resistant *Staphylococcus aureus* by a component of tea (*Camellia sinensis*): a study by electron microscopy. *FEMS Microbiol. Lett. 176*, 463-469.

[98] Neuhaus, F.C., and Baddiley, J. (2003). A continuum of anionic charge: structures and functions of D-alanyl-teichoic acids in Gram-positive bacteria. *Microbiol. Molec. Biol. Rev. 67*, 686-723.

[99] Scott, W.J. (1953). Water relations of *Staphylococcus aureus* at 30°C. *Aust. J. Biol. Sci. 6*, 549-564.

[100] Stapleton, P.D., Gettert, J., and Taylor, P.W. (2006). Epicatechin gallate, a component of green tea, reduces halotolerance in *Staphylococcus aureus*. *Int. J. Food Microbiol. 111*, 276-279.

[101] Sugai, M., Komatsuzawa, H., Akiyama, T., Hong, Y.-M., Oshida, T., Miyake, Y., Yamaguchi, T., and Suginaka, H. (1995). Identification of endo-β-*N*-acetylglucosaminidase and *N*-acetylmuramyl-L-alanine amidase as cluster-dispersing enzymes in *Staphylococcus aureus. J. Bacteriol. 177*, 1491-1496.

[102] Lichenstein, H.S., Hastings, A.E., Langley, K.E., Mendiaz, E.A., Rohde, M.F., Elmore, R., and Zukowski, M.M. (1990). Cloning and nucleotide sequence of the N-acetylmuramidase M1-encoding gene from *Streptomyces globisporus. Gene 88*, 81-86.

[103] Bernal, P., Zloh, M., and Taylor, P.W. (2009). Disruption of D-alanyl esterification of Staphylococcus aureus cell wall teichoic acid by the β-lactam resistance modifier (-)-epicatechin gallate. *J. Antimicrob. Chemother. 63*, 1156-1162.

[104] Gross, M., Cramton, S.E., Götz, F., and Peschel, A. (2001). Key role of teichoic acid net charge in *Staphylococcus aureus* colonization of artificial surfaces. *Infect. Immun. 69*, 3423-3426.

[105] Peschel, A., Otto, M., Jack, R.W., Kalbacher, H., Jung, G., and Götz, F. (1999). Inactivation of the *dlt* operon in *Staphylococcus aureus* confers sensitivity to defensins, protegrins, and other antimicrobial peptides. *J. Biol. Chem. 274*, 8405-8410.

[106] Peschel, A., Vuong, C., Otto, M., and Götz, F. (2000). The D-alanine residues of *Staphylococcus aureus* teichoic acids alter the susceptibility to vancomycin and the activity of autolytic enzymes. *Antimicrob. Agents Chemother. 44*, 2845-2847.

[107] Wecke, J., Madela, K., and Fischer, W. (1997). The absence of D-alanine from lipoteichoic acid and wall teichoic acid alters surface charge, enhances autolysis and increases susceptibility to methicillin in *Bacillus subtilis. Microbiology 143*, 2953-2960.

[108] Pinho, M.G., and Errington, J. (2003). Dispersed mode of *Staphylococcus aureus* cell wall synthesis in the absence of the division machinery. *Molec. Microbiol. 50*, 871-881.

[109] Pinho, M.G., Errington, J. (2005). Recruitment of penicillin-binding protein PBP2 to the division site of *Staphylococcus aureus* is dependent on its transpeptidation substrates. *Molec. Microbiol. 55*, 799-807.

[110] Sieradski, K., and Tomasz, A. (2003). Alterations of cell wall structure and metabolism accompany reduced susceptibility to vancomycin in an isogenic series of clinical isolates of *Staphylococcus aureus. J. Bacteriol. 185*, 7103-7110.

[111] Alksne, L.E., and Projan, S.J. (2000). Bacterial virulence as a target for antimicrobial chemotherapy. *Curr. Opin. Biotechnol. 11*, 625-636.

[112] Projan, S.J., and Novick, R.P. (1997). The molecular basis of pathogenicity. In K.B. Crossley and G.L. Archer (Eds.), The Staphylococci in Human Disease (pp55-81). New York: Churchill Livingstone.

[113] Diep, B.A., and Otto, M. (2008). The role of virulence determinants in community-associated MRSA pathogenesis. *Trends Microbiol. 16*, 361-369.

[114] Balaban, N., Goldkorn, T., Nhan, R.T., Dang, L.B., Scott, S., Ridgley, R.M., Rasooly, A., Wright, S.C., Larrick, J.W., Rasooly, R., and Carlson, J.R. (1998). Autoinducer of virulence as a target for vaccine and therapy against *Staphylococcus aureus. Science 280*, 438-440.

[115] Rasko, D.A., Moreira, C.G., Li, D.R., Reading, N.C., Ritchie, J.M., Waldor, M.K., Williams, N., Taussig, R., Wei, S., Roth, M., Hughes, D.T., Huntley, J.F., Fina, M.W.,

Falck, J.R., and Sperandio, V. (2008). Targeting QseC signaling and virulence for antibiotic development. *Science 321*, 1078-1080.

[116] Liautard, J.-P., Jubier-Maurin, V., Boigegrain, R.-A., and Köhler, S. (2006). Antimicrobials: targeting virulence genes necessary for intracellular multiplication. *Trends Microbiol. 14*, 109-113.

[117] Cegelski, L., Marshall, G.R., Eldridge, G.R., and Hultgren, S.J. (2008). The biology and future prospects of antivirulence therapies. *Nature Rev. Microbiol. 6*, 17-27.

[118] Williams, P. (2007). Quorum sensing, communication and cross-kingdom signaling in the bacterial world. *Microbiology 153*, 3923-3938.

[119] Scott, R.J., Lian, L.Y., Muharram, S.H., Cockayne, A., Wood, S.J., Bycroft, B.W., Williams, P., and Chan, W.C. (2003). Side-chain-to-tail thiolactone peptide inhibitors of the staphylococcal quorum-sensing system. *Bioorg. Med. Chem. Lett. 13*, 2449-2253.

[120] Wu, H., Song, Z., Hentzer, M., Andersen, J.B., Molin, S., Givskov, M., and Høiby, N. (2004). Synthetic furanones inhibit quorum-sensing and enhance bacterial clearance in *Pseudomonas aeruginosa* lung infection in mice. *J. Antimicrob. Chemother. 53*, 1054-1061.

[121] Bjarnsholt, T., and Givskov, M. (2007). Quorum-sensing blockade as a strategy for enhancing host defences against bacterial pathogens. *Phil. Trans. Royal Soc. B. 362*, 1213-1222.

[122] Avery, O.T., and Dubos, R. (1930). The specific action of a bacterial enzyme on pneumococci of type III. *Science 72*, 151-152.

[123] Dubos, R., and Avery, O.T. (1931). Decomposition of the capsular polysaccharide of pneumococci type III by a bacterial enzyme. *J. Exp. Med. 54*, 51-71.

[124] Avery, O.T., and Dubos, R. (1931). The protective action of a specific enzyme against type III pneumococcus infection in mice. *J. Exp. Med. 54*, 73-89.

[125] Goodner, K., Dubos, R., and Avery, O.T. (1932). The action of a specific enzyme upon the dermal infection of rabbits with type III pneumococcus. *J. Exp. Med. 55*, 393-404.

[126] Harvey, D., Holt, D.E., and Bedford, H. (1999). Bacterial meningitis in the newborn: a prospective study of mortality and morbidity. *Semin. Perinatol. 23*, 218-225.

[127] Robbins, J.B., McCracken, G.H., Gotschlich, E.C., Ørskov, F., Ørskov, I., and Hanson, L.A. (1974). *Escherichia coli* K1 polysaccharide associated with neonatal meningitis. *N. Eng. J. Med. 290*, 1216-1220.

[128] Polin, R.A., and Harris, M.C. (2001). Neonatal bacterial meningitis. *Semin. Neonatol. 6*, 157-172.

[129] Nassif, X., Bourdoulous, S., Eugène, E., and Couraud, P.-E. (2002). How do extracellular pathogens cross the blood-brain barrier? *Trends Microbiol. 10*, 227-232.

[130] Parkkinen, J., Korhonen, T.K., Pere, A., Hacker, J., and Soinila, S. (1988). Binding sites in the rat brain for *Escherichia coli* S fimbriae associated with neonatal meningitis. *J. Clin. Invest. 81*, 860-865.

[131] Sarff, L.D., McCracken, G.H., Schiffer, M.S., Glode, M.P., Robbins, J.B., Ørskov, I., and Ørskov, F. (1975). Epidemiology of *Escherichia coli* K1 in healthy and diseased newborns. *Lancet i*, 1099-1104.

[132] Obata-Yasuoka, M., Ba-Thein, W., Tsukamoto, T., Yoshikawa, H., and Hayashi, H. (2002). Vaginal *Escherichia coli* share common virulence factor profile, serotypes and phylogeny with other extraintestinal *E. coli*. *Microbiology 148*, 2745-2752.

[133] de Louvois, J. (1994). Acute bacterial meningitis in the newborn. *J, Antimicrob. Chemother. 34(Suppl. A)*, 61-73.

[134] Bot, A., Antohi, S., and Bona, C. (1997). Immune response of neonates elicited by somatic transgene vaccination with naked DNA. *Front. Biosci. 2*, 173-188.

[135] Furrie, E. (2007). A molecular revolution in the study of intestinal microflora. *Gut 55*, 141-143.

[136] Palmer, C., Bik, E.M., DiGuilio, D.B., Relman, D.A., and Brown, P.O. (2007). Development of the human infant intestinal microbiota. *PLoS Biol. 5*, 1556-1573.

[137] Tomlinson, S., and Taylor, P.W. (1985). Neuraminidase associated with coliphage E that specifically depolymerizes the *Escherichia coli* K1 capsular polysaccharide. *J. Virol. 55*, 374-378.

[138] Long, G.S., Bryant, J.M., Taylor, P.W., and Luzio, J.P. (1995). Complete nucleotide sequence of the gene encoding bacteriophage E endosialidase: implications for K1E endosialidase structure and function. *Biochem. J. 309*, 543-550.

[139] Leggate, D.R., Bryant, J.M., Redpath, M.B., Head, D., Taylor, P.W., and Luzio, J.P. (2002). Expression, mutagenesis and kinetic analysis of recombinant K1E endosialidase to define the site of proteolytic processing and requirements for catalysis. *Molec. Microbiol. 44*, 749-760.

[140] Mushtaq, N., Redpath, M.B., Luzio, J.P., and Taylor, P.W. (2004). Prevention and cure of systemic *Escherichia coli* K1 infection by modification of the bacterial phenotype. *Antimicrob. Agents Chemother. 48*, 1503-1508.

[141] Mushtaq, N., Redpath, M.B., Luzio, J.P., and Taylor, P.W. (2005). Treatment of experimental *Escherichia coli* infection with recombinant bacteriophage-derived capsule depolymerase. *J. Antimicrob. Chemother. 56*, 160-165.

[142] Taylor, P.W. (1983). Bactericidal and bacteriolytic activity of serum against Gram-negative bacteria. *Microbiol. Rev. 47*, 46-83.

[143] Glode, M.P., Sutton, A., Moxon, E.R., and Robbins, J.B. (1977). Pathogenesis of neonatal *Escherichia coli* meningitis: induction of bacteremia and meningitis in infant rats fed *E. coli* K1. *Infect. Immun. 16*, 75-80.

[144] Pluschke, G., Mercer, A., Kusećek, B., Pohl, A., and Achtman, M. (1983). Induction of bacteremia in newborn rats by *Escherichia coli* K1 is correlated with only certain O (lipopolysaccharide) antigen types. *Infect. Immun. 39*, 599-608.

[145] Martindale, J., Stroud, D., Moxon, E.R., and Tang, C.M. (2000). Genetic analysis of *Escherichia coli* K1 gastrointestinal colonization. *Molec. Microbiol. 37*, 1293-1305.

[146] Zelmer, A., Bowen, M., Jokilammi, A., Finne, J., Luzio, J.P., and Taylor, P.W. (2008). Differential expression of the polysialyl capsule during blood-to-brain transit of neuropathogenic *Escherichia coli* K1. *Microbiology 154*, 2522-2532.

[147] Bonacorsi, S., and Bingen, E. (2005). Molecular epidemiology of *Escherichia coli* causing neonatal meningitis. *Int. J. Med. Microbiol. 295*, 373-381.

[148] Deszo, E.L., Steenbergen, S.M., Freedberg, D.I., and Vimr, E.R. (2005). *Escherichia coli* K1 polysialic acid *O*-acetyltransferase gene, *neuO*, and the mechanism of capsule form variation involving a mobile contingency locus. *Proc. Natl. Acad. Sci. U.S.A. 102*, 5564-5569.

[149] Jokilammi, A., Ollikka, P., Korja, M., Jakobsson, E., Loimaranta, V., Haataja, H., and Finne, J. (2004). Construction of antibody mimics from a noncatalytic enzyme – detection of polysialic acid. *J. Immunol. Methods 295*, 149-160.

[150] Sunil, V.R., Patel, K.J., Nilsen-Hamilton, M., Heck, D.E., Laskin, J.D., and Laskin, D.L. (2007). Acute endotoxemia is associated with upregulation of lipocalin 24p3/Lcn2 in lung and liver. *Exp. Molec. Pathol. 83*, 177-187.

[151] Mock, M., and Fouet, A. (2001). Anthrax. *Ann. Rev. Microbiol. 55*, 647-671.

[152] Stepanov, A.V., Marinin, L.I., Pomerantsev, A.P., and Staritsin, N.A. (1996). Development of novel vaccines against anthrax in man. *J. Biotechnol. 44*, 155-160.

[153] Inglesby, T.V., Henderson, D.A., Bartlett, J.G., Ascher, M.S., Eitzen, E., Friendlander, A.M., Hauer, J., McDade, J., Osterholm, M.T., O'Toole, T., Parker, G., Perl, T.M., Russell, P.K., and Tonat, K. (1999). Anthrax as a biological weapon: medical and public health management. *J. Amer. Med. Assoc. 281*, 1735-1745.

[154] Read, T.D., Peterson, S.N., Tourasse, N., Baillie, L.W., Paulsen, I.T., Nelson, K.E., Tettelin, H., Fouts, D.E., Eisen, J.A., Gill, S.R., Holtzapple, E.K., Okstad, O.A., Helgason, E., Rilstone, J., Wu, M., Kolonay, J.F., Beanan, M.J., Dodson, R.J., Brinkac, L.M., Gwinn, M., DeBoy, R.T., Madpu, R., Daugherty, S.C., Durkin, A.S., Haft, D.H., Nelson, W.C., Peterson, J.D., Pop, M., Khouri, H.M., Radune, D., Benton, J.L., Mahamoud, Y., Jiang, L., Hance, I.R., Weidman, J.F., Berry, K.J., Plaut, R.D., Wolf, A.M., Watkins, K.L., Nierman, W.C., Hazen, A., Cline, R., Redmond, C., Thwaite, J.E., White, O., Salzberg, S.L., Thomason, B., Friedlander, A.M., Koehler, T.M., Hanna, P.C., Kolstø, A.B., and Fraser, C.M. (2003). The genome sequence of *Bacillus anthracis* Ames and comparison to closely related bacteria. *Nature 423*, 81-86.

[155] Koehler, T.M. (2002). *Bacillus anthracis* genetics and virulence gene regulation. *Curr. Top. Microbiol. Immunol. 271*, 143-164.

[156] Candela, T. and Fouet, A. (2005). *Bacillus anthracis* CapD, belonging to the γ-glutamyltranspeptidase family, is required for the covalent anchoring of capsule to peptidoglycan. *Molec. Microbiol. 57*, 717-726.

[157] Uchida, I., Makino, S., Sasakawa, C., Yoshikawa, M., Sugimoto, C., and Terakado, N. (1993). Identification of a novel gene, *dep*, associated with depolymerization of the capsular polymer of *Bacillus anthracis*. *Molec. Microbiol. 9*, 487-496.

[158] Ivins, B.E., Ezzell, J.W., Jemski, J., Hedlund, K.W., Ristoph, J.D., and Leppla, S.H. (1986). Immunization studies with attenuated strains of *Bacillus anthracis*. *Infect. Immun. 52*, 454-458.

[159] Welkos, S.L., Vietri, N.J. and Gibbs, P.H. (1993). Non-toxigenic derivatives of the Ames strain of *Bacillus anthracis* are fully virulent for mice: role of plasmid pXO2 and chromosome in strain-dependent virulence. *Microb. Pathogen. 14*, 381-388.

[160] Drysdale, M., Heninger, S., Hutt, J., Chen, Y., Lyons, C.R., and Koehler, T.M. (2005). Capsule synthesis by *Bacillus anthracis* is required for dissemination in murine inhalation anthrax. *EMBO J. 24*, 221-227.

[161] Scorpio, A., Chabot, D.J., Day, W.A., O'Brien, D.K., Vietri, N.J., Itoh, Y., Mohamadzadeh, M., and Friedlander, A.M. (2007). Poly-γ-glutamate capsule-degrading enzyme treatment enhances phagocytosis and killing of encapsulated *Bacillus anthracis*. *Antimicrob. Agents Chemother. 51*, 215-222.

[162] Scorpio, A., Tobery, S.A., Ribot, W.J., and Friedlander, A.M. (2008). Treatment of experimental anthrax with recombinant capsule depolymerase. *Antimicrob. Agents Chemother. 52*, 1014-1020.

In: Antibiotic Resistance: Causes and Risk Factors
Editors: A. R. Bonilla and K. P. Muniz

ISBN 978-1-60741-623-4
© 2009 Nova Science Publishers, Inc.

Chapter V

Performance to Antibiotics in *Staphylococcus aureus*, *Streptococcus agalactiae* and *Enterococcus* spp.

*Antonio Sorlózano[1], José Gutiérrez[*1], Eva Román[4], Juan de Dios Luna[2], Juan Román[3], Estrella Martín[5], José Liébana[3], José Luis García[5], Samuel Bernal[5] and Pilar Morales[5]*

[1]Departments of Microbiology and [2]Biostatistics, University of Granada, Spain
Microbiology[3] and Pharmacy[4] Services, San Cecilio University Hospital.
Granada, Spain
[5]Microbiology Service, Valme University Hospital,
Seville, Spain

Abstract

Staphylococcus aureus, *Streptococcus agalactiae* and *Enterococcus* spp. are bacteria with a high capacity for acquiring determinants of resistance to antibiotics, giving rise to multi-resistance problems. It is assumed that this is related to consumption of antibiotics. The study objectives were to determine the antibiotic susceptibility of these three species in two Spanish hospitals and establish the relationship between consumption of antibiotics and their activity. The activity of antibiotics was evaluated against 1000 clinical isolates of *S. aureus*, *Enterococcus* spp. and *S. agalactiae* identified in the Microbiology Services of San Cecilio Hospital in Granada and Valme Hospital in Seville, determining the relationship between the consumption of antibiotics and susceptibility findings. Glycopeptides and linezolid were the only antibiotics active against 100% of clinical isolates of *S. aureus*, with cotrimoxazole and rifampicin also showing excellent activity. All isolates of *S. agalactiae* were susceptible to ampicillin,

* Correspondence: Dr. José Gutiérrez, Departamento de Microbiología, Facultad de Medicina, Avda. de Madrid 11.
E-18012 Granada, Spain. Tfn: 34-958 24 20 71; Fax: 34-958 24 61 19; E-mail: josegf@ugr.es

cefotaxime, vancomycin and linezolid, with an excellent activity for levofloxacin. All enterococci were susceptible to ampicillin, glycopeptides and linezolid. Finally, a statistically significant inverse relationship was found for the whole set of antibiotics between their consumption and the susceptibility to them of *S. aureus*. The three species retained susceptibility to glycopeptides and linezolid. A good susceptibility was also shown by *S. aureus* to cotrimoxazole and rifampicin and by enterococci and *S. agalactiae* to ampicillin. There was a significant association between antibiotic consumption and rates of resistance to *S. aureus*.

Keywords: *Staphylococcus aureus*, *Enterococcus* spp., *Streptococcus agalactiae*, susceptibility, defined daily dose.

Introduction

Staphylococcus aureus is one of the most common causes of hospital as well as community infections. As a result of its high frequency and the presence of methicillin-resistant isolates (MRSA), it is considered one of the world's most important nosocomial pathogens [1]. The dissemination of this microorganism is especially frequent in certain hospital areas, like Intensive Care Units, among others, and it is an important cause of morbimortality [2].

S. aureus is a bacterium with a high capacity for acquiring determinants of resistance to antibiotics, giving rise to significant multi-resistance problems. Thus, MRSA strains, in addition to being resistant to beta-lactams, can also be resistant to tetracyclines, macrolides, lincosamides, chloramphenicol, aminoglycosides or quinolones, among others, sometimes offering scant therapeutic options [3]. Moreover, in recent years we have witnessed a significant increase in community infections of this bacterium. This, together with the description of MRSA strains with reduced susceptibility to glycopeptides [4], and even with high-level resistance to vancomycin [5], leads to the need for correct detection and therapeutic control of this bacterial species.

Streptococcus agalactiae forms part of the normal flora of the human gastrointestinal and urogenital tracts. It is the primary cause of neonatal sepsis and is a major infectious agent in expectant mothers and an agent of systemic infections in adults with basic diseases [6]. Beta-lactams are still the antibiotics of choice in the treatment and prophylaxis of *S. agalactiae* infections. The intrapartum administration of penicillin G or ampicillin as prophylaxis for neonatal infection by this bacterium is recommended for all women identified as vaginal or rectal carriers during pregnancy [7]. However, there are less and less empirical therapeutic options every day for allergic patients, since the current rates of resistance to erythromycin of *S. agalactiae* in Spain are situated around 18% [8]. In these cases, the options can be vancomycin, tigecycline [9] or linezolid.

For their part, enterococci are major opportunistic nosocomial pathogens. Reduced susceptibility has been described to a large number of antibiotics, including beta-lactams, lincosamides, aminoglycosides and cotrimoxazole. In addition, they also present a high capacity to acquire new resistance. In Spain, most *Enterococcus faecalis* isolates preserve their susceptibility to ampicillin [10]. However, strains that are resistant to glycopeptides [11] or oxazolidinones [12] have been described, reducing current therapeutic alternatives.

The main reason for bacterial resistance to antibiotics to be generated and expand is their excessive use [13]. It has classically been assumed that the appearance of resistance following the therapeutic use of an antibiotic is just a matter of time [14]. In this regard, Spain is one of the developed countries with the highest consumption of antibiotics and bacterial resistance rates, particularly in community-originating pathogens [15].

As a result of all of the foregoing, the objectives of our study were to comparatively determine the antibiotic susceptibility of recent clinical isolates of the *S. aureus*, *Enterococcus* spp. and *S. agalactiae* species in two level-3 Spanish hospitals, and determine the relationship between the consumption of antibiotics and susceptibility findings.

Material and Methods

Bacterial Isolates

The study was conducted on 1000 bacterial isolates obtained from clinical samples processed at the Clinical Microbiology Services of the San Cecilio University Hospital in Granada (HSC) and the Valme University Hospital in Seville (HV), from January 2005 to September 2006 at HSC, and from March to September 2006 at HV. The total isolates for each bacterial species and corresponding hospital (HSC/HV) were: *S. aureus* (280/87), *E. faecalis* (52/133), *E. faecium* (7/0) and *S. agalactiae* (303/138).

Each service performed microorganism identification by means of the regular procedures used at each of them. Once the isolates were classified, they were then kept at −20° C until the susceptibility study was conducted.

Susceptibility Study

All isolates were subjected to susceptibility tests to various antibiotics (table 1) that are regularly used against aerobic grampositive microorganisms, by means of a standardised microdilution procedure [16], with a wide range of dilutions.

In order to detect methicillin resistance, and considering the possibility of conflicting results when determining the *in vitro* susceptibility among beta-lactam antibiotics, in addition to repeating the microdilution procedure, a diffusion procedure with oxacillin (1 μg) and cefoxitin (30 μg) disks in Mueller-Hinton agar (BioMérieux, France) was performed [17]. In addition, a disk of amoxicillin/clavulanic acid (20/10 μg) was added to 15 mm of the oxacillin disk to detect any possible hyperproduction of beta-lactamase. The isolate was considered MRSA when the diameters of the growth inhibition halos were ≤12 mm for oxacillin and ≤17 mm for cefoxitin and no synergy occurred with the amoxicillin/clavulanic acid, and it was considered susceptible to methicillin when the halos were ≥13 mm for oxacillin and ≤18 mm for cefoxitin.

Table 1. MIC$_{50}$, MIC$_{90}$ values (in μg/ml) and percentage of susceptible isolates for each species under study in both hospitals

Antibiotic	*S. aureus*					
	San Cecilio Hospital			Valme Hospital		
	MIC$_{50}$	MIC$_{90}$	Susceptible isolates (%)	MIC$_{50}$	MIC$_{90}$	Susceptible isolates (%)
Penicillin	> 4	> 4	7.5	> 4	> 4	4.6
Ampicillin						
Oxacillin	1	> 32	65.7	0.25	> 32	80.5
Amoxicillin/ clavulanic acid	4/2	64/32	65.7	2/1	64/32	80.5
Cefazolin	1	> 256	65.7	0.5	64	80.5
Cefotaxime						
Vancomycin	0.25	0.5	100	0.5	0.5	100
Teicoplanin	0.125	1	100	0.5	1	100
Gentamycin	0.5	64	77.9	1	2	93.1
Tobramycin	4	> 256	62.5	1	> 256	77
Kanamycin	4	> 512	62.5	2	> 512	77
Erythromycin	0.5	> 64	58.9	0.125	> 64	75.9
Clindamycin	0.125	> 64	73.2	≤ 0.03	0.25	90.8
Telithromycin	0.06	> 64	70.4	≤ 0.03	0.125	93.1
Levofloxacin	1	16	61.8	0.125	4	82.8
Cotrimoxazole	0.06/1.19	0.5/9.5	95.7	0.06/1.19	0.125/2.4	100
Rifampicin	≤ 0.015	0.03	98.9	≤ 0.015	≤ 0.015	98.9
Linezolid	2	4	100	2	2	100

Antibiotic	*Enterococcus* spp.					
	San Cecilio Hospital			Valme Hospital		
	MIC$_{50}$	MIC$_{90}$	Susceptible isolates (%)	MIC$_{50}$	MIC$_{90}$	Susceptible isolates (%)
Penicillin						
Ampicillin	0.125	1	100	1	2	100
Oxacillin						
Amoxicillin/ clavulanic acid						
Cefazolin						
Cefotaxime						
Vancomycin	1	2	100	0.5	1	100
Teicoplanin	≤ 0.03	0.125	100	≤ 0.03	0.125	100
Gentamycin	16	> 2048	NA	16	> 2048	NA
Tobramycin						
Kanamycin						
Erythromycin						
Clindamycin						
Telithromycin						
Levofloxacin	2	32	61	1	64	74.4
Cotrimoxazole						
Rifampicin						
Linezolid	2	2	100	2	2	100

Table 1. Continued)

| Antibiotic | S. agalactiae | | | | | |
| | San Cecilio Hospital | | | Valme Hospital | | |
	MIC$_{50}$	MIC$_{90}$	Susceptible isolates (%)	MIC$_{50}$	MIC$_{90}$	Susceptible isolates (%)
Penicillin						
Ampicillin	0.06	0.125	100	0.03	0.06	100
Oxacillin						
Amoxicillin/ clavulanic acid						
Cefazolin						
Cefotaxime	0.03	0.06	100	0.03	0.03	100
Vancomycin	0.5	1	100	1	1	100
Teicoplanin	≤ 0.004	0.125	NA	0.008	0.125	NA
Gentamycin	4	8	NA	4	8	NA
Tobramycin						
Kanamycin						
Erythromycin	≤ 0.03	> 64	77.2	≤ 0.03	> 64	81.3
Clindamycin	≤ 0.03	> 64	78.5	≤ 0.03	> 64	84
Telithromycin						
Levofloxacin	0.5	1	98	0.5	0.5	99.3
Cotrimoxazole						
Rifampicin						
Linezolid	1	2	100	1	1	100

NA: The CLSI does not define the cut points for this antibiotic in this species.

In parallel to the microdilution method, a diffusion procedure was also followed for the *S. aureus* and *S. agalactiae* isolates with a double disk of erythromycin (15 µg) and clindamycin (2 µg) in order to determine the resistance phenotype to macrolides, lincosamides and streptogramins (MLSb), according to CLSI recommendations [18].

S. aureus ATCC 29213 and *E. faecalis* ATCC 29212 reference strains were used in all the tests [16].

Determination of the Defined Daily Dose (DDD)

This study also linked the susceptibility of the clinical isolates of *S. aureus* obtained in 2005 at the HSC Microbiology Service to consumption figures (in DDD) of the most representative active ingredients of each group between 2004 and 2005.

Two consumption parameters were used, depending on the scope: DDD/1000 inhabitants-day in reference to out-of-hospital consumption, and DDD/100 stays in the case of in-hospital consumption. The DDD/1000 inhabitants-day values were obtained using the pharmacy office prescription dispensing software of the Andalusian Health System, called MicroStrategy®. This software also provided us with separate data for the two health districts (Granada District and Metropolitan District) into which the HSC's area of influence is divided, as well as data regarding prescriptions made in HSC outpatient visits.

For the consumption of antibiotics within the HSC, the DDD/100 stays were obtained for the same period of time using the Farmatools® software system. Unlike MicroStrategy®, this system provides us with total milligrams of antibiotic consumed in-hospital. The number of hospital stays during the time frame of the study was provided by the Archinet® software system of the hospital's Admissions Service.

Statistical Tests

Fisher's exact test is used for tables r x s to compare the susceptibility of isolates from the HSC and those obtained at the HV, for each of the species under study. This comparison was performed both in terms of clinical categories (considering susceptible *vs.* some degree of resistance) and considering the distribution of MICs for all the isolates of a species, for each of the tested antibiotics. To determine the relationship between the DDD values for 2004 and 2005, and the percentage of *S. aureus* isolates susceptible to each group of antibiotics obtained in 2005 at the HSC, a point cloud was used, and prior to transforming consumption data using the base 10 logarithm, the straight line was calculated per squared minimums and Pearson's correlation coefficient.

Table 2. Results of Fisher's exact test comparing the distribution of the isolates of each species according to clinical category (CC) and MIC value between both hospitals

Antibiotic	*S. aureus*		*Enterococcus* spp.		*S. agalactiae*	
	p (CC)	p (MIC)	p (CC)	p (MIC)	p (CC)	p (MIC)
Penicillin	0.4675	0.4308				
Ampicillin			1.0000	0.0000	1.0000	0.0003
Oxacillin	0.0112	0.0000				
Amoxicillin/ clavulanic acid	0.0112	0.0001				
Cefazolin	0.0112	0.0017				
Cefotaxime					1.0000	0.7127
Vancomycin	1.0000	0.0606	1.0000	0.3948	1.0000	0.9407
Teicoplanin	1.0000	0.0000	1.0000	0.9033	NA	0.0000
Gentamycin	0.0008	0.2920	NA	0.8816	NA	0.7967
Tobramycin	0.0138	0.1056				
Kanamycin	0.0138	0.0659				
Erythromycin	0.005	0.0004			0.3837	0.8536
Clindamycin	0.0004	0.0000			0.2435	0.9946
Telithromycin	0.0000	0.0000				
Levofloxacin	0.0002	0.0000	0.0862	0.0260	0.4423	0.0014
Cotrimoxazole	0.0769	0.0002				
Rifampicin	1.0000	0.3188				
Linezolid	1.0000	0.0053	1.0000	0.0828	1.0000	0.0000

NA: The CLSI does not define the cut points for this antibiotic in this species.

Table 3. Distribution of MIC values as accrued percentages for those antibiotics where there were differences in the comparison per clinical category and MIC distribution

Species	Antibiotic (Hospital)	≥64	32	16	8	4	2	1	0.5	0.25	0.125	0.06	0.03	0.015	0.008	≤0.004
S. aureus	Teicoplanin (HSC)					100	99.3	95.7	87.9	71.4	50.3	25.4	16.4	0	0	0
	Teicoplanin (HV)						100	98.9	87.4	48.3	19.5	9.2	3.4	0	0	0
	Cotrimoxazole* (HSC)	100	98.6	97.1	96.4	95.7	95.7	95	90.7	81.8	69.6	54.6	31.8	0	0	0
	Cotrimoxazole* (HV)									100	96.6	71.3	40.2	0	0	0
	Linezolid (HSC)					100	73.2	17.9	1.4	0.7	0.4	0	0	0	0	0
	Linezolid (HV)						100	17.2	0	0	0	0	0	0	0	0
Enterococcus spp.	Ampicillin (HSC)				100	98.3	94.9	93.2	84.7	69.5	66.1	42.4	16.7	0	0	0
	Ampicillin (HV)					100	99.2	77.4	12.8	0	0	0	0	0	0	0
	Levofloxacin (HSC)	100	91.5	72.9	62.7	61	61	37.3	23.7	5.1	1.7	0	0	0	0	0
	Levofloxacin (HV)	100	89.5	80.5	77.4	74.4	74.4	66.2	39.8	11.3	0.8	0	0	0	0	0
S. agalactiae	Ampicillin (HSC)									100	99.7	85.8	33.3	5	0.3	0
	Ampicillin (HV)										100	92.8	50	8.7	2.2	0
	Teicoplanin (HSC)								100	99	96	88.4	81.2	77.6	75.6	74.9
	Teicoplanin (HV)								100	99.3	91.3	80.4	72.5	63	55.1	47.1
	Levofloxacin (HSC)		100	99.7	99.7	99.3	98	95	80.9	25.1	1	0	0	0	0	0
	Levofloxacin (HV)				100	99.3	99.3	97.8	90.6	35.5	5.1	0.7	0	0	0	0
	Linezolid (HSC)						100	68	7.9	0	0	0	0	0	0	0
	Linezolid (HV)						100	94.9	15.2	0	0	0	0	0	0	0

HSC: San Cecilio Hospital (Granada); HV: Valme Hospital (Seville).

*Only the MIC value referring to the concentration of trimetoprim is shown.

Results

Table 1 shows the MIC_{50} and MIC_{90} values and the percentage of susceptible isolates obtained after performing the microdilution test on the 1000 clinical isolates. Table 2 shows the results of Fisher's exact test comparing the susceptibility of the isolates from both hospitals, in terms of clinical category and MIC distribution. Table 3 shows the distribution of MIC values as accrued percentages for those antibiotics where there were differences, according to Fisher's exact test, in the comparison per clinical category and MIC distribution.

Staphylococcus aureus

Glycopeptides and linezolid were the only antibiotics active against 100% of clinical isolates of *S. aureus*, with cotrimoxazole and rifampicin also showing excellent activity. The least active antibiotic against them was penicillin.

For *S. aureus* there were no significant differences in susceptibility of the isolates to penicillin, vancomycin and rifampicin between the two hospitals (table 2). There were significant differences in susceptibility to oxacillin, amoxicillin/clavulanic acid, cefazoline, erythromycin, clindamycin, telithromycin and levofloxacin (table 2). For these antibiotics, *S. aureus* isolates from the HV were more susceptible than those from the HSC.

Although no significant differences were found with regard to the activity of teicoplanin, cotrimoxazole and linezolid, analysed per clinical category, there were significant differences from the point of view of MIC distribution (table 2). Thus, the isolates showed lower teicoplanin MICs at the HSC than at the HV, and vice-versa for the other two antibiotics (table 3).

Gentamycin was the most active among the aminoglycosides. Analysing the activity of this group, significant differences were observed in terms of clinical category. However, from the point of view of how the MICs were distributed, it was seen that the three antibiotics behaved the same at both hospitals.

After performing the susceptibility test, there were 33 *S. aureus* isolates presenting *in vitro* discordance between results for oxacillin, amoxicillin/clavulanic acid and cefazoline: all were resistant to oxacillin, 15 were susceptible to amoxicillin/clavulanic acid and to cefazoline, and the other 18 were resistant to amoxicillin/clavulanic acid and susceptible to cefazoline. After repeating the microdilution procedure and performing the diffusion with disks, the 33 isolates showed resistance to the three antibiotics, and synergy was not observed between oxacillin and amoxicillin/clavulanic acid in any case.

Finally, the resistance phenotype to macrolides, lincosamides and streptogramins of these isolates at the HSC and HV was, respectively: susceptible, 58.6% and 75.9%; cMLSb, 26.4% and 9.2%; iMLSb, 4.3% and 8%; phenotype M 10.3% and 6.9%, phenotype L, 0.4% and 0%. Of note is the small percentage of *S. aureus* isolates with inducible versus constitutive phenotype in both hospitals.

Streptococcus agalactiae

For *S. agalactiae* we observed that 100% were susceptible to ampicillin, cefotaxime, vancomycin and linezolid. Levofloxacin also showed excellent activity. There were no significant differences in susceptibility of the isolates to cefotaxime, gentamycin, erythromycin and clindamycin between the two hospitals (table 2).

In addition, although no significant differences were found with regard to the activity of ampicillin, teicoplanin, levofloxacin and linezolid analysed per clinical category, there were significant differences from the point of view of MIC distribution (table 2). Thus, the isolates showed lower teicoplanin MICs at the HSC than at the HV, and vice-versa for the other three antibiotics (table 3).

The resistance phenotype to macrolides, lincosamides and streptogramins of these isolates at the HSC and HV was, respectively: susceptible, 77.2% and 81.3%; cMLSb, 21.1% and 15.9%; iMLSb, 1% and 1.4%; phenotype M 0.7% and 1.4%. Once again, like with *S. aureus*, of note is the small percentage of isolates with inducible phenotype against the constituting agent in both hospitals.

Enterococcus spp.

The activity of the antibiotics tested on *Enterococcus* spp. from the HSC, as compared to those from the HV, was similar. Most significantly, differences in the distribution of MICs in ampicillin and levofloxacin can be observed, with lower values at the HV (table 3).

Relationship between DDD and Antibiotic Susceptibility in *S. aureus*

In 2005, 225 *S. aureus* isolates were identified only at the HSC. Just 7 of these isolates were susceptible to all the tested antibiotics. The remaining 218 (96.9%) presented resistance to at least one antibiotic. Table 4 shows the accumulated resistance figures to the various antibiotics in these isolates.

Tables 5 and 6 list consumption of different groups of antibiotics (defined for the most representative active ingredients) at the HSC and in the health district dependent on this hospital in 2004 and 2005, as well as the percentage of isolates susceptible to each antibiotic group in the 225 *S. aureus* isolates identified in 2005.

Figures 1 and 2 shows the relationship between in-hospital and out-of-hospital consumption, respectively, of the different groups of antibiotics (expressed in $\log_{10}$ of the DDD) and the percentage of susceptibility of the 225 *S. aureus* isolates. The values of the correlation coefficient were r = - 0.798 (*p=0.01*) when in-hospital consumption was assessed, and r = - 0.818 (*p=0.007*) when out-of-hospital consumption was assessed. In both cases we can see that a statistically significant inverse relationship exists for the whole set of antibiotics between their consumption and the susceptibility to them of *S. aureus*: the more antibiotics consumed, the lower the percentage of isolates susceptible to them.

Table 4. Accrued resistance to various antibiotics in the clinical isolates of *S. aureus* from the San Cecilio Hospital, identified in 2005

Resistance to different antibiotics	Number of isolates	Total isolates
P	77	79
L	2	
P, O	1	24
P, G	1	
P, L	3	
P, E	14	
P, TS	2	
L, E	1	
E, C	1	
E, TS	1	
P, O, L	4	19
P, L, E	1	
P, L, C	2	
P, T, E	2	
P, E, C	8	
K, To, E	1	
L, E, C	1	
P, O, L, E	3	20
P, O, E, TS	1	
P, G, K, To	2	
P, K, To, L	1	
P, K, To, TS	1	
P, L, T, C	1	
P, L, E, C	3	
P, T, E, C	8	
P, O, K, To, L	2	14
P, O, L, T, E	1	
P, O, L, E, C	5	
P, G, K, To, T	1	
P, K, To, T, E	1	
P, K, To, E, C	1	
P, K, To, E, TS	1	
P, L, T, E, C	1	
G, K, To, C, TS	1	
P, O, G, K, To, L	3	16
P, O, K, To, L, E	10	
P, G, K, To, T, E	1	
P, L, T, E, C, TS	1	
K, To, L, T, E, C	1	
P, O, G, K, To, L, E	1	8
P, O, G, K, To, E, C	1	
P, O, K, To, L, T, E	1	
P, O, K, To, L, E, C	1	
P, G, K, To, L, E, C	2	
P, G, K, To, T, E, C	1	
P, G, K, To, E, C, TS	1	

Resistance to different antibiotics	Number of isolates	Total isolates
P, O, G, K, To, L, E, C	5	10
P, O, K, To, L, T, E, C	5	
P, O, G, K, To, L, T, E, C	25	26
P, O, K, To, L, T, E, C, TS	1	
P, O, G, K, To, L, T, E, C, R	1	1
P, O, G, K, To, L, T, E, C, TS, R	1	1

P: Penicillin, O: Oxacillin, G: Gentamycin, K Kanamycin, To: Tobramycin, L: Levofloxacin, T: Telithromycin, E: Erythromycin, C: Clindamycin, TS: Trimetoprim-sulfamethoxazole, R: Rifampicin.

Table 5. Antibiotic consumption at San Cecilio Hospital in 2004 and 2005 (in DDD/100 stays) and percentage of susceptible *S. aureus* isolates in 2005

Group	Antibiotic	DDD/100 stays 2004	DDD/100 stays 2005	Total group DDD	Susceptibility percentage
Beta-lactams	Penicillin	0.929	0.963	146.315	7.1
	Amoxicillin	3.385	2.632		
	Ampicillin	1.288	1.898		
	Amoxicillin/ clavulanic acid	25.692	62.295		
	Cloxacillin	2.384	2.315		
	Cefazolin	19.460	23.666		
Macrolides	Clarithromycin	1.473	1.197	5.548	48.4
	Erythromycin	0.756	0.791		
	Azithromycin	0.483	0.803		
	Spiramycin	0.036	0.009		
Lincosamides	Clindamycin	1.433	1.937	3.37	65.3
Aminoglycosides	Tobramycin	1.614	1.063	8.645	78.7
	Gentamycin	2.752	2.312		
	Amikacin	0.519	0.385		
Fluoroquinolones	Ciprofloxacin	7.582	6.479	33.05	59.6
	Norfloxacin	1.087	0.925		
	Levofloxacin	6.508	8.455		
	Moxifloxacin	1.1	0.914		
Glycopeptides	Vancomycin	0.861	1.466	6.913	100
	Teicoplanin	2.928	1.658		
Oxazolidinones	Linezolid	3.606	1.18	4.786	100
Rifamycins	Rifampicin	0.533	0.808	1.341	98.2
	Cotrimoxazole	0.877	2.09	2.967	94.7

Table 6. Antibiotic consumption in the health district dependent on San Cecilio Hospital in 2004 and 2005 (in DDD/1000 inhabitants) and percentage of susceptible *S. aureus* isolates in 2005

Group	Antibiotic	DDD/1000 inhabitants 2004	DDD/1000 inhabitants 2005	Total group DDD	Susceptibility percentage
Beta-lactams	Penicillin	24598	20935	4551187	7.1
	Amoxicillin	681478	614712		
	Ampicillin	2351	1224		
	Amoxicillin/ clavulanic acid	1310547	1479446		
	Cloxacillin	32376	32384		
	Cefuroxime	187786	163350		
Macrolides	Clarithromycin	161060	129137	694580	48.4
	Roxithromycin	7924	5300		
	Erythromycin	43631	39438		
	Azithromycin	134960	128213		
	Acetylspiramycin	6788	5600		
	Spiramycin	1890	1882		
	Josamycin	12215	7864		
	Midecamycin	5141	3537		
Ketolides	Telithromycin	18575	16500	35075	72.4
Lincosamides	Clindamycin	14949	16144	31093	65.3
Aminoglycosides	Amikacin	107	1	13176	78.7
	Tobramycin	1115	607		
	Gentamycin	6172	5174		
Fluoroquinolones	Ciprofloxacin	152770	160828	713735	59.6
	Norfloxacin	61676	50854		
	Ofloxacin	23305	19995		
	Levofloxacin	57040	75330		
	Moxifloxacin	56828	55109		
Glycopeptides	Vancomycin	55	25	80	100
Rifamycins	Rifampicin	2746	3728	6474	98.2
	Cotrimoxazole	37479	41910	79389	94.7

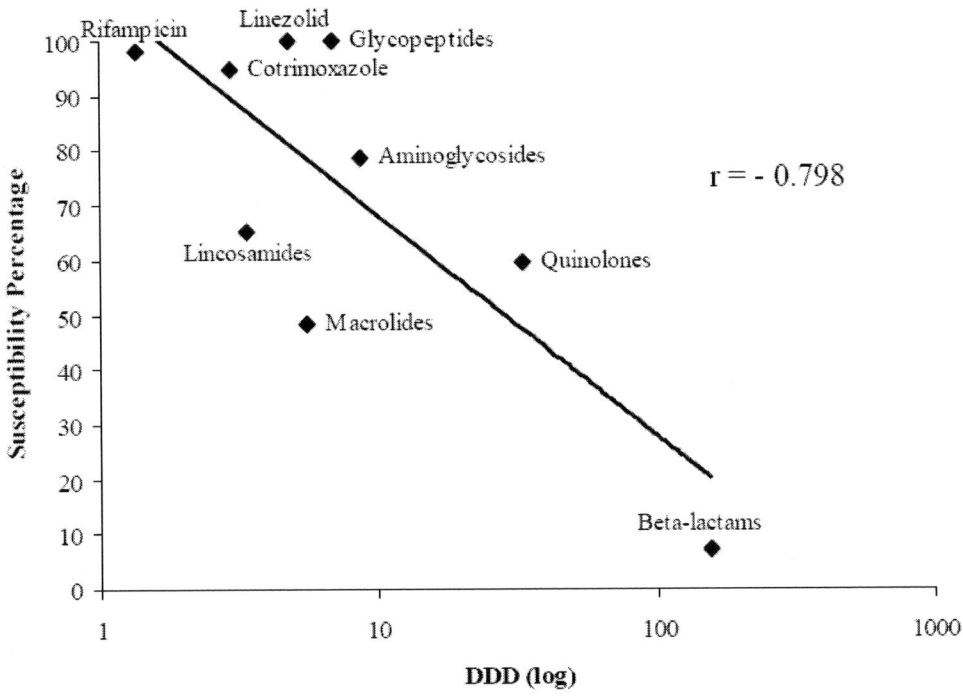

Figure 1. Relationship between in-hospital consumption of antibiotics in 2004 and 2005 and the susceptibility of *S. aureus* isolates in 2005.

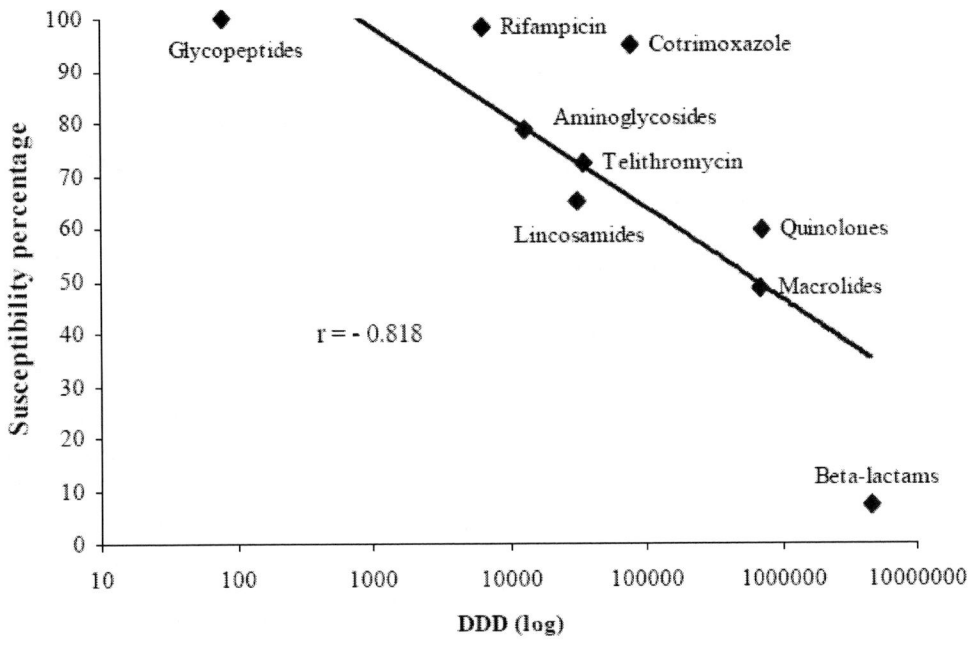

Figure 2. Relationship between out-of-hospital consumption of antibiotics in 2004 and 2005 and the susceptibility of *S. aureus* isolates in 2005.

Discussion

The San Cecilio Hospital in Granada and Valme Hospital in Seville are two general speciality hospitals, which are comparable in terms of their healthcare, number of beds and the population they serve. Moreover, both are located in the Autonomous Community of Andalusia. It can be assumed that the data on susceptibility between microorganisms identified in both hospitals should also be similar, and that microbiological differences, if any, should not be due to the nature of the healthcare activity. For this reason, it was decided to perform a comparative study of the activity of various antibiotics on a significant number of clinical isolates of grampositive cocci, particularly *S. aureus*, with significant multi-resistance rates.

Prior studies conducted in Spain have documented a considerable increase in the detection of MRSA isolates in recent years. Thus, an increase from 1.5% to 31.2% was observed between 1986 and 2002 at Gregorio Marañón Hospital in Madrid [19]. In the Spanish multi-centre study on Antimicrobial Resistance Surveillance (VIRA) [20], average MRSA prevalence values of 29% were obtained, closer to those obtained at the HSC than those found for the HV.

Comparing our susceptibility results for other antibiotics with those of the aforementioned study, we observed that, in general, the susceptibility of *S. aureus* to glycopeptides and linezolid was maintained, although the same was also true for rifampicin and cotrimoxazole. The results obtained for aminoglycosides are also similar. In the case of macrolides and lincosamides, we found a greater percentage of susceptible isolates in both hospitals in the present study, with a greater percentage of isolates with constitutive MLSb phenotype as compared to inducible MLSb phenotype, as shown in other studies [21]. As for telithromycin, other studies [22] find a similar percentage of activity to that obtained at the HSC, but lower than that found at the HV. Finally, resistance figures to levofloxacin at the HSC are far higher than those detected at the HV and in other studies in our sphere [23].

S. agalactiae continues to be susceptible to ampicillin and, in general, to beta-lactams, with no resistant strain having been described as yet. As can be seen from our study and others [24], *S. agalactiae* has a good level of susceptibility to fluoroquinolones, glycopeptides and linezolid. On the other hand, the resistance to macrolides and lincosamides has increased, with current resistance figures around 15%. The greater presence of strains with cMLSb phenotype versus iMLSb phenotype, as described by other authors [8], is especially characteristic. Although beta-lactams are considered to be the antibiotics of choice in intrapartum prophylaxis of colonised women, they should be considered as alternatives in allergic patients as well. If, due to their high resistance rate to macrolides and lincosamides, we were to discard levofloxacin and rifampicin (which are restricted in the case of pregnant women) as well as vancomycin (currently being questioned due to its complexity of administration and toxicity), the utilisation of linezolid may be useful. In addition, new formulations of this antibiotic that facilitate their out-of-hospital use are now available.

In a recent multi-centre study [25] on *E. faecalis* and *E. faecium* isolates obtained from 41 Spanish hospitals, rates of resistance (*E. faecalis* - *E. faecium*) to ampicillin, vancomycin and linezolid of 1.3% - 65.1%; 0.4% - 3.9%; 0.7% - 0%, were obtained, respectively, noting a major increase in the resistance of *E. faecium* to ampicillin, which in our case, given the scant number of isolates of this species, we have not found, nor have we found resistances to vancomycin or linezolid in either of the two hospitals. For levofloxacin, resistance figures at the HSC are similar to those detected in other Spanish studies [23], and higher than those detected at the HV.

As for the relationship between antibiotic consumption and susceptibility to antibiotics in clinical isolates of *S. aureus*, given the fact that bacterial resistance evolves over a lengthy period of time, our study period should have been longer. However, no consumption information exists before 2004, since the Farmatools® programme was not installed until then. In any case, the inverse relationship between consumption and susceptibility is obvious.

In this regard, several studies show that Spain is one of the European countries with the highest antibiotic prescription rates and antibiotic resistance rates, particularly with regard to community pathogens [15,26]. Most antibiotics are prescribed in primary care, where they are handled differently from what occurs at the hospital level. Irrational prescription, inappropriate dispensing, incorrect use, the absence of advisory committees at the out-of-hospital level, etc. are some of the problems that facilitate the appearance of resistance [27].

In conclusion, the isolated grampositive cocci from clinical samples in the study hospitals are uniformly susceptible to glycopeptides and linezolid. *S. aureus* remains susceptible to cotrimoxazole and rifampicin, and enterococci and *S. agalactiae* continue to be susceptible to ampicillin. In the present study, the isolates from the Valme Hospital were shown, in general, to be slightly more susceptible than those from the San Cecilio Hospital. In any case, the findings for the two hospitals are similar to those obtained in other studies of the same characteristics conducted in our country. Finally, we obtained an inverse relationship between consumption and susceptibility, demonstrating that the greater the consumption of antibiotics, the higher the rates of resistance.

References

[1]   Westh H, Zinn CS, Rosdahl VT. An international multicenter study of antimicrobial consumption and resistance in *Staphylococcus aureus* isolates from 15 hospitals in 14 countries. *Microb. Drug Resist.*, 2004; 10: 169-76.

[2]   Zinn CS, Westh H, Rosdahl VT, et al. An international multicenter study of antimicrobial resistance and typing of hospital *Staphylococcus aureus* isolates from 21 laboratories in 19 countries or states. *Microb. Drug Resist.*, 2004; 10: 160-8.

[3]   Sorlózano A, Gutiérrez J, Salmerón A, et al. Activity of tigecycline against clinical isolates of S*taphylococcus aureus* and extended-spectrum β-lactamase-producing *Escherichia coli* in Granada, Spain. *Int. J. Antimicrob. Agents*, 2006; 28: 532-6.

[4]   Cartolano GL, Cheron M, Benabid D, et al. Methicillin-resistant *Staphylococcus aureus* (MRSA) with reduced susceptibility to glycopeptides (GISA) in 63 French general hospitals. *Clin. Microbiol. Infect.*, 2004; 10: 448-51.

[5]   Weigel LM, Donlan RM, Shin DH, et al. High-level vancomycin-resistant *Staphylococcus aureus* isolates associated with a polymicrobial biofilm. *Antimicrob. Agents Chemother.*, 2007; 51: 231-8.

[6] Mollerach A, Mëndez E, Massa R, et al. *Streptococcus agalactiae* isolated in Santa Fe, Argentina: antibiotic susceptibility and erythromycin-clindamycin resistance mechanisms. *Enferm. Infecc. Microbiol. Clin.*, 2007; 25: 67-8.

[7] The Spanish Society of Obstetrics and Gynecology, The Spanish Society of Neonatology, The Spanish Society of Infectious Diseases and Clinical Microbiology, et al. Prevention of perinatal group B streptococcal disease. Spanish revised guidelines. *Enferm. Infecc. Microbiol. Clin.*, 2003; 21: 417-23.

[8] Betriú C, Culebras E, Gómez M, et al. Erythromycin and clindamycin resistance and telithromycin susceptibility in *Streptococcus agalactiae*. *Antimicrob. Agents Chemother.*, 2003; 47: 1112-4.

[9] Sorlózano A, Gutiérrez J, Román E, et al. A comparison of the activity of tigecycline against multiresistant clinical isolates of *Staphylococcus aureus* and *Streptococcus agalactiae*. *Diagn. Microbiol. Infect. Dis.*, 2007; 58: 487-9.

[10] Causse M, Franco-Álvarez de Luna F, García-Mayorgas AD, et al. Antimicrobial susceptibility of *Enterococcus faecalis* isolated from patients in Córdoba (Spain). *Rev. Esp. Quimioter.*, 2006; 19: 140-3.

[11] Maciá MD, Juan C, Oliver A, et al. Molecular characterization of a glycopeptide-resistant *Enterococcus faecalis* outbreak in an intensive care unit. *Enferm. Infecc. Microbiol. Clin.*, 2005; 23: 460-3.

[12] Sánchez-Gómez JC, Fraile-Malmierca F, Valverde-Romero AD, et al. Linezolid-resistant *Enterococcus faecalis*: first report in Spain. *J. Chemother.,* 2006; 18: 440-2.

[13] Bronzwaer SL, Cars O, Buchholz U, et al. A European study on the relationship between antimicrobial use and antimicrobial resistance. *Emerg. Infect. Dis.*, 2002; 8: 278-82.

[14] Linares-Rodríguez JF, Martínez-Menéndez JL. Antimicrobial resistance and bacterial virulence. *Enferm. Infecc. Microbiol. Clin.*, 2005; 23: 86-93.

[15] Palop V, Melchor A, Martínez I. Reflections on the use of antibiotics in primary care. *Aten. Primaria.,* 2003; 32: 42-7.

[16] Clinical and Laboratory Standards Institute. Methods for dilution antimicrobial susceptibility tests for bacteria that grow aerobically. Approved Standard CLSI Publication M7-A7 (7th ed.). Wayne (PA): Clinical and Laboratory Standards Institute, 2006.

[17] Swenson JM, Lonsway D, McAllister S, et al. Detection of *mecA*-mediated resistance using reference and commercial testing methods in a collection of *Staphylococcus aureus* expressing borderline oxacillin MICs. *Diagn. Microbiol. Infect. Dis.*, 2007; 58: 33-9.

[18] Clinical and Laboratory Standards Institute. Performance standards for antimicrobial susceptibility testing; seventeenth informational supplement. CLSI publication M100-S17., Wayne (PA), 2006.

[19] Cuevas O, Cercenado E, Vindel A, et al. Evolution of the antimicrobial resistance of *Staphylococcus* spp. in Spain: Five nationwide prevalence studies, 1986 to 2002. *Antimicrob. Agents Chemother.,* 2004; 48: 4240-5.

[20] Picazo JJ, Betriú C, Rodríguez-Avial I, et al. Antimicrobial resistance surveillance: VIRA study 2006. *Enferm. Infecc. Microbiol. Clin.*, 2006; 24: 617-28.

[21] Millán L, Cerdá P, Rubio MC, et al. In vitro activity of telithromycin, quinupristin/dalfopristin, linezolid and comparator antimicrobial agents against *Staphylococcus aureus* clinical isolates. *J. Chemother.*, 2004; 16: 230-7.

[22] Cantón R, Loza E, Morosini MI, et al. Antimicrobial resistance amongst isolates of *Streptococcus pyogenes* and *Staphylococcus aureus* in the PROTEKT antimicrobial surveillance programme during 1999-2000. *J. Antimicrob. Chemother.*, 2002; 50: 9-24.

[23] Loza E, Cantón R, Pascual A, et al. Comparative in vitro activity of garenoxacin (BMS-284756). Sentry program, Spain (1999-2000). *Enferm. Infecc. Microbiol. Clin.*, 2003; 21: 404-9.

[24] González JJ, Andreu A. Susceptibility of vertically transmitted Group B streptococci to antimicrobial agents. Multicenter study. *Enferm. Infecc. Microbiol. Clin.*, 2004; 22: 286-91.

[25] Oteo J, Cuevas O, Navarro C, et al. Trends in antimicrobial resistance in 3469 enterococci isolated from blood (EARSS experience 2001-06, Spain): increasing ampicillin resistance in *Enterococcus faecium. J. Antimicrob. Chemother.*, 2007; 59: 1044-5.

[26] Goossens H, Ferech M, Vander Stichele R, et al. Outpatient antibiotic use in Europe and association with resistance: a cross-national database study. *Lancet*, 2005; 365: 579-87.

[27] Pastor-Sánchez R. Alteraciones del nicho ecológico: resistencias bacterianas a los antibióticos. *Gac. Sanit.*, 2006; 20: 175-81.

In: Antibiotic Resistance: Causes and Risk Factors
Editors: A. R. Bonilla and K. P. Muniz

ISBN 978-1-60741-623-4
© 2009 Nova Science Publishers, Inc.

Chapter VI

Microbiological and Pharmacological Principles of Recent Antibiotic Therapy

*Cristina Carrasco[a], Antonio Sorlózano[a], José Cabeza[b],
Gonzalo Piédrola[a] and José Gutiérrez[a]**

[a]Department of Microbiology, School of Medicine, University of Granada, Spain
[b]Service of Pharmacy, San Cecilio University Hospital, Granada, Spain

Introduction

The past few years have seen a major rise in resistance to antibiotics among Gram-negative bacteria (beta-lactamase [ESBL]-producing enterobacteria, carbapenem-resistant *P. aeruginosa* and *A. baumannii* …) [1] and, especially, among Gram-positive bacteria (methicillin-resistant *S. aureus* [MRSA], glycopeptide-intermediate [GISA] or resistant *S. aureus* [GRSA], vancomycin-resistant enterococci [VRE], multi-drug resistant *S. pneumoniae* [MDRSP]) [2]. This trend has considerably reduced therapeutic options and brought about a need for novel antibiotics, which have been approved by the Food and Drugs Administration (FDA) since 2000.

The first of these was linezolid, an oxazolidinone for the treatment of nosocomial and community-acquired pneumonias and skin and soft tissue infections caused by Gram-positive bacteria, including MRSA, GRSA, VRE, and MDRSP [3]. The cephalosporin cefditoren pivoxil was approved to treat community-acquired respiratory infections (upper and lower airways) and uncomplicated infections of skin and soft tissues produced by Gram-positive or -negative bacteria that are not resistant to this group of antibiotics [4].

The carbapenem ertapenem is indicated for the treatment of intra-abdominal, skin and soft tissue infections, and community acquired pneumonia caused by Gram-positive or-negative microorganisms and is especially indicated for infections produced by ESBL-producing enterobacteria [5]. Doripenem is a new carbapenem that can be used against intra-

* Correspondence: Dr. José Gutiérrez, Departamento de Microbiología, Facultad de Medicina, Avda. de Madrid 11. E-18012 Granada, Spain. Tfn: 34-958 24 20 71; Fax: 34-958 24 61 19; E-mail: josegf@ugr.es

abdominal and urinary infections due to Gram-negative or -positive microorganisms at a lower dose than required for other antibiotics in this group [6].

Daptomycin is a useful antibiotic for monotherapy of bacteremia and skin and soft tissue infections caused by Gram-positive multiresistant bacteria (MRSA, GISA, GRSA) [7].

Gemifloxacin is a new quinolone for treating respiratory infections (e.g., community pneumonia or bronchitis) caused by Gram-positive and –negative bacteria, including MDRSP [8]. Telithromycin offers an alternative treatment for community-acquired pneumonia due to Gram-positive and –negative microorganisms, including MDRSP [9].

Tigecycline was approved for intra-abdominal, skin, and soft tissue infections caused by Gram-positive and–negative bacteria, including multi-resistant bacteria (ESBL, MRSA) [10].

Retapamulin is used topically for impetigo produced by Gram-positive microorganisms [11].The objective of our study will be to review the *in vitro* antibiotic activity, action mechanisms, and resistance (if reported) of the above antibiotics and to describe their pharmacokinetic and pharmacodynamic properties.

Linezolid

Structure

Linezolid or N-[[3-[3-fluoro-4-(4-morpholinyl)phenyl]-2-oxo-5-oxazolidinyl]-methyl]-acetamide ($C_{16}H_{20}FN_3O_4$), is a tricyclic structure molecule with one oxazolidinone ring, one methylacetamide radical, and one fluorine atom in meta position [12].

Mechanism of Action

Oxazolidinones exert their antibiotic effect by the inhibition of protein synthesis, similar to macrolides, lincosamides, chloramphenicol, and tetracyclines [13]. However, unlike these antibiotics, its action is based on blockage of the initiation complex [13-15]. Specifically, linezolid acts by binding to subunit 50S, probably in domain V of the 23S peptidyl-transferase center, which would interfere with the binding of aminoacyl-tRNA to this area [16].

Spectrum of Activity

Linezolid shows excellent *in vitro* activity against the main Gram-positive pathogens such as staphylococci, streptococci, and enterococci, including isolates resistant to other antibiotics [13,15]. It is also active against *Corynebacterium* spp., *Bacillus* spp., *L. monocytogenes*, *Rhodococcus* spp., and *E. rhusopathiae*; anaerobic Gram-positives such as *Clostridium* spp. and *Peptostreptococcus* spp.; mycobacteria (*M. tuberculosis*, *M. marinum*, *M. avium-intracellulare*, *M. fortuitum*, *M. chelonae,* and *M. abscessus*) and *Nocardia* spp. [14,15,17].

Nonetheless, the majority of Gram-negative bacteria are resistant (*Enterobacteriaceae, Pseudomonas* spp., *Acinetobacter* spp., among others), probably because of the presence of active expulsion systems [13,15,18]. Linezolid is active against anaerobic Gram-negatives such as *B. fragilis, F. nucleatum,* and *Prevotella* spp. and presents moderate activity against *H. influenzae, M. catarrhalis, Legionella* spp., and *Neisseria* spp. [13-15,17].

Table 1 depicts the *in vitro* activity of linezolid against different microorganisms and the corresponding MIC_{50} and MIC_{90} values in published studies [19-21].

Table 1. *In vitro* activity of linezolid against various microorganisms [19-21]

Microorganism	MIC_{50} (in µg/ml)	MIC_{90} (in µg/ml)
S. aureus		
MSSA	1-2	1-4
MRSA	1-2	1-4
Coagulase-negative staphylococci		
Methicillin-susceptible	0.5-1	1-4
Methicillin-resistant	0.5	1-2
S. pneumoniae		
Penicillin-susceptible	0.5-1	1
Penicillin-resistant	0.5-1	1
Beta-hemolytic streptococci	0.5-1	1-2
Enterococcus spp.		
Vancomycin-susceptible	1-4	1-4
Vancomycin-resistant	1-4	2-4
Corynebacterium spp.	0.25	1
L. monocytogenes	2	2
Rhodococcus spp.	2	2
M. tuberculosis	0.01	1
Nocardia spp.	2	4
H. influenzae	4	4-16
B. pertussis	2	4
M. catarrhalis	4	4-8
Legionella spp.	2	4-16
N. gonorrhoeae	4	32
H. pylori	16	32
P. multococida	2	2
B. fragilis	0.5-4	2-4
Prevotella spp.	1	4
Peptostreptococcus spp.	0.5-1	2
Fusobacterium spp.	0.5	1-8
Porphyromonas spp.	1	2
C. perfringens	0.5-2	2-4
C. difficile	1-4	2-8

Mechanisms of Resistance

Since its introduction, there have been some sporadic cases of resistance to linezolid, mainly in *S. aureus*, coagulase-negative staphylococci, *E. faecalis,* and *E. faecium* [22-24]. This resistance is usually mediated by mutations in domain V of the 23S region of rRNA [25,26] or other ribosomal proteins, such as riboprotein L4 [27].

G2576T mutation is the most frequent cause of resistance to linezolid found in clinical isolates of *Enterococcus* spp. and *Staphylococcus* spp. [28,29]. Other reported mutations include G2447T and T2500A in *S. aureus*, C2534T in *S. epidermidis*, G2505A in *E. faecium,* and C2512T, G2513T, and C2610G in *E. faecalis* [30,31]. Some microorganisms such as *S. aureus* have several copies of the gene that encodes domain V of the 23S region of rRNA, and a large number of copies with the mutation may confer high levels of resistance to the antibiotic (MIC>4 µg/ml). Therefore, the level of resistance depends on the number of mutated copies, which has been associated with the dose and time of exposure to linezolid [25,26,29].

In *S. pneumonia* isolates, deletion of 6 pb in the gene that codifies for riboprotein L4 confers resistance to oxazolidinones, macrolides, and chloramphenicol. This is because, although these antibiotics possess different action mechanisms, the binding site to the large subunit of the ribosome is the same and riboprotein L4 is part of this region [27].

Cases of resistance to linezolid mediated by plasmid *cfr* (*chloramphenicol-florfenicol resistance*) were also recently published, initially reported in an isolate of *S. sciuri* from a veterinary sample [32]. This plasmid encodes a methyltransferase that confers resistance against linezolid and chloramphenicol by methylation in position A2503 of region 23S of rRNA. The presence of this resistance determinant has been verified in MRSA isolates obtained from human clinical samples and, unlike in animal samples, it is included in the bacterial chromosome and may have been part of a plasmid [33]. It forms the *mlr* (*modification of the large ribosomal unit*) transcriptional unit along with the *erm(B)* gene, which in turn encodes a methylase that confers resistance to macrolides, lincosamides, and streptogramin B. Hence, the expression of the operon in an isolate would confer resistance to all antibiotics that act at the level of ribosomal subunit 50S [25].

Although mutations in domain V of the 23S region of rRNA would contribute to a slow dissemination of resistance to linezolid, concerns have been expressed that horizontal transmission of plasmid *cfr* between bacterial isolates would permit a faster propagation of resistance and would increase resistance to the above antibiotics [25,34].

Pharmacology

Table 2 shows the most relevant pharmacokinetic parameters in healthy individuals after a single dose of 600 mg or repeated doses of 600 mg every 12 hrs [35].

Absorption

Linezolid achieves total bioavailability after oral administration. At the usual therapeutic doses, it gives plasma concentrations above the MIC_{90} of the majority of susceptible microorganisms [36,37], and its C_{max} is reached at 1-2 h after oral administration. In the case of multiple doses, the administration of 600 mg every 12 h yields mean C_{max} and C_{min} values of 21.2 μg/ml and 6.1 μg/ml, respectively. The predictive pharmacodynamic value of linezolid is based on maintaining the concentration of the pharmaceutical above the MIC during ≥ 40% of the dose interval [35].

Table 2. Mean values (standard deviation) of pharmacokinetic parameters of linezolid in healthy adults [35]

Dose	C_{max} (mg/l)	C_{min} (mg/l)	T_{max} (h)	AUC^a (mg*h/l)	CL (ml/min)	$T_{1/2}$ (h)
400 mg oral						
Single dose	8.10 (1.83)		1.52 (1.01)	55.10 (25.00)	146 (67)	5.20 (1.50)
Every 12 h	11.00 (4.37)	3.08 (2.25)	1.12 (0.47)	73.40 (33,50)	110 (49)	4.69 (1.70)
600 mg oral						
Single dose	12.6 (4.0)		1.3 (0.66)	91.4 (39.30)	127 (48)	4.3 (1.65)
Every 12 h	21.2 (5.78)	6.1 (2.94)	1.0 (0.62)	138.0 (42.10)	80 (29)	5.4 (2.06)
600 mg intravenous						
Single dose	12.9 (1.60)		0.5 (0.10)	80.2 (33.30)	138 (39)	4.4 (2.40)
Every 12 h	15.1 (2.52)	3.7 (2.36)	0.5 (0.03)	138.0 (42.10)	123 (40)	4.8 (1.70)
600 mg in oral suspension						
Single dose	11.0 (2.76)		1.0 (0.88)	80.8 (35.10)	142 (45)	4.6 (1.71)

Cmax: maximum plasma concentration; Cmin: minimum plasma concentration; Tmax: time for Cmax; AUC^a: area under concentration-time curve (AUC for single dose = AUC0-∞; for multiple-dose = AUC0-₍₀-τ₎); CL: systemic clearance; T1/2: mean elimination half-life.

Oral bioavailability of this antibiotic is not altered by the combined administration of antacids that contain aluminium and magnesium [38] or by concomitant enteral nutrition [39]. Welshman et al. concluded that the C_{max} is reduced when linezolid is administered in combination with food but its clinical efficacy is not affected [40].

Distribution

It spreads rapidly in well-perfused tissue. The distribution volume of linezolid is approximately equivalent to the total body water. The binding to plasma proteins is 35% and is independent from the concentration of the antibiotic, explaining why no pharmacological interactions result from the displacement of linezolid from its binding sites to proteins [35].

Linezolid penetration in soft tissue after a single dose of 600 mg produces an area under the curve (AUC) at 8 h of 1.4 ± 0.3 mg*h/l for plasma and of 1.3 ± 0.4 mg*h/l for muscle and adipose tissue. Multiple doses produce AUC values at 8 h of 0.9 ± 0.2 mg*h/l and 1.0 ± 0.5 mg*h/l, respectively. Therefore, linezolid rapidly penetrates adipose and musculoskeletal tissue, reaching adequate concentrations to inhibit the growth of the majority of bacteria against which it presents activity [41].

Metabolism

Linezolid primarily metabolizes by oxidation to two inactive metabolites: aminoethoxy acetic acid and hydroxyethyl glycine. The formation of these inactive metabolites depends on the duration and concentration of linezolid. It is not metabolized by cytochrome CYP450 and does not therefore interact with pharmaceuticals dependent on this system [35].

Elimination

The mean elimination half-life ($T_{1/2}$) is 5-7 h, therefore administration every 12 hrs provides a concentration in steady-state within the therapeutic range [42]. Total clearance of linezolid is approximately 120 ml/min and takes place by renal and extrarenal pathways, with the latter representing 65% of the total. In the plateau stage, approximately 30% of the administered dose appears in non-metabolized urine and 50% in the form of the two inactive metabolites. Elimination by feces is minimal, with only 9% of the administered dose appearing as inactive metabolites [35].

Pharmacokinetics in Specific Situations

There are no differences in the pharmacokinetic parameters between young adults (18-45 yrs) and the elderly (> 65 yrs), indicating that the dose does not have to be adjusted for elderly patients. However, children under 12 yrs present a lower AUC, a more rapid clearance and a shorter mean elimination half-life in comparison to adults. Clearance decreases progressively until adolescence, when it equals that of adults [43,44]. The distribution volume of females is slightly lower than that of males, explaining the higher C_{max} and approximately 38% lower mean clearance in females than in males [45]. There are no significant differences in mean elimination half-life between the sexes, therefore it is not necessary to adjust the dose for the sex of the patient.

Linezolid elimination does not appear to be affected in mild hepatic insufficiency, or in moderate (creatinine clearance of 30-80 ml/min) or even severe (creatinine clearance of 10-29 ml/min) renal insufficiency, therefore it does not appear necessary to adjust the dose for these patients [35]. However, because inactive metabolites of linezolid can accumulate in patients with renal insufficiency, the use of linezolid in these patients must take account of the potential risks of this accumulation. However, there have been reports of linezolid accumulation in patients on hemodialysis [46].

The concentration that linezolid can reach in bone at 5 h after intravenous perfusion of 600 mg linezolid is below the MIC_{90} for staphylococci, and continuous perfusion or more frequent administrations may be required for bone diseases [47]. The plasma linezolid concentration after oral dosage of 600 mg every 12 h provides adequate levels of the antibiotic in the tissue of the diabetic foot [48], despite the reduced blood flow caused by the disease [49]. In patients with mechanical ventilation-associated pneumonia, the plasma concentration in lung parenchyma is around 100%, achieving sufficient activity to treat microorganisms with a high MIC_{90} [50]. In patients with cystic fibrosis treated with oral linezolid, sputum concentrations achieved are above the MIC_{90} for bacteria such as MRSA during most of the inter-dose interval [51].

Pharmacokinetic and pharmacodynamic parameters of antibiotics are significantly altered in critically ill septic patients. There is a risk of prolonged periods during which the antibiotic concentration remains below MIC_{90} and of an inadequate AUC/MIC relationship. Whitehouse et al. analyzed the pharmacokinetic characteristics of linezolid in critical patients and concluded that a dose of 600 mg every 12 h is appropriate and that the dose does not need adjustment according to the renal function [52]. However, Adembri et al. compared the continuous administration of linezolid with the usual regimen of 600 mg every 12 h and found that plasma levels were significantly more stable with continuous administration [53].

Adverse Effects

In general, linezolid has good tolerance, both in oral and intravenous administration [14,17]. During phase III of linezolid development, clinical, controlled, and comparative trials with other antibiotics such as oxacillin, dicloxacillin, clarithromycin, vancomycin, ceftriaxone, and cefpodoxime showed that certain adverse effects were slightly more frequent in linezolid-treated individuals than in those treated with the other antibiotics, including diarrhea (4.3% of study subjects), nausea (3.4%) and cephalalgia (2.2%) [14,54,55]. The appearance of these side effects was independent of the administration pathway. Other symptoms observed in both experimental groups included taste changes, vomiting, vaginitis caused by candida, and liver function abnormalities.

The incidence of the most severe side effects was similar between linezolid-treated patients and those treated with the other antibiotics, and the most severe symptom was thrombocytopenia. Hypertension, severe vomiting, temporary ischemic processes, liver function abnormalities, pancreatitis and renal failure were observed in 0.4% of individuals [55]. Alterations found in biochemical and hematological markers (transaminase alterations, thrombocytopenia, etc.) may have been due to the high doses applied or to the prolongation of treatment for more than two weeks, and normal values were reestablished after the therapy [14,17,54,55]. After the commercialization of linezolid, some adverse effects were reported that had not been observed during preclinical trials, adding further effects to its known myelotoxicity, such as neurotoxicity (optic and peripheral neuropathies, and reversible posterior leukoencephalopathy) [56-64], lactic acidosis [63,65-68], serotoninergic syndrome [68-73], facial paralysis [74], tongue discoloration [75], and bradycardia [76].

Biochemical and hematological alterations continue to appear during prolonged treatment with linezolid [66,77-79]. Inhibition of mitochondrial protein synthesis would be the cause of severe effects such as various pancytopenias (anemia and thrombocytopenia) [58,65]. Spellberg et al. reported a clinical improvement in patients with linezolid-induced pancytopenias after administration of vitamin B_6, since pyridoxine is required in the synthesis of d-aminolevulinic acid, precursor of the heme group [78]. Nevertheless, this finding was not confirmed in subsequent studies [77,79]. However, it has been verified that the combined administration of linezolid and rifampicin decreases the rates of adverse hematologic effects [77].

The onset of neuropathies has been related to long exposure to linezolid, generally in treatments of > 28 days [58-64], although some cases appeared during the first week of treatment [56,57]. The mechanism of this effect has yet to be determined, but it has been proposed that linezolid inhibits the protein synthesis of the mitochondria through its affinity to bind with 16S mitochondrial rRNA [63,67]. In the case of optic neuropathy, energy deficit in the macula would cause axonal destruction and the consequent visual symptoms, as observed in situations of nutritional deficit [56-58,60,64,65,67]. Another hypothesis is based on the activity of this antibiotic as inhibitor of monoamino oxidase (MAO), an enzyme involved in the synthesis of neurotransmitters [57]. At any rate, withdrawal of the antibiotic treatment reverts optic (but not peripheral) neuropathy in the majority of patients [56,57,64].

More recently, one case of reversible posterior leukoencephalopathy has been reported [62], and the most plausible mechanism would be alteration of the blood brain barrier by inhibition of mitochondrial protein synthesis. However, other toxicity mechanisms are not rules out.

Linezolid was initially developed as an antidepressant but was finally commercialized as antibiotic. Nonetheless, the Food and Drug Administration (FDA) did not contraindicate the combined administration of linezolid with antidepressive pharmaceuticals. Experiments conducted with venlafaxine, citalopram, fluoxetine, paroxetine and sertraline and some isolated cases of hypertensive crisis secondary to the combination of bupropion and linezolid suggest the need to correct this guideline [72]. Because of its structural similarity to toloxatone, linezolid acts as reversible and unspecific inhibitor of MAO, hence its combined administration with SSRIs (*serotonin reuptake inhibitors*) could trigger the onset of a serotoninergic syndrome [69-73], whose initial first symptoms were observed after a few days of administration in young patients [71]. The best option is to withdraw linezolid treatment and reestablish the antidepressive therapy after two weeks [72]. Nonetheless, if the clinical situation of the individual requires it, linezolid can be combined with SSRIs as long as the treatment does not exceed 14 days and the patient is monitored at all times.

Clinical Indications

Based on the results obtained in phase III of the trial, the FDA approved in 2000 the use of linezolid to treat the infections listed below [35]:

- Infections caused by vancomycin-resistant *E. faecium* (endocarditis, post-neurosurgery meningitis, peritonitis, cholangitis and some types of abscesses, including liver abscesses).
- Community-acquired pneumonia due to *S. pneumoniae* (including multi-resistant strains) or by *S. aureus* (only MSSA).
- Nosocomial pneumonia due to *S. aureus* (MSSA and MRSA) or due to S. *pneumoniae* (including MDRSP).
- Complicated skin and soft tissue infections caused by *S. aureus* (MSSA and MRSA), *S. pyogenes,* or *S. agalactiae*
- Non-complicated skin and soft tissue infections caused by *S. aureus* (only MSSA) or by *S. pyogenes*.

Specific indications were not determined at the time of linezolid commercialization for certain population groups (children, pregnant women or breastfeeding mothers) due to the lack of experimental data. However, since it was classified by the FDA as category C fetal risk, the use of linezolid in pregnant women is only justified if the benefit outweighs the risk to the fetus [14,17,55]. It is not recommended to administer linezolid during breastfeeding because there are no studies on its excretion in colostrum [17,55].

Indications for adults are considered appropriate for pediatric age groups [80]. However, according to Ventakesh et al., linezolid is only recommended for children and newborns who are intolerant to vancomycin or who require an oral therapy because of its adverse effects and the longer time on intravenous therapy in comparison to vancomycin [81]. In contrast, other studies underline the safety and effectiveness of treatment with linezolid [82]. It has been observed that thrombocytopenia is a much more frequent adverse effect in adults than in children [81,82], who most commonly suffer from diarrhea, nausea, vomiting, transaminase elevation, or skin eruptions [81].

At any rate, most studies stress the need to revise the initial indications and to increase knowledge on the behavior of the antibiotic in specific population groups. Finally, linezolid should not be the first choice antibiotic in many of these infections but rather a therapeutic alternative in cases of difficult treatment or infections caused by multi-resistant microorganisms [15,17,83].

Cefditoren Pivoxil

Structure

This new third generation cephalosporin, 2,2-dimethyl-propionyloxymethyl-7-[(Z)-2-(2-aminothiazole-4-yl)-2-ethoxyiminoacetamide]-3-[(Z)-2-(4-methylthiazole-5-yl)ethenyl]-8-oxo-5-thia-1-azabicyclo[4.2.0]oct-2-ene-2-carboxylate) ($C_{25}H_{28}N_6O_7S_3$), presents various structural differences in relation to other antibiotics in its group, which confer it exclusive properties [84,85]. Even though the mechanism of action is the same and based on the presence of the β-lactamic ring, cefditoren also has three new radicals located at the ends of the molecule: the aminothiazole and methylthiazole groups are responsible for the broad spectrum of activity shown by this antibiotic against Gram-negative and -positive microorganisms, respectively, and the pivoxil group improves its oral absorption and bioavailability [86].

Mechanism of Action

As with other β-lactam antibiotics, cefditoren pivoxil acts through the inhibition of the cellular wall synthesis through the binding to the PBPs (*penicillin-binding proteins*), causing bacterial lysis and subsequent death [84,85]. Its distinguishing trait is its greater affinity for these proteins in comparison with other β-lactam antibiotics. Thus, for example, cefditoren shows a high affinity for *S. aureus* PBPs 1, 2 and 3; *S. pneumoniae* PBPs 1A, 2X and 2B; *E. coli* PBPs 1A, 1B and 3 and *H. influenzae* PBP4 [84,87].

Spectrum of Activity

In vitro studies prior to the marketing of this antibiotic showed a high level of cefditoren activity against MSSA isolates (including β-lactamase producers), but not against MRSA isolates [88]. *Enterococcus* spp. and *Listeria* spp. isolates did not show susceptibility either [84,89].

Regarding streptococci, penicillin-susceptible *S. pneumoniae* isolates were also susceptible to this antibiotic [84,86,87]. It has since been proven after its marketing that cefditoren may also inhibit the growth of penicillin-resistant *S. pneumoniae*, even at concentrations lower than other β-lactam antibiotics [90] and independently from resistance to other antibiotics, such as macrolides or fluoroquinolones [91]. Data obtained during test trials against *S. agalactiae,* streptococci groups C and G and *Streptococcus* of the *viridans* group (including samples with intermediate susceptibility to penicillin) showed a good activity of cefditoren against these pathogens [84,85]. The highest microbiologic eradication rates produced in the treatment of pharyngo-amygdalitis caused by *S. pyogenes* bacteria currently correspond, according to certain authors, to cefditoren [92].

Among Gram-negative bacteria, cefditoren shows good activity against *H. influenzae, H. parainfluenzae* and *M. catarrhalis*, including β-lactamase producing isolates [86,93-95]. Cefditoren is the most active cephalosporin against *H. influenzae* and it may become an excellent alternative to the treatment of infections caused by this pathogen, especially against the BLNAR (*β-lactamase-negative ampicillin-resistant*) phenotype [94].

Compared to other antibiotics, both β- and non-β-lactam, it is equally active against *E. coli* [90,96]. Actually, according to Lerma et al., cefditoren was the most active oral antibiotic against the isolates of this species obtained in urine samples, except for ESBLs producers, against which amoxicillin-clavulanic acid showed MIC_{90} values lower than those of cefditoren [96]. This fact is especially interesting considering the possibility of administering cefditoren against urinary tract infections caused by *E. coli* [90]. Other Gram-negative bacteria, such as *Klebsiella* spp., *P. mirabilis* and *Salmonella* spp., also proved to be very susceptible to the action of this cephalosporin in the previous trials ($MIC_{90} \leq 1$ μg/ml), in contrast with the values obtained for *Citrobacter* spp., *Enterobacter* spp., *M. morganii*, *Providencia* spp. and *S. marcescens* ($MIC_{90} > 16$ μg/ml) [89]. However, it has no activity against Gram-negative aerobic bacteria such as *P. aeruginosa, Acinetobacter* spp. or *S. maltophilia*, amongst others [86,89].

It is more active against *N. gonorrhoeae* and *N. meningitidis* than other third-generation cephalosporins (like ceftriaxone or ceftazidime) and it remains active against isolates with alterations of PBP2 or β-lactamase-producing isolates. The long lateral chain present in the C3 position of the molecule allows it to maintain its affinity for these proteins, in spite of their being altered [97].

Cefditoren is also active against some anaerobic bacteria such as *Peptostreptococcus* spp. and *Clostridium* spp., although with variable MICs depending on the species, with the lowest being the susceptibility of the various *Bacteroides* spp [87].

Table 3 shows the *in vitro* activity of this antibiotic against different pathogens [84,85,88,89,91,93-96].

Table 3. *In vitro* **activity of cefditoren pivoxil in different bacterial species**
[84,85,88,89,91,93-96]

Microorganism	MIC$_{50}$ (in μg/ml)	MIC$_{90}$ (in μg/ml)
S. aureus		
Methicillin-susceptible	0.5	0.39-3.13
Methicillin-resistant	>64	50-128
S. pneumoniae		
Penicillin-susceptible	≤0.015	≤0.06-0.78
Penicillin-intermediate	0.12	0.5-10
Penicillin-resistant	0.25	0.39-2
S. pyogenes	0.03	≤0.006-0.06
S. agalactiae	0.03	0.025-0.05
Viridans group streptococci		
Penicillin-susceptible	-	0.25
Penicillin-intermediate	-	2
Penicillin-resistant	-	8
Enterococcus spp.	>16	>16
H. influenzae		
Beta-lactamase-positive	≤0.008-0.015	0.015-0.06
Beta-lactamase-negative	≤0.008-0.03	0.008-0.03
Beta-lactamase-negative, ampicillin-susceptible	-	0.06
Beta-lactamase-negative, ampicillin-resistant	0.03	0.125-0.25
H. parainfluenzae	-	0.06
M. catarrhalis		
Beta-lactamase-positive	0.12	0.25-1
Beta-lactamase-negative	≤0.008	≤0.008-0.06
E. coli	0.06-0.25	0.125-3.13
Quinolone-resistant	0.125	0.25
Penicillinase-positive	0.06	0.125
Penicillinase hyperproduction	4	16
Inhibitor resistant TEM (IRT)	0.06	0.5
ESBLs-producing	8	32
K. pneumoniae	0.12	0.12-64
K. oxytoca	0.06	0.12-1
Salmonella spp.	0.25	0.2-4
Shigella spp.	-	0.1-1
P. mirabilis	0.03	0.12
Citrobacter spp.	1	>16
Enterobacter spp.	0.5-1	0.78-25
M. morganii	0.12	>16
Providencia spp.	-	0.2-2
P. vulgaris	-	0.78-16
P. rettgeri	-	1.56-4
S. marcescens	1	>16
Acinetobacter spp.	>16	>16
P. aeruginosa	>16	>16
S. maltophilia	>16	>16
N. gonorrhoeae	-	≤0.006-0.06

Mechanism of Resistance

The production of β-lactamases is the most common mechanism of bacterial resistance to β-lactam antibiotics. These enzymes may be coded by plasmids or chromosomally and they inactivate these antibiotics by hydrolyzing the amide bond of the β-lactam ring which is common to all of them. However, cefditoren is stable against the majority of the chromosomal and plasmidic β-lactamases that are most frequent in Gram-positive and Gram-negative pathogens [84-87,90], therefore it is active against isolates that produce this type of enzymes in species such as *S. aureus, H. influenzae, H. parainfluenzae, M. catarrhalis, K. pneumoniae* and *E. coli*. However, like the other cephalosporins, it is hydrolyzed by ESBLs [87,88,96]. The overproduction of chromosomal β-lactamase that may be induced by *Enterobacter* spp., *Citrobacter* spp., *Morganella* spp. and *Serratia* spp. also causes resistance in these bacteria [89].

In Gram-positive bacteria, the modification of PBPs is the most frequent resistance mechanism to β-lactam antibiotics, such as in MRSA and in penicillin-resistant *S. pneumoniae*. Cefditoren is active against penicillin-resistant *S. pneumoniae*, given that its lateral C3 chain maintains its affinity against PBP2X, showing MIC_{50} values that are similar to those of amoxicillin and cefuroxime [87,98], but it shows no activity against MRSA isolates [88].

Pharmacology

Cefditoren pivoxil is a prodrug hydrolyzed by gastrointestinal sterases after it is orally administered and it passively diffuses through the intestinal membrane. The prodrug is not detected in the plasma and it has no microbiology activity [99].

Its pharmacokinetics has been studied in healthy volunteers and in patients with kidney and liver failure [86]. Table 4 shows the most relevant pharmacokinetic parameters of cefditoren in healthy individuals, after a single dose of 200 and 400 mg, or after multiple doses of 400 mg every 12 hours for 7 days.

Table 4. Pharmacokinetic of cefditoren administered after the meal in healthy volunteers [86]

Parameter	Single doses		Multiple doses
	200 mg	**400 mg**	**400 mg/12 h**
C_{max} (mg/l)	2.7	3.8 – 4.6	3.9 – 4.9
T_{max} (h)	1.8	2.4 – 3.1	2.1 – 2.7
AUC (mg*h/l)	10.8	11.4 – 17.4	11.4 – 15.7
$T_{1/2}$ (h)	1.4	1.4 – 1.7	1.5
Cl_r (l/h)	-	3.8-5.0	4.1 – 5.6

C_{max}: maximum plasma concentration: T_{max}: time to C_{max}; AUC: area under concentration-time curve; $T_{1/2}$: elimination half-time; Cl_r: renal clearance.

Absorption

The bioavailability of cefditoren is 15-20% before breakfast. The ingestion of food, especially with fatty content, promotes its absorption and doubles its bioavailability, so that C_{max} and AUC increase between 50% and 70%, in comparison to it being administered before breakfast [86].

In the studies carried out in healthy volunteers, single doses of 200 or 400 mg and multiple doses of 400 mg/12 h or 400 mg/8 h, always administered 30 minutes after eating, achieved a value of C_{max} of 2.5, 4.1, 3.27 and 3.77 mg/l, respectively. Both the 8-hour and the 12-hour administration pattern maintained levels that exceeded MIC_{50} and MIC_{90} for at least 40% of the time and the half-life of the antibiotic were 1.36 ± 0.2 h and 1.9 ± 0.2 h for each of the patterns, respectively [100].

Cefditoren shows a linear pharmacokinetic, with a good relation between AUC_∞ and C_{max} after two single doses of 200 and 400 mg. Evidence of linearity was also shown with 100 and 300 mg doses [100].

Distribution

The average volume of distribution of cefditoren in steady-state is 9.3 ± 1.6 l, and its binding to plasmatic proteins is 88% [99]. Similar to the other cephalosporins, it is distributed both in the vascular and in the interstitial compartments. It penetrates in the bronchial mucosa, the epithelial coating fluid, the skin ampoule fluid and the amygdalar tissue [86].

Some works have been published studying how the high binding to plasma proteins affects the therapeutic effect of cefditoren. Thus, a study entailing the administration of a single dose of 400 mg before breakfast found that the probability of obtaining a bacteriostatic response is lower than 90% for MICs over 0.03 mg/l. This provoked uncertainty, since the currently admitted cutting point for cefditoren remains at 0.125 mg/l [101]. However, these results are yet to be confirmed by other *in vitro* studies that have shown antibiotic activity on strains with MICs between 0.25 and 0.5 mg/l in culture media with an albumin concentration similar to the physiological levels [102].

Metabolism

The metabolism of cefditoren pivoxil occurs mainly in the intestine, where it is hydrolyzed to cefditoren [86]. AUC_∞ and C_{max} with doses of 400 mg/12 h and 400 mg/8 h are similar on different days and similar to those obtained after the administration of a single dose, thus indicating that cefditoren does not accumulate [100].

Elimination

The non-absorbed fraction, which nearly amounts to 80%, is excreted with faeces, in which it appears as inactive metabolites. Up to 18% of the dosage administered is recovered through urine, unmetabolized [103]. The urine level of cefditoren reaches its maximum level of 154.5 mg/l in the 400 mg/12 h pattern and 185.6 mg/l in the 400 mg/8 h pattern [100]. The half-life of the antibiotic in plasma is approximately 1 to 1.5 h. Total clearance adjusted by bioavailability is 25-30 l/h and renal clearance is 80-90 ml/min, approximately [86].

Pharmacokinetics in Specific Situations

There are statistically significant differences amongst the pharmacokinetics on the basis of age and sex. Studies on healthy volunteers with ages between 25 and 40 years compared with patients aged over 65 years who received multiple doses of 400 mg/12 h for 7 days showed C_{max} and AUC in the latter as 26% and 33%, above, respectively, and a 16% longer $T_{1/2}$. This is explained by the fact that old aged patients show a creatinine clearance 26% lower than young people [86]. On the other hand, women showed 13% lower kidney clearance than men, such that their C_{max} and AUC are 14% and 16% higher, respectively [99]. However, such variations are not clinically relevant and therefore dosage-adjustment is not necessary.

In patients with moderate kidney failure (creatinine clearance of 30-50 ml/min) or severe kidney failure (creatinine clearance below 30 ml/min), the values of C_{max} and AUC are between 1 and 3 times higher than in patients with normal kidney function. In patients with moderate kidney failure the maximum doses should be 200 mg/12 h and, for patients with severe kidney failure, the maximum daily dosage should not exceed 200 mg [86].

Plasma levels of cefditoren are not significantly altered in patients with slight or moderate liver failure (Child-Pugh A or B) and therefore dosage adjustment is not required. There are no data available for patients with severe liver failure and therefore, in principle, its use is not advisable [86,99].

Adverse Effects

The most common secondary effects, documented during the phase of the clinical trials, were gastrointestinal problems (with a frequency exceeding 10%), mainly diarrhoea, nausea, abdominal pain and dyspepsia; followed by headaches and vaginal candidiasis in 1-10% of the cases [84,85,87,104]. Their intensity and frequency, specially that of diarrhoea, were dose-dependent and, in most cases, slight or moderate, and self-limited [87,104]. With a frequency of over 1% were sleep disorders, allergic reactions, anorexia, fungal infections, respiratory problems, alteration of the hepatic function, fever and cytopaenias, which occurred regardless of the dosage that had been administered [85].

On the other hand, several cases of carnitine deficit were described in patients that had received long-term treatment with antibiotics containing pivalic acid, such as cefditoren [105,106]. Carnitine is essential in the processes of fatty acid oxidation and in the formation of ketonic bodies in the periods before breakfast, and its deficit is linked to the loss of appetite, hypoglycaemia, loss of consciousness and seizures. It is thought that after 1 to 2 weeks of treatment with these types of antibiotics, the levels of serum carnitine are reduced by 25%. Makino et al. advise carnitine supplements in patients that are to undergo cefditoren treatment for more than 2 weeks [106].

Clinical Indications

In 2001 the FDA approved the use of cefditoren pivoxil as treatment for the following infectious processes, be them slight or moderate, in adults and children over 12-years [99]:

- Acute exacerbation of chronic bronchitis or community-acquired pneumonia by *H. influenzae, H. parainfluenzae* and *M. catarrhalis* (including β-lactamase-producing isolates), as well as *S. pneumoniae* (only penicillin-susceptible isolates).
- Pharyngitis caused by *S. pyogenes*.
- Non-complicated infections of skin and soft tissues due to MSSA isolates (including β-lactamase-producing isolates) or *S. pyogenes*.

Once launched on the market, cefditoren proved to be equally effective in the treatment of infections caused by penicillin-resistant *S. pneumoniae* isolates, especially in community-acquired pneumonia [104]. In addition, in some countries cefditoren is used in the treatment of non-complicated urinary tract infections caused by non-ESBL-producing *E. coli* [85].

There are no studies of cefditoren in children younger than 12 years old, pregnant women or breastfeeding mothers. It is considered as an antibiotic belonging to the B category of faetal risk, since definite data on whether it can cross the placenta are lacking. It is also unknown whether it reaches mother's milk, so it is also unadvisable during lactancy [84,85,99].

It is also contraindicated in patients allergic to β-lactamic and in patients with carnitine deficit or with congenital alterations in their metabolism [87,99]. Like with other antibiotics, the prolonged treatment with cefditoren is linked to excess growth of non-susceptible microbiota, such as enterococci, *C. difficile* or *Candida* spp. [85,87,99].

Ertapenem

Structure

Ertapenem or [4R-[3(3S,5S),4α,5β,6β(R)]]3-[[5-[[(3-carboxyphenyl)amino]carbonyl]-3-pyrrolinidyl]thio]-6-(1-hydroxyethyl)-4-methyl-7-oxo-1-azabiciclo[3.2.0]hept-2-ene-2-carboxylic acid monosodium salt ($C_{22}H_{24}N_3NaO_7S$) is a carbapenem aimed for parenteral administration [107-110].

Its molecular structure was specifically developed to be active against community pathogens and to improve the pharmacokinetic properties of its group predecessors (imipenem and meropenem) [111]. Thus, it shares a trans-hydroxyethyl group in position 6 with the previous ones which confers it stability against β-lactamases [109]; however, it differs from meropenem solely in its 2' substituent, where it carries a *meta*-substituted benzoic acid group, which confers it a high capacity of binding to plasma proteins [109,111]. In addition and similar to meropenem (not imipenem), it has a 1-beta-methyl group which protects the antibiotic from hydrolysis by renal dehydropeptidase-1 [108,109].

Mechanism of Action

Like other β-lactam drugs, ertapenem inhibits the synthesis of the cell wall by binding to PBPs [108,111]. Above all, it presents a high affinity for *E. coli* PBP2 and PBP3 [108-110]. In fact, this carbapenem has between 30 to 40 times more affinity for PBP2 than other β-lactam agents. In the case of PBP3, the affinity is equal to that of cephalosporins, but approximately 70 times higher than that of imipenem [112]. Like other β-lactam agents, it shows no affinity for *Staphylococcus* spp. PBP2a [111] and, because of its anionic nature, as well as its high molecular weight and lypophility, this antibiotic does not show a high affinity for porine OprD [111].

Spectrum of Activity

Like other carbapenems, ertapenem is known for its wide spectrum of activity against both aerobic and anaerobic Gram-positive and Gram-negative bacteria. However, activity against non fermenting Gram-negative bacilli, such as *Pseudomonas* spp., *Acinetobacter* spp., *B. cepacia* and *S. maltophillia* is very limited [108-110,113-119].

As regards Gram-positive microorganisms, it is active against *Staphylococcus* spp. (except against methicillin-resistant isolates, although it is deemed that therapeutic success may be obtained if administered in combination with linezolid) [120], *S. pneumoniae* (although its activity against penicillin-resistant isolates is reduced) and other streptococci such as *S. agalactiae* and *S. pyogenes*. It is not active against the *Streptococcus* group *viridans* [109,114,117] or against enterococci [110,113-115,119].

However, it is very active against *Enterobacteriaceae* isolates, including AmpC or ESBLs β-lactamase producers [115-117] and it also shows excellent activity against *Haemophilus* spp., *Moraxella* spp., *Neisseria* spp. or *Pasteurella* spp., amongst others [108,109,117]. Regarding activity against anaerobic bacteria, it is active against *Bacteroides* spp., *Clostridium* spp. (except for *C. difficile*), *Eubacterium* spp., *Fusobacterium* spp., *Peptostreptococcus* spp., *Porphyromonas* spp., *Prevotella* spp. and *Propionibacterium* spp. [108,109,113,117].

Table 5 shows a summary of ertapenem's activity against several microorganisms of clinical interest [116,117,119-133].

Table 5. *In vitro* activity of ertapenem against various microorganisms [116,117,119-133]

Microorganism	MIC_{50} (in µg/ml)	MIC_{90} (in µg/ml)
S. aureus		
MSSA	0.12-0.25	0.25-0.5
MRSA	4- >32	16- >32
Coagulase-negative staphylococci		
Methicillin-susceptible	0.12	0.5
Methicillin-resistant	8	>16
Microorganism	**MIC_{50} (in µg/ml)**	**MIC_{90} (in µg/ml)**
S. pneumoniae		
Penicillin-susceptible	0.016-0.03	0.03-0.06
Penicillin-resistant	0.5-1	1-2
S. agalactiae	≤0.03-0.06	≤0.03-0.125
S. pyogenes	≤0.008-0.03	0.016-0.06
Viridans group streptococci	8	2-16
E. faecalis	8-16	16- >64
E. faecium	16- >64	16- >64
Citrobacter spp.	≤0.008-0.12	<0.03-0.5
E. aerogenes	0.06	0.25-1
E. cloacae	≤0.03-0.06	0.06-1
E. coli		
Non ESBL-producing	≤0.008-0.03	≤0.015-0.12
ESBL producing	≤0.03	0.03- 0.125
K. oxytoca	0.008-0.03	≤0.03-0.06
K. pneumoniae		
Non ESBL-producing	0.008-0.12	<0.015-0.5
ESBL producing	0.06	0.25
M. morganii	≤0.015-0.03	0.03-8
P. mirabilis	≤0.015-0.03	≤0.015-0.06
P. vulgaris	≤0.015-0.06	<0.03-0.25
Providencia spp.	≤0.015-0.12	0.03-0.25
Salmonella spp.	≤0.008	≤0.008-0.03
Serratia spp.	≤0.03-0.06	0.06-0.12
Shigella spp.	≤0.008	≤0.008-0.015
H. influenzae	0.06	0.06-0.25
H. parainfluenzae	0.03	0.125
P. aeruginosa	4-8	16- >64
A. baumannii	2	4- >16
B. cepacia	8	>16
S. maltophilia	16- >64	16- >64
Aeromonas spp.	0.06-0.5	0.25- >16
M. catarrhalis	≤0.008-0.016	≤0.015-0.03
Betalactamase-positive	≤0.0075	0.03
Betalactamase-negative	≤0.0075	0.015
Microorganism	**MIC_{50} (in µg/ml)**	**MIC_{90} (in µg/ml)**
N. meningitidis	≤0.008	0.008-0.016
Bacteroides spp.	0.125-0.25	1-2
Clostridium spp.	0.126-0.5	2-4
Peptostreptococcus spp.	0.06-0.125	0.5-1
Propionibacterium spp.	0.06-0.25	0.12-0.5
Fusobacterium spp.	≤0.015	≤0.015-0.03
Porphyromonas spp.	≤0.015	≤0.015-0.125
Prevotella spp.	0.06-0.125	0.125-0.5

Mechanisms of Resistance

Methicillin-resistant staphylococci, enterococci and, to a certain degree, penicillin-resistant *S. pneumoniae* are resistant to ertapenem, due to its lack of affinity for the PBPs present in these bacteria [109].

It is stable to hydrolysis by the majority of β-lactamases, including penicillinases, cephalosporinases and ESBLs, so that, like the rest of carbapenems, it maintains activity against ESBLs and AmpC producing *Enterobacteriaceae* [107,109,110,134,135]. It is, however, hydrolysable, mainly by metallo-β-lactamases (MBL) such as IMP or VIM and, to a lesser degree, by some enzymes of Ambler's classes A (such as KPC carbapenemases) and D (such as those of OXA type) [108,111,119,136]. KPC carbapenemases have been described in *K. pneumoniae, K. oxytoca, Enterobacter* spp., *E. coli, Salmonella* spp., *C. freundii, P. mirabilis, Serratia* spp. or *P. aeruginosa* [137-139], while OXA-type carbapenemases have mainly been described in *A. baumannii* isolates [140].

However, the presence of carbapenemases is not the only mechanism of resistance against this antibiotic in *Enterobacteriaceae*, but others may be present, such as the reduction in permeability, a reduction of the expression of porines or the overexpression of efflux systems. In addition, these mechanisms are frequently associated to the production of ESBLs and/or AmpC β-lactamases [110,119,136,141-145]. Thus, for example, ESBLs and/or AmpC-producing *K. pneumoniae* or *E. coli* isolates that are resistant to ertapenem through deficiency of porines OmpK36/OmpK35 and OmpC/OmpF, respectively, have been described [146,147]. Resistance to this antibiotic by means of the reduction of OmpF and OmpD porines associated to the expression of active efflux systems has also been described in *E. cloacae* [148]. Lastly, the expression of an extended-spectrum AmpC (ESAC) β-lactamase has been recently described in *E. coli*, associated to the reduction of OmpC and OmpF porine expression, which confers the isolate a high degree of resistance to ertapenem and reduced susceptibility to imipenem [149]. It is, therefore, generally clear that several mechanisms must participate in order for resistance to this antibiotic to be expressed [108].

Amongst other mechanisms, resistance to ertapenem in non-fermenting Gram-negative bacteria is related to the hyperproduction of AmpC chromosomal β-lactamase, the presence of OXA-type carbapenemase, scarce penetration and/or expulsion through efflux systems [150-152].

Pharmacology

The pharmacokinetics of ertapenem have been analyzed in healthy volunteers and in some special populations, such as the old-aged and patients with different degrees of renal failure, and the administration of both single and multiple doses has been assessed. The main pharmacokinetic parameters are shown in table 6 [153,154].

C_{max} after 1 g intravenous perfusion for 30 minutes in healthy young adults is approximately 150 mg/l (end of the perfusion). There is evidence that, in dosage ranging from 0.5 to 2 g, the AUC increase in adults is almost proportional to the dosage. There is no accumulation of ertapenem after multiple IV doses between 0.5 and 2 g per day. From 2 g dose onwards, the free fraction increases in a non-proportional manner, and this lack of linearity appears when the total level of ertapenem is >150 mg/l [153].

Table 6. Pharmacokinetic of ertapenem in healthy adults [153,154]

Parameters	Mean ± standar deviation
C_{max} (mg/l)	103 ± 26.3
C_{min} (mg/l)	1.2 ± 0.6
AUC_{0-24} (mg*h/l)	539.7 ± 66.5
Vd_{ss} (l/kg)	8.2 ± 1.5
CL (ml/h/kg)	29.5 ± 3.4
$T_{1/2}$ (h)	3.8 ± 0.6

C_{max}: maximum plasma concentration; AUC: area under concentration-time curve, Vd_{ss}: apparent volume of distribution at steady state; CL: systemic clearance. $T_{1/2}$: elimination half-time.

Absorption

Ertapenem is completely absorbed when administered intramuscularly. A study carried out on 26 healthy volunteers, administered 1 g of intramuscular ertapenem, showed an approximate bioavailability of 92%. Plasma levels achieved after intramuscular administration are similar to the ones achieved intravenously. AUC is also comparable, with values of 591.4 mg*h/l for intramuscular administration and 541.8 mg*h/l for intravenous administration. There is a slight difference in the time when plasma levels exceed 4 mg/l (18.1 h intramuscularly and 16.9 h intravenously). In addition, ertapenem does not accumulate after multiple intramuscular doses [155].

Distribution

The distribution volume of total ertapenem is 0.11 l/kg and that of free ertapenem is 1.8-2.9 l/kg [156]. Binding to plasma proteins is inversely dependent on plasma concentration in a range that goes from 96% at a concentration of 10 mg/l to 84% at a concentration of 300 mg/l. Ertapenem levels in healthy volunteers administered 1 g in IV perfusion during 30 minutes were 150 mg/l at the end of the perfusion, 10 mg/l at 12 h, 4 mg/l at 17 h and 1-2 mg/l at 24 h. On the other hand, the level of free ertapenem was 15 mg/l at the end of the perfusion, 1.7 mg/l at 6 h, 1.1 mg/l at 8 h and 0.5 mg/l at 12 h [156].

The distribution of ertapenem in the interstitial space of the skeletal muscle and subcutaneous adipose tissue is much lower than in plasma, and the C_{max} of free ertapenem obtained are 6.7 ± 4.1 mg/l and 4.0 ± 1.6 mg/l, respectively. This penetration is consistent with the degree of concentration-dependent plasma protein binding. AUC in muscle and adipose tissues shows low values: 39.7 ± 24.8 mg*h/l and 18.6 ± 4.6 mg*h/l, respectively. However, the level of free ertapenem in the interstitial fluid exceeds MIC_{90} for the most important pathogens at 7 h (subcutaneous tissue) and 10 h (muscular tissue) [154].

The penetration of ertapenem has been studied in various tissues of intraabdominal localization in patients who underwent abdominal surgery. The tissue/plasma level rate obtained is 0.19 for the colon, 0.17 for the small intestine, 0.17 for the biliary vesicle, 0.08 for the liver and 0.095 for the pancreas [157]. The penetration in the bone and in the synovial fluid after the administration of a dosage of 1 g of ertapenem IV for 30 minutes has also been studied. The tissue/plasma level rate in the spongy bone tissue is 0.19, in the cortical bone tissue, 0.13 and in the synovial fluid it is 0.41 [158].

Ertapenem is detected in breastfeeding milk up to 5 days after the interruption of treatment. The concentration is 0.38 ml/l before 24 h after the last dosage [159]. It is not known whether ertapenem can penetrate the cerebrospinal fluid or cross the placental barrier.

Metabolism

Approximately 40% of the dosage administered appears unaltered in the urine. A study with radiolabelled ertapenem found that the terminal half-life of ertapenem is 4 h, almost 40% of radioactivity is recovered in urine as unaltered ertapenem, and another 40% as inactive metabolite, while about 10% is recovered in faeces [156]. Hepatic metabolism plays a small role in the elimination of ertapenem and studies show it does not inhibit metabolism mediated by any of the six main isoforms of CYP [160].

Elimination

Renal clearance of unaltered ertapenem is 12.8 ml/min compared with a total clearance of 28.4 ml/min. The kidneys are responsible for about 80% of total clearance of ertapenem; average renal clearance of free ertapenem is 207 ml/min, which is reduced to 98 ml/min when administered in combination with probenecid, a fact that indicates that tubular excretion greatly contributes to the renal elimination of ertapenem [156].

Pharmacokinetics in Specific Situations

There are no significant differences in AUC between men and women. In women, ertapenem shows a lower distribution volume, a higher C_{max} and a slightly shorter half life. These values lack clinical significance, so no adjustment is required depending on the gender [153]. Plasma level and half life of ertapenem are slightly higher in old people than in young adults. This difference is justified by the age-related reduction of the kidney function and it lacks clinical significance, so no adjustment of dosage is required in healthy old patients. No data is available on paediatric population [161].

In patients with slight renal failure (creatinine clearance between 60 and 90 ml/min/1.7 m^2) total ertapenem AUC is not altered; in patients with moderate renal failure (30-60 ml/min/1.7 m^2), AUC is increased by 1.5 times, while in patients with advanced kidney failure (10-30 ml/min/1.7 m^2) and in its final stages (renal clearance lower than 10 ml/min/1.7 m^2), the AUC is up to 2 times that of the AUC in healthy volunteers. The effect of renal failure on free ertapenem AUC is slightly higher than on the levels of total ertapenem [162]. Since it lacks significant liver metabolism, hepatic failure should not alter ertapenem's pharmacokinetics. Thus, no adjustment of the dosage is recommended in patients with hepatic problems [156].

Adverse Effects

Generally, ertapenem is a well tolerated antibiotic [163] and its secondary effects are not too different from those observed with other β-lactam agents [164]. However, adverse reactions have been referred in approximately 20% of patients treated with ertapenem. The most common, in different clinical trials, were gastrointestinal problems, such as diarrhoea (1.7-14.3%, with a low incidence of pseudomembranous colitis), nausea (0.8-5.7%) and vomiting (1-3.3%) [163]. Also frequent were the appearance of phlebitis and thrombophlebitis (0.8-12.2%), followed by erythema and pain at the site of the injection [159,165,166-171]. Less frequent were cephaleas (0.4-4.7%) [159,167,168] and candidiasis (1.3-2.9%) [165,168], amongst others. Alterations were also observed in the enzymes of the liver function, both in transaminases [115,159,165,166-171], as well as in alkaline phosphatase [115,159,166-169], and there were alterations in the leukocyte and platelet counts [166-168].

The possibility of seizures [163,172] is noticeable amongst the most serious effects, although these have been related to possible pre-existing factors such as central nervous system disorders, previous treatments with anticonvulsants and kidney failure [172-174] since, in most cases, they disappear after the interruption of the treatment, without any need for specific therapy [167]. Sets of symptoms of gastric ulcer, colitis and cholecystitis may also appear [118].

Clinical Indications

In 2001 the FDA approved the use of ertapenem for the treatment of the following infectious processes [175]:

- Complicated intraabdominal infections caused by *E. coli*, *C. clostridioforme*, *E. lentum*, *Peptostreptococcus* spp., *B. fragilis*, *B. distasonis*, *B. ovatus*, *B. thetaiotaomicron* or *B. uniformis*.
- Complicated skin and soft tissue infections caused by *S. aureus* (only MSSA isolates), *S. pyogenes*, *E. coli* or *Peptostreptococcus* spp.
- Community acquired pneumonia caused by *S. pneumoniae* (only penicillin-susceptible isolates), *H. influenzae* (only negative β-lactamase isolates) or *M. catarrhalis*.
- Complicated infections of the urinary tract, pyelonephritis included, caused by *E. coli* or *K. pneumoniae*.
- Acute pelvic and gynaecology infections caused by *S. agalactiae*, *E. coli*, *B. fragilis*, *P. asaccharolytica*, *Peptostreptococcus* spp. or *P. bivia*.
- For the prophylaxis of surgical opening infections after programmed (colorectal or gynaecological) abdominal surgery in adults.

However, in Europe it is not indicated in the treatment of complicated urinary tract infections and its use has only been approved in the prophylaxis after a colorectal surgery [160]. Ertapenem is counterindicated in persons with hypersensitivity to β-lactam agents. There are not enough data available on its effect on pregnant women, so precaution is advised in its use. In addition, it is excreted in calostrum, so breastfeeding should be interrupted if the mother needs treatment with this antibiotic [108,175]. Equally so, its administration is not advised in children under 3 months of age, although the indications for adults may be extended to the paediatric population as from 3 months onwards [176]. The good safety and absence of pharmacology interactions make ertapenem an antibiotic adequate for its use in over 65 years-old patients [108], especially in the treatment of community acquired pneumonia [177].

Doripenem

Structure

Doripenem or (4R, 5S, 6S)-6-[(1R)-1-1hydroxyethyl]-4-methyl-7-oxo-3[[(3S, 5S)-S-(sulfamoylaminomethyl)-pyrrolidin-3-yl]-thio]-1-azabicyclo-[3.2.0]-hept-2-ene-2-carboxylic acid monohydrate) is a carbapenem for parenteral use [126]. Its chemical structure is similar to that of meropenem and ertapenem, all of which, contrary to imipenem, include a 1-beta-methyl lateral chain that makes them resistant to the action of the renal dehydropeptidase-1 [126,178-180]. In addition, the novelty offered by this molecule regarding the other components of the group is based on the fact that it has a sulfamoylaminomethyl group substituting the dimethylcarbamoyl lateral chain [178].

Mechanism of Action

Like other β-lactam agents, doripenem acts by inhibiting the synthesis of the bacterial cell wall by means of its binding to PBPs [181,182]. It has a great affinity, especially for *P. aeruginosa* PBP2 and 3 and for *E. coli* PBP2 [181,183].

Spectrum of Activity

Doripenem shows the spectrum of activity of the predecessors of its group (imipenem, meropenem and ertapenem) both against Gram-positive and Gram-negative bacteria [126,178,179]. It also has a slightly higher activity against certain pathogens than other carbapenems [178].

Among Gram-positive pathogens, it shows good activity against *S. aureus* and coagulase-negative staphylococci (only methicillin-susceptible isolates), *S. pneumoniae, S. agalactiae, S. constellatus, S. intermedius* and others [178,180,184]. It is not active against methicillin-resistant staphylococci isolates, although a certain synergy is observed when administered in combination with vancomycin or teicoplanin [185]. Neither is it active against enterococci [178,181], like the rest of carbapenems.

Like other carbapenems, it is active against Gram-negative bacteria, including enterobacteria such as *E. cloacae, E. aerogenes, C. freundii, M. morganii, Providencia* spp.,

Table 7. *In vitro* activity of doripenem against various microorganisms
[126,127,179,184,188-192]

Microorganism	MIC$_{50}$ (in µg/ml)	MIC$_{90}$ (in µg/ml)
S. aureus		
MSSA	0.03-0.06	0.03-0.06
MRSA	0.5-1	4-32
S. epidermidis (methicillin-resistant)	0.03	0.03-0.06
S. pneumoniae		
Penicillin-susceptible	≤0.008	≤0.008-1
Penicillin-resistant	0.5	1
S. pyogenes		
Penicillin-susceptible	≤0.008	0.008-0.03
Macrolide-susceptible	≤0.008	≤0.008
Viridans group streptococci		
Penicillin-susceptible	0.03	0.06
Penicillin-resistant	1-2	4
E. faecalis		
Vancomycin-susceptible	4	8
E. faecium		
Vancomycin-susceptible	32	>32
Vancomycin-resistant	>32	>32
C. freundii	0.03-0.06	0.06-0.12
E. aerogenes	0.06	0.12
E. cloacae	0.03	0.25
E. coli		
Non ESBL-producing	0.03	≤0.015-0.06
ESBL producing	≤0.015-0.03	0.03-0.06
K. oxytoca	0.03	0.06
K. pneumoniae		
Non ESBL-producing	0.03-0.06	0.03-0.12
ESBL producing	0.03-0.12	0.06-0.12
M. morganii	0.25	0.5
P. mirabilis	0.5	2
Providencia spp.	0.06-0.125	0.5
Salmonella spp.	0.03-0.12	0.06-0.12
S. marcescens	0.12	0.5
H. influenzae	0.06-0.12	0.25-1
P. aeruginosa	0.25-0.5	0.5-8
Carbapenem-resistant	8	>32
Metallobetalactamase-producer	>32	>32
Acinetobacter spp.	0.5	1-32
Carbapenem-resistant	8	>32
B. cepacia	0.5-8	4-32
Aeromonas spp.	0.03-0.5	1
M. catarrhalis	≤0.015	0.03
S. maltophilia	>16	> 16
B. fragilis	0.25-0.5	0.25-1
B. thetaiotaomicron	0.25-0.5	1
Prevotella spp.	0.06-0.12	0.125-0.5
Peptostreptococcus spp.	0.06-0.12	0.25
Porphyromonas spp.	≤0.015-0.03	0.03-0.05
C. difficile	≤0.015-1	0.03-2
P. acnes	0.06-0.12	0.125-0.25

Serratia spp., *Salmonella* spp., *Shigella* spp., *P. mirabilis*, *Klebsiella* spp. and *E. coli* (including AmpC and ESBLs β-lactamase producing isolates) [180,181]. It also shows excellent activity against multi-resistant non-fermenting bacilli such as *P. aeruginosa*, *B. cepacia* and *Acinetobacter* spp. [178,180,182], probably because of the sulfamoylaminomethyl-pyrrolidin-yl-thio lateral chain in position 2 [186,187]. However, as with other carbapenems, doripenem is not active against *S. maltophilia*, due to its instability against this bacteria's L1 (MBL) enzyme [179-181].

Additionally, doripenem has activity against most clinically relevant anaerobic pathogens such as *Bacteroides* spp., *Prevotella* spp., *Peptostreptococcus* spp., *Porphyromonas* spp. and *Propionibacterium* spp. [126,178,188]. The study of Wexler et al. shows doripenem as the most active carbapenem against *C. difficile* [189].

Table 7 shows *in vitro* MIC$_{50}$ and MIC$_{90}$ values obtained against several microorganisms of clinical interest [126,127,179,184,188-192].

Mechanism of Resistance

Mechanisms of bacterial resistance to doripenem include inactivation through carbapenemases, PBPs mutation, reduction of the external membrane permeability and active efflux. It has a lower capacity of resistant mutant selection than other carbapenems [178,193,194]. According to Mushtaq et al., this would be due to the fact that bacteria have not yet undergone sufficient exposure to develop specific resistance, since this is a new antibiotic [193], a reason for which it is, potentially, a strategy to prevent the spread of carbapenem-resistant isolates [194].

Carbapenems cross the external membrane of *P. aeruginosa* using OprD-type porines [181]. Thus, the loss or reduction of their expression will entail a reduction in carbapenem activity, especially of imipenem [194]. However, in order for the activity of meropenem, ertapenem or doripenem to be affected up to high levels of resistance, another mechanism of resistance, such as the overexpression of active efflux pumps, must also be present. Doripenem is a substrate of several efflux systems, such as MexAB-OprM, MexCD-OprJ and MexXY-OprM [195] and so these isolates, defective in OprD and overproducers of efflux pumps, will be markedly resistant to doripenem and meropenem. The problem is that, unlike isolates with exclusive loss of OprD porin, they are also resistant to other non-β-lactam antibiotics, such as fluorquinolones [194,196,197]. According to Huynh et al., concurrent administration of doripenem with an aminoglycoside would prevent the appearance of resistance in this pathogen [186]. Equally so, the selection of doripenem-resistant mutants through bmeB1 and bmeB11 efflux systems overexpression has been proven in *B. fragilis* [198].

Regarding enzymatic resistance, doripenem is stable against the action of most β-lactamases of Ambler's A, C and D classes, including ESBLs and AmpC [179,184]. However, this antibiotic may be hydrolyzed by class B β-lactamases (IMP, VIM, SPM or GIM metallo-β-lactamases) present in non-fermenting Gram-negative pathogens such as *Pseudomonas* spp., *A. baumannii* and *S. maltophilia*, amongst others [181], some class A β-lactamases (SPE, NMC-A, IMI-1, KPC) and some class D (OXA-10) [179,180,194]. Current worries are based on the fact that mobile elements that codify metallo-β-lactamases, observed until now in non-fermenting bacilli, have also started appearing among *Enterobacteriaceae* [199].

Pharmacology

The pharmacokinetics of doripenem have been studied after the single administration of a 250 and 500 mg dose in 1 hour perfusion and after multiple doses in healthy volunteers and in renal failure patients. Its main pharmacokinetic parameters after the administration of single doses are shown in table 8 [200].

Table 8. Pharmacokinetic of doripenem in healthy adults after administration of a single dose of 250 and 500 mg in 1 h infusion [200]

Parameter	250 mg	500 mg
C_{max} (mg/l)	18.1	23.0
AUC (mg*h/l)	20.26	34.4
Vd_{ss} (l/h)	-	16.8
Cl_p (l/h)	-	15.9
Cl_r (l/h)	-	10.8
$T_{1/2}$ (h)	0.9	0.86

C_{max}: maximum plasma concentration; AUC: area under concentration-time curve, Vd_{ss}: apparent volume of distribution at steady state; CL_p: plasmatic clearance; Cl_r: renal clearance; $T_{1/2}$: elimination half-time.

Absorption

There is no data available on the absorption of doripenem.

Distribution

The pharmacokinetics of doripenem are linear over a dose range of 125 mg to 1 g, administered as a single dose through intravenous perfusion for 30 to 60 minutes. Doripenem does not accumulate after several intravenous perfusions of 500 mg or 1 g administered every 8 hours for 7 to 10 days [200].

The volume of distribution at steady state is 16.8 l. The binding of doripenem to plasma proteins is low (approx. 8%) and independent of the plasma concentration of the drug [201]. It is mainly distributed in the extracellular space, which involves penetration in a great variety of tissues. Amongst others, after a single dose of 250 or 500 mg, doripenem is detected in the peritoneal fluid, gallbladder tissue, bile, urine, dermal tissues, uterine tissue, middle ear, palatine tonsil tissue, aqueous humour and gingival tissue [200].

After a 500 mg dose of doripenem, an $AUC_{0-\infty}$ of 49.3 ± 6.5 mg*h/l in peritoneal fluid and a peritoneal fluid/plasma relation of 0.53 ± 0.17 are obtained. Average free doripenem exposure time (91% of the dose) is 78.2% for MICs of 1 mg/l, 41.5% for 4 mg/l and 13.1% for 16 mg/l. The probability of obtaining 40% of the dose administration interval with levels higher than MIC is higher in the peritoneal fluid than in plasma. To achieve a probability equal to or exceeding 90% of the pharmakodynamics objective in the peritoneal fluid a dose between 250 and 500 mg is required three times a day for *E. coli*, *Klebsiella* spp. and *E. cloacae*; however, *P. aeruginosa* requires the infusion of 1 g in 30 minutes perfusion three times a day [202-204].

Metabolism

Doripenem is relatively stable and most of the dosage administered remains unaltered. Its metabolization occurs through dehydropeptidase-1 and it does not undergo any CYP450-mediated metabolism.

Elimination

Doripenem is excreted unaltered and mainly through the kidneys. Its average plasma terminal excretion half life in healthy and young adults is approximately 1 hour and plasma clearance is approximately 15.9 l/h. When administered in combination with probenecid, excretion is significantly reduced, which suggests that elimination occurs through active tubular secretion and glomerular filtration. In studies with radiolabelled doripenem 71% of the dosage was recovered in urine as unaltered active ingredient and 15% as inactive metabolite. In addition, less than 1% of radioactivity was recovered in the faeces [201].

Pharmacokinetics in Specific Situations

Pharmacokinetic parameters of doripenem are not altered by age, sex or race. Its pharmacokinetics have not been determined in liver failure patients, but it is probable that it is not altered due to the low hepatic metabolism it shows [200]. Renal failure increases elimination terminal average life and systemic exposure time to the drug. After a single dose of 500 mg in patients with slight renal failure (creatinine clearance of 50-79 ml/min), AUC is increased 1.6 times; in moderate renal failure patients (creatinine clearance of 31-50 ml/min), AUC is increased 2.8 times and, in severe renal failure patients (creatinine clearance ≤ 30 ml/min) AUC is increased 5.1 times in comparison with persons with normal renal function. Adjustment of the dosage is thus required in moderate and severe renal failure patients [200]. Patients under haemodialysis to which doripenem is administered immediately after the session show an AUC increased 7.8 times in comparison with persons with normal renal function. 52% of the dose of doripenem is recovered 4 hours after the session (46% unaltered). No data is available on dose adjustment for these patients [200].

Adverse Effects

During phase III clinical trials on doripenem, the most common adverse events were nausea, vomiting, diarrhoea, phlebitis, skin rashes, cephalea and anaemia, observed in 2-7%

of patients treated. Other less frequent effects (0-2%) were oral candidiasis and increase of liver function enzymes, amongst others [205]. Other effects have been described after its commercialization, such as Stevens-Johnson syndrome, toxic skin necrolysis, interstitial pneumonia, pseudomembranous diarrhoea and seizures [181,206]. Regarding the latter, and due to the low affinity this antibiotic has shown towards GABA receptors (in comparison with other β-lactam drugs) and to the lower basic nature of the lateral chain of the molecule, doripenem has one of the lowest excitatory potentials of the group of carbapenems [184,187,207]. Recent trials have shown that only 1.1% of patients treated with doripenem suffered this type of effects, in comparison with 3.8% of those treated with imipenem [208].

Clinical Indications

The FDA approved the use of doripenem in 2007 as treatment for the following infectious processes in adults [206]:

- Complicated intraabdominal infections caused by *E. coli*, *K. pneumoniae*, *P. aeruginosa*, *B. fragilis*, *B. caccae*, *B. thetaiotaomicron*, *B. uniformis*, *B. vulgatus*, *S. intermedius*, *S. constellatus* and *P. micros*.
- Complicated urinary tract infections (pyelonephritis included) caused by *E. coli*, *K. pneumoniae*, *P. mirabilis*, *P. aeruginosa* and *A. baumannii*.

Subsequently, the European Medicines Agency (EMEA) also authorized the use of this antibiotic for the treatment of nosocomial pneumonia (including pneumonia associated with mechanic ventilation) [201]. Doripenem is counterindicated in persons with hypersensitivity to β-lactam agents. It is classified as foetal risk B category so, due to the absence of experimental data in pregnant women, infants and children under 18, caution is advised when using it in these population groups [206].

Daptomycin

Structure

Daptomycin or N-decanoyl-L-tryptophyl-L-asparaginyl-L-aspartyl-L-threonylglycyl-L-ornithyl-L-aspartyl-D-alanyl-L-aspartylglycyl-D-seryl-threo-3-methyl-L-glutamyl-3-anthraniloyl-L-alanine-lactone is currently the only representative of a new group of antibiotics, the cyclic lipopeptides, and is derived from *Streptomyces roseosporus* fermentation products [209]. Its structure is made up of 13 aminoacids, 10 of which make up a central cyclic structure through ester unions, while the remaining three constitute a small lateral peptidic chain that presents an N-decanoil rest in the last aminoacid and is responsible for the antibiotic activity of the molecule [210,211].

Mechanism of Action

The mechanism of action of daptomycin is not currently clear as yet, and several models have been proposed. At first the hypothesis was that this antibiotic may work by inhibiting the synthesis of lipoteichoic acids [212]. However, works carried out on *S. aureus* or *E. faecalis* did not manage to prove this hypothesis [213].

Thus, for the first time, Silverman et al. proposed a plausible model of action for daptomycin using previous evidence on the dissipation of the membrane potential produced by the antibiotic [214]. For this author, daptomycin would insert itself in the bacterial membrane, in which it would form pore-like structures, alter the integrity of the membrane and produce a massive liberation of ions such as K^+ from inside the cell, with the subsequent bacterial death. Some authors consider this mechanism to explain the fast bactericide effect of daptomycin [215].

Starting from the model proposed by Silverman, Jung et al. established that this was a calcium ion-dependent process, so that Ca^{2+} and daptomycin would previously be bound in solution, thus producing a conformational change that would allow the antibiotic to reduce its negative charge and increase its amphipatic properties [216,217]. This would promote interaction with cytoplasmatic membranes and its insertion in them through the triptophan residue present in the lipid tail of this antibiotic. Jung thinks the error in Silverman's model is thinking that bacterial death is a result of depolarization, when, actually, bacterial death precedes it in the experiments. Therefore, for this and other authors, based on experimental evidence, the loss of bacterial viability is not only a consequence of the depolarization of the membrane, but also of other phenomena yet to be determined, which may alter the integrity and permeability of this structure [218].

The main advantage of daptomycin in relation to its exclusive mechanism of action is that, unlike other antibiotics, it is active against bacteria in growth and in stationary phases [219]. In addition, the bactericide effect of daptomycin is characterized by not provoking bacterial lysis, thus preventing the liberation of proinflammatory cytokines which would provoke self aggression mediated by the immune system in the individual [211,219,220].

Spectrum of Activity

Daptomycin is active against Gram-positive microorganisms, both aerobic and anaerobic, multi-resistant isolates included [210,215]. It does not have any activity against Gram-negative bacteria, since it is unable to penetrate their external membrane [210,221].

It has bactericide effect on multi-resistant bacteria such as meticillin-resistant *S. aureus*; glycopeptide resistant *S. aureus* (GISA or GRSA); *S. pneumoniae* (including penicillin-resistant isolates), *S. agalactiae*, *S. pyogenes*, *S. viridans* or *S. bovis*; *Enterococcus* spp. (including VRE isolates) [210,211,215,222,223]. *In vitro,* it is also active against *Corynebacterium* spp., *Listeria* spp. and *Bacillus* spp., as well as anaerobic bacteria (*C. perfrigens*, *Peptrostreptococcus* spp., *Propionibacterium* spp.) [210,211,224,225]. Table 9 shows daptomycin MIC_{50} and MIC_{90} values in various *in vitro* sensitivity trials against Gram-positive bacteria [210,215,224,226-229].

**Table 9. *In vitro* activity of daptomycin in different bacterial species
[210,215,224,226-229]**

Microorganism	MIC_{50} (in µg/ml)	MIC_{90} (in µg/ml)
S. aureus		
MSSA	0.25	0.25-0.62
MRSA	0.44	0.5-1
GISA	-	0.125-0.5
Coagulase-negative staphylococci		
CoNS methicillin-susceptible	0.12-0.25	0.24-0.5
CoNS methicillin-resistant	0.24	0.44
S. pneumoniae	0.24	0.25-0.5
Penicillin-resistant	-	0.25
S. agalactiae	0.09	0.12-0.5
S. pyogenes	≤0.12	0.25-0.5
Viridans group streptococci	0.25-0.5	0.5-1
E. faecalis	1	1-2
VSE	1	1-2
VRE	1	1-4
E. faecium	1-4	2-8
VSE	2	4
VRE	2	2-4
Bacillus spp.	1	2
Corynebacterium spp.	≤0.03	1
C. perfrigens	0.5	2
P. acnes	0.5	1
Listeria spp.	2	2

Several studies show that daptomycin MICs against MRSA isolates do not exceed 0.5 or 0.75 µg/ml [230,231]. However, some authors have proved that there is an increase in daptomycin MIC values in *S. aureus* isolates with reduced sensitivity to glycopeptides, in which values equal to or exceeding 2 µg/ml are achieved and which, following current criteria, may be considered isolates with reduced sensitivity to daptomycin [232,233]. In the case of enterococci with VanA or VanB phenotypes, a slight increase of daptomycin MIC has been observed (1 µg/ml to 8 µg/ml), a reason for which the FDA declared that its use may only be approved in the case of vancomycin-susceptible *E. faecalis* [234], while the EMEA did not refer to this fact [235].

Mechanism of Resistance

The mechanism of resistance against daptomycin is not totally proven, but various hypotheses have risen over the last years.

Kaatz et al. produced *in vitro* mutants of *S. aureus* that were resistant to daptomycin through the alteration of the composition of the bacterial membrane [236]. Thus, the loss of an 81 kDa membrane protein with activity similar to a chaperone protein increased MIC values against this antibiotic. For this author, several membrane proteins may be involved in resistance against daptomycin, so that the degree of resistance in an isolate would be related to the number of non-expressed proteins.

Friedman et al. described daptomycin-resistant clinical isolates through point mutations in the *mprF* gene or through the insertion of a nucleotide in the *yycF* gene, amongst others [237]. These genes codify a lysil-fosfatidil-glycerol-synthetase enzyme (involved in regulating the surface electrostatic load of the cell membrane) and a histidine-synthetase (involved in the synthesis of membrane fatty acids), respectively, such that the depolarization caused by daptomycin does not occur in isolates with these mutations. More recently, Murthy et al. described a new mutation that is present in the *mrpF* gene (T345A), also associated with resistance against daptomycin in MRSA [238].

Cui et al. stated for the first time the possible existence of a cross-resistance mechanism between glycopeptides and daptomycin in *S. aureus* [232]. The thickened wall presented by VISA isolates may also prevent the entry and action of daptomycin, a molecule with greater molecular weight. Julian et al. observed that there was a reduction of the degree of murein cross-linking on VISA isolate cellular walls with reduced susceptibility to daptomycin [239]. In addition, a point mutation was observed in the *mprF* gene which may affect antibiotics that act at the bacterial wall level, such as glycopeptides or daptomycin.

Jones et al. stated that the mechanism of resistance to daptomycin includes several related processes and that, when any of the previous processes occurs in isolation, it causes a reduction in the susceptibility, but all the resistance mechanisms are required (alteration of membrane proteins, reduction of depolarization and thickening of the membrane) for obtaining isolates that are clearly resistant to daptomycin [240].

Equally so, daptomycin-resistant *E. faecalis* isolates are being detected. For Hidron et al., in spite of the lack of conclusive data, the daptomycin-resistance mechanisms present in that species may be similar to those described in *S. aureus* [241].

Pharmacology

Daptomycin pharmacokinetics has been studied in healthy volunteers and in patients suffering from Gram-positive infections. Pharmacokinetics is linear up to a 6 mg/kg of body weight dose and slightly non-linear in the AUC with the 8 mg/kg dosage administered via 30 minutes/24 hours IV infusion for 7-14 days [242]. The main pharmacokinetic parameters are shown in table 10 [243].

Absorption
Studies in animals showed that daptomycin is not absorbed in significant amounts after oral administration.

Distribution
Daptomycin binds reversibly to plasma proteins in about 90%. Said binding is independent of the dosage administered [242] a fact which, together with the high molecular weight of daptomycin, indicates that distribution must be limited to plasma and interstitial fluid [243]. The distribution volume in steady state was approximately 0.1 l/kg in healthy adult volunteers. It is mainly distributed through tissues that are very vascularized. Total

penetration of daptomycin in inflammatory fluid (measured as the inflammatory fluid's AUC_{0-24} compared with that of plasma) is 68.4% [244].

Table 10. Pharmacokinetic of daptomycin at the therapeutic dose (4 mg/kg) [243]

Parameter	Mean ± standar deviation
C_{max} (mg/l)	57.8 ± 3.0
C_{min} (mg/l)	5.9 ± 1.6
AUC_{0-24} (mg*h/l)	494 ± 75.0
Vd_{ss} (l/kg)	0.09
CL (ml/h/kg)	7.1 - 8.3
$T_{1/2}$ (h)	8.1 - 9

C_{max}: maximum plasma concentration; AUC: area under concentration-time curve, Vdss: apparent volume of distribution at steady state; CL: systemic clearance; $T_{1/2}$: elimination half-time.

Metabolism

In vitro studies on human hepatocytes have not shown any important involvement of the CYP450 system on the metabolism of daptomycin. Systemic metabolism is very small or non-existent [245].

Elimination

Daptomycin is mainly excreted via the kidneys, and the renal function is the parameter that most influences the variability of daptomycin pharmacokinetic parameters. A study with radiolabelled daptomycin recovered 78% of radioactivity in urine and 5% in faeces [246]. After a single dose of 4 mg/kg of body weight, an average of 53% of the unaltered dosage was recovered in urine in the first 24 h. Urinary excretion is about 50-60% in 24 hours and it does not seem to be dependent on the dosage administered [243].

There are no data available on the excretion of daptomycin in breast milk. Animal studies have not shown penetration of daptomycin in the hematoencephalic (blood-brain) barrier [243].

Pharmacokinetics in Specific Situations

The influence of gender on the pharmacokinetics of daptomycin has been studied, but the difference (approximately 20%) lacks clinical significance [242]. With regards to age, a study carried out on groups of children aged 12 to 17, 7 to 11 and 2 to 6, who were administered a 4 mg/kg dose, showed that daptomycin clearance is faster in the youngest group. Estimated total body exposure in adolescents is comparable to that of adults. Elimination half-life is 6.7 h in adolescents, 5.6 h in children aged 7 to 11 and 5.3 h in children under 6 years [247].

Dose adjustment is not required exclusively on the basis of age; however, renal function must be assessed and dosage reduced if there is evidence of severe renal failure [248].

The influence of body weight has been studied in moderately obese healthy volunteers (body mass index between 25 and 40 kg/m^2) or morbidly obese (body mass index over

40 kg/m^2). Obesity does not alter plasma half-life parameters, fraction of unaltered daptomycin excreted in urine and absolute renal clearance. The distribution volume and plasma clearance is higher in obese than in normal weight patients. Obese individuals show an exposure to daptomycin higher than non-obese individuals, but no dose-adjustment is considered necessary only on the basis of obesity [249].

Renal function is the main conditioner of inter-individual variability in daptomycin clearance. Clearance in dialyzed patients is approximately 1/3 of healthy volunteers (0.27 versus 0.81 l/h) [250]. The doses recommended for patients with creatinine clearance lower than 30 ml/min is 4 mg/kg every 48 h. Patients subject to haemodialysis should receive doses after the haemodialysis session [243].

In patients with moderate liver failure (Child-Pugh B), the binding to plasma proteins, total clearance, renal clearance and distribution volume are similar to those of healthy volunteers. No dose adjustment is required in this group of patients. No data is available in patients with severe liver failure (Child-Pugh C), but since hepatic metabolism has not been shown, dose adjustment does not seem to be required [243].

On the other hand, in studies in which daptomycin was combined with gentamicine with the aim of increasing its bactericide action, no alteration was observed in the pharmacokinetic profile of the latter [251].

The need to administer doses higher than the therapeutic dosage in severe infections caused by resistant microorganisms led to the study of the pharmacokinetic parameters of daptomycin at doses higher than the usual. A study in 36 healthy volunteers administered multiple doses higher than those approved in the product data sheet showed that half-life was approximately 8 hours, plasma clearance normalized by weight was about 9-10 ml*h/l, the distribution volume was 100 ml/kg and binding to plasma proteins was 90-93%. All those parameters were independent of the dosage [252].

Adverse Effects

Daptomycin is a generally well-tolerated antibiotic. Although initial clinical studies showed effects on skeletal muscles, such as myopathy and CPK serum elevations, it was shown that a dosage of the antibiotic once a day every 12 h prevented the appearance of this unwanted effect [215].

The most frequent secondary effects observed (>5%) were: constipation, nausea, reaction at the site of the injection, headaches and diarrhoea. Between 1-5% of the patients suffered insomnia, vomiting, itching, rashes, liver function alterations, CPK elevation, *Candida* spp. infections, urinary tract infections, low blood pressure, dizziness, anaemia, dyspnoea and fever [235]. The effects are, however, reversible [211]. Authors such as Katz et al. report at least a slight adverse effect in 41.7% of treated patients, the most common being nausea and CPK elevation, frequently accompanied by weakness and muscular pain [253].

Clinical Indications

The FDA approved the use of daptomycin in 2003 as treatment for the following infectious processes [245]:

- Complicated skin and soft tissue infections caused by *S. aureus* (including methicillin-resistant isolates), *S. pyogenes*, *S. agalactiae*, *S. dysgalactiae* subsp. *equisimilis* and *E. faecalis* (only vancomycin-susceptible isolates).
- In 2006, the treatment of bacteraemia caused by *S. aureus* (including MSSA and MRSA), whether or not associated with right-side infectious endocarditis, was included.

In addition, several studies were carried out to assess the application of daptomycin for cases of endocarditis caused by multi-resistant enterococci, meningitis (pneumococcal or staphylococcal) and community-acquired pneumonia. It yielded no satisfactory results in the latter infection, since lung surfactant may interfere with the action of the antibiotic [254].

Due to lack of experimental data, daptomycin is counterindicated in patients with hypersensitivity to this antibiotic, as well as in pregnant women (foetal risk B category), infants and children under 18 years old [245].

Gemifloxacin

Structure

Gemifloxacin or 7-[(4Z)-3-(aminomethyl)-4-(methoxyimino)-1-pyrrolidinyl]-1-cyclopropyl-6-fluoro-1,4-dihydro-4-oxo-1,8-naphthyridine-3-carboxylic acid is a new fluor quinolone that maintains the original bicyclic nucleus of nalidixic acid [255]. It is characterized by a cyclopropyl group in position 1, determinant of the activity against Gram-negative bacteria; a hydrogen in position 5, determining activity against Gram-positive bacteria; 3-aminomethyl and 4-methyloximino substituents in position 7, responsible of the low toxicity on the central nervous system and of the marked activity of this antibiotic against *S. pneumoniae*; and one nitrogen in position 8, which confers it activity against anaerobic bacteria [255,256].

Mechanism of Action

Quinolone antibiotics act by inhibiting bacterial DNA replication, reparation and transcription through binding to topoisomerase II (or DNA gyrase) and topoisomerase IV enzymes involved in these bacterial processes [257]. Although most quinolones have affinity for both enzymes, their chemical structure determines a preferred target, preferences that could be reflected in a higher affinity of the different drugs for the respective primary target of quinolone action, which is DNA gyrase in Gram-negative organisms and topoisomerase IV in Gram-positive bacteria [258]. Notwithstanding, gemifloxacin is a quinolone able to indistinctly join both topoisomerases, as an effect of the presence of the methoxy group [259].

Bacteriostatic action of quinolones occurs through the formation of a quinolone-enzyme-DNA complex which reversibly blocks cell replication and growth. On the contrary, the bactericide effect of gemifloxacin against pathogens such as *E. coli*, *S. aureus* or *S. pneumoniae* is a consequence of the liberation of free DNA ends from these ternary complexes [260]. Lastly, it may be noted that gemifloxacin, like the majority of quinolones, is able to achieve good concentrations inside polymorphonuclear (PMN) leukocytes while maintaining its activity against various intracellular pathogens [261].

Spectrum of Activity

New generations of quinolones have been developed with the aim of improving activity against Gram-positive bacteria, but without loss of activity against Gram-negative bacteria, which molecules such as ciprofloxacin possess. Thus, generation IIIb, to which gemifloxacin belongs, is characterized by a marked activity against Gram-positive bacteria, such as *S. pneumoniae*, including penicillin-resistant and/or ciprofloxacin-resistant isolates, together with a good activity against Gram-negative bacteria and against respiratory pathogens such as *C. pneumoniae*, *L. pneumophila* and *M. pneumonie* [256,262].

Gemifloxacin is more active than ciprofloxacin against *S. aureus* (including ciprofloxacin-resistant, MSSA and MRSA isolates), against coagulase-negative staphylococci, against β-haemolytic streptococci (*S. pyogenes* and *S. agalactiae*) and particularly against *S. pneumoniae* (including MDRSP isolates) [257,263-272], and its activity against *E. faecalis* is higher than against *E. faecium* [273].

Activity against Gram-negative bacteria is similar to that shown by ciprofloxacin [255]. Thus, it is active against most of the species belonging to the *Enterobacteriaceae* family, such as *E. coli*, *E. cloacae*, *E. aerogenes*, *C. freundii*, *K. pneumoniae*, *K. oxytoca*, *M. morganii*, *Proteus* spp., *Providencia* spp., *S. marcescens*, species of non-typhi *Salmonella*, *Shigella* spp. and *Yersinia* spp. [266,271,273-275]. It is also active against *Aeromonas* spp., *Pasteurella* spp. [275], *N. meningitidis* [264,276] and *N. gonorrhoeae*, especially against ciprofloxacin-resistant isolates [277].

Gemifloxacin also shows excellent activity against respiratory pathogens such as *L. pneumophila*, *C. pneumoniae*, *H. influenzae* and *M. catarrhalis* [257,260,263,264, 266,273,278-282]. In this sense, it is more active than erythromycin against all *L. pneumophila* serogroups and other species of the same gender, reason for which some authors propose gemifloxacin as treatment of choice against legionellosis [282,283].

On the contrary, activity against non-fermenting Gram-negative bacilli is lower. For example, ciprofloxacin is more active than gemifloxacin against *P. aeruginosa* [265]. Similarly, MIC values are higher in *Acinetobacter* spp. and *S. maltophilia* [264].

The activity of gemifloxacin against anaerobic bacteria is similar to that of other quinolones like levofloxacin and trovafloxacin, although variable depending on the microorganism [268]. Activity is limited against *Bacteroides* spp., *Clostridium* spp. (*C. difficile* is the less susceptible species) and *Prevotella* spp. It is however more active against

Peptostreptococcus spp., *Porphyromonas* spp., *Fusobacterium* spp. and *Veillonella* spp. [265,275,284-289].

Lastly, gemifloxacin shows excellent activity against *L. monocytogenes*, *Nocardia* spp., *H. pylori*, *Mycoplasma* spp. and *Ureaplasma* spp., including quinolone-resistant isolates [260,278,290-295].

Table 11 summarizes gemifloxacin *in vitro* activity against several microorganisms [271-275,279-305].

Table 11. *In vitro* activity of gemifloxacin against various microorganisms [271-275,279-305]

Microorganism	MIC_{50} (in µg/ml)	MIC_{90} (in µg/ml)
S. aureus		
Ciprofloxacin-susceptible	0.03	0.03
Ciprofloxacin-resistant	4	8
MSSA	0.5	8
MRSA	0.03-4	1->128
Coagulase-negative staphylococci		
Ciprofloxacin-susceptible	0.016	0.03
Ciprofloxacin-resistant	2-1	4
Methicillin-susceptible	0.03	0.12
Methicillin-resistant	0.12	1
S. pneumoniae		
Penicillin-susceptible	0.015-0.03	0.015-0.06
Penicillin-resistant	0.008-0.03	0.015-0.06
Quinolone-susceptible	0.06	0.06
Quinolone-resistant	0.03-0.25	0.06-1
S. agalactiae	0.015-0.06	0.03-0.25
S. pyogenes	0.015-0.06	0.015-0.25
Enterococcus spp.		
Vancomycin-resistant	2-16	>16
Vancomycin-susceptible	0.06-0.12	2-4
Ciprofloxacin-susceptible	0.06	0.25
Ciprofloxacin-resistant	8	32
L. monocytogenes	0.125	0.125-0.25
Nocardia spp.	1	4
Enterobacteriaceae		
Quinolone-susceptible	≤0.03	0.25
Quinolone-resistant	16	64
Haemophilus spp.		
Quinolone-susceptible	≤0.008	0.06
Quinolone-resistant	0.25	1
P. aeruginosa		
Quinolone-susceptible	0.25	1
Quinolone-resistant	32	>128
H. pylori	0.06	0.13
B. cepacia	1	8
Aeromonas spp.	≤0.015-0.03	0.03-0.25
Legionella spp.	0.015	0.03
Bacteroides spp.	0.5	>16
Mycoplasma spp.	0.12	0.25
Ureaplasma spp.	0.125	0.25

Mechanism of Resistance

Basically, bacterial resistance to fluoroquinolones derives from mutations in QRDR (*quinolone resistance-determining region*) of genes *gyrA/gyrB* and *parC/parE* of the DNA gyrase and of topoisomerase IV, respectively. In spite of the fact that primary targets vary depending on the drug [306], the appearance of mutations in these genes implies a reduction of the activity of all fluoroquinolones [307].

The reduction of permeability also conditions resistance to quinolones [308]. In relation to this, alterations have been described in Gram-negative bacteria such as *E. coli* [309] and *P. aeruginosa* [310]. Also, the active expulsion of the antibiotic through efflux pumps determines resistance to quinolones in *P. aeruginosa* [311], *S. aureus* [312] and *S. pneumoniae* [313].

Due to the double affinity of gemifloxacin for both bacterial topoisomerases, the probability of selection of resistant mutants during treatment is very low [257,260,305,314]. In the case that one of the targets suffers a mutation, the antibiotic could always bind and block the other to act on the bacteria and prevent the appearance of high levels of resistance [257]. Thus, gemifloxacin becomes an excellent therapeutic option when the prevalence of multiresistant isolates is high or in patients in which previous treatments with other quinolones have already selected resistances [263].

In relation to resistance to gemifloxacin, one of the most extensively studied case is that of *S. pneumoniae*. Isolates carrying mutations in *gyrA* and *parC* are active against gemifloxacin. However, the appearance of new spontaneous mutations in any of the genes would confer resistance against this antibiotic to the isolate [260,263,315]. Generally, resistance to gemifloxacin starts with a mutation in the *gyrA* gene and, once this first mutation has taken place, the probability of a second mutation in *parC* occurring is very high [259,263]. Unlike the case with other fluoroquinolones, gemifloxacin maintains activity against these double mutants (even with a third mutation in *parE*) which, however, are resistant to ciprofloxacin [259,263,278,315,316]. In addition, resistance to fluoroquinolones in *S. pneumoniae* may be mediated by efflux systems, such as the PmrA multidrug transporter [260,317]. The combination of the overexpression of this system with mutations in the topoisomerase genes will provide the bacteria with higher levels of resistance to gemifloxacin [316].

In *E. coli* and *S. aureus*, mutations in topoisomerases would affect MIC values for gemifloxacin, but without reaching resistance levels. Besides, for significant resistance to gemifloxacin to exist in *E. coli*, the concurrence of a mutation in the *Mar*-controlled drug extrusion system [258,318] would be necessary. In *S. aureus*, the overexpression of the NorA expulsion system does not seem to influence sensitivity to gemifloxacin either, probably due to the fact that the voluminous substituents in position 7 of gemifloxacin prevent it from being a good substrate for the efflux pump [318].

Lastly, the reduction of permeability in some microorganisms does not seem to be an important mechanism of resistance to gemifloxacin. Thus, the mutations in the *nalB*, *nfxB* and *nfxC* genes, related with permeability in *P. aeruginosa*, a pathogen that is intrinsically less susceptible to gemifloxacin than to ciprofloxacin, do not entail an important variation in its susceptibility [258].

Pharmacology

The main pharmacokinetic parameters are shown in table 12 [319-324].

Table 12. Pharmacokinetic of gemifloxacin after multiple doses [319-324]

Parameters	Mean ± standar deviation
C_{max} (mg/l)	1.61 ± 0.51
T_{max} (min)	30-120
AUC (mg*h/l)	9.93 ± 3.07
Vd_{ss} (l/kg)	4.18
CL (ml/h/kg)	160
$T_{½}$ (h)	6-8

C_{max}: maximum plasma concentration; T_{max}: time to C_{max}; AUC: area under concentration-time curve, Vd_{ss}: apparent volume of distribution at steady state; CL: total clearance; $T_{½}$: elimination half-time.

Absorption

Pharmacokinetic studies have shown that gemifloxacin is quickly absorbed, with a bioavailability of 70%. Maximum concentrations are achieved approximately one hour after administration [319]. Both C_{max} and AUC are linear and dose-dependent and they are maintained basically stable after repeated administration at 24 hour intervals. These parameters are not altered due to the presence of fatty foods [320,324].

Distribution

It shows a very high volume of distribution, 4.18 l/kg for a dosage of 320 mg, a value that suggests a great distribution in the tissues, something important for the assessment of the effectiveness of the antibiotic in the treatment of intracellular bacterial infections [320]. Animal studies have shown that maximum concentration is achieved in organs such as liver, stomach, intestines and kidneys, with values between 9 and 25 times higher than plasma levels [323]. It achieves sufficient urine concentrations to eliminate most of the bacteria responsible for urinary tract infections [321]. Binding to plasma protein is about 70% and is not altered by age or kidney function [320,322,324].

Metabolism

Liver metabolism is very limited. CYP450 system does not play an important role in the metabolism of gemifloxacin [323].

Elimination

Gemifloxacin is eliminated in urine and faeces. Half-life is between 6 and 8 hours. Renal clearance is 160 ml/min after sole and multiple doses. About 20% to 35% of the dosage administered is excreted unaltered in urine 24 hours later, and data suggest the participation of active tubular excretion [320,321,324]. Faecal excretion occurs through biliary and gastrointestinal pathways [323].

Pharmacokinetics in Specific Situations

Age does not affect the pharmacokinetics of gemifloxacin in adults and there are no significant differences between men and women when differences in body weight are considered. Population pharmacokinetic studies show that after the administration of 320 mg of gemifloxacin, AUC values were 10% higher in healthy women than in healthy men; however, no gender-based dosage adjustment is necessary [325].

There were no significant changes in the plasma elimination half life in patients with slight, moderate or severe liver failure, so dosage adjustment is not recommended in any case [325]. In patients with renal failure, the results of the studies with repeated doses of 320 mg indicate that clearance of gemifloxacin is reduced and plasma clearance is prolonged, resulting in about 70% increase in AUC values. Pharmacokinetic studies show that gemifloxacin C_{max} was not significantly altered in subjects with renal failure. It is not necessary to adjust the dosage in patients with creatinine clearance above 40 ml/min. Dosage modification is recommended in patients with creatinine clearance equal to or less than 40 ml/min [325].

Adverse Effects

Gemifloxacin is a generally well tolerated antibiotic and may be compared to other fluorquinolones [257,263,326] when it comes to safety. The most common adverse effects observed in the various clinical trials, although with less than 10% incidence, were diarrhoea, skin rashes, headaches, abdominal pain, nausea, vomiting, dizziness, rhinitis, insomnia, arthralgias, myalgias, taste alteration and eye pain. Symptoms were slight or moderate and disappeared without any need for treatment [319,320,326-331].

In the clinical trials carried out by Vousden et al. the phototoxic dose-dependent effect of glemifloxacin was comparable to that which occurred in the placebo group and, in any case, very similar to the one produced by ciprofloxacin [332]. On the other hand, the incidence of phototoxicity was 0.04% in the trials carried out by Ball et al., there were only 0.1% cases of reversible tendinitis, no case of spontaneous rupture of tendons and no cases of angioedema, erythema multiforme, toxic skin necrolysis or Stevens-Johnson syndromes [328]. The 3-aminomethyl and 4-methyloximino substituents in position 7 are the groups responsible for the low incidence of neurotoxic effects [257].

Unlike other fluoroquinolones, gemifloxacin does not produce hypoglycaemia, so it may be coadministered with hypoglycaemic agents or with insulin [328]. Moderate alterations of hepatic transaminases have been observed, although their basal levels are recovered after the interruption of treatment [320,328]. There were no significant changes in the creatinine or urea levels in plasma, and the levels of N-acetylglucosamine and □2-microglobulin were within normalcy. Appearance of crystaluria was only referred in one individual [320]. No important changes were observed in the QT interval or in other electrocardiographic parameters [320,328]. In any case, the incidence of these effects was lower than in other quinolones and is comparable to what occurs with levofloxacin. Notwithstanding, precaution is recommended in the use of gemifloxacin in patients with risk factors like cardiac disease, hypokalaemia, and hypomagnesaemia, and in patients undergoing antiarrhythmic treatments or prior treatments with macrolides [257].

The incidence of skin reactions was directly related to the duration of the treatment, occurring most frequently in post-menopausal women undergoing hormone replacement therapy [263,328]. However, no relationship seems to exist between the incidence of this adverse event and the systemic exposure to gemifloxacin or N-acetyl gemifloxacin, its main metabolite [278]. Neither does it seem to produce any serious systemic effect, such as Stevens-Johnson syndrome or skin toxic necrolysis [333].

The same adverse events observed in clinical trials have been observed since the commercialization of gemifloxacin in 2003. Acute renal failure, gastritis and ventricular extrasystoles have been observed amongst the most serious adverse events related to the treatment [329]. Treatment with gemifloxacin may also cause pseudomembranous colitis [325].

In addition, gemifloxacin is able to strongly inhibit cytokine production (mainly IL-1a, IL-1b, IL-6, IL-10 and TNF-α) in monocytes. Although this phenomenon only occurs after a prolonged antibiotic treatment, its effects on the modulation of the immune system should be considered [334].

Clinical Indications

The FDA approved the use of gemifloxacin in 2003 as treatment for the following infectious processes [325]:

- Acute exacerbation of chronic bronchitis by *S. pneumoniae*, *H. influenzae*, *H. parainfluenzae* or *M. catarrhalis*.
- Slight to moderate community acquired pneumonia caused by *S. pneumoniae* (including MDRSP isolates), *H. influenzae*, *M. catarrhalis*, *M. pneumoniae*, *C. pneumoniae* or *K. pneumoniae*.

Some of the possible uses not considered by the FDA are diabetic foot infections (especially if there is a suspicion of a polymicrobial aetiology), otitis media, meningitis caused by *N. meningitidis* in children, intraabdominal infections and bone infections [257].

Gemifloxacin is counterindicated in patients who are hypersensitive to quinolones. Since no studies have been carried out in pregnant women (although it has been classified as foetal risk C category), breast-feeding mothers and children under 18 years, its use is not recommended except if the potential benefit surpasses the risk. On the contrary, no counterindication exists in the geriatric population, even in that with concomitant medication [325,328].

Telithromycin

Structure

Telithromycin is a semisynthetic derivative of erythromycin and the first component of the ketolide group, which in turn belongs to the family of macrolides [335,336]. The presence of the keto group in position 3 of the macrolide ring, in place of the cladinose sugar present in erythromycin is responsible for the fact that, unlike macrolides of 14 and 15 atoms, ketolides do not induce MLS_B type of resistance. The additional presence of a carbamate substituent in position C11-C12 allows the evasion of active efflux systems [335-337]. In addition, telithromycin is characterised by its butyl-imidazolyl-pyridinyl chain linked to the carbamate residue, which is responsible for increasing the affinity for the bacterial ribosome [335,337,338]. Lastly, and like clarithromycin, the chemical structure of telithromycin is completed with a methyl group in position C6 which results in a great stability at the gastrointestinal level (i.e., at acid pH), in addition to preventing the internal hemiketalization process [335,337].

Mechanism of Action

Ketolides share their mechanism of action with macrolides: they inhibit protein synthesis by preventing mRNA translation [336,339,340]. To accomplish this, they bind to the uppermost portion of the peptidic exit channel, close to the peptidyltransferase center of ribosomal subunit 50S, specifically, they interact with certain nucleotides in the II and V domains of subunit 23S of the rRNA. Telithromycin protects residues A2058, A2059 and G2505, localized in the central loop of domain V, and also residue A752 of domain II, from chemical modification, a fact that indicates there is direct contact between these nucleotides and the molecule of the antibiotic [341,342]. The presence of the butyl-imidazolyl-pyridinyl chain bound to the C11-C12 carbamate group in the structure of telithromycin is responsible for the high binding affinity for bacterial ribosome, higher than macrolides (10 times higher than erythromycin and 6 times higher than clarithromycin) [343]. According to Douthwaite et al., nucleotide A752 of domain II and nucleotides A2058, A2059 and G2505 of domain V limit the exit of the peptidic channel of subunit 50S by forming a pocket within which one single molecule interacts with both domains at the same time. This way the translation of mRNA as well as the growth of the emerging peptide are prevented, thus impeding its exit through the corresponding ribosomal channel, which has been blocked by the action of the drug [341].

In addition, telithromycin inhibits the assembly of the large ribosomal subunit. Its interaction with the 50S subunit precursors blocks this process and favours the degradation of said non-bound precursor particles by cell ribonucleases [335,337,338,343].

Spectrum of Activity

Telithromycin shows *in vitro* activity against Gram-positive and some Gram-negative bacteria, as well as against atypical respiratory pathogens, intracellular pathogens and protozoa. It is active against *Staphylococcus* spp., including MSSA isolates and macrolide-sensitive isolates. Although it maintains its activity against isolates expressing inducible MLS_B resistance, it is inactive against isolates with constituent MLS_B resistance [343-348]. It is also not considered active against MRSA isolates, since most of them carry the *erm* gene [337,343,347].

It is also active against *S. pneumoniae*, regardless of its susceptibility or resistance to penicillin, and it maintains a good activity against macrolide resistant isolates, either by alteration of the target or by active expulsion mechanisms [349]. It shows activity against erythromycin-susceptible *S. agalactiae* and *S. pyogenes*, inducible *ermB*⁺ and both inducible and constituent *ermTR*⁺, and against streptococci of the viridans group (including macrolide-resistant isolates) [349-356].

In spite of being the most active macrolide against macrolide-susceptible *Enterococcus* spp., it is not active against resistant isolates, such that its therapeutic use is not recommended for the treatment of infections caused by clinical isolates of this genus [347]. Other susceptible Gram-positive bacteria are *Lactobacillus* spp., *Pediococcus* spp., *Leuconostoc* spp., *E. rhusopathiae*, *Listeria* spp., *Micrococcus* spp. and *Stomatococcus* spp. [335].

As regards Gram-negative bacteria, it is active against respiratory pathogens such as *H. influenzae* and *M. catarrhalis* (β-lactamase-producing isolates, BRO-1 and -2 phenotypes and other β-lactam-resistant isolates), in a way similar to azithromycin, the most effective macrolide against these pathogens [357-359]. *B. pertussis*, *C. jejuni*, *H. ducreyi*, *G. vaginalis* and *Neisseria* spp. are also susceptible (including β-lactamase-producing isolates) [335,359]. However, it shows no activity against *Enterobacteriaceae* or non-fermenting bacilli [337,343,359,360]. Telithromycin has also proven to have *in vitro* activity against Gram-negative intracellular pathogens such as *L. pneumophila*, *C. pneumoniae*, *C. psitacii*, *C. trachomatis*, *Rickettsia* spp., *Bartonella* spp., *F. turalensis*, *B. burgdorferi*, *C. burnetti* and *R. equii* [335,337,343,348,361,362]. Other susceptible pathogens are *M. pneumoniae* and *U. urealyticum* [363,364].

Studies on the activity of telithromycin against anaerobic pathogens have revealed various results on the microorganism, since good results against *Propionibacterium* spp., *Peptostreptococcus* spp., *Porphyromonas* spp., *Prevotella* spp. and some species of *Clostridium* spp. such as *C. perfrigens* have been observed; however, its action is reduced against *C. difficile*, *Bacteroides* group *fragilis* and *Fusobacterium* spp., due to impermeability of the bacterial wall which prevents the diffusion of the macrolide [335,343,365,366].

In addition, telithromycin is moderately active against protozoa such as *T. gondii*, *Cryptosporidium* spp. and *Plasmodium* spp. and it shows variable activity against rapidly growing mycobacteria, although very small against those of slow growth [367].

Table 13 shows the *in vitro* activity of telithromycin against some of the abovementioned pathogens [344-370].

Table 13. *In vitro* activity of telithromycin against various microorganisms [344-370]

Microorganism	MIC_{50} (in µg/ml)	MIC_{90} (in µg/ml)
S. aureus		
Erythromycin-susceptible	0.06-0.25	0.25-2
Erythromycin-resistant		
Inducible	0.125	0.125
Constitutive	>128	>128
Methicillin-susceptible		
Erythromycin-S/Clindamycin-S	0.06	0.12
Erythromycin-R/Clindamycin-S	0.12	0.12
Erythromycin-R/Clindamycin-R	>64	>64
Methicillin-resistant		
Erythromycin-S/Clindamycin-S	0.5	-
Erythromycin-R/Clindamycin-S	0.12	0.12
Erythromycin-R/Clindamycin-R	>64	>64
Coagulase-negative staphylococci		
Methicillin-susceptible		
Erythromycin-S/Clindamycin-S	0.06	0.12
Erythromycin-R/Clindamycin-S	0.12	0.25
Erythromycin-R/Clindamycin-R	>64	>64
Methicillin -resistant		
Erythromycin-S/Clindamycin-S	0.06	0.12
Erythromycin-R/Clindamycin-S	0.06	0.25
Erythromycin-R/Clindamycin-R	>64	>64
S. pneumoniae		
Erythromycin susceptible	≤0.008-0.016	0.008-0.03
Erythromycin resistant		
mef$^+$	0.063-0.125	0.125-0.5
ermB$^+$	0.01-0.06	0.06-0.5
Erythromycin-S/Clindamycin-S	0.03	0.03
Erythromycin-R/Clindamycin-S	0.12-0.25	0.25-0.5
Erythromycin-R/Clindamycin-R	0.06	0.5-1
S. pyogenes		
Macrolide-susceptible	≤0.015	0.06
Macrolide-resistant		
erm (TR)$^+$ inducible	0.06	0.06
erm (B)$^+$ constitutive	8	64
mef (A)$^+$	0.06-0.5	0.25-1
Viridans group streptococci		
Erythromycin-susceptible	≤0.03	≤0.03
Erythromycin-resistant	0.06-0.12	1
S. agalactiae	0.016-0.12	0.016-0.05
H. influenzae	1-2	2
H. ducreyi	0.015	0.015
L. pneumophila	0.03	0.12
H. pylori	0.25	0.25
B. pertussis	0.03	0.06
C. jejuni	1	4
C. pneumoniae	0.06	0.125
M. catarrhalis	0.06	0.06-0.12
Neisseria spp.	0.015	0.12
Actinomyces spp.	≤0.03	≤0.03

Microorganism	MIC$_{50}$ (in µg/ml)	MIC$_{90}$ (in µg/ml)
Eubacterium spp.	≤0.03-0.5	>32
Propionibacterium spp	≤0.015	≤0.03
Peptostreptococcus spp.	0.01-0.12	0.06-4
Fusobacterium spp.	2-64	4->64
Prevotella spp.	0.06-0.25	0.25-4
Porphyromonas spp.	0.12	0.25
Bacteroides spp.	1-8	4- >64
M. pneumoniae	≤0.015	≤0.015
Ureaplasma spp.	0.03	0.25

Mechanism of Resistance

The mechanisms to resist macrolides include the modification of the target through methylase action, rRNA 23S and/or ribosomal protein mutation, inactivation of the antibiotic and its active efflux.

The first of these mechanisms is due to the action of the *erm* (*erythromycin resistance methylase*) gene codified methylases. These enzymes methylate the A2058 nucleotide and provoke a conformational change of the ribosome, thus reducing the affinity of the antibiotic for the 50S subunit. Its expression is characterized by cross-resistance to macrolides, lincosamides, and streptogramines B (MLS$_B$ resistance phenotype). The degree of resistance of MLS$_B$ isolates is dependant on the effectiveness in the rRNA methylation process [371]. Depending on the codifying gene, the methylase may incorporate one or two methyl groups to the nucleotide. Thus, monomethylation confers low to intermediate degree resistance to macrolides and B streptogramins, but a high degree of resistance to lincosamides; while dymethylation confers high degrees of resistance to all three groups and, in addition, resistance to telithromycin [340,367,371]. On the other hand, the expression of MLS$_B$ resistance may be constitutive (cMLS$_B$) or inducible (iMLS$_B$). When it is constitutive, isolates are resistant to all macrolides, lincosamides and streptogramines B. If the expression is inducible, isolates are resistant to 14 and 15 atom macrolides, while 16-atom macrolides, lincosamides and streptogramines, continue to be active. This dissociation of the resistance is due to the different inducing capacity of the antibiotics in this group, such that only 14 and 15-atom macrolides induce methylase synthesis [372]. Ketolides cannot induce this type of resistance, since they lack cladinose sugar in its molecular structure [336,338,343,347,367]. Notwithstanding, the capacity of telithromycin to transform *erm*(A)$^+$ staphylococci with iMLS$_B$ phenotype in cMLS$_B$ has been proven [373].

Other mechanisms of resistance that involve the modification of the rRNA structure were identified. Mutations or deletions in the II and V domains of the 23S rRNA [374] or in the L4 and L22 ribosomal proteins, which are close to the point of action of macrolides, i.e., adjacent to nucleotides A2058, A2059 and A752, confer resistance to those antibiotics mainly in *S. pneumoniae* isolates, but this was also observed in micoplasms, mycobacteria, *H. influenzae* and *H. pylori* [375-382]. Generally, due to a greater capacity of binding to the ribosome as a result of the presence of the butyl-imidazolyl-pyridinyl chain linked to the carbamate group, ketolides maintain their activity against this type of isolates [338,376].

Garza-Ramos et al. described a mutation in the 2609 position of the rRNA which confers resistance to ketolides, but not to macrolides, which contain cladinose in their molecule [383].

Another mechanism of resistance to macrolides is based on enzymatic inactivation of the antibiotic, either by sterase-mediated hydrolysis of the lactone ring or by phosphorilation/glycosilation in position C2' (place of desosamine sugar binding to rRNA 23S) [343,367]. The presence of phosphotransferases confers resistance to 14 and 15-atom macrolides, while the presence of sterases confers resistance to 16-carbon-atom macrolides. In *S. aureus*, sterase mph(C) also inactivates telithromycin [384].

Two types of macrolide efflux systems have been described as active expulsion mechanisms of the antibiotic: MS and M. The first appears in staphylococci and is characterized by resistance to 14-atom macrolides and to streptogramines B due to the expression of the *msr* (*macrolide streptogramin resistance*) gene. The M phenotype which appears in streptococci is, however, characterized by resistance to 14 and 15-atom macrolides as a consequence of the expression of an efflux pump codified by the *mef* (*macrolide efflux*) gene [375,376,]. Although ketolides act as inductors of both families of genes, they are not good substrates for active expulsion pumps, due to the presence of the carbamate group [343].

Lastly, Tripathi et al. described a mechanism conferring resistance to ketolides and macrolides through short peptides (3 to 6 aminoacids) codified by regions localized in subunit 23S of the rRNA. The expression of these genes may occur through mutation or degradation of the rRNA or by activation of these silent genes in the ribosome. Translation occurs in ribosomes and short peptides that emerge and expel the antibiotic from the ribosome. Peptides specifically interact with the molecular structure of the drug, so much that various sequences have been described amongst those that confer resistance to erythromycin, clarithromycin and telithromycin [385].

Pharmacology

The pharmacokinetics of telithromycin after administration of single and multiple once daily 800 mg doses to healthy adult subjects are shown in table 14 [386].

Table 14. Pharmacokinetic of telithromycin after administration of single and multiple once daily 800 mg doses to healthy adult subjects [386]

Parameter	Single dose	Multiple dose
C_{max} (mg/l)	1.9 (0.80)	2.27 (0.71)
AUC (mg*h/l)	8.25 (2.6)	12.5 (5.4)
CL_{24h} (mg/l)	0.03 (0.013)	0.07 (0.051)
$T_{1/2}$ (h)	7.16 (1.3)	9.81 (1.9)
T_{max} (h)	1.0 (0.5-4.0)	1.0 (0.5-3.0)

C_{max}: maximum plasma concentration; AUC: area under concentration-time curve, CL_{24h}: plasma concentration at 24 hours post-dose; $T_{1/2}$: elimination half-time; T_{max}: time to C_{max}.

Absorption

The absorption rate is fast, with a T_{max} of 1 hour [387]. C_{max} at the usual clinical dosages of 1.9 mg/l, increased in a manner proportional to the dose. Pharmacokinetic parameters are not modified due to the concomitant administration of the drug with food. A slight increase of the AUC has even been described in said situation [388].

It has an absolute bioavailability of 57% in both young and elderly subjects. Following oral dosing, the mean terminal elimination half-life of telithromycin is 10 hours [386].

Distribution

Total *in vitro* protein binding is approximately 60% to 70% [386]. Telithromycin (and macrolides) shows a wide penetration in body tissues and fluids. The volume of distribution of telithromycin after intravenous infusion is 2.9 l/kg. The plasma C_{max} is shown as reduced due to the fact that its rapid and large quantity diffusion to the tissues amounts to its fast disappearance from plasma although it shows an adequate bioavailability. A high volume of distribution of telithromycin suggests that this antibiotic suffers from significant tissular and, most probably, intracellular, incorporation with a high presence in macrophages and polymorphonuclear leukocytes [389]. Probably the slow exit of the drug towards the exterior of polymorphonuclear leukocytes and its high levels, maintained in time, in fibroblasts and macrophages, may suggest an explanation to the effective concentrations present at the place of the infection [390].

Mean white blood cell concentrations of telithromycin peaked at 72.1 μg/ml at 6 hours, and remained at 14.1 μg/ml 24 hours after 5 days of repeated dosing of 600 mg once daily. After 10 days, repeated dosing of 600 mg once daily, white blood cell concentrations remained at 8.9 μg/ml 48 hours after the last dose [386].

Metabolism

In total, metabolism accounts for approximately 70% of the dose. In plasma, the main circulating compound after administration of an 800 mg radiolabeled dose was parent compound, representing 56.7% of the total radioactivity. Approximately 37% of the dosage administered is metabolized in the liver by the action of isoenzimes CYP3A4 and CYP2D6 [391]. The main metabolite is an alcohol, RU-76363, which presents an *in vitro* activity between 4 and 16 times lower than the original molecule. The main metabolite represented 12.6% of the AUC of telithromycin. Three other plasma metabolites were quantified, each representing 3% or less of the AUC of telithromycin [386].

Elimination

93% of telithromycin dosage is eliminated in the faeces, although only 20% as the original molecule and about 12-17% of the dosage is eliminated unmetabolized in urine [390].

Pharmacokinetics in Specific Situations

The C_{max} and AUC values of telithromycin slightly increase in old-aged patients as a consequence of a reduction of the drug's clearance [392]. However, $T_{1/2}$ is not modified, so no dosage adjustment is needed in the absence of tolerance problems, in old-aged patients [386].

The administration of telithromycin in patients with slight or moderate kidney failure takes place with an increase in the C_{max} and AUC values amounting to 37% and 40-50%, respectively. Thus, it is recommended that patients with severe renal failure (creatinine clearance lower than 30 ml/min), with or without associated hepatic failure, be administered half of the dosage [386].

In spite of the compensating increase in renal clearance that occurs, the administration of telithromycin in patients with hepatic failure allows for the observation of a statistically significant increase in $T_{1/2}$ and C_{min} of the antibiotic. However, the scarce repercusion of these modifications does not actually require dosage adjustment [386].

Adverse Effects

Telithromycin is a generally well tolerated antibiotic. During phase III clinical trials, adverse effects were infrequent (0.2-2%) and slight to moderate in nature [393-402]. The most frequent effects were gastrointestinal and hepatic, such as diarrhoea (1.8-16.6%), vomiting (2.3-5.2%), nausea (1.8-10.5%), dyspepsia, dysgeusia, flatulence, anorexia, oral candidiasis, glositis, stomatitis, ALT and AST elevation (8.4%), hepatitis with or without jaundice (0.07%). Neurologic effects have also been described, such as somnolence, insomnia, anxiety, vertigo, cephalea o parestesias; skin effects such as rashes, eczema, pruritus, urticaria or multiform erythema, and visual effects such as blurred vision, diplopia or difficulty focusing. Other unwanted effects were bradychardia, low blood pressure, thrombocytosis (2.5-5.5%) [393,397], serum elevation of bilirubin and alkaline phosphatase and an increase in eosinophils and platelet counts [394].

After the commercialization of telithromycin, some severe effects have also been described, such as allergic reactions (including angioedema and anaphylaxis) [403], pill-induced esophagitis [404], pancreatitis, hepatotoxicity (including fulminant hepatitis) [405-408], kidney failure (severe acute interstitial nephritis) [409], cardiovascular alterations (atrial arrhythmias, palpitations, QTc prolongation), musculoskeletal alterations (muscle cramps, rare reports of exacerbation of myasthenia gravis) and nervous alterations (loss of consciousness) [410].

Clinical Indications

The FDA approved the use of telithromycin in 2004 for the treatment of community-acquired pneumonia (of mild to moderate severity) due to *S. pneumoniae*, (including MDRSP), *H. influenzae, M. catarrhalis, C. pneumoniae,* or *M. pneumoniae,* for patients 18 years old and above [386].

Telithromycin is counterindicated in patients hypersensitive to macrolides, as well as in patients with myasthenia gravis, or with a history of hepatitis and/or jaundice after treatment with macrolides [348,386]. Like with other antibiotics, treatment with telithromycin is associated to pseudomembranous cholitis [386].

Finally, it may be noted that telithromycin may result in QT interval prolongation in specific patients, with subsequent risk of ventricular arrhythmias. Thus, it is recommended that its usage be avoided in individuals with congenital prolongation of said interval, patients suffering from hypopotassemia or hypomagnesemia, clinically significant bradycardia, and in patients receiving antiarrhythmic agents [348,386]. In addition to this, and due to the visual alterations and loss of consciousness that may result because of treatment with telithromycin, it is advised that certain activities, such as motor vehicle driving, hard machinery handling or any other dangerous action, be avoided [386].

Tigecycline

Structure

Tigecycline or 9-t-butylglycylamido-minocycline ($C_{29}H_{39}N_5O_8$) is semisynthetically derived from minocycline [411]. Its was developed within a new group of antibiotics, glycylcyclines, to bypass the bacterian mechanisms to resist tetracyclines, both through ribosomal protection and through the expulsion of the antibiotic by means of efflux systems [412-414]. The presence of the N,N-dymethylglycylamide in position 9 of the minocycline molecule makes this feature of tigecycline possible, in addition to widening its spectrum of action [413-415].

Mechanism of Action

Tigecycline enters the cell through diffusion in Gram-positive microorganisms, but possibly through porins in Gram-negative bacteria, although several studies have shown that the loss of porins does not modify the activity of the antibiotic [416]. In the citoplasm, it reaches the 30S ribosomal unit and blocks protein synthesis [414,415,417-420]. The binding to the ribosome is reversible, something that would explain the bacteriostatic effect of this antibiotic on most bacteria, except for *S. pneumoniae*, *H. influenzae* and *N. gonorrhoeae*, against which it shows bactericide activity [415,421].

The activity of tigecycline and, above all, protection against the mechanisms of resistance against tetracyclines, would possibly be based on the fact that the binding to subunit 30S takes place with an orientation that is slightly different from that of other antibiotics of this same group, or that the configuration of the ribosome is altered to fit the volume of the 9-t-butylgycylamido group which is characteristic of this molecule [415].

Spectrum of Activity

Tigecycline shows excellent activity against most of the Gram-positive cocci and aerobic Gram-negative bacilli [421-424]. Amongst the Gram-positive pathogens, it is active against *S. aureus* (both MSSA and MRSA isolates, as well as GISA and GRSA), *S. epidermidis* and

S. haemolyticus (both susceptible and resistant to methicillin); against *S. pneumoniae* (including penicillin-resistant strains), *S. agalactiae*, *S. pyogenes* and the *S. anginosus* group; against *Enterococcus* spp., both susceptible and resistant to vancomycin, and against other Gram-positive bacteria, such as *L. monocytogenes* [414,415].

Table 15 summarizes the *in vitro* activity of tigecycline against different microorganisms, as well as their corresponding MIC_{50} and MIC_{90} in different studies [414,417,423,425-427,429].

**Table 15. *In vitro* activity of tigecycline in different bacterial species
[414,417,423,425-427,429]**

Microorganism	MIC_{50} (in µg/ml)	MIC_{90} (in µg/ml)
S. aureus		
Methicillin-susceptible	≤0.13-0.5	0.25-0.5
Methicillin-resistant	≤0.13-0.5	0.25-1
Vancomycin-intermediate	0.25	0.5
Vancomycin-resistant	0.125	0.125-0.5
Coagulase-negative sthaphylococci		
Methicillin-susceptible	0.25-0.5	0.25-1
Methicillin-resistant	0.5-1	0.25-1
Enterococcus spp.		
E. faecalis	0.06-0.25	0.125-0.5
E. faecium	0.06-0.25	0.06-0.25
E. avium	0.06	0.06
E. casseliflavus	0.13-0.25	0.13-0.25
E. gallinarum	0.13	0.13-0.25
E. raffinosus	0.06	0.13
S. pneumonie		
Penicillin-susceptible	0.03-0.25	0.06-0.25
Penicillin-intermediate	0.03-0.25	0.06-0.5
Penicillin-resistant	0.06-0.25	0.13-0.25
Tetracycline-susceptible	0.03	0.03
Tetracycline-resistant	0.03	0.03
Group A streptococci	0.06-0.13	0.06-0.25
Group B streptococci	0.06-0.13	0.06-0.25
Viridans group streptococci		
Penicillin-susceptible	0.06	0.25
Penicillin-resistant	0.03	0.06
Tetracycline-susceptible	0.03	0.06
Tetracycline-resistant	0.06	0.13
Enterobacteriaceae		
E. coli		
Non-ESBL producing	0.12-0.5	0.25-1
ESBL producing	0.13-0.25	0.5-1
Ciprofloxacin-susceptible	0-06-1	0-125-1
Cirpofloxacin-resistant	0.125-1	0.125-1
K. pneumoniae		

Non-ESBL producing	0.25-1	1-2
ESBL producing	0.25-1	1-4
K. oxytoca	0.5-1	1
M. morganii	2-4	4
P. mirabilis	2-4	4-8
P. vulgaris	4	4
Providencia spp.	4	8
Shigella spp.	0.25	0.5
Salmonella spp.	1	1
Citrobacter spp.	0.125-1	0.25-2
Enterobacter spp.	0.25- 1	0.5-2
S. marcencens	0.5-4	1-4
Gram-negative non-*Enterobactericeae*		
S. maltophilia	0.5-2	2-4
P. aeruginosa	8- >16	16-32
A. baumannii	0.5-4	1-8
B. cepacia	2-4	4-32
Gram-negative respiratory pathogens		
H. influenza	0.25-1	0.5-2
Moraxella spp.	0.06-0.13	0.13-0.25
N. gonorrhoeae		
Tetracycline-susceptible	0.06	0.13
Tetracycline-intermediate	0.13	0.25
Tetracycline-resistant	0.25	0.5
B. fragilis	0.13-4	0.13-8
C. perfringens	0.03-0.5	0.25-1
C. difficile	$\leq$0.06-0.13	0.03-0.125
P. acnes	0.03	0.06
Peptostreptococcus spp.	0.03-0.12	0.03-0.25
Fusobacterium spp.	0.02-0.06	0.06
Prevotella spp.	0.03-0.5	0.06-1
Porphyromonas spp.	0.03-0.06	0.06
M. abscessus		
Tetracycline-susceptible	$\leq$0.13	0.25
Tetracycline-resistant	$\leq$0.13	0.25
M. chelonae		
Tetracycline-susceptible	$\leq$0.06	$\leq$0.13
Tetracycline-resistant	$\leq$0.06	$\leq$0.13
M. fortuitum group		
Tetracycline-susceptible	$\leq$0.06	$\leq$0.13
Tetracycline-resistant	$\leq$0.06	$\leq$0.13
M. avium complex	$\geq$32	$\geq$32
M. lentiflavum	$\geq$32	$\geq$32
M. marinum	2-16	3-16
M. kansaii	16	32
C. pneumoniae	0.13	0.13
M. hominis		
Tetracycline-susceptible	0.25	0.5
Tetracycline-resistant	0.25	0.5
M. pneumoniae	0.13	0.25
U. urealyticum	4	8

It also shows remarkable *in vitro* activity against Gram-negative bacteria, including ESBL or carbapenemase producers, since it does not show cross-resistance with other antibiotic groups. It is active against *E. coli, K. pneumoniae, K. oxytoca, E. cloacae, C. freundii, S. marcescens, A. hydrophila, H. influenzae, M. catarrhalis, P. multocida* and *E. corrodens*, as well as against some non-fermenting bacilli, such as *A. baumannii, S. maltophilia, B. cepacia, B. pseudomallei* and *B. thailandensis* [414,417,423,425-427]. However, the susceptibility of certain active-expulsion system producing species, such as *P. aeruginosa* and others belonging to the *Proteus* spp. and *Providencia* spp., is reduced [414,415,428].

Its spectrum of activity also encompasses anaerobic bacteria, such as *B. fragilis, B. ovatus, B. distasonis, B. thetaiotaomicron, B. uniformis, B. vulgatus, Fusobacterium* spp., *Gemella* spp., *Peptostreptococcus* spp., *Porphyromonas* spp., *Prevotella* spp., *Propionibacterium* spp., *C. perfringens* or *C. difficile* [414,415,428].

Lastly, tigecycline is also active against *C. pneumoniae, C. trachomatis, M. pneumoniae, U. urealyticum* and *L. pneumophila*, in addition to atypical micobacteria such as *M. abscessus, M. chelonae* and *M. fortuitum* (both susceptible and resistant to tetracyclines). On the other hand, *M. avium-intracellulare, M. kansasii* and *M. marinum* show less susceptibility to this antibiotic [414,415,428].

Mechanism of Resistance

The tet(M) protein, coded at one transposon, when present in Gram-positive bacteria (such as streptococci, staphylococci and enterococci, mainly) or in *Neisseria* spp., prevents the binding of tetracyclines to the 30S ribosomal subunit and thus confers resistance to the bacteria [415,430]. However, the fact that tigecycline binds to the same region as the rest of tetracyclines, but with a different orientation and a greater affinity, results in making these microorganisms susceptible to this antibiotic, although they may express said resistance determinant [422,431].

Tet(A-E) proteins are active efflux pumps, specific for macrolydes and tetracyclines which are mainly present in *Enterobacteriaceae* and *Acinetobacter* spp. On the other hand, the presence of this type of pumps has also been described in *S. aureus*, although in this case they are codified by *tetK* [415,422,430-433]. Tigecycline is also able to avoid these resistance mechanisms because it is not an adequate substrate for this type of pumps, since the butylgycylamido group, part of the molecule, interferes with its expulsion outside the cell [434].

But the really worrying aspect nowadays, in relation to the spread of the resistance to tigecycline, is the overproduction of multidrug efflux systems, already observed in *S. aureus* (*multidrug and toxic-compound extrusion* or "MATE" family), or in Gram-negative bacteria [430,432,435-437]. Thus, the *ramA* [435] has been described in *K. pneumoniae,* which may be involved in the reduction of the sensitivity of this bacteria to tigecycline through the expression of the multidrug system AcrAB. The sensitivity to tigecycline may also be reduced in other Gram-negative microorganisms by different types of pumps, such as the

MexXY system in *P. aeruginosa* or AdeABC and AdeIJK in *A. baumannii* [422,428,432,435,437-439].

Lastly, the presence of the tet(X) protein has been described in *B. fragilis*, a flavine-dependent monooxygenase that incorporates a hydroxyl group to change into tigecycline and the result, hydroxy-tigecycline, is a molecule that is less active than its precursor. However, there are currently no clinical isolates with this type of resistance to tigecycline [440].

Pharmacology

Clinical studies have been carried out comparing a single dose (from 12.5 to 300 mg) against multiple doses (25, 50 or 100 mg every 12 hours), and, at the same time, volume and infusion rates to assess safety, tolerability and pharmacokinetics of the antibiotic [441]. The data relating to the pharmacokinetics of tigecycline come both from clinical trials carried out on healthy volunteers [442], and from phase III clinical trials on the treatment of skin and soft tissue infections (SSTIs) and complicated intraabdominal infections [443]. The final approved dosage was of 100 mg intravenously as loading dosage followed by a 50 mg perfusion every 12 hours [444].

The mean pharmacokinetic parameters of tigecycline after single and multiple intravenous doses based on pooled data from clinical pharmacology studies are summarized in table 16. Intravenous infusions of tigecycline were administered over approximately 30 to 60 minutes [444].

Table 16. Pharmacokinetic of tigecycline [444]

Dose	C_{max}[b] (mg/l)	C_{max}[c] (mg/l)	C_{min} (mg/l)	AUC (mg*h/l)	CL (l/h)	$T_{1/2}$ (h)
Single dose (100 mg)	1.45	0.90	-	5.19	21.8	27.1
Multiple dose[a]	0.87	0.63	0.13	-	23.8	42.4

[a] 100 mg initially, followed by 50 mg every 12 hours; [b] 30 minute infusion; [c] 60 minute infusion. C_{max}: maximum plasma concentration; C_{min}: minimum plasma concentration ; AUC: area under concentration-time curve; CL: systemic clearance; $T_{1/2}$: elimination half-time.

Absorption
Tigecycline is administered intravenously and, therefore, has a bioavailability of 100%.

Distribution
It binds to plasmatic protein in a range that goes from 71%, at a plasma level of 0.1 mg/l, up to 89% at a concentration of 1.0 mg/l [444].

The tissue distribution volume of tigecycline is wide (>10 l/kg) and the antibiotic reaches high levels in various tissues [445]. Thus, 4 hours after a single endovenous dosage of 100 mg, concentrations in the biliary vesicle, lungs and colon were 38, 8.6, and 2.1 times higher than the plasma levels, respectively, while the synovial fluid or the bones showed lower levels (0.58 and 0.35 times, respectively) than those of plasma [446]. The level of tigecycline in these tissues has not been studied after the administration of multiple doses.

In the case of healthy individuals being administered a 100 mg dosage followed by a perfusion of 50 mg every 12 hours, a C_{max} of 15.2 µg/ml, an AUC_{0-12} of 134 mg*h/l (77.5 times higher than the AUC_{0-12} in the serum of these individuals) and a $T_{1/2}$ of 23.7 hours was achieved in alveolar cells [447]. The level of tigecycline in alveolar cells is therefore much higher than in serum, which explains its usefulness in the treatment of infections in the lower respiratory airways. Additionally, a study on skin blisters (flictenas) showed the AUC_{0-12} (1.61 mg*h/ml) of tigecycline in blister fluid to be approximately 26% lower than the ABC_{0-12} in the serum of these individuals [448].

Metabolism

Tigecycline shows scarce metabolism. Healthy male volunteers who received radiolabelled tigecycline expelled the substance in urine and faeces, but some products of its metabolism such as a glucuronid, an N-acetyl metabolite and a tigecycline epimer were also expelled (each of them in no more than 10% of the administered dosage) [449].

Elimination

Using radio-marked tigecycline it was shown that 59% of administered tigecycline is eliminated by means of biliary/faecal excretion, mostly unaltered, and 33% through urinary excretion [441,449]. Tigecycline is excreted unaltered in urine (15% of the total) and renal clearance is less than 20% of total clearance [441,448]. In practice, tigecycline pharmacokinetics is not affected by renal function or by haemodialysis, and also not significantly affected by meals [445].

Pharmacokinetics in Specific Situations

The effect of age and sex on tigecycline pharmacokinetics has been studied in healthy volunteers from three different age groups (18 to 50 years, 65 to 75 years and over 75 years). When administered a sole dosage of 100 mg in 1 hour infusion, C_{max} is equivalent in all groups (0.85-1 mg/l), while AUC is lowest in under 50-year-old males and highest in over-75 year old males [448]. Adjustment of doses according to age or sex is not necessary [450].

In cases of complicated intraabdominal infection and complicated skin and soft tissue infections caused by *S. aureus* and streptococci, the predictor of tigecycline response is the rate at steady-state of AUC and MIC (AUC/MIC). The cutting point of AUC/MIC is 6.96 for microbiology response ($p=0.0004$) in the case of intraabdominal infection [451] and of 17.9 ($p=0.0001$) in Gram-positive bacteria infections [452].

In sole dosage studies no alteration of tigecycline pharmacokinetics has been observed in patients with slight liver failure. However, in patients with moderate to severe liver failure, the half-life of elimination increases in about 23-43% and clearance is reduced in 25-55%, respectively [453]. Based on the pharmacokinetic profile of tigecycline, adjustment of the dosage is not justified for patients with slight to moderate liver failure (Child-Pugh A or B).

However, in severe liver failure patients (Child-Pugh C) the dosage of tigecycline should be reduced to 100 mg followed later by 25 mg every 12 hours.

In patients with creatinine clearance lower than 30 ml/min, pharmacokinetic parameters of tigecycline are not altered. In patients with severe kidney failure, the AUC increases in about 30% with regards to individuals with normal renal function. Adjustment of the dosage is not necessary in patients with kidney failure or undergoing haemodialysis [443].

Adverse Effects

The most common adverse events observed during the clinical trials were gastrointestinal (nausea and vomiting), with a frequency exceeding 10% of the individuals [414,415,418,428,431,454-459]. Said symptoms were slight and disappeared with the interruption of the antibiotic treatment in most cases [431]. In addition, it was observed that the appearance of these events was dose-related and they were more frequent in women than in men [455,458]. Other, less frequent, adverse events included vertigo, phlebitis, abdominal pain, dyspepsia, anorexia, pruritus, headaches or transaminase abnormalities [454].

Studies carried out after the commercialization of tigecycline have shown the appearance of other adverse events, such as the possibility of pseudomembranous colitis or acute pancreatitis episodes [458,459]. This last process is recognized as an adverse event derived from tetracycline therapy, but not from that of tigecycline. However, in 2007 and for the first time, 24 cases of acute pancreatitis were described after an average of 8.5 days of tigecycline treatment [460]. More recently, Gilson et al. has published another acute pancreatitis case after 13 days of treatment with this antibiotic [455]. This author points out that the possibility of affecting the pancreas may be related to the preferred elimination of this antibiotic through the biliary system, a level at which it reaches a concentration that is 500 times higher than that of plasma.

Clinical Indications

The FDA approved the use of tigecycline in 2005 as treatment for the following infectious processes [444]:

- Complicated skin and soft tissue infections produced by *S. aureus* (MSSA and MRSA isolates), *E. faecalis* (only vancomycin-sensitive isolates), *S. agalactiae*, the *S. anginosus* group (including *S. anginosus, S. intermedius* and *S. constellatus*), *S. pyogenes*, *E. coli* and *B. fragilis.*
- Complicated intraabdominal infections caused by *E. coli*, *K. pneumoniae*, *K. oxytoca*, *C. freundii*, *E. cloacae*, *E. faecalis* (only vancomycin-sensitive isolates), *S. aureus* (only MSSA isolates), the *S. anginosus* group, *B. fragilis, B. thetaiotaomicron, B. uniformis*, *B. vulgatus*, *C. perfringens* and *P. micros* group.

Regarding these clinical indications, the most important application of this antibiotic would be to treat the infection of deep injuries after an abdominal surgery (usually produced by pathogens such as MRSA, *Enterobacteriaceae*, streptococci and anaerobic pathogens) and for the treatment of skin and soft tissue infections caused by MRSA and/or Gram-negative bacteria [431]. However, the administration of tigecycline would not be indicated in patients with uncomplicated infections at these locations or in those where other therapeutic alternatives are available [456].

Neither is its use recommended as treatment against serious infections caused by *P. aeruginosa* or *Proteus* spp. [414,415], against which activity has not been shown. Also, since it shows mainly biliary elimination, it is not indicated for the treatment of urinary tract infections, due to the scarce concentration achieved in the urine [431,442].

Some recent studies show the efficacy of tigecycline against other type of infections initially not included, such as community-acquired pneumonias [461] or other infections caused by multi-resistant microorganisms [462].

In this sense, treatment against community-acquired pneumonias caused by *S. pneumoniae* has traditionally included the administration of fluoroquinolones and β-lactam agents in conjunction with macrolides. However, the appearance of pneumococci isolates resistant to these antibiotics [463] has resulted in the search for alternative therapies, thus marking the start of the use of tigecycline against this pathogen, since its capacity to penetrate the pulmonary tissue is also known to be good. According to Tanaseanu et al. monotherapy with tigecycline is as effective as treatment with levofloxacine in community-acquired pneumonias caused by *S. pneumoniae*, and even by less frequent microorganisms such as *H. influenzae*, *M. catarrhalis*, *C. pnemoniae*, *M. pneumoniae* or *L. pneumophila* [461].

The same reasons are used to consider using tigecycline against multi-resistant pathogens. Thus, this antibiotic has shown adequate activity in tests carried out against the different species of *Acinetobacter* spp., including carbapenemase-producing isolates [462]. However, these results were received with caution, since more studies are deemed necessary to determine whether tigecycline is a good therapeutic alternative against multi-resistant pathogen infections [422].

Lastly, this antibiotic is contraindicated for patients that are hypersensitive to tetracyclines and for pregnant women, due to the risk of fetal damage [457]. As with the rest of tetracyclines, it may have a damaging effect on ossification and dentition so it is also not recommended for breastfeeding mothers or patients under 18 years of age [415].

Retapamulin

Structure

Retapamulin or (3S,4R,5S,6S,8R,9R,10R)-6-ethenyl-5-hydroxy-4,6,9,10-tetramethyl-1-oxodecahydro-3,9-propano-3-cyclopenta[8]annulen-8-yl{[(1R,3s,5S)-8-methyl-8-azabicyclo[3.2.1]oct-3-yl]sulfanyl}acetate is the first semisynthetic pleuromutilin adequate for topic use in humans [464-467]. It was developed as a sulfanyl-acetate derivative of pleuromutilin, a natural product obtained from the fermentation of the fungus *Pleurotus mutilus* (now called *Clitopilus scyphoides*) and it is characterized by its wide spectrum of action, although its bioavailability is limited [468].

Mechanism of Action

Pleuromutilins are a group of antibiotics which, until the appearance of retapamulin, were restricted to veterinary use [464,469]. They act by inhibiting bacterial protein synthesis, specifically preventing the formation of peptidic links. To achieve this, pleuromutilins interact with the subunit 50S of the bacterial ribosome thus preventing peptidic transfer, but in a manner different from that of other antibiotics that also act at this level, like macrolides, mupirocin or fusidic acid, such that it does not show cross-resistance with them [468-474].

Spectrum of Activity

Retapamulin presents excellent *in vitro* activity against microorganisms responsible for skin and soft tissue infections, especially against Gram-positive bacteria such as *S. aureus* (both MRSA and MSSA isolates), coagulase-negative staphylococci, *S. pyogenes*, *S. agalactiae*, *S. viridans* group, *Corynebacterium* spp. or *Micrococcus* spp. It is also active against some respiratory pathogens, such as *S. pneumoniae*, *H. influenzae* or *M. catarrhalis*, including those isolates resistant to other antibiotics (such as β-lactams, macrolides, quinolones, fusidic acid or mupirocin) [464-466,471-476]. It also shows activity against anaerobic bacteria such as *Propionibacterium* spp., including isolates resistant to cotrimoxazole, erythromycin, clindamycin and tetracycline; *B. fragilis* group, including β-lactamase-producing isolates, clindamycin-resistant *C. clostridioforme*, *Prevotella* spp., *Porphyromonas* spp. and *Fusobacterium* spp. [471,472]. On the contrary, activity against enterococci is minimal, as against non-fermenting and Gram-negative pathogens such as *Enterobacteriaceae* [473].

It should be noted that *in vitro* susceptibility of MRSA to retapamulin does not correspond to results obtained *in vivo*. Thus, its clinical application is not recommended in patients with infections caused by these isolates, due to the possibility of therapeutic failure, a phenomenon that may be due to the presence of several virulence factors, such as Panton-Valentine leukocidin (PVL) in *S. aureus* isolates [477].

Table 17 summarizes the activity of retapamulin against different microorganisms in terms of MIC_{50} and MIC_{90} [464,466,471-473].

Mechanism of Resistance

Retapamulin shows a low capacity of resistance selection [466,470]. It has been proven in *S. aureus* and *S. pyogenes* that the capacity to select retapamulin resistance is lower than that produced by mupirocin or by fusidic acid, two topic antibiotics commonly used in the treatment of skin and soft tissue infections [476].

Table 17. *In vitro* activity of retapamulin against various microorganisms
[464,466,471-473]

Microorganism	MIC$_{50}$ (in µg/ml)	MIC$_{90}$ (in µg/ml)
S. aureus		
MSSA	0.06-0.12	0.12
MRSA	0.06-0.12	0.12
Mupirocin-susceptible	0.06	0.12
Mupirocin-resistant	0.06	0.12
Coagulase-negative staphylococci		
Methicillin-susceptible	0.12	4
Methicillin-resistant	0.06	0.12
Mupirocin-susceptible	≤0.03	0.06
Mupirocin-resistant	≤0.03	0.06
S. pneumoniae	0.06	0.12
S. agalactiae	0.016-0.03	0.03
S. pyogenes	0.08-0.016	0.016-0.03
Enterococcus spp.	64	128
H. influenzae	0.5	2
M. catarrhalis	0.3	0.3
B. fragilis	0.25	64
Clostridium spp.	0.5	64
Fusobacterium spp.	≤0.015	2
Prevotella spp.	≤0.015	0.03
Porphyromonas spp.	≤0.015	≤0.015
Propionibacterium spp.	≤0.015-0.125	0.25

Two of the main mechanisms causing resistance to pleuromutilins are mutations of the *rplC* gene, which codifies ribosomal protein L3 of subunit 50S, as well as the presence of unspecified efflux systems in the bacteria, such as the ABC-type efflux transporter vga(Av) system, which is also responsible for the reduction of susceptibility to lincosamides and streptogramin A [469,473,478]. In addition, susceptibility to pleuromutilins may be affected by the presence of a Cfr-rRNA methyltransferase [469,473].

Pharmacology

Table 18 shows the main pharmacokinetic parameters of retapamulin in healthy volunteers who were administered ointment 1% once a day for at least 7 days on whole skin or on abrasions [477,479].

Absorption

The value of C_{max} after the daily application of ointment 1% (and subsequent coverage of the area using a drape) on 800 cm^2 of whole skin surface was 3.5 ng/ml on day 7 (range of 1.2 to 7.8 ng/ml), and after the application on 200 cm^2 of eroded skin it was 9.0 ng/ml (range of 6.7 to 12.8 ng/ml). The absorption of retapamulin depends on the skin surface exposed to the drug and on whether the skin is whole or has suffered abrasions. C_{max} is higher when occlusive or semi-occlusive bandages are used than when they are not used [477,479].

Table 18. Pharmacokinetic of retapamulin after application on whole skin and abrasions, in healthy volunteers [477,479]

Parameter	Mean (range)	
	Whole skin	Skin abrasions
C_{max} (ng/ml)	3.5 (1.2-7.8)	9.0 (6.7-12.8)
AUC (ng*h/ml)	49.9	134.9
T_{max} (h)	22.4 (16.0-24.0)	22.5 (0.0-22.6)

C_{max}: maximum plasma concentration; AUC: area under concentration-time curve; T_{max}: time to C_{max}.

Distribution

About 94% of retapamulin binds to plasma proteins, regardless of the concentration. Apparent volume distribution has not been determined in humans [477,479].

Metabolism

Studies have shown that retapamulin metabolizes extensively through cytochrome P450, mainly through the mono-oxygenation and N-demethylation pathways [477,479].

Elimination

The elimination of retapamulin is unknown due to the low systemic exposure to the drug after topical application [477,479].

Pharmacokinetics in Specific Situations

The pharmacokinetic characteristics of retapamulin have not been studied in patients younger than 2 years old or in patients with renal or hepatic failure [477,479].

Adverse Effects

Adverse effects derived from treatment with retapamulin and described during the clinical trial period have been scarce and slight to moderate in nature. Irritation, skin rash or local pains (on the site of application) may be noted, with a frequency similar to that observed after the application of mupirocin (1.4-6.5% of cases). Other effects with lower incidence were nasopharyngitis (3%), headaches (2%), skin dryness (0.7%) and paresthesias (0.7%) [465,476,480].

Clinical Indications

Retapamulin was approved in 2007 by the FDA for topical treatment of superficial skin infections, such as impetigo caused by *S. aureus* (only MSSA isolates) or *S. pyogenes*, small infected lacerations, abrasions and sutured lesions [477]. In Europe it has also been granted license for the treatment of open-wound infections caused by the same microorganisms [479].

Currently several studies are underway to determine the usefulness of this antibiotic against other skin and soft tissue infections, especially those caused by MRSA isolates [473].

Retapamulin is counterindicated in people with hypersensitivity to said antibiotic or to any of its excipients, such as butylated hydroxytoluene, possible cause of local skin reactions, and ocular or mucosa irritation. No data is available on the use of this antibiotic on infants or on pregnant women (it is considered a class B foetal risk), a reason for which caution is advised in its prescription, even though it may be administered to such patients if a systemic antibiotic is deemed unadvisable.

References

[1]   Slama TG. Gram-negative antibiotic resistance: There is a price to pay. *Crit. Care*, 2008; 12 (Suppl 4): S4.

[2]   Aksoy DY, Unal S. New antimicrobial agents for the treatment of Gram-positive bacterial infections. *Clin. Microbiol. Infect.*, 2008; 14: 411-20.

[3]   Chien JW, Kucia ML, Salata RA. Use of linezolid, an oxazolidinone, in the treatment of multidrug-resistant gram-positive bacterial infections. *Clin. Infect. Dis.*, 2000; 30: 146-51.

[4]   Balbisi EA. Cefditoren, a new aminothiazolyl cephalosporin. *Pharmacotherapy*, 2002; 22: 1278-93.

[5]   Odenholt I. Ertapenem: A new carbapenem. *Expert Opin. Investig. Drugs*, 2001; 10: 1157-66.

[6]   Limited AI. Doripenem: S4661. *Drugs R.D.*, 2003; 4: 363-5.

[7]   Tally FP, DeBruin MF. Development of daptomycin for gram-positive infections. *J. Antimicrob. Chemother.*, 2000; 46: 523-6..

[8]   Lowe MN, Lamb HM. Gemifloxacin. *Drugs*, 2000; 59: 1137-47.

[9]   Wellington K, Noble S. Telithromycin. *Drugs*, 2004; 64: 1683-94.

[10]   Rubinstein E, Vaughan D. Tigecycline: A novel glycylcycline. *Drugs*, 2005; 65: 1317-36.

[11]   Yang LP, Keam SJ. Retapamulin: A review of its use in the management of impetigo and other uncomplicated superficial skin infections. *Drugs*, 2008; 68: 855-73.

[12]   Brickner SJ, Hutchinson DK, Barbachyn MR, Manniner PR, Ulanowicz DA, Garmon SA, et al. Synthesis and antibacterial activity of U-100592 and U-100766, two oxazolidinone antibacterial agents for the potential treatment of multidrug-resistant gram-positive bacterial infections. *J. Med. Chem.*, 1996; 39: 673-9.

[13]   Livermore DM. Linezolid in vitro: mechanism and antibacterial spectrum. *J. Antimicrob. Chemother.*, 2003; 51 (Suppl 2): ii9–16.

[14]   Carmona PM, Romá E, Monte E, García J, Gobernado M. Role of linezolid in antimicrobial therapy. *Enferm. Infecc. Microbiol. Clin.*, 2003; 21: 30-41

[15]   Moellering RC. Linezolid: The first oxazolidinone antimicrobial. *Ann. Intern. Med.*, 2003; 138: 135-42.

[16] Leach KL, Swaney SM, Colca JR, McDonald WG, Blinn JR, Thomasco LM, et al. The site of action of oxazolidinone antibiotics in living bacteria and in human mitochondria. *Mol. Cell.*, 2007; 26: 393-402.

[17] Pigrau C. Oxazolidinones and Glycopeptides. *Enferm. Infecc. Microbiol. Clin.*, 2003; 21: 157-65.

[18] Schumacher A, Trittler R, Bohnert JA, Kümmerer K, Pagès JM, Kern WV. Intracellular accumulation of linezolid in *Escherichia coli*, *Citrobacter freundii* and *Enterobacter aerogenes*: role of enhanced efflux pump activity and inactivation. *J. Antimicrob. Chemother.*, 2007; 59: 1261-4

[19] Cercenado E, García-Garrote F, Bouza E. In vitro activity against multiply resistant Gram-positive clinical isolates. *J. Chemother.*, 2001; 47: 77-81.

[20] Diekema DJ, Jones RN. Oxazolidinone antibiotics. *Lancet*, 2001; 358: 1975–82.

[21] Zhanel GG, DeCorby M, Nichol KA, Wierzbowski A, Baudry PJ, Karlowsky JA, et al. Antimicrobial susceptibility of 3931 organisms isolated from intensive care units in Canada: Canadian National Intensive Care Unit Study, 2005/2006. *Diagn. Microbiol. Infect. Dis.*, 2008; 62: 67–80.

[22] Tarazona RE, Padilla TP, Gomez JC, Sanchez JE, Hernandez MS. First report in Spain of linezolid non-susceptibility in a clinical isolate of *Staphylococcus haemolyticus*. *Int. J. Antimicrob. Agents*, 2007; 30: 277-8.

[23] Tsiodras S, Gold HS, Sakoulas G, Eliopoulos GM, Wennersten C, Venkataraman L, et al. Linezolid resistance in a clinical isolate of *Staphylococcus aureus*. *Lancet*, 2001; 358: 207-8

[24] Werner G, Strommenger B, Klare I, Witte W. Molecular detection of linezolid resistance in *Enterococcus faecium* and *Enterococcus faecalis* by use of 5' nuclease real-time PCR compared to a modified classical approach. *J. Clin. Microbiol.*, 2004; 42: 5327-31.

[25] Arias CA, Vallejo M, Reyes J, Panesso D, Moreno J, Castañeda E, et al. Clinical and microbiological aspects of linezolid resistance mediated by the *cfr* gene encoding a 23S rRNA methyltransferase. *J. Clin. Microbiol.*, 2008; 46: 892-6.

[26] Scheetz MH, Knechtel SA, Malczynski M, Postelnick MJ, Qi C. Increasing incidence of linezolid-intermediate or -resistant, vancomycin-resistant *Enterococcus faecium* strains parallels increasing linezolid consumption. *Antimicrob. Agents Chemother.*, 2008; 52: 2256-9.

[27] Wolter N, Smith AM, Farrell DJ, Schaffner W, Moore M, Whitney CG, et al. Novel mechanism of resistance to oxazolidinones, macrolides, and chloramphenicol in ribosomal protein L4 of the pneumococcus. *Antimicrob. Agents Chemother.*, 2005; 49: 3554-7.

[28] Hong T, Li X, Wang J, Sloan C, Cicogna C. Sequential linezolid-resistant *Staphylococcus epidermidis* isolates with G2576T mutation. *J. Clin. Microbiol.*, 2007; 45: 3277–80.

[29] Saager B, Rohde H, Timmerbeil BS, Franke G, Pothmann W, Dahlke J, et al. Molecular characterisation of linezolid resistance in two vancomycin-resistant (Van B) *Enterococcus faecium* isolates using Pyrosequencing™. *Eur. J. Clin. Microbiol. Infect. Dis.*, 2008; 27: 873-8.

[30]   Kelly S, Collins J, Maguire M, Gowing C, Flanagan M, Donnelly M, et al. An outbreak of colonization with linezolid-resistant *Staphylococcus epidermidis* in an intensive therapy unit. *J. Antimicrob. Chemother.*, 2008; 61: 901–7.

[31]   Meka VG, Pillai SK, Sakoulas G, Wennersten C, Venkataraman L, DeGirolami PC, et al. Linezolid resistance in sequential *Staphylococcus aureus* isolates associated with a T2500A mutation in the 23S rRNA gene and loss of a single copy of rRNA. *J. Infect. Dis.*, 2004; 190: 311-7.

[32]   Schwarz S, Werckenthin C, Kehrenberg C. Identification of a plasmid-borne chloramphenicol-florfenicol resistance gene in *Staphylococcus sciuri*. *Antimicrob. Agents Chemother.*, 2000; 44: 2530-3.

[33]   Toh SM, Xiong L, Arias CA, Villegas MV, Lolans K, Quinn J, et al. Acquisition of a natural resistance gene renders a clinical strain of methicillin-resistant *Staphylococcus aureus* resistant to the synthetic antibiotic linezolid. *Mol. Microbiol.*, 2007; 64: 1506-14.

[34]   Mendes RE, Deshpande LM, Castanheira M, DiPersio J, Saubolle MA, Jones RN. First report of *cfr*-mediated resistance to linezolid in human staphylococcal clinical isolates recovered in the United States. *Antimicrob. Agents Chemother.*, 2008; 52: 2244-6.

[35]   Zyvox™ [package insert]. Kalamazoo, MI: Pharmacia and Upjohn Company, 2000.

[36]   Stalker DJ, Jungbluth GL, Hopkins NK, Batts DH. Pharmacokinetics and tolerance of single- and multiple-dose oral or intravenous linezolid, an oxazolidinone antibiotic, in healthy volunteers. *J. Antimicrob. Chemother.*, 2003; 51: 1239-46.

[37]   Stalker DJ, Jungbluth GL. Clinical pharmacokinetics of linezolid, a novel oxazolidinone antibacterial. *Clin. Pharmacokinet.*, 2003; 42: 1129-40.

[38]   Grunder G, Zysset-Aschmann Y, Vollenweider F, Maier T, Krähenbühl S, Drewe J. Lack of pharmacokinetic interaction between linezolid and antacid in healthy volunteers. *Antimicrob. Agents Chemother.*, 2006; 50: 68-72.

[39]   Beringer P, Nguyen M, Hoem N, Louie S, Gill M, Gurevitch M, et al. Absolute bioavailability and pharmacokinetics of linezolid in hospitalized patients given enteral feedings. *Antimicrob. Agents Chemother.*, 2005; 49: 3676-81.

[40]   Welshman IR, Sisson TA, Jungbluth GL, Stalker DJ, Hopkins NK. Linezolid absolute bioavailability and the effect of food on oral bioavailability. *Biopharm. Drug Dispos.*, 2001; 22: 91-7.

[41]   Dehghanyar P, Bürger C, Zeitlinger M, Islinger F, Kovar F, Müller M, et al. Penetration of linezolid into soft tissues of healthy volunteers after single and multiple doses. *Antimicrob. Agents Chemother.*, 2005; 49: 2367-71.

[42]   Slatter JG, Stalker DJ, Feenstra KL, Welshman IR, Bruss JB, Sams JP, et al. Pharmacokinetics, metabolism, and excretion of linezolid following an oral dose of [(14)C] linezolid to healthy human subjects. *Drug Metab. Dispos.*, 2001; 29: 1136-45.

[43]   Jungbluth GL, Welshman IR, Hopkins NK. Linezolid pharmacokinetics in pediatric patients: an overview. *Pediatr. Infect. Dis. J.*, 2003; 22: S153-7.

[44]   Lyseng-Williamson KA, Goa KL. Linezolid: in infants and children with severe Gram-positive infections. *Paediatr. Drugs*, 2003; 5: 419-29; discussion 430-1.

[45]   Sisson TL, Jungbluth GL, Hopkins NK. Age and sex effects on the pharmacokinetics of linezolid. *Eur. J. Clin. Pharmacol.*, 2002; 57: 793-7.

[46] Tsuji Y, Hiraki Y, Mizoguchi A, Hayashi W, Kamohara R, Kamimura H, et al. Pharmacokinetics of repeated dosing of linezolid in a hemodialysis patient with chronic renal failure. *J. Infect. Chemother.*, 2008; 14: 156-60.

[47] Metallidis S, Nikolaidis J, Lazaraki G, Koumentaki E, Gogou V, Topsis D, et al. Penetration of linezolid into sternal bone of patients undergoing cardiopulmonary bypass surgery. *Int. J. Antimicrob. Agents*, 2007; 29: 742-4.

[48] Majcher-Peszynska J, Haase G, Sass M, Mundkowski R, Pietsch A, Klammt S, et al. Pharmacokinetics and penetration of linezolid into inflamed soft tissue in diabetic foot infections. *Eur. J. Clin. Pharmacol.*, 2008; 64: 1093-100.

[49] Stein GE, Schooley S, Peloquin CA, Missavage A, Havlichek DH. Linezolid tissue penetration and serum activity against strains of methicillin-resistant *Staphylococcus aureus* with reduced vancomycin susceptibility in diabetic patients with foot infections. *J. Antimicrob. Chemother.*, 2007; 60: 819-23.

[50] Boselli E, Breilh D, Rimmelé T, Djabarouti S, Toutain J, Chassard D, et al. Pharmacokinetics and intrapulmonary concentrations of linezolid administered to critically ill patients with ventilator-associated pneumonia. *Crit. Care Med.*, 2005; 33: 1529-33.

[51] Saralaya D, Peckham DG, Hulme B, Tobin CM, Denton M, Conway S, et al. Serum and sputum concentrations following the oral administration of linezolid in adult patients with cystic fibrosis. *J. Antimicrob. Chemother.*, 2004; 53: 325-8.

[52] Whitehouse T, Cepeda JA, Shulman R, Aarons L, Nalda-Molina R, Tobin C, et al. Pharmacokinetic studies of linezolid and teicoplanin in the critically ill. *J. Antimicrob. Chemother.*, 2005; 55: 333-40.

[53] Adembri C, Fallani S, Cassetta MI, Arrigucci S, Ottaviano A, Pecile P, et al. Linezolid pharmacokinetic/pharmacodynamic profile in critically ill septic patients: intermittent versus continuous infusion. *Int. J. Antimicrob. Agents*, 2008; 31: 122-9.

[54] Ament PW, Jamshed N, Horne JP. Linezolid: its role in the treatment of Gram-positive, drug-resistant bacterial infections. *Am. Fam. Physician*, 2002; 65: 663-70.

[55] French G. Safety and tolerability of linezolid. *J. Antimicrob. Chemother.*, 2003; 51: Suppl 2, ii45–ii53.

[56] Azamfirei L, Copotoiu SM, Branzaniuc K, Szederjesi J, Copotoiu R, Berteanu C. Complete blindness after optic neuropathy induced by short-term linezolid treatment in a patient suffering from muscle dystrophy. *Pharmacoepidemiol. Drug Saf*, 2007; 16: 402-4.

[57] Bressler AM, Zimmer SM, Gilmore JL, Somani J. Peripheral neuropathy associated with prolonged use of linezolid. *Lancet Infect. Dis.*, 2004; 4: 528-31.

[58] Ferry T, Ponceau B, Simon M, Issartel B, Petiot P, Boibieux A, et al. Possibly linezolid-induced peripheral and central neurotoxicity: report of four cases. *Infection*, 2005; 33: 151-4.

[59] Frippiat F, Bergiers C, Michel C, Dujardin JP, Derue G. Severe bilateral optic neuritis associated with prolonged linezolid therapy. *J. Antimicrob. Chemother.*, 2004; 53: 1114-5.

[60] Lee E, Burger S, Shah J, Melton C, Mullen M, Warren F, et al. Linezolid-associated toxic optic neuropathy: A report of 2 cases. *Clin. Infect. Dis.*, 2003; 37: 1389-91.

[61] Legout L, Senneville E, Gomel JJ, Yazdanpanah Y, Mouton Y. Linezolid-induced neuropathy. *Clin. Infect. Dis.*, 2004; 38: 767-8.

[62] Nagel S, Köhrmann M, Huttner HB, Storch-Hagenlocher B, Schwab S. Linezolid-induced posterior reversible leukoencephalopathy síndrome. *Arch. Neurol.*, 2007; 64: 746-8.

[63] Narita M, Tsuji BT, Yu VL. Linezolid-associated peripheral and optic neuropathy, lactic acidosis, and serotonin syndrome. *Pharmacotherapy*, 2007; 27: 1189-97.

[64] Saijo T, Hayashi K, Yamada H, Wakakura M. Linezolid-induced optic neuropathy. *Am. J. Ophthalmol.*, 2005; 139: 1114-6.

[65] Carson J, Cerda J, Chae JH, Hirano M, Maggiore P. Severe lactic acidosis associated with linezolid use in a patient with the mitochondrial DNA A2706G polymorphism. *Pharmacotherapy*, 2007; 27: 771-4.

[66] Kopterides P, Papadomichelakis E, Armaganidis A. Linezolid use associated with lactic acidosis. *Scand. J. Infect. Dis.*, 2005; 37: 153-4.

[67] Palenzuela L, Hahn NM, Nelson RP, Arno JN, Schobert C, Bethel R, et al. Does linezolid cause lactic acidosis by inhibiting mitochondrial protein synthesis? *Clin. Infect. Dis.*, 2005; 40: e113-6.

[68] Wiener M, Guo Y, Patel G, Fries BC. Lactic acidosis after treatment with linezolid. *Infection*, 2007; 35: 278-81.

[69] Lawrence KR, Adra M, Gillman PK. Serotonin toxicity associated with the use of linezolid: A review of postmarketing data. *Clin. Infect. Dis.*, 2006; 42: 1578-83.

[70] Miller DG, Lovell EO. Antibiotic-induced serotonin síndrome. *J Emerg Med*, 2008; May 1 [Epub ahead of print] doi:10.1016/j.jemermed.2007.10.072.

[71] Morales-Molina JA, Mateu-de Antonio J, Marín-Casino M, Grau S. Linezolid-associated serotonin syndrome: what we can learn from cases reported so far. *J. Antimicrob. Chemother.*, 2005; 56: 1176-8.

[72] Packer S, Berman SA. Serotonin syndrome precipitated by the monoamine oxidase inhibitor linezolid. *Am. J. Psychiatry*, 2007; 164: 246-7.

[73] Taylor JJ, Wilson JW, Estes LL. Linezolid and serotonergic drug interactions: A retrospective survey. *Clin. Infect. Dis.*, 2006; 43: 180-7.

[74] Thai XC, Bruno-Murtha LA. Bell's palsy associated with linezolid therapy: Case report and review of neuropathic adverse events. *Pharmacotherapy*, 2006; 26: 1183-9.

[75] Amir KA, Bobba RK, Clarke B, Nagy-Agren S, Arsura EL, Balogun SA, et al. Tongue discoloration in an elderly kidney transplant recipient: Treatment-related adverse event? *Am. J. Geriatr. Pharmacother.*, 2006; 4: 260-3.

[76] Tartarone A, Gallucci G, Iodice G, Romano G, Coccaro M, Vigliotti ML, et al. Linezolid-induced bradycardia: a case report. *Int. J. Antimicrob. Agents*, 2004; 23: 412-3.

[77] Soriano A, Ortega M, García S, Peñarroja G, Bové A, Marcos M, et al. Comparative study of the effects of pyridoxine, rifampin, and renal function on hematological adverse events induced by linezolid. *Antimicrob. Agents Chemother.*, 2007; 51: 2559-63.

[78] Spellberg B, Yoo T, Bayer AS. Reversal of linezolid-associated cytopenias, but not peripheral neuropathy, by administration of vitamin B6. *J Antimicrob Chemother*, 2004; 54: 832-5.

[79] Youssef S, Hachem R, Chemaly RF, Adachi J, Ying J, Rolston K, et al. The role of vitamin B6 in the prevention of haematological toxic effects of linezolid in patients with cancer. *J. Antimicrob. Chemother.*, 2008; 61: 421-4.

[80] Cuzzolin L, Fanos V. Linezolid: A new antibiotic for newborns and children? *J. Chemother.*, 2006; 18: 573-81.

[81] Venkatesh MP, Placencia F, Weisman LE. Coagulase-negative staphylococcal infections in the neonate and child: An update. *Semin. Pediatr. Infect. Dis.*, 2006; 17: 120-7.

[82] da Silva PS, Monteiro Neto H, Sejas LM. Successful treatment of vancomycin-resistant enterococcus ventriculitis in a child. *Braz. J. Infect. Dis.*, 2007; 11: 297-9.

[83] Manfredi R. Update on the appropriate use of linezolid in clinical practice. *Ther. Clin. Risk Manag.*, 2006; 2: 455-64.

[84] Guay RP. Review of cefditoren, an advanced-generation, broad-spectrum oral cephalosporin. *Clin. Ther.*, 2001; 23: 1924-37.

[85] Hernandez-Martín J, Roma E, Salavert M, Domenech L, Poveda JL. Cefditoren pivoxil: A new oral cephalosporin for skin, soft tissue and respiratory tract infections. *Rev. Esp. Quimioterap.*, 2006; 19: 231-46.

[86] Wellington K, Curran MP. Cefditoren pivoxil: A review of its use in the treatment of bacterial infections. *Drugs*, 2004; 64: 2597-618.

[87] Darkes MJ, Plosker GL. Cefditoren pivoxil. *Drugs*, 2002; 62: 319-36.

[88] Lee MY, Ko KS, Oh WS, Park S, Lee JY, Baek JY, et al. In vitro activity of cefditoren: Antimicrobial efficacy against major respiratory pathogens from Asian countries. *Int. J. Antimicrob Agents*, 2006; 28: 14-8.

[89] Jones RN, Biedenbach DJ, Johnson DM. Cefditoren activity against nearly 1000 non-fastidious bacterial isolates and the development of in vitro susceptibility test methods. *Diagn. Microbiol. Infect. Dis.*, 2000; 37: 143-6.

[90] Gimenez MJ, Gomez-Lus ML, Valdes L, Aguilar L. The role of the third-generation oral cephalosporin cefditoren pivoxil in the treatment of community-acquired infection in adults. *Rev Esp Quimioterap*, 2005; 18: 210-6.

[91] Seral C, Suarez L, Rubio-Calvo C, Gomez-Lus R, Gimeno M, Coronel P, et al. In vitro activity of cefditoren and other antimicrobial agents against 288 *Streptococcus pneumoniae* and 220 *Haemophilus influenzae* clinical strains isolated in Zaragoza, Spain. *Diagn. Microbiol. Infect. Dis.*, 2008; 62: 210-5.

[92] Granizo JJ, Gimenez MJ, Barberan J, Coronel P, Gimeno M, Aguilar L. Efficacy of cefditoren in the treatment of upper respiratory tract infections: A pooled analysis of six clinical trials. *Rev. Esp. Quimioter.*, 2008; 21: 14-21.

[93] Johnson DM, Biedenbach DJ, Beach ML, Pfaller MA, Jones RN. Antimicrobial activity and in vitro susceptibility test development for cefditoren against *Haemophilus influenzae*, *Moraxella catarrhalis*, and *Streptococcus* species. *Diagn. Microbiol. Infect. Dis*, 2000; 37: 99-105.

[94] Biedenbach DJ, Jones RN, Fritsche TR. Antimicrobial activity of cefditoren tested against contemporary (2004–2006) isolates of *Haemophilus influenzae* and *Moraxella catarrhalis* responsible for community-acquired respiratory tract infections in the United States. *Diagn. Microbiol. Infect. Dis.*, 2008; 61: 240-4.

[95] Gracia M, Díaz C, Coronel P, Gimeno M, García-Rodas R, del Prado G, et al. Antimicrobial susceptibility of *Haemophilus influenzae* and *Moraxella catarrhalis* isolates in eight Central, East and Baltic European countries in 2005–06: results of the Cefditoren Surveillance Study. *J. Antimicrob. Chemother.*, 2008; 61: 1180-5.

[96] Lerma M, Cebrian L, Gimenez MJ, Coronel P, Gimeno M, Aguilar L, García de Lomas et al. β-lactam susceptibility of *Escherichia coli* isolates from urinary tract infections exhibiting different resistance phenotypes. *Rev. Esp. Quimioter.*, 2008; 21: 149-52.

[97] Vazquez JA, Galarza P, Gimenez MJ, Coronel P. In vitro susceptibility of Spanish isolates of *Neisseria gonorrhoeae* to cefditoren and five other antimicrobial agents. *Int. J. Antimicrob. Agents*, 2007; 29: 473-4.

[98] Yamada M, Watanabe T, Miyara T, Baba N, Saito J, Takeuchi Y, et al. Crystal structure of cefditoren complexed with *Streptococcus pneumoniae* penicillin-binding protein 2X: Structural basis for its high antimicrobial activity. *Antimicrob. Agents Chemother.*, 2007; 51: 3902-7.

[99] Spectracef™ [package insert]. Lake Forest, IL: TAP Pharmaceuticals, 2001.

[100] Sadaba B, Azanza JR, Quetglas EG, Campanero MA, Honorato J, Coronel P, et al. Pharmacokinetic/pharmacodynamic serum and urine profile of cefditoren following single-dose and multiple twice- and thrice-daily regimens in healthy volunteers: A phase I study. *Rev. Esp. Quimioter.*, 2007; 20: 51-60.

[101] Lodise TP, Kinzig-Schippers M, Drusano GL, Loos U, Vogel F, Bulitta J, et al. Use of population pharmacokinetic modeling and Monte Carlo simulation to describe the pharmacodynamic profile of cefditoren in plasma and epithelial lining fluid. *Antimicrob. Agents Chemother.*, 2008; 52:1945-51.

[102] Sevillano D, Aguilar L, Alou L, Gimenez MJ, Gonzalez N, Torrico M, et al. High protein binding and cidal activity against penicillin-resistant *Streptococcus pneumoniae*: A cefditoren in vitro pharmacodynamic simulation. *PLoS ONE*, 2008; 3: e2717.

[103] Martin SI, Kaye KM. Beta-lactam antibiotics: Newer formulations and newer agents. *Infect. Dis. Clin. N Am.*, 2004; 18: 603-19.

[104] Fogarty CM, Cyganowski M, Palo WA, Horn RC, Craig WA. A comparison of cefditoren pivoxil and amoxicillin-clavulanate in the treatment of community-acquired pneumonia: A multicenter, prospective, randomized, investigator-blinded, parallel-group study. *Clin. Ther.*, 2002; 24: 1854-70.

[105] Brass EP, Mayer MD, Mulford DJ, Stickler TK, Hoppel CL. Impact on carnitine homeostasis of short-term treatment with the pivalate prodrug cefditoren pivoxil. *Clin. Pharmacol. Ther.*, 2003; 73: 338-47.

[106] Makino Y, Sugiura T, Ito T, Sugiyama N, Koyama N. Carnitine-associated encephalopathy caused by long-term treatment with an antibiotic containing pivalic acid. *Pediatrics*, 2007; 120: 739-41.

[107] Brink AJ, Feldman C, Grolman DC, Muckart D, Pretorius J, Richards GA, et al. Appropriate use of the carbapenems. *S. Afr. Med. J.*, 2004; 94: 857-61.

[108] Gobernado M, Acuña C. Ertapenem. *Rev Esp Quimioterap*, 2007; 20: 277-99.

[109] Livermore DM, Sefton AM, Scott GM. Properties and potential of ertapenem. *J. Antimicrob. Chemother.*, 2003; 52: 331-44.

[110] Shah PM, Isaacs RD. Ertapenem, the first of a new group of carbapenems. *J. Antimicrob. Chemother.*, 2003; 52: 538-42.

[111] Hammond ML. Ertapenem: A group 1 carbapenem with distinct antibacterial and pharmacological properties. *J Antimicrob Chemother*, 2004; 53 (Suppl S2): ii7-ii9.

[112] Kohler J, Dorso KL, Young K, Hammond GG, Rosen H, Kropp H, et al. In vitro activities of the potent, broad-spectrum carbapenem MK-0826 (L-749,345) against broad-spectrum β-lactamase and extended-spectrum β-lactamase-producing *Klebsiella pneumoniae* and *Escherichia coli* clinical isolates. *Antimicrob Agents Chemother*, 1999; 43: 1170-6.

[113] Goldstein EJC, Citron DM, Merriam CV, Warren YA, Tyrrell KL, Fernandez H. Comparative in vitro activities of ertapenem (MK-0826) against 469 less frequently identified anaerobes isolated from human infections. *Antimicrob Agents Chemother*, 2002; 46: 1136-40.

[114] Friedland IR, Isaacs R, Mixson LA, Motyl M, Woods GL. Use of surrogate antimicrobial agents to predict susceptibility to ertapenem. *Diagn Microbiol Infect Dis*, 2002; 43: 61-4.

[115] Jiménez-Cruz F, Jasovich A, Cajigas J, Jiang Q, Imbeault D, Woods GL, et al. A prospective, multicenter, randomized, double-blind study comparing ertapenem and ceftriaxone followed by appropriate oral therapy for complicated urinary tract infections in adults. *Urology*, 2002; 60: 16-22.

[116] Livermore DM, Oakton KJ, Carter MW, Warner M. Activity of ertapenem (MK- 0826) versus *Enterobacteriaceae* with potent β-lactamases. *Antimicrob Agents Chemother*, 2001; 45: 2831-7.

[117] Loza E, Morosini MI, Canton R, Almaraz F, Reig M, Baquero F. Comparative *in vitro* activity of ertapenem against aerobic and anaerobic bacteria. *Rev Esp Quimioterp*, 2003; 16: 209-15.

[118] Vetter N, Cambronero-Hernandez E, Rohlf J, Simon S, Carides A, Oliveria T, et al. A prospective, randomized, double-blind multicenter comparison of parenteral ertapenem and ceftriaxone for the treatment of hospitalized adults with community-acquired pneumonia. *Clin Ther*, 2002; 24: 1770-85.

[119] Wexler HM. In vitro activity of ertapenem: review of recent studies. *J Antimicrob Chemother*, 2004; 53 (Suppl S2): ii11–ii21.

[120] Jacqueline C, Caillon J, Grossi O, Le Mabecque V, Miegeville AF, Bugnon D, et al. In vitro and in vivo assessment of linezolid combined with ertapenem: A highly synergistic combination against methicillin-resistant *Staphylococcus aureus*. *Antimicrob Agents Chemother*, 2006; 50: 2547-9.

[121] Fuchs PC, Barry AL, Brown SD. In vitro activities of ertapenem (MK-0826) against clinical bacterial isolates from 11 North American medical centers. *Antimicrob Agents Chemother*, 2001; 45: 1915-8.

[122] Goldstein EJC, Citron DM, Merriam CV, Warren YA, Tyrrell KL. Comparative in vitro activities of ertapenem (MK-0826) against 1,001 anaerobes isolated from human intra-abdominal infections. *Antimicrob Agents Chemother*, 2000; 44: 2389-94.

[123] Goldstein EJC, Citron DM, Merriam CV, Warren YA, Tyrrell KL. Comparative in vitro activity of ertapenem and 11 other antimicrobial agents against aerobic and anaerobic pathogens isolated from skin and soft tissue animal and human bite wound infections. *J Antimicrob Chemother*, 2001; 48: 641-51.

[124] Hicks PS, Pelak B, Woods GL, Bartizal KF, Motyl M. Comparative in vitro activity of ertapenem against bacterial pathogens isolated from patients with lower respiratory tract infections. *Clin. Microbiol. Infect.*, 2002; 8: 753-7.

[125] Hoellman DB, Kelly LM, Credito K, Anthony L, Ednie LM, Jacobs MR, et al. In vitro antianaerobic activity of ertapenem (MK-0826) compared to seven other compounds. *Antimicrob. Agents Chemother.*, 2002; 46: 220-4.

[126] Jones RN, Huynh HK, Biedenbach DJ, Fritsche TR, Sader HS. Doripenem (S-4661), a novel carbapenem: comparative activity against contemporary pathogens including bactericidal action and preliminary in vitro methods evaluations. *J. Antimicrob. Chemother.*, 2004; 54: 144-54.

[127] Jones RN, Sader HS, Fritsche TR. Comparative activity of doripenem and three other carbapenems tested against Gram-negative bacilli with various β-lactamase resistance mechanisms. *Diagn. Microbiol. Infect. Dis.*, 2005; 52: 71-4.

[128] Ling TKW, Xiong J, Yu Y, Lee CC, Ye H, Hawkey PM, et al. Multicenter antimicrobial susceptibility survey of gram-negative bacteria isolated from patients with community-acquired infections in the People's Republic of China *Antimicrob. Agents Chemother.*, 2006; 50: 374-8.

[129] Marchese A, Gualco L, Schito AM, Debbia EA, Schito GC. In vitro activity of ertapenem against selected respiratory pathogens. *J. Antimicrob. Chemother.*, 2004; 54: 944-51.

[130] Pelak BA, Bartizal K, Woods GL, Gesser RM, Motyl M. Comparative in vitro activities of ertapenem against aerobic and facultative bacterial pathogens from patients with complicated skin and skin structure infections. *Diagn. Microbiol. Infect. Dis.*, 2002; 43: 129-33.

[131] Rolston KVI, LeBlanc BM, Streeter H, Ho DH. In vitro activity of ertapenem against bacterial isolates from cancer patients. *Diagn. Microbiol. Infect. Dis.*, 2002; 43: 219-23.

[132] Song JH, Ko KS, Lee MY, Park S, Baek JY, Lee JY, et al. In vitro activities of ertapenem against drug-resistant *Streptococcus pneumoniae* and other respiratory pathogens from 12 Asian countries. *Diagn. Microbiol. Infect. Dis.*, 2006; 56: 445-50.

[133] Sorlózano A, Gutiérrez J, Romero JM, Luna JD, Damas M, Piédrola G. Activity *in vitro* of twelve antibiotics against clinical isolates of extended-spectrum beta-lactamase producing *Escherichia coli. J. Basic. Microbiol.*, 2007; 47: 413-6.

[134] Friedland I, Stinson L, Ikaiddi MM, Harm S, Woods GL. Resistance in *Enterobacteriaceae*: Results of a multicenter surveillance study, 1995–2000. *Infect. Control. Hosp. Epidemiol.*, 2003; 24: 607-12.

[135] Girlich D, Poirel L, Nordmann P. Do CTX-M β-lactamases hydrolyse ertapenem? *J. Antimicrob. Chemother.*, 2008; 62: 1155-6.

[136] Mena A, Plasencia V, García L, Hidalgo O, Ayestarán JI, Alberti S, et al. Characterization of a large outbreak by CTX-M-1-producing *Klebsiella pneumoniae* and mechanisms leading to in vivo carbapenem resistance development. *J. Clin. Microbiol.*, 2006; 44: 2831-7.

[137] Anderson KF, Lonsway DR, Rasheed JK, Biddle J, Jensen B, McDougal LK, et al. Evaluation of methods to identify the *Klebsiella pneumoniae* carbapenemase in *Enterobacteriaceae. J. Clin. Microbiol.*, 2007; 45: 2723-5.

[138] Cai JC, Zhou HW, Zhang R, Chen GX. Emergence of *Serratia marcescens, Klebsiella pneumoniae*, and *Escherichia coli* isolates possessing the plasmid-mediated carbapenem-hydrolyzing β-lactamase KPC-2 in intensive care units of a chinese hospital. *Antimicrob. Agents Chemother.*, 2008; 52: 2014-8.

[139] Tibbetts R, Frye JG, Marschall J, Warren D, Dunne W. Detection of KPC-2 in a clinical isolate of *Proteus mirabilis* and first reported description of carbapenemase resistance caused by a KPC β-lactamase in *Proteus mirabilis. J. Clin. Microbiol.*, 2008; 46: 3080-3.

[140] Naas T, Levy M, Hirschauer C, Marchandin H, Nordmann P. Outbreak of carbapenem-resistant *Acinetobacter baumannii* producing the carbapenemase OXA-23 in a tertiary care hospital of Papeete, French Polynesia. *J. Clin. Microbiol.*, 2005; 43: 4826-9.

[141] Aschbacher R, Doumith M, Livermore DM, Larcher C, Woodford N. Linkage of acquired quinolone resistance (qnrS1) and metallo-□-lactamase (blaVIM-1) genes in multiple species of *Enterobacteriaceae* from Bolzano, Italy. *J. Antimicrob. Chemother.*, 2008; 61: 515-23.

[142] Lartigue MF, Poirel L, Poyart C, Réglier-Poupet H, Nordmann P. Ertapenem resistance of *Escherichia coli. Emerg. Infec.t Dis.*, 2007; 13: 315-7.

[143] Livermore DM, Carter MW, Bagel S, Wiedemann B, Baquero F, Loza E, et al. In vitro activities of ertapenem (MK-0826) against recent clinical bacteria collected in Europe and Australia. *Antimicrob. Agents Chemother.*, 2001; 45: 1860-7.

[144] Martínez-Martínez L, Pascual A, Hernández-Allés S, Alvarez-Díaz D, Suárez AI, Tran J, et al. Roles of β-lactamases and porins in activities of carbapenems and cephalosporins against *Klebsiella pneumoniae. Antimicrob. Agents Chemother.*, 1999; 43: 1669-73.

[145] Woodford N, Dallow JWT, Hill RLR, Palepou MFI, Pike R, Ward ME, et al. Ertapenem resistance among *Klebsiella* and *Enterobacter* submitted in the UK to a reference laboratory. *Int. J. Antimicrob. Agents*, 2007; 29: 456-9.

[146] Jacoby GA, Mills DM, Chow N. Role of β-lactamases and porins in resistance to ertapenem and other β-lactams in *Klebsiella pneumoniae. Antimicrob. Agents Chemother.*, 2004; 48: 3203-6.

[147] Oteo J, Delgado-Iribarren A, Vega D, Bautista V, Rodríguez MC, Velasco M, et al. Emergence of imipenem resistance in clinical *Escherichia coli* during therapy. *Int. J. Antimicrob. Agents*, 2008; 32: 534-7.

[148] Szabo D, Silveira F, Hujer AM, Bonomo RA, Hujer KM, Marsh JW, et al. Outer membrane protein changes and efflux pump expression together may confer resistance to ertapenem in *Enterobacter cloacae. Antimicrob Agents Chemother*, 2006; 50: 2833-5.

[149] Mammeri H, Nordmann P, Berkani A, Eb F. Contribution of extended-spectrum AmpC (ESAC) β-lactamases to carbapenem resistance in *Escherichia coli*. *FEMS Microbiol. Lett.*, 2008; 282: 238-40.

[150] Fraenkel CJ, Ullberg M, Bernander S, Ericson E, Larsson P, Rydberg J, et al. In vitro activities of three carbapenems against recent bacterial isolates from severely ill patients at Swedish hospitals. *Scand. J. Infect. Dis.*, 2006; 38: 853-9.

[151] Livermore DM, Mushtaq S, Warner M. Selectivity of ertapenem for *Pseudomonas aeruginosa* mutants cross-resistant to other carbapenems. *J. Antimicrob. Chemother.*, 2005; 55: 306-11.

[152] Quale J, Bratu S, Gupta J, Landman D. Interplay of efflux system, *ampC*, and *oprD* expression in carbapenem resistance of *Pseudomonas aeruginosa* clinical isolates. *Antimicrob. Agents Chemother.*, 2006; 50: 1633-41.

[153] Majumdar AK, Musson DG, Birk KL, Kitchen CJ, Holland S, McCrea J, et al. Pharmacokinetics of ertapenem in healthy young volunteers. *Antimicrob. Agents Chemother.*, 2002; 46: 3506-11.

[154] Burkhardt O, Brunner M, Schmidt S, Grant M, Tang Y, Derendorf H. Penetration of ertapenem into skeletal muscle and subcutaneous adipose tissue in healthy volunteers measured by in vivo microdialysis. *J. Antimicrob. Chemother.*, 2006; 58: 632-6.

[155] Musson DG, Majumdar A, Birk K, Holland S, Wickersham P, Li SX, et al. Pharmacokinetics of intramuscularly administered ertapenem. *Antimicrob. Agents Chemother.*, 2003; 47: 1732-5.

[156] Nix DE, Majumdar AK, DiNubile MJ. Pharmacokinetics and pharmacodynamics of ertapenem: An overview for clinicians. *J. Antimicrob. Chemother.*, 2004; 53 (Suppl 2): ii23-8.

[157] Wittau M, Wagner E, Kaever V, Koal T, Henne-Bruns D, Isenmann R. Intraabdominal tissue concentration of ertapenem. *J. Antimicrob. Chemother.*, 2006; 57: 312-6.

[158] Boselli E, Breilh D, Djabarouti S, Bel JC, Saux MC, Allaouchiche B. Diffusion of ertapenem into bone and synovial tissues. *J. Antimicrob. Chemother.*, 2007; 60: 893-6.

[159] Roy S, Higareda I, Angel-Muller E, Ismail M, Hague C, Adeyi B, et al. Ertapenem once a day versus piperacillin–tazobactam every 6 hours for treatment of acute pelvic infections: A prospective, multicenter, randomized, double-blind study. *Infect. Dis. Obstet. Gynecol.*, 2003; 11: 27-7.

[160] European Medicines Agency (EMEA). EPAR H-389-PI report on ertapenem. Available: http://www.emea.europa.eu/humandocs/PDFs/EPAR/invanz/H-389-PI-ES.pdf (consulted on December 5, 2008).

[161] Musson DG, Majumdar A, Holland S, Birk K, Xi L, Mistry G, et al. Pharmacokinetics of total and unbound ertapenem in healthy elderly subjects. *Antimicrob. Agents Chemother.*, 2004; 48: 521-4.

[162] Mistry GC, Majumdar AK, Swan S, Sica D, Fisher A, Xu Y, et al. Pharmacokinetics of ertapenem in patients with varying degrees of renal insufficiency and in patients on hemodialysis. *J. Clin. Pharmacol.*, 2006; 46: 1128-38.

[163] Teppler H, Gesser RM, Friedland IR, Woods GL, Meibohm A, Herman G, et al. Safety and tolerability of ertapenem. *J. Antimicrob. Chemother.*, 2004; 53 (Suppl S2): ii75-ii81.

[164] Tice AD. Ertapenem: A new opportunity for outpatient parenteral antimicrobial therapy. *J. Antimicrob. Chemother.*, 2004; 53 (Suppl S2): ii83–ii86.

[165] Gesser RM, McCarroll KA, Woods GL. Evaluation of outpatient treatment with ertapenem in a double blind controlled clinical trial of complicated skin/skin structure infections. *J. Infect.*, 2004; 48: 32-8.

[166] Graham DR, Lucasti C, Malafaia O, Nichols RL, Holtom P, Quintero Perez N, et al. Ertapenem once daily versus piperacillin-tazobactam 4 times per day for treatment of complicated skin and skin-structure infections in adults: Results of a prospective, randomized, double-blind multicenter study. *Clin. Infect. Dis.*, 2002; 34: 1460-8.

[167] Ortiz-Ruiz G, Caballero-Lopez J, Friedland IR, Woods GL, Carides A, the Protocol 018 ertapenem community-acquired pneumonia Study Group. A study evaluating the efficacy, safety, and tolerability of ertapenem versus ceftriaxone for the treatment of community-acquired pneumonia in adults. *Clin. Infect. Dis.*, 2002; 34: 1076-83.

[168] Ortiz-Ruiz G, Vetter N, Isaacs R, Carides A, Woods GL, Friedland I. Ertapenem versus ceftriaxone for the treatment of community-acquired pneumonia in adults: combined analysis of two multicentre randomized, double-blind studies. *J. Antimicrob. Chemother.*, 2004; 53 (Suppl S2): ii59–ii66.

[169] Solomkin JS, Yellin AE, Rotstein OD, Christou NV, Dellinger EP, Tellado JM, et al. Ertapenem versus piperacillin/tazobactam in the treatment of complicated intraabdominal infections results of a double-blind, randomized comparative Phase III trial. *Ann. Surg.*, 2003; 237: 235-45.

[170] Tomera KM, Burdmann EA, Reyna OG, Jiang Q, Wimmer WM, Woods GL, et al. Ertapenem versus ceftriaxone followed by appropriate oral therapy for treatment of complicated urinary tract infections in adults: Results of a prospective, randomized, double-blind multicenter study. *Antimicrob. Agents Chemother.*, 2002; 46: 2895-900.

[171] Wells WG, Woods GL, Jiang Q, Gesser RM. Treatment of complicated urinary tract infection in adults: combined analysis of two randomized, double-blind, multicentre trials comparing ertapenem and ceftriaxone followed by appropriate oral therapy. *J. Antimicrob. Chemother.*, 2004; 53 (Suppl S2): ii67–ii74.

[172] Ong C, Chua AC, Tambyah PA. Seizures associated with ertapenem. *Int. J. Antimicrob. Agents*, 2008; 31: 290-8.

[173] Fica AE, Abusada NJ. Seizures associated with ertapenem use in patients with CNS disorders and renal insufficiency. *Scand. J. Infect. Dis.*, 2008; 40: 983-5.

[174] Lunde JL, Nelson RE, Storandt HF. Acute seizures in a patient receiving divalproex sodium after starting ertapenem therapy. *Pharmacotherapy*, 2007; 27: 1202-5.

[175] Invanz™ [package insert]. Whitehouse Station, NJ: Merck Sharp and Dohme, 2005.

[176] Arguedas A, Cespedes J, Botet FA, Blumer J, Yogev R, Gesser R, et al. Safety and tolerability of ertapenem versus ceftriaxone in a double-blind study performed in children with complicated urinary tract infection, community-acquired pneumonia or skin and soft-tissue infection. *Int. J. Antimicrob. Agents*, 2009; 33: 163-7.

[177] Woods GL, Isaacs RD, McCarroll KA, Friedland IR. Ertapenem therapy for community-acquired pneumonia in the elderly. *J. Am. Geriatr. Soc.*, 2003; 51: 1526-32.

[178] Anderson DL. Doripenem. *Drugs Today (Barc)*, 2006; 42: 399-404.

[179] Fritsche TR, Stilwell MG, Jones RN. Antimicrobial activity of doripenem (S-4661): A global surveillance report (2003). *Clin. Microbiol. Infect.*, 2005; 11: 974-84.

[180] Walsh F. Doripenem: A new carbapenem antibiotic a review of comparative antimicrobial and bactericidal activities. *Ther. Clin. Risk Manag.*, 2007; 3: 789-94.

[181] Greer NG. Doripenem (Doribax): The newest addition to the carbapenems. *Proc. (Bayl Univ. Med. Cent.)*, 2008; 21: 337-41.

[182] Vergidis PI, Falagas ME. New antibiotic agents for bloodstream infections. *Int. J. Antimicrob. Agents*, 2008; 32: 60-5.

[183] Davies TA, Shang W, Bush K, Flamm RK. Affinity of doripenem and comparators to penicillin-binding proteins in *Escherichia coli* and *Pseudomonas aeruginosa*. *Antimicrob. Agents Chemother.*, 2008; 52: 1510-2.

[184] Dalhoff A, Janjic N, Echols R. Redefining penems. *Biochem. Pharmacol.*, 2006; 71: 1085-95.

[185] Kobayashi Y. Study of the synergism between carbapenems and vancomycin or teicoplanin against MRSA, focusing on S-4661, a carbapenem newly developed in Japan. *J. Infect. Chemother.*, 2005; 11: 259-61.

[186] Huynh HK, Biedenbach DJ, Jones RN. Delayed resistance selection for doripenem when passaging *Pseudomonas aeruginosa* isolates with doripenem plus an aminoglycoside. *Diagn. Microbiol. Infect. Dis.*, 2006; 55: 241-3.

[187] Tsuji M, Ishii Y, Ohno A, Miyazaki S, Yamaguchi K. In vitro and in vivo antibacterial activities of S-4661, a new carbapenem. *Antimicrob. Agents Chemother.*, 1998; 42: 94-9.

[188] Goldstein EJC, Citron DM, Merriam CV, Warren YA, Tyrrell KL, Fernandez HT. In vitro activities of doripenem and six comparator drugs against 423 aerobic and anaerobic bacterial isolates from infected diabetic foot wounds. *Antimicrob Agents Chemother*, 2008; 52: 761-6.

[189] Wexler HM, Engel AE, Glass D, Li C. In vitro activities of doripenem and comparator agents against 364 anaerobic clinical isolates. *Antimicrob. Agents Chemother.*, 2005; 49: 4413-7.

[190] Chen Y, Garber E, Zhao Q, Ge Y, Wikler MA, Kaniga K, et al. In vitro activity of doripenem (S-4661) against multidrug-resistant Gram-negative bacilli isolated from patients with cystic fibrosis. *Antimicrob. Agents Chemother.*, 2005; 49: 2510-1.

[191] Ge Y, Wikler MA, Sahm DF, Blosser-Middleton RS, Karlowsky JA. In vitro antimicrobial activity of doripenem, a new carbapenem. *Antimicrob. Agents Chemother.*, 2004; 48: 1384-96.

[192] Jones RN, Huynh HK, Biedenbach DJ. Activities of doripenem (S-4661) against drug-resistant clinical pathogens. *Antimicrob. Agents Chemother.*, 2004; 48: 3136-40.

[193] Mushtaq S, Ge Y, Livermore DM. Doripenem versus *Pseudomonas aeruginosa* in vitro: Activity against characterized isolates, mutants, and transconjugants and resistant selection potential. *Antimicrob. Agents Chemother.*, 2004; 48: 3086-92.

[194] Sakyo S, Tomita H, Tanimoto K, Fujimoto S, Ike Y. Potency of carbapenems for the prevention of carbapenem-resistant mutants of *Pseudomonas aeruginosa*. The high potency of a new carbapenem doripenem. *J. Antibiot.*, 2006; 59: 220-8.

[195] Masuda N, Sakagawa E, Ohya S, Gotoh N, Tsujimoto H, Nishino T. Substrate specificities of MexAB-OprM, MexCD-OprJ, and MexXY-OprM efflux pumps in *Pseudomonas aeruginosa. Antimicrob. Agents Chemother.*, 2000; 44: 3322-7.

[196] Köhler T, Michea-Hamzehpour M, Epp SF, Pechere JC. Carbapenem activities against *Pseudomonas aeruginosa*: Respective contributions of OprD and efflux systems. *Antimicrob. Agents Chemother.*, 1999; 43: 424-7.

[197] Livermore DM. Of Pseudomonas, porins, pumps and carbapenems. *J. Antimicrob. Chemother.*, 2001; 47: 247-50.

[198] Pumbwe L, Glass D, Wexler HM. Efflux pump overexpression in multiple-antibiotic-resistant mutants of *Bacteroides fragilis. Antimicrob. Agents Chemother.*, 2006; 50: 3150-3.

[199] Luzzaro F, Docquier JD, Colinon C, Endimiani A, Lombardi G, Amicosante G, et al. Emergence in *Klebsiella pneumoniae* and *Enterobacter cloacae* clinical isolates of the VIM-4 metallo-beta-lactamase encoded by a conjugative plasmid. *Antimicrob. Agents Chemother.*, 2004; 48: 648-50.

[200] Keam SJ. Doripenem: A review of its use in the treatment of bacterial infections. *Drugs*, 2008; 68: 2021-57.

[201] European Medicines Agency (EMEA). Summary of product characteristics: Doribax. Available: http://www. emea.europa.eu/humandocs/Humans/EPAR/doribax/ doribax. htm (consulted on December 15, 2008).

[202] Ikawa K, Morikawa N, Urakawa N, Ikeda K, Ohge H, Sueda T. Peritoneal penetration of doripenem after intravenous administration in abdominal-surgery patients. *J. Antimicrob. Chemother.*, 2007; 60: 1395-7.

[203] Ikawa K, Morikawa N, Ikeda K, Ohge H, Sueda T. Development of breakpoints of carbapenems for intraabdominal infections based on pharmacokinetics and pharmacodynamics in peritoneal fluid. *J. Infect. Chemother.*, 2008; 14: 330-2.

[204] Ikawa K, Morikawa N, Ikeda K, Ohge H, Sueda T. Pharmacodynamic assessment of doripenem in peritoneal fluid against Gram-negative organisms: use of population pharmacokinetic modeling and Monte Carlo simulation. *Diagn. Microbiol. Infect. Dis.*, 2008; 62: 292-7.

[205] Lucasti C, Jasovich A, Umeh O, Jiang J, Kaniga K, Friedland I. Efficacy and tolerability of IV doripenem versus meropenem in adults with complicated intra-abdominal infection: A phase III, prospective, multicenter, randomized, double-blind, noninferiority study. *Clin. Ther.*, 2008; 30: 868-83.

[206] Doribax™ [package insert]. Raritan, NJ: Ortho-McNeil Pharmaceutical Inc, 2007.

[207] Horiuchi M, Kimura M, Tokumura M, Hasebe N, Arai T, Abe K. Absence of convulsive liability of doripenem, a new carbapenem antibiotic, in comparison with β-lactam antibiotics. *Toxicology*, 2006; 222: 114-24.

[208] Chastre J, Wunderink R, Prokocimer P, Lee M, Kaniga K, Friedland I. Efficacy and safety of intravenous infusion of doripenem versus imipenem in ventilator-associated pneumonia: A multicenter, randomized study. *Crit. Care Med.*, 2008; 36: 1089-96.

[209] McHenney MA, Hosted TJ, Dehoff BS, Rosteck PR Jr, Baltz RH. Molecular cloning and physical mapping of the daptomycin gene cluster from *Streptomyces roseosporus. J. Bacteriol.*, 1998; 180: 143-51.

[210] Cottagnoud P. Daptomycin: a new treatment for insidious infections due to gram-positive pathogens. *Swiss Med. Wkly*, 2008; 138: 93-9.

[211] Hernández V, Romá E, Salavert M, Bosó V, Poveda JL. Daptomycin: revitalizing a former drug due to the need of new active agents against grampositive multirresistant bacterias. *Rev. Esp. Quimioterap.*, 2007; 20: 261-76.

[212] Canepari P, Boaretti M, Lle MM, Satta G. Lipoteichoic acid as a new target for activity of antibiotics: Mode of action of daptomycin (LY146032). *Antimicrob. Agents Chemother.*, 1990; 34: 1220-6.

[213] Laganas V, Alder J, Silverman JA. In vitro bactericidal activities of daptomycin against *Staphylococcus aureus* and *Enterococcus faecalis* are not mediated by inhibition of lipoteichoic acid biosynthesis. *Antimicrob. Agents Chemother.*, 2003; 47: 2682-84.

[214] Silverman JA, Perlmutter NG, Shapiro HM. Correlation of daptomycin bactericidal activity and membrane depolarization in *Staphylococcus aureus. Antimicrob. Agents Chemother.*, 2003; 47: 2538-44.

[215] Shoemaker DM, Simou J, Roland WE. A review of daptomycin for injection (Cubicin) in the treatment of complicated skin and skin structure infections. *Ther. Clin. Risk Manag.*, 2006; 2: 169-74.

[216] Jung D, Rozek A, Okon M, Hancock REW. Structural transitions as determinants of the action of the calcium-dependent antibiotic daptomycin. *Chem. Biol.*, 2004; 11: 949-57.

[217] Jung D, Powers JP, Straus SK, Hancock REW. Lipid-specific binding of the calcium-dependent antibiotic daptomycin leads to changes in lipid polymorphism of model membranes. *Chem. Phys. Lipids*, 2008; 154: 120-8.

[218] Hobbs JK, Miller K, O'Neill AJ, Chopra I. Consequences of daptomycin-mediated membrane damage in *Staphylococcus aureus. J. Antimicrob. Chemother.*, 2008; 62: 1003-8.

[219] Hancock, REW. Mechanisms of action of newer antibiotics for gram-positive pathogens. *Lancet Infect. Dis.*, 2005; 5: 209-18.

[220] Cotroneo N, Harris R, Perlmutter N, Beveridge T, Silverman JA. Daptomycin exerts bactericidal activity without lysis of *Staphylococcus aureus. Antimicrob. Agents Chemother.*, 2008; 52: 2223-5.

[221] Carpenter CF, Chambers HF. Daptomycin: Another novel agent for treating infections due to drug-resistant gram-positive pathogens. *Clin. Infect. Dis.*, 2004; 38: 994-1000.

[222] Diederen BM, Van Duijn I, Willemse P, Kluytmans JA. In vitro activity of daptomycin against methicillin-resistant *Staphylococcus aureus*, including heterogeneously glycopeptides-resistant strains. *Antimicrob. Agents Chemother.*, 2006; 50: 3189-91.

[223] Fluit AC, Schmitz FJ, Verhoef J, Milatovic D. In vitro activity of daptomycin against grampositive European clinical isolates with defined resistance determinants. *Antimicrob. Agents Chemother.*, 2004; 48: 1007-11.

[224] Steenbergen JN, Alder J, Thorne GM, Tally FP. Daptomycin: a lipopeptide antibiotic for the treatment of serious gram-positive infections. *J. Antimicrob. Chemother.*, 2005; 55: 283-8.

[225] Tyrrell KL, Citron DM, Warren YA, Fernandez HT, Merriam CV, Goldstein EJ. In vitro activities of daptomycin, vancomycin, and penicillin against *Clostridium difficile*,

Clostridium perfringens, Finegoldia magna, and *Propionibacterium acnes. Antimicrob. Agents Chemother.*, 2006; 50: 2728-31.

[226] Biedenbach DJ, Bell JM, Sader HS, Fritsche TR, Jones RN, Turnidge JD. Antimicrobial susceptibility of gram-positive bacterial isolates from the Asia–Pacific region and an in vitro evaluation of the bactericidal activity of daptomycin, vancomycin, and teicoplanin: a SENTRY Program Report (2003–2004). *Int. J. Antimicrob. Agents,* 2007; 30: 143-9.

[227] Critchley IA, Draghi1 DC, Sahm1 DF, Thornsberry C, Jones ME, Karlowsky1 JA. Activity of daptomycin against susceptible and multidrug-resistant gram-positive pathogens collected in the SECURE study (Europe) during 2000–2001. *J. Antimicrob. Chemother.,* 2003; 51: 639-49.

[228] Jones RN, Fritsche TR, Sader HS, Rossa JE. LEADER surveillance program results for 2006: An activity and spectrum analysis of linezolid using clinical isolates from the United States (50 medical centers). *Diagn. Microbiol. Infect. Dis.,* 2007; 59: 309-17.

[229] Malli E, Spiliopoulou I, Kolonitsiou F, Klapsa D, Giannitsioti E, Pantelidi K, et al. In vitro activity of daptomycin against gram-positive cocci: The first multicentre study in Greece. *Int. J. Antimicrob. Agents,* 2008; 32: 525-8.

[230] Denis O, Deplano A, Nonhoff C, Hallin M, De Ryck R, Vanhoof R, et al. In vitro activities of ceftobiprole, tigecycline, daptomycin, and 19 other antimicrobials against methicillin-resistant *Staphylococcus aureus* strains from a national survey of Belgian hospitals. *Antimicrob. Agents Chemother.,* 2006; 50: 2680-5..

[231] Jorgen B, Merckoll P, Melby KK. Susceptibility to daptomycin, quinupristin/dalfopristin and linezolid and some other antibiotics in clinical isolates of methicillin-resistant and methicillin-sensitive *Staphylococcus aureus* from the Oslo area. *Scand. J. Infect. Dis.,* 2007; 39: 1059-62.

[232] Cui L, Tominaga E, Neoh HM, Hiramatsu K. Correlation between reduced daptomycin susceptibility and vancomycin resistance in vancomycin-intermediate *Staphylococcus aureus. Antimicrob Agents Chemother,* 2006; 50: 1079-82.

[233] Petersen P, Bradford P, Weiss W, Murphy TM, Sum PE, Projan SJ. In vitro and in vivo activities of tigecycline (GAR-936), daptomycin, and comparative antimicrobial agents against glycopeptide-intermediate *Staphylococcus aureus* and other resistant grampositive pathogens. *Antimicrob. Agents Chemother.,* 2002; 46: 2595-601.

[234] Food and Drug Administration (FDA). CDER N021572 report on daptomycin. September 2003. Available: http://www.fda.gov/cder/rdmt/nmecy2003.htm (consulted on December 2, 2008).

[235] European Medicines Agency (EMEA). EPAR H-637-II-05-AR report on daptomycin. July 2007. Available: http://www.emea.europa.eu/humandocs/PDFs/EPAR /cubicin /EMEA-H-637-II-05-AR (consulted on December 2, 2008).

[236] Kaatz GW, Lundstrom TS, Seo SM. Mechanisms of daptomycin resistance in *Staphylococcus aureus. Int. J. Antimicrob. Agents,* 2006; 28: 280-7.

[237] Friedman L, Alder JD, Silverman JA. Genetic changes that correlate with reduced susceptibility to daptomycin in *Staphylococcus aureus. Antimicrob. Agents Chemother.,* 2006; 50: 2137-45.

[238] Murthy MH, Olson ME, Wickert RW, Fey PD, Jalali Z. Daptomycin non-susceptible meticillin-resistant *Staphylococcus aureus* USA 300 isolate. *J. Med. Microbiol.*, 2008; 57: 1036-8.

[239] Julian K, Kosowska-Shick K, Whitener C, Roos M, Labischinski H, Rubio A, et al. Characterization of a daptomycin-nonsusceptible vancomycin-intermediate *Staphylococcus aureus* strain in a patient with endocarditis. *Antimicrob. Agents Chemother.*, 2007; 51: 3445-8.

[240] Jones T, Yeaman MR, Sakoulas G, Yang SJ, Proctor RA, Sahl HG, et al. Failures in clinical treatment of *Staphylococcus aureus* infection with daptomycin are associated with alterations in surface charge, membrane phospholipid asymmetry, and drug binding. *Antimicrob. Agents Chemother.*, 2008; 52: 269-78.

[241] Hidron AI, Schuetz AN, Nolte FS, Gould CV, Osborn MK. Daptomycin resistance in *Enterococcus faecalis* prosthetic valve endocarditis. *J. Antimicrob. Chemother.*, 2008; 61: 1394-6.

[242] Dvorchik BH, Brazier D, DeBruin MF, Arbeit RD. Daptomycin pharmacokinetics and safety following administration of escalating doses once daily to healthy subjects. *Antimicrob. Agents Chemother.*, 2003; 47: 1318-23.

[243] Schriever CA, Fernandez C, Rodvold KS, Danziger LH. Daptomycin: a novel cyclic lipopeptide antimicrobial. *Am. J. Health Syst. Pharm.*, 2005; 62: 1145-58.

[244] Wise R, Gee T, Andrews JM, Dvorchik B, Marshall G. Pharmacokinetics and inflammatory fluid penetration of intravenous daptomycin in volunteers. *Antimicrob. Agents Chemother.*, 2002; 46: 31-3.

[245] Cubicin™ [package insert]. Lexington, MA: Cubist Pharmaceuticals Inc., 2003.

[246] Woodworth JR, Nyhart EH Jr, Brier GL, Wolny JD, Black HR. Single-dose pharmacokinetics and antibacterial activity of daptomycin, a new glipopeptide antibiotic, in healthy volunteers. *Antimicrob. Agents Chemother.*, 1992; 36: 318-25.

[247] Abdel-Rahman SM, Benziger DP, Jacobs RF, Jafri HS, Hong EF, Kearns GL. Single-dose pharmacokinetics of daptomycin in children with suspected or proved gram-positive infections. *Pediatr. Infect. Dis. J.*, 2008; 27: 330-4.

[248] Dvorchik B, Damphousse D. Single-dose pharmacokinetics of daptomycin in young and geriatric volunteers. *J. Clin. Pharmacol.*, 2004; 44: 612-20.

[249] Dvorchik BH, Damphousse D. The pharmacokinetics of daptomycin in moderately obese, morbidly obese, and matched nonobese subjects. *J. Clin. Pharmacol.*, 2005; 45: 48-56.

[250] Dvorchik B, Arbeit RD, Chung J, Liu S, Knebel W, Kastrissios H. Population pharmacokinetics of daptomycin. *Antimicrob. Agents Chemother.*, 2004; 48: 2799-807.

[251] DeRyke CA, Sutherland C, Zhang B, Nicolau DP, Kuti JL. Serum bactericidal activities of high-dose daptomycin with and without coadministration of gentamicin against isolates of *Staphylococcus aureus* and *Enterococcus* species. *Antimicrob. Agents Chemother.*, 2006; 50: 3529-34.

[252] Benvenuto M, Benziger DP, Yankelev S, Vigliani G. Pharmacokinetics and tolerability of daptomycin at doses up to 12 milligrams per kilogram of body weight once daily in healthy volunteers. *Antimicrob. Agents Chemother.*, 2006; 50: 3245-9.

[253] Katz DE, Lindfield KC, Steenbergen JN, Benziger DP, Blackerby KJ, Knapp AG, et al. A pilot study of high-dose short duration daptomycin for the treatment of patients with complicated skin and skin structure infections caused by gram-positive bacteria. *Int. J. Clin. Pract.*, 2008; 62: 1455-64.

[254] Silverman JA, Mortin LI, Vanpraagh AD, Li T, Alder J. Inhibition of daptomycin by pulmonary surfactant: In vitro modeling and clinical impact. *J. Infect. Dis.*, 2005; 191: 2149-52.

[255] Ball P. Quinolone generations: Natural history or natural generation? *J. Antimicrob. Chemother.*, 2000; 46: 17-24.

[256] Appelbaum PC, Hunter PA. The fluoroquinolone antibacterials: past, present and future perspectives. *Int. J. Antimicrob. Agents*, 2000; 16: 5-15.

[257] Saravolatz LD, Leggett J. Gatifloxacin, gemifloxacin, and moxifloxacin: the role of 3 newer fluoroquinolones. *Clin. Infect. Dis.*, 2003; 37: 1210-5.

[258] Schulte A, Heisig P. In vitro activity of gemifloxacin and five other fluoroquinolones against defined isogenic mutants of *Escherichia coli, Pseudomonas aeruginosa* and *Staphylococcus aureus. J. Antimicrob. Chemother.*, 2000; 46: 1037-8.

[259] Oncu S. Treatment of community-acquired pneumonia, with special emphasis on gemifloxacin. *Ther. Clin. Risk Manag.*, 2007; 3: 441-8.

[260] Ferrara AM. New fluoroquinolones in lower respiratory tract infections and emerging patterns of pneumococcal resistance. *Infection*, 2005; 33: 106-14.

[261] Garcia I, Pascual A, Ballesta S, Joyanes P, Perea EJ. Intracellular penetration and activity of gemifloxacin in human polymorphonuclear leukocytes. *Antimicrob. Agents Chemother.*, 2000; 44: 3193-5.

[262] Hong CY, Kim YK, Chang JH, Kim SH, Choi H, Nam DH, et al. Novel fluoroquinolone antibacterial agents containing oxime-substituted (aminomethyl)pyrrolidines: Synthesis and antibacterial activity of 7-(4-(aminomethyl)-3-(methoxyimino)pyrrolidin-1-yl)-1-cyclopropyl-6-fluoro-4-oxo- 1,4-dihydro[1,8] naphthyridine-3-carboxylic acid (LB20304). *J. Med. Chem.*, 1997; 40: 3584-93.

[263] Appelbaum PC, Gillespie SH, Burley CJ, Tillotson GS. Antimicrobial selection for community-acquired lower respiratory tract infections in the 21st century: a review of gemifloxacin. *Int J Antimicrob Agents*. 2004; 23: 533-46.

[264] Blondeau JM, Hansen G, Metzler KL, Borsos S, Irvine LB, Blanco L. In vitro susceptibility of 4903 bacterial isolates to gemifloxacin an advanced fluoroquinolone. *Int. J. Antimicrob. Agents*, 2003; 22: 147-54.

[265] Cormican MG, Jones RN. Antimicrobial activity and spectrum of LB20304, a novel fluoronaphtyridone. *Antimicrob. Agents Chemother.*, 1997; 41: 204-11.

[266] Erwin ME, Jones RN. Studies to establish quality control ranges for SB-265805 (LB20304) when using National Committee for Clinical Laboratory Standards Antimicrobial Susceptibility Test Methods. *J. Clin. Mmicrobiol.*, 1999; 37: 279-80.

[267] Hardy D, Amsterdam D, Mandell LA, Rotstein C. Comparative in vitro activities of ciprofloxacin, gemifloxacin, grepafloxacin, moxifloxacin, ofloxacin, sparfloxacin, trovafloxacin, and other antimicrobial agents against bloodstream isolates of gram-positive cocci. *Antimicrob. Agents Chemother.*, 2000; 44: 802-5.

[268] Jones RN, Erwin ME, Biedenbach DJ, Johnson DM, Pfaller MA. Development of in vitro susceptibility testing methods for gemifloxacin (formerly LB20304a or SB-265805), an investigational fluoronaphthyridone. *Diagn. Microbiol. Infect. Dis.*, 1999; 35: 227-34.

[269] Leonard SN, Kaatz GW, Rucker LR, Rybak MJ. Synergy between gemifloxacin and trimethoprim/sulfamethoxazole against community-associated methicillin-resistant *Staphylococcus aureus*. *J. Antimicrob. Chemother.*, 2008; 62: 1305-10.

[270] McCloske L, Moore T, Niconovich N, Donald B, Broskey J, Jakielaszek C, et al. In vitro activity of gemifloxacin against a broad range of recent clinical isolates from the USA. *J. Antimicrob. Chemother.*, 2000; 45: 13-21.

[271] Oh JI, Paek KS, Ahn MJ, Kim MY, Hong CY, Kim IC, et al. In vitro and in vivo evaluations of LB20304, a new fluoronaphthyridone. *Antimicrob. Agents Chemother.*, 1996; 40: 1564-8.

[272] Wise R, Andrews JM. The in-vitro activity and tentative breakpoint of gemifloxacin, a new fluoroquinolone. *J. Antimicrob. Chemother.*, 1999; 44: 679-88.

[273] Yong DE, Cheong HJ, Kim YS, Park YJ, Kim WJ, Woo JH, et al. In vitro activity of gemifloxacin against recent clinical isolates of bacteria in Korea. *J. Korean Med. Sci.*, 2002; 17: 737-42.

[274] Bouchillon SK, Hoban DJ, Johnson JL, Johnson BM, Butler DL, Saunders KA, et al. In vitro activity of gemifloxacin and contemporary oral antimicrobial agents against 27247 Gram-positive and Gram-negative aerobic isolates: A global surveillance study. *Int. J. Antimicrob. Agents*, 2004; 23: 181-96.

[275] Fuchs PC, Barry AL, Brown SD. In vitro activity of gemifloxacin against contemporary clinical bacterial isolates from eleven North American medical centers, and assessment of disk diffusion test interpretive criteria. *Diagn. Microbiol. Infect. Dis.*, 2000; 38: 243-53.

[276] Vazquez JA, Berron S, Gimenez MJ, de la Fuente L, Aguilar L. In vitro susceptibility of *Neisseria meningitidis* isolates to gemifloxacin and ten other antimicrobial agents. *Eur. J. Clin. Microbiol. Infect. Dis.*, 2001; 20:150-1.

[277] Jones RN, Deshpande LM, Erwin ME, Barrett MS, Beach ML. Anti-gonococcal activity of gemifloxacin against fluoroquinolone-resistant strains and a comparison of agar dilution and Etest methods. *J. Antimicrob. Chemother.*, 2000; 45: 67-70.

[278] Blondeau JM, Tillotson G. Role of gemifloxacin in the management of community-acquired lower respiratory tract infections. *Int J Antimicrob Agents*, 2008; 31: 299-306.

[279] Deshpande LM, Jones RN. Antimicrobial activity of advanced-spectrum fluoroquinolones tested against more than 2000 contemporary bacterial isolates of species causing community-adquired respiratory tract infections. *Diagn. Microbiol. Infect. Dis.*, 2000; 37: 139-42.

[280] Garcia-Garrote F, Cercenado E, Martin-Pedroviejo J, Cuevas O, Bouza E. Comparative in vitro activity of the new quinolone gemifloxacin (SB-265805) with other fluoroquinolones against respiratory tract pathogens. *J. Antimicrob. Chemother.*, 2001; 47: 681-4.

[281] Hammerschlag MR. Activity of gemifloxacin and other new quinolones against *Chlamydia pneumoniae*: A review. *J. Antimicrob. Chemother.* 2000; 45: 35-9.

[282] Stout JE, Sens K, Mietzner S, Obman A, Yu VL. Comparative activity of quinolones, macrolides and ketolides against *Legionella* species using in vitro broth dilution and intracellular susceptibility testing. *Int. J. Antimicrob. Agent*s, 2005; 25: 302-7.

[283] Dubois J, St-Pierre C. Comparative in vitro activity and post-antibiotic effect of gemifloxacin against *Legionella* spp. *J. Antimicrob. Chemother.*, 2000; 45: 41-6.

[284] Fernandez-Roblas R, Cabria F, Esteban J, Lopez JC, Gadea I, Soriano F. In vitro activity of gemifloxacin (SB-265805) compared with 14 other antimicrobials against intestinal pathogens. *J. Antimicrob. Chemother.*, 2000; 46: 1023-7.

[285] Goldstein EJ, Citron DM, Merriam CV, Tyrrell K, Warren Y. Activities of gemifloxacin (SB 265805, LB20304) compared to those of other oral antimicrobial agents against unusual anaerobes. *Antimicrob. Agents Chemother.*, 1999; 43: 2726-30.

[286] Goldstein EJ, Conrads G, Citron DM, Merriam CV, Warren Y, Tyrrell K. In vitro activity of gemifloxacin compared to seven other oral antimicrobial agents against aerobic and anaerobic pathogens isolated from antral sinus puncture specimens from patients with sinusitis. *Diagn. Microbiol. Infect. Dis.*, 2002; 42: 113-8.

[287] King A, May J, French G, Phillips I. Comparative in vitro activity of gemifloxacin. *J. Antimicrob. Chemother.*, 2000; 45: 1-12.

[288] Kleinkauf N, Ackermann G, Schaumann R, Rodloff AC. Comparative in vitro activities of gemifloxacin, other quinolones, and nonquinolone antimicrobials against obligately anaerobic bacteria. *Antimicrob. Agents Chemother.*, 2001; 45:1896-9.

[289] Mortensen JE, Rodgers GL. In vitro activity of gemifloxacin and other antimicrobial agents against isolates of *Bordetella pertussis* and *Bordetella parapertussis*. *J. Antimicrob. Chemother.*, 2000; 45: 47-9.

[290] Duffy LB, Crabb D, Searcey K, Kempf MC. Comparative potency of gemifloxacin, new quinolones, macrolides, tetracycline and clindamycin against *Mycoplasma* spp. *J. Antimicrob. Chemother.*, 2000; 45: 29-33.

[291] Hansen G, Swanzy S, Gupta R, Cookson B, Limaye AP. In vitro activity of fluoroquinolones against clinical isolates of *Nocardia* identified by partial 16S rRNA sequencing. *Eur. J. Clin. Microbiol. Infect. Dis.*, 2008; 27: 115-20.

[292] Marco F, Almela M, Nolla-Salas J, Coll P, Gasser I, Ferrer MD, et al. In vitro activities of 22 antimicrobial agents against *Listeria monocytogenes* strains isolated in Barcelona, Spain. *Diagn. Microbiol. Infect. Dis.*, 2000; 38: 259-61.

[293] Martinez-Martinez L, Joyanes P, Suarez AL, Perea EJ. Activities of gemifloxacin and five other antimicrobial agents against *Listeria monocytogenes* and coryneform bacteria isolated from clinical samples. *Antimicrob. Agents Chemother.*, 2001; 45: 2390-2.

[294] Minehart HW, Chalker AF. In vitro activity of gemifloxacin against *Helicobacter. pylori*. *J. Antimicrob. Chemother.*, 2001; 47: 360-1.

[295] Pereyre S, Renaudin H, Bebear C, Bebear CM. In vitro activities of the newer quinolones garenoxacin, gatifloxacin, and gemifloxacin against human mycoplasmas. *Antimicrob. Agents Chemother.*, 2004; 48: 3165-8.

[296] Berron S, Vazquez JA, Gimenez MJ, de la Fuente L, Aguilar L. In vitro susceptibilities of 400 spanish isolates of *Neisseria gonorrhoeae* to gemifloxacin and 11 other antimicrobial agents. *Antimicrob. Agents Chemother.*, 2000; 44: 2543-4.

[297] Biedenbach DJ, Jones RN. Evaluation of in vitro susceptibility testing criteria for gemifloxacin when tested against *Haemophilus influenzae* strains with reduced susceptibility to ciprofloxacin and ofloxacin. *Diagn. Microbiol. Infect. Dis.*, 2002; 43: 323-6.

[298] Davies TA, Kelly LM, Pankuch GA, Credito KL, Jacobs MR, Appelbaum PC. Antipneumococcal activities of gemifloxacin compared to those of nine other agents. *Antimicrob. Agents Chemother.*, 2000; 44: 304-10.

[299] Goldstein EJ, Citron DM, Warren Y, Tyrrell K, Merriam CV. In vitro activity of gemifloxacin (SB 265805) against anaerobes. *Antimicrob. Agents Chemother.*, 1999; 43: 2231-5.

[300] Gonullu N, Aktas Z, Salcioglu M, Bal C, Ang O. Comparative in vitro activities of five quinolone antibiotics, including gemifloxacin, against clinical isolates. *Clin. Microbiol. Infect.*, 2001; 7: 499-503.

[301] Higgins PG, Coleman K, Amyes SG. Bactericidal and bacteriostatic activity of gemifloxacin against *Acinetobacter* spp. in vitro. *J. Antimicrob. Chemother.*, 2000; 45: 71-7.

[302] Hoban DJ, Bouchillon SK, Karlowsky JA, Johnson JL, Butler DL, Miller LA, et al. A comparative in vitro surveillance study of gemifloxacin activities against 2,632 recent *Streptococcus pneumoniae* isolates from across Europe, North America, and South America. The Gemifloxacin Surveillance Study Research Group. *Antimicrob. Agents Chemother.*, 2000; 44: 3008-11.

[303] Ieven M, Goossens W, De Wit S, Goossens H. In vitro activity of gemifloxacin compared with other antimicrobial agents against recent clinical isolates of streptococci. *J. Antimicrob. Chemother.*, 2000; 45: 51-3.

[304] Marco F, Barrett MS, Jones RN. Antimicrobial activity of LB20304, a fluoronaphthyridone, tested against anaerobic bacteria. *J. Antimicrob. Chemother.*, 1997; 40: 605-7.

[305] Pottumarthy S, Fritsche TR, Jones RN. Activity of gemifloxacin tested against *Neisseria gonorrhoeae* isolates including antimicrobial-resistant phenotypes. *Diagn. Microbiol. Infect. Dis.*, 2006; 54: 127-34.

[306] Davies TA, Evangelista A, Pfleger S, Bush K, Sham DF, Goldschmidt R. Prevalence of single mutations in topoisomerase type II genes among levofloxacin-susceptible clinical strains of *Streptococcus pneumoniae* isolated in the United States in 1992 to 1996 and 1999 to 2000. *Antimicrob. Agents Chemother.*, 2002; 46: 119-24.

[307] Davidson R, Cavalcanti R, Brunton JL, Bast DJ, de Azavedo JCS, Kisbey P, et al. Resistance to levofloxacin and failure of treatment of pneumococcal pneumonia. *N. Engl. J. Med.*, 2002; 346: 747-50.

[308] Legakis NJ, Tzouvelekis LS, Makris A, Kotsifaki H. Outer membrane alterations in multirresistant mutants of *Pseudomonas aeruginosa* selected by ciprofloxacin. *Antimicrob. Agents Chemother.*, 1989; 33: 124-7.

[309] Pages JM, Bolla JM, Bernadec A, Fourel D. Immunological approach of assembly and topology of OmpF, an outer membrane protein of *Escherichia coli. Biochimie*, 1990; 72: 169-76.

[310] Jones RN. Resistance patterns among nosocomial pathogens: Trends over the past few years. *Chest*, 119: 397-404.

[311] Gotoh N. Antibiotic resistance caused by membrane impermeability and multidrug efflux systems. *Nippon Rinsho*, 2001; 59: 712-8.

[312] Kaatz GW, Seo SM, Ruble CA. Eflux-mediated fluoroquinolone resistance in *Staphylococcus aureus. Antimicrob. Agents Chemother.*, 1993; 37: 1086-94.

[313] Gill MJ, Brenwald NP, Wise R. Identification of an efflux pump gene, *pmrA*, associated with fluoroquinolone resistance in *Streptococcus pneumoniae. Antimicrob. Agents Chemother.*, 1999; 43: 187-9.

[314] Blondeau JM, Missaghi B. Gemifloxacin: A new fluoroquinolone. *Expert Opin. Pharmacother.*, 2004; 5: 1117-52.

[315] Heaton VJ, Ambler JE, Fisher LM. Potent antipneumococcal activity of gemifloxacin is associated with dual targeting of gyrase and topoisomerase IV, an in vivo target preference for gyrase, and enhanced stabilization of cleavable complexes in vitro. *Antimicrob. Agents Chemother.*, 2000; 44: 3112-7.

[316] Azoulay-Dupuis E, Bedos JP, Mohler J, Moine P, Cherbuliez C, Peytavin G, et al. Activity of gemifloxacin against quinolone-resistant *Streptococcus pneumoniae* strains in vitro and in a mouse pneumonia model. *Antimicrob Agents Chemother.*, 2005; 49: 1046-54.

[317] Brenwald NP, Appelbaum P, Davies T, Gill MJ. Evidence for efflux pumps, other than PmrA, associated with fluoroquinolone resistance in *Streptococcus pneumoniae. Clin. Microbiol. Infect.*, 2003; 9: 140-3.

[318] Ince D, Zhang X, Silver LC, Hooper DC. Topoisomerase targeting with and resistance to gemifloxacin in *Staphylococcus aureus. Antimicrob. Agents Chemother.*, 2003; 47: 274-82.

[319] Allen A, Bygate E, Oliver S, Johnson M, Ward C, Cheon AJ, et al. Pharmacokinetics and tolerability of gemifloxacin (SB-265805) after administration of single oral doses to healthy volunteers. *Antimicrob. Agents Chemother.*, 2000; 44: 1604-8.

[320] Allen A, Bygate E, Vousden M, Oliver S, Johnson M, Ward C, et al. Multiple-dose pharmacokinetics and tolerability of gemifloxacin administered orally to healthy volunteers. *Antimicrob. Agents Chemother.*, 2001; 45: 540-5.

[321] Bhavnani SM, Andes DR. Gemifloxacin for the treatment of respiratory tract infections: In vitro susceptibility, pharmacokinetics and pharmacodynamics, clinical efficacy, and safety. *Pharmacotherapy*, 2005; 25: 717-40.

[322] Seo MK, Lee YH, Kim IC, Lee SH, Jeong YN, Lee S, et al. Pharmacokinetics of LB20304, a new fluoroquinolone, in rats and dogs. *Arch. Pharm. Res.*, 1996; 19: 359-67.

[323] Yoo BK, Triller DM, Yong CS, Lodise TP. Gemifloxacin: A new fluoroquinolone approved for treatment of respiratory infections. *Ann. Pharmacother.*, 2004; 38: 1226-35.

[324] Zhanel GG, Noreddin A. Pharmacokinetics and pharmacodynamics of the new fluoroquinolones: Focus on respiratory infections. *Curr. Opinion. Pharmacol.*, 2001; 1: 459-63.

[325] Factive™ [package insert]. Seoul, Korea: Genesoft Pharmaceuticals, 2003.

[326] Ferguson BJ, Anon J, Poole MD, Hendrick K, Gilson M, Seltzer EG. Short treatment durations for acute bacterial rhinosinusitis: Five days of gemifloxacin versus 7 days of gemifloxacin. *Otolaryngol. Head Neck. Surg.*, 2002; 127: 1-6.

[327] Ball P, Wilson R, Mandell L, Brown J, Henkel T, the 069 Clinical Study Group. Efficacy of gemifloxacin in acute exacerbactions of chronic bronchitis: a randomised, double-blind comparison with trovafloxacin. *J. Chemother.*, 2001; 13: 288-98.

[328] Ball P, Mandell L, Patou G, Dankner W, Tillotson G. A new respiratory fluoroquinolone, oral gemifloxacin: A safety profile in context. *Int. J. Antimicrob. Agents*, 2004; 23: 421-9.

[329] File TM Jr, Mandell LA, Tillotson G, Kostov K, Georgiev O. Gemifloxacin once daily for 5 days versus 7 days for the treatment of community-acquired pneumonia: A randomized, multicentre, double-blind study. *J. Antimicrob. Chemother.*, 2007; 60: 112-20.

[330] Léophonte P, File T, Feldman C. Gemifloxacin once daily for 7 days compared to amoxicillin/clavulanic acid thrice daily for 10 days for the treatment of community-acquired pneumonia of suspected pneumococcal origin. *Respir Med*, 2004, 98: 708-20.

[331] Lode H, File TM Jr, Mandell L, Ball P, Pypstra R, Thomas M, et al. Oral gemifloxacin versus sequential therapy with intravenous ceftriaxone/oral cefuroxime with or without a macrolide in the treatment of patients hospitalized with community-acquired pneumonia: A randomized, open-label, multicenter study of clinical efficacy and tolerability. *Clin. Ther.*, 2002; 24: 1915-36.

[332] Vousden M, Ferguson J, Richards J, Bird N, Allen A. Evaluation of phototoxic potential of gemifloxacin in healthy volunteers compared with ciprofloxacin. *Chemotherapy*, 1999; 45: 512-20.

[333] Iannini P, Mandell L, Patou G, Shear N. Cutaneous adverse events and gemifloxacin: Observations from the clinical trial program. *J. Chemother.*, 2006; 18: 3-11.

[334] Araujo F, Slifer T, Li S, Kuver A, Fong L, Remington J. Gemifloxacin inhibits cytokine secretion by lipopolysaccharide stimulated human monocytes at the post-transcriptional level. *Clin. Microbiol. Infect.*, 2004; 10: 213-9.

[335] Bryskier A. Ketolides-telithromycin, an example of a new class of antibacterial agents. *Clin. Microbiol. Infect.*, 2000; 6: 661-9.

[336] Leclercq R. Overcoming antimicrobial resistance: Profile of a new ketolide antibacterial, telithromycin. *J Antimicrob Chemother*, 2001; 48: 9-23.

[337] Nguyen M, Chung EP. Telithromycin: The first ketolide antimicrobial. *Clin Ther*, 2005; 27: 1144-63.

[338] Douthwaite S, Champney WS. Structures of ketolides and macrolides determine their mode of interaction with the ribosomal target site. *J. Antimicrob. Chemother.*, 2001; 48: 1-8.

[339] Capobianco JO, Cao ZS, Shortidge VD, Ma Z, Flamm RK, Zhong P. Studies of the novel ketolide ABT-773: Transport, binding to ribosomes, and inhibition of protein synthesis in *Streptococcus pneumoniae. Antimicrob. Agents Chemother.*, 2000; 44: 1562-7.

[340] Lonks JR, Goldmann DA. Telithromycin: A ketolide antibiotic for treatment of respiratory tract infections. *Clin. Infect. Dis.*, 2005; 40: 1657-64.

[341] Douthwaite S, Hansen LH, Mauvais P. Macrolide-ketolide inhibition of MLS resistant ribosomes is improved by alternative drug interaction with domain II of 23S rRNA. *Mol. Microbiol.*, 2000; 36: 183-93.

[342] Xiong L, Shah S, Mauvais P, Mankin AS. A ketolide resistance mutation in domain II of 23S rRNA reveals the proximity of hairpin 35 to the peptidyl transferase centre. *Mol. Microbiol.*, 1999; 31: 633-9.

[343] Ackermann G, Rodloff AC. Drugs of the 21st century: Telithromycin (HMR 3647)--the first ketolide. *J. Antimicrob. Chemother.*, 2003; 51: 497-511.

[344] Barry AL, Fuchs PC, Brown SD. Relative potency of telithromycin, azithromycin and erythromycin against recent clinical isolates of gram-positive cocci. *Eur. J. Clin. Microbiol. Infect. Dis.*, 2001; 20: 494-7.

[345] Okamoto H, Miyazaki S, Tateda K, Ishii Y, Yamaguchi K. Comparative in vitro activity of telithromycin (HMR 3647), three macrolides, amoxycillin, cefdinir and levofloxacin against gram-positive clinical isolates in Japan. *J. Antimicrob. Chemother.*, 2000; 46: 797-802.

[346] Schmitz FJ, Petridou J, Milatovic D, Verhoef J, Fluit AC, Schwarz S. In vitro activity of new ketolides against macrolide-susceptible and –resistant *Staphylococcus aureus* isolates with defined resistance gene status. *J. Antimicrob. Chemother.*, 2002; 49: 573-84.

[347] Tran MP. Telithromycin: A novel agent for the treatment of community-acquired upper respiratory infections. *Proc (Bayl Univ Med Cent)*. 2004; 17: 475-9.

[348] Turner M, Corey GR, Abrutyn E. Telithromycin. *Ann. Intern. Med.*, 2006; 144: 447-8.

[349] Morosini MI, Canton R, Loza E, Negri MC, Galan JC, Almaraz F, et al. In vitro activity of telithromycin against Spanish *Streptococcus pneumoniae* isolates with characterized macrolide resistance mechanisms. *Antimicrob. Agents Chemother.*, 2001; 45: 2427-31.

[350] Alcaide F, Benitez MA, Carratala J, Gudiol F, Linares J, Martin R. In vitro activities of the new ketolide HMR 3647 (telithromycin) in comparison with those of eight other antibiotics against viridans group streptococci isolated from blood of neutropenic patients with cancer. *Antimicrob. Agents Chemother.*, 2001; 45: 624-6.

[351] Giovanetti E, Montanari MP, Marchetti F, Varaldo PE. In vitro activity of ketolides telithromycin and HMR 3004 against italian isolates of *Streptococcus pyogenes* and *Streptococcus pneumoniae* with different erythromycin susceptibility. *J. Antimicrob. Chemother.* 2000; 46: 905-8.

[352] Jalava J, Kataja J, Seppala H, Huovinen P. In vitro activities of the novel ketolide telithromycin (HMR 3647) against erythromycin-resistant *Streptococcus* species. *Antimicrob. Agents Chemother.*, 2001; 45: 789-93.

[353] Kozlov RS, Bogdanovitch TM, Appelbaum PC, Ednie L, Stratchounski LS, Jacobs MR, et al. Antistreptococcal activity of telithromycin compared with seven other drugs in relation to macrolide resistance mechanisms in Russia. *Antimicrob. Agents Chemother.*, 2002; 46: 2963-8.

[354] Malhotra-Kumar S, Lammens C, Martel A, Mallentjer C, Chapelle S, Verhoeven J, et al. Oropharyngeal carriage of macrolide-resistant viridans group streptococci: a

prevalence study among healthy adults in Belgium. *J. Antimicrob. Chemother.*, 2004; 53: 271-6.

[355] Tomas I, Alvarez M, Lopez-Melendez C, Limeres J, Tomas M, Diz P. In vitro activity of telithromycin against *mef*A and *erm*B erythromycin-resistant viridans streptococci isolated from bacteremia of oral origin in Spain. *Oral. Microbiol. Immunol.*, 2005; 20: 35-8.

[356] Ubukata K, Iwata S, Sunakawa K. In vitro activities of new ketolide, telithromycin, and eight other macrolide antibiotics against *Streptococcus pneumoniae* having *mef*A and *erm*B genes that mediate macrolide resistance. *J. Infect. Chemother.*, 2003; 9: 221-6.

[357] Buxbaum A, Forsthuber S, Graninger W, Georgopoulos A. Comparative activity of telithromycin against typical community-acquired respiratory pathogens. *J. Antimicrob. Chemother.*, 2003; 52: 371-4.

[358] Dohar J, Canton R, Cohen R, Farrell DJ, Felmingham D. Activity of telithromycin and comparators against bacterial pathogens isolated from 1,336 patients with clinically diagnosed acute sinusitis. *Ann. Clin. Microbiol. Antimicrob.*, 2004; 3:15.

[359] Felmingham D, Farrell DJ. In vitro activity of telithromycin against Gram-negative bacterial pathogens. *J. Infect.*, 2006; 52: 178-80.

[360] Goldstein EJ, Citron DM, Merriam CV, Warren Y, Tyrrel KL, Fernandez H. In vitro activities of telithromycin and 10 oral agents against aerobic and anaerobic pathogens isolated from antral puncture specimens from patients with sinusitis. *Antimicrob. Agents Chemother.*, 2003; 47: 1963-7.

[361] Miyashita N, Fukano H, Niki Y, Matsushima T. In vitro activity of telithromycin, a new ketolide, against *Chlamydia pneumoniae*. *J. Antimicrob. Chemother.*, 2001; 48: 403-5.

[362] Rolain JM, Maurin M, Bryskier A, Raoult D. In vitro activities of telithromycin (HMR 3647) against *Rickettsia rickettsii*, *Rickettsia conorii*, *Rickettsia africae*, *Rickettsia typhi*, *Rickettsia prowazekii*, *Coxiella burnetii*, *Bartonella henselae*, *Bartonella quintana*, *Bartonella bacilliformis*, and *Ehrlichia chaffeensis*. *Antimicrob. Agents Chemother.*, 2000; 44: 1391-3.

[363] Bebear CM, Renaudin H, Bryskier A, Bebear C. Comparative activities of telithromycin (HMR 3647), levofloxacin, and other antimicrobial agents against human mycoplasmas. *Antimicrob. Agents Chemother.*, 2000; 44: 1980-2.

[364] Kenny GE, Cartwright FD. Susceptibilities of *Mycoplasma hominis*, *Mycoplasma pneumoniae*, and *Ureaplasma urealyticum* to GAR-936, dalfopristin, dirithromycin, evernimicin, gatifloxacin, linezolid, moxifloxacin, quinupristin-dalfopristin, and telithromycin compared to their susceptibilities to reference macrolides, tetracyclines, and quinolones. *Antimicrob. Agents Chemother.*, 2001; 45: 2604-8.

[365] Tomas I, Tomas M, Alvarez M, Velasco D, Potel C, Limeres J, et al. Susceptibility of oral obligate anaerobes to telithromycin, moxifloxacin and a number of commonly used antibacterials. *Oral Microbiol. Immunol.*, 2007; 22: 298-303.

[366] Wexler HM, Molitoris E, Molitoris D, Finegold SM. In vitro activity of telithromycin (HMR 3647) against 502 strains of anaerobic bacteria. *J. Antimicrob. Chemother.*, 2001; 47: 467-9.

[367] Mensa J, Garcia-Vazquez E, Vila J. Macrolides, ketolidos and streptogramins. *Enferm Infecc. Microbiol. Clin.*, 2003; 21: 200-8.

[368] Morosini MI, Canton R, Loza E, del Campo R, Almaraz F, Baquero F. *Streptococcus pyogenes* isolates with characterized macrolide resistance mechanisms in Spain: In vitro activities of telithromycin and cethromycin. *J. Antimicrob. Chemother.*, 2003; 52: 50-5.

[369] Ackermann G, Schaumann R, Pless B, Claros MC, Rodloff AC. In vitro activity of telithromycin (HMR 3647) and seven other antimicrobial agents against anaerobic bacteria. *J. Antimicrob. Chemother.*, 2000; 46: 115-9.

[370] Fernandez-Roblas R, Esteban J, Cabria F, Lopez JC, Jimenez MS, Soriano F. In vitro susceptibilities of rapidly growing mycobacteria to telithromycin (HMR 3647) and seven other antimicrobials. *Antimicrob. Agents Chemother.*, 2000; 44: 181-2.

[371] Liu M, Douthwaite S. Activity of the ketolide telithromycin is refractory to Erm monomethylation of bacterial rRNA. *Antimicrob. Agents Chemother.*, 2002; 46: 1629-33.

[372] Weisblum B. Insights into erythromycin action from studies of its activity as inducer of resistance. *Antimicrob. Agents Chemother.*, 1995; 39: 797-805.

[373] Schmitz FJ, Petridou J, Jagusch H, Astfalk N, Scheuring S, Schwarz S. Molecular characterization of ketolide-resistant *erm* (A)-carrying *Staphylococcus aureus* isolates selected in vitro by telithromycin, ABT-773, quinupristin and clindamycin. *J. Antimicrob. Chemother.*, 2002; 49: 611-7.

[374] Vester B, Douthwaite S. Macrolide resistance conferred by base substitutions in 23S rRNA. *Antimicrob. Agents Chemother.*, 2001; 45: 1-12.

[375] Canu A, Malbruny B, Coquemont M, Davies TA, Appelbaum PC, Leclercq R. Diversity of ribosomal mutations conferring resistance to macrolides, clindamycin, streptogramin, and telithromycin in *Streptococcus pneumoniae*. *Antimicrob. Agents Chemother.*, 2002; 46: 125-31.

[376] Edelstein PH. Pneumococcal resistance to macrolides, lincosamides, ketolides, and streptogramin B agents: Molecular mechanisms and resistance phenotypes. *Clin. Infect. Dis.*, 2004; 38: S322–7.

[377] Hisanaga T, Hoban DJ, Zhanel GG. Mechanisms of resistance to telithromycin in *Streptococcus pneumoniae*. *J. Antimicrob. Chemother.*, 2005; 56: 447-50.

[378] Horii T, Notake S, Yoda Y, Yanagisawa, H. Emergence of telithromycin resistance in *Haemophilus influenzae* in Japan. *J. Med. Microbiol.*, 2007; 56: 1705-6.

[379] Pereyre S, Guyot C, Renaudin H, Charron A, Bebear C, Bebear CM. In vitro selection and characterization of resistance to macrolides and related antibiotics in *Mycoplasma pneumoniae*. *Antimicrob. Agents Chemother.*, 2004; 48: 460-5.

[380] Tait-Kamradt A, Davies T, Cronan M, Jacobs MR, Appelbaum PC, Sutcliffe J. Mutations in 23S rRNA and ribosomal protein L4 account for resistance in pneumococcal strains selected in vitro by macrolide passage. *Antimicrob. Agents Chemother.*, 2000; 44: 2118-25.

[381] Walsh F, Willcock J, Amyes S. High-level telithromycin resistance in laboratory-generated mutants of *Streptococcus pneumoniae*. *J. Antimicrob. Chemother.*, 2003; 52: 345-53.

[382] Yusupov MM, Yusupova GZ, Baucom A, Lieberman K, Earnest TN, Cate JH. Crystal structure of the ribosome at 5.5 A resolution. *Science*, 2001; 292: 883-96.

[383] Garza-Ramos G, Xiong L, Zhong P, Mankin A. Binding site of macrolide antibiotics on the ribosome: New resistance mutation identifies a specific interaction of ketolides with rRNA. *J. Bacteriol.*, 2001; 183: 6898-907.

[384] Chesneau O, Tsvetkova K, Courvalin P. Resistance phenotypes conferred bymacrolide phosphotransferases. *FEMS Microbiol. Lett.*, 2007; 269: 317-22.

[385] Tripathi S, Kloss PS, Mankin AS. Ketolide resistance conferred by short peptides. *J. Biol. Chem.*, 1998; 273: 20073-7.

[386] Ketek™ [package insert]. Bridgewater, NJ: Sanofi-Aventis US LLC, 2007.

[387] Namour F, Wessels DH, Pascual MH, Reynolds D, Sultan E, Lenfant B. Pharmacokinetics of the new ketolide telithromycin (HMR 3647) administered in ascending single and multiple doses. *Antimicrob. Agents Chemother.*, 2001; 45: 170-5.

[388] Lenfant B, Perret C, Pascual MH. The bioavailability of HMR 3647, a new once-daily ketolide antimicrobial, is unaffected by food. *J. Antimicrob. Chemother.*, 1999; 44: 55.

[389] Mtairag EM, Abdelghaffar H, Douhet C, Labro MT. Role of extracellular calcium in in vitro uptake and intraphagocytic location of macrolides. *Antimicrob. Agents Chemother.*, 1995; 39: 1676-82.

[390] Azanza Perea JR, Garcia Quetglas E, Sádaba Díaz de Rada B. Telithromycin: Pharmacokinetic and clinical implications. *Arch. Bronconeumol.*, 2003; 39: 9-15.

[391] Barman Balfour J, Figgitt D. Telithromycin. *Drugs*, 2001; 61: 815-30.

[392] Perret C, Wessels DH. Oral bioavailability of the ketolide telithromycin (HMR 3647) is similar in both elderly and young subjects. *Clin. Microb. Infect.*, 2000; 6: 203-4.

[393] Carbon C, Moola S, Velancsics I, Leroy B, Rangaraju M, Decosta P. Telithromycin 800 mg once daily for seven to ten days is an effective and well-tolerated treatment for community-acquired pneumonia. *Clin. Microbiol. Infect.*, 2003; 9: 691-703.

[394] Dunbar LM, Hassman J, Tellier G. Efficacy and tolerability of once-daily oral telithromycin compared with clarithromycin for the treatment of community-acquired pneumonia in adults. *Clin. Ther.*, 2004; 26: 48-62.

[395] Ferguson BJ, Guzzetta RV, Spector SL, Hadley JA. Efficacy and safety of oral telithromycin once daily for 5 days versus moxifloxacin once daily for 10 days in the treatment of acute bacterial rhinosinusitis. *Otolaryngol. Head Neck Surg.*, 2004; 131: 207-14.

[396] Fogarty CM, Patel TC, Dunbar LM, Leroy BP. Efficacy and safety of telithromycin 800 mg once daily for 7 days in community-acquired pneumonia: An open-label, multicenter study. *BMC Infect. Dis.*, 2005; 5:43.

[397] Hagberg L, Torres A, van Rensburg D, Leroy B, Rangaraju M, Ruuth E. Efficacy and tolerability of once-daily telithromycin compared with high-dose amoxicillin for treatment of community-acquired pneumonia. *Infection*, 2002; 30: 378-86.

[398] Norrby SR, Quinn J, Rangaraju M, Leroy B. Evaluation of 5-day therapy with telithromycin, a novel ketolide antibacterial, for the treatment of tonsillopharyngitis. *Clin. Microbiol. Infect.*, 2004; 10: 615-23.

[399] Quinn J, Ruoff GE, Ziter PS. Efficacy and tolerability of 5-day, once-daily telithromycin compared with 10-day, twice-daily clarithromycin for the treatment of

group A beta-hemolytic streptococcal tonsillitis/pharyngitis: A multicenter, randomized, double-blind, parallel-group study. *Clin. Ther.*, 2003; 25: 422-43.

[400] Tellier G, Niederman MS, Nusrat R, Patel M, Lavin B. Clinical and bacteriological efficacy and safety of 5 and 7 day regimens of telithromycin once daily compared with a 10 day regimen of clarithromycin twice daily in patients with mild to moderate community-acquired pneumonia. *J. Antimicrob. Chemother.* 2004; 54: 515-23.

[401] Van Rensburg DJ, Matthews PA, Leroy B. Efficacy and safety of telithromycin in community-acquired pneumonia. *Curr. Med. Res. Opin.*, 2002; 18: 397-400.

[402] Zervos MJ, Heyder AM, Leroy B. Oral telithromycin 800 mg once daily for 5 days versus cefuroxime axetil 500 mg twice daily for 10 days in adults with acute exacerbations of chronic bronchitis. *J. Int. Med. Res.*, 2003; 31: 157-69.

[403] Bottenberg MM, Wall GC, Hicklin GA. Apparent anaphylactoid reaction treatement with a single dose of telithromycin. *Ann. Allergy Asthma Immunol.*, 2007; 98: 89-91.

[404] Buyukberber M, Demirci F, Savas MC, Kis C, Gulsen MT, Koruk M. Pill esophagitis caused by telithromycin: A case report. *Turk J. Gastroenterol.*, 2006; 17: 113-5.

[405] Brinker AD, Wassel RT, Lyndly J, Serrano J, Avigan M, Lee WM, et al. Telithromycin-associated hepatotoxicity: Clinical spectrum and causality assessment of 42 cases. *Hepatology*, 2009; 49: 250-7.

[406] Clay KD, Hanson JS, Pope SD, Rissmiller RW, Purdum PP, Banks PM. Brief communication: Severe hepatotoxicity of telithromycin: three case reports and literature review. *Ann. Intern. Med.*, 2006; 144: 415-20.

[407] Dore DD, DiBello JR, Lapane KL. Telithromycin use and spontaneous reports of hepatotoxicity. *Drug. Saf.*, 2007; 30: 697-703.

[408] Onur O, Guneysel O, Denizbasi A, Celikel C. Acute hepatitis attack after exposure to telithromycin. *Clin. Ther.*, 2007; 29: 1725-9.

[409] Tintillier M, Kirch L, Almpanis C, Cosyns JP, Pochet JM, Cuvelier C. Telithromycin-induced acute interstitial nephritis: A first case report. *Am J Kidney Kis*, 2004; 44: 25-7.

[410] Hatanaka Y, Zamami Y, Koyama T, Hobara N, Jin X, Kitamura Y, et al. A ketolide antibiotic, telithromycin, inhibits vascular adrenergic neurotransmission in the rat mesenteric vascular bed. *Br. J. Pharmacol.*, 2008; 155: 826-36.

[411] Petersen PJ, Jacobus NV, Weiss WJ, Sum PE, Testa RT. In vitro and in vivo antibacterial activities of a novel glycylcycline, the 9-t-butylglycylamido derivative of minocycline (GAR-936). *Antimicrob. Agents Chemother.*, 1999; 43: 738-44.

[412] Biedenbach DJ, Beach ML, Jones RN. In vitro antimicrobial activity of GAR-936 tested against antibiotic resistant gram-positive blood stream infection isolates and strains producing extended-spectrum beta-lactamases. *Diagn. Microbiol. Infect. Dis.*, 2001; 40: 173-7.

[413] Fritsche TR, Kirby JT, Jones RN. In vitro activity of tigecycline (GAR-936) tested against 11,859 recent clinical isolates associated with community-acquired respiratory tract and Gram-positive cutaneous infections. *Diagn. Microbiol. Infect. Dis.*, 2004; 49: 201-9.

[414] Noskin GA. Tigecycline: A new glycylcycline for treatment of serious infections. *Clin. Infect. Dis.*, 2005; 41(Suppl 5): S303-14.

[415] Gobernado M. Bacterial resistance and a new antibiotic: tigecycline. *Rev. Esp. Quimioter.*, 2006; 19: 209-9.

[416] Conejo MC, Hernández JR, Pacual A. Effect of porin loss on the activity of tigecycline against *Klebsiella pneumoniae* producing extended-spectrum beta-lactamases or plasmid-mediated AmpC-type beta-lactamases. *Diagn. Microbiol. Infect. Dis.*, 2008; 61: 343-5.

[417] Betriú C, Rodríguez-Avial I, Gómez M, Culebras E, López F, Álvarez J, et al. Antimicrobial activity of tigecycline against clinical isolates from Spanish medical centers. Second multicenter study. *Diagn. Microbiol. Infect. Dis.*, 2006; 56: 437-44.

[418] Bradford PA, Weaver-Sands DT, Petersen PJ. In vitro activity of tigecycline against isolates from patients enrolled in phase 3 clinical trials of treatment for complicated skin and skin-structure infections and complicated intra-abdominal infections. *Clin. Infect. Dis.*, 2005; 41(Suppl 5): S315-32.

[419] Fritsche TR, Strabala PA, Sader HS, Dowzicky MJ, Jones RN. Activity of tigecycline tested against a global collection of *Enterobacteriaceae*, including tetracycline-resistant isolates. *Diagn. Microbiol. Infect. Dis.*, 2005; 52: 209-13.

[420] Mercier RC, Kennedy C, Meadows C. Antimicrobial activity of tigecycline (GAR-936) against *Enterococcus faecium* and *Staphylococcus aureus* used alone and in combination. *Pharmacotherapy*, 2002; 22: 1517-23.

[421] Zinner SH. Overview of antibiotic use and resistance: Setting the stage for tigecycline. *Clin. Infect. Dis.*, 2005; 41(Suppl. 5): S289-92.

[422] Kelesidis T, Karageorgopoulos DE, Kelesidis I, Falagas ME. Tigecycline for the treatment of multidrug-resistant *Enterobacteriaceae*: a systematic review of the evidence from microbiological and clinical studies. *J. Antimicrob. Chemother.*, 2008; 62: 895-904.

[423] Sorlózano A, Gutiérrez J, Salmerón A, Luna JD, Martínez-Checa F, Román J, et al. Activity of tigecycline against clinical isolates of *Staphylococcus aureus* and extended-spectrum-betalactamase-producing *Escherichia coli* in Granada, Spain. *Int. J. Antimicrob. Agents*, 2006; 28: 532-6.

[424] Sorlózano A, Gutiérrez J, Román E, Luna JD, Román J, Liébana J, et al. A comparison of the activity of tigecycline against multiresistant clinical isolates of *Staphylococcus aureus* and *Streptococcus agalactiae*. *Diagn. Microbiol. Infect. Dis.*, 2007; 58: 487-9.

[425] Doan TL, Fung HB, Mehta D, Riska PE. Tigecycline: A glycylcycline antimicrobial agent. *Clin. Ther.*, 2006; 28: 1079-106.

[426] Pankey GA. Tigecycline. *J. Antimicrob. Chemother.*, 2005; 56: 470-80.

[427] Reinert RR, Low DE, Rossi F, Zhang X, Wattal C, Dowzicky MJ. Antimicrobial susceptibility among organisms from the Asia/Pacific Rim, Europe and Latin and North America collected as part of TEST and the in vitro activity of tigecycline. *J. Antimicrob. Chemother.*, 2007; 60: 1018-29.

[428] Guay DRP. Oritavancin and tigecycline: Investigational antimicrobials for multidrug-resistant bacteria. *Pharmacotherapy*, 2004; 24: 58-68.

[429] Katsandri A, Avlamis A, Pantazatou A, Petrikkos GL, Legakis NJ, Papaparaskevas J, et al. In vitro activities of tigecycline against recently isolated Gram-negative anaerobic

bacteria in Greece, including metronidazole-resistant strains. *Diagn. Microbiol. Infect. Dis.*, 2006; 55: 231-6.

[430] Keeney D, Ruzin A, McAleese F, Murphy E, Bradford PA. MarA-mediated overexpression of the AcrAB efflux pump results in decreased susceptibility to tigecycline in *Escherichia coli*. *J. Antimicrob. Chemother.*, 2008; 61: 46-53.

[431] Livermore DM. Tigecycline: what is it, and where should it be used? *J. Antimicrob. Chemother.*, 2005; 56: 611-4.

[432] Livermore DM. Introduction: the challenge of multiresistance. *Int. J. Antimicrob. Agents*, 2007; 29(Suppl. 3): S1–S7.

[433] Werner G, Gfrörer S, Fleige C, Witte W, Klare I. Tigecycline-resistant *Enterococcus faecalis* strain isolated from a German intensive care unit patient. *J. Antimicrob. Chemother.*, 2008; 61: 1182-3.

[434] Dean CR, Visalli MA, Projan SJ, Sum PE, Bradford PA. Efflux-mediated resistance to tigecycline (GAR-936) in *Pseudomonas aeruginosa* PAO1. *Antimicrob. Agents Chemother.*, 2003; 47: 972-8.

[435] Bratu S, Landman D, Martin DA, Georgescu C, Quale J. Correlation of antimicrobial resistance with β-lactamases, the OmpA-like porin, and efflux pumps in clinical isolates of *Acinetobacter baumannii* endemic to New York City. *Antimicrob. Agents Chemother.*, 2008; 52: 2999-3005.

[436] Fluit AC, Florijn A, Verhoef J, Milatovic D. Presence of tetracycline resistance determinants and susceptibility to tigecycline and minocycline. *Antimicrob. Agents Chemother.*, 2005; 49: 1636-8.

[437] Reid GE, Grim SA, Aldeza CA, Janda WM, Clark NM. Rapid development of *Acinetobacter baumannii* resistance to tigecycline. *Pharmacotherapy*, 2007; 27: 1198-201.

[438] Damier-Piolle L, Magnet S, Brémont S, Lambert T, Courvalin P. AdeIJK, a resistance-nodulation-cell division pump effluxing multiple antibiotics in *Acinetobacter baumannii*. *Antimicrob. Agents Chemother.*, 2008; 52: 557-62.

[439] Naesens R, Ursi JP, Van Schaeren J, Jeurissen A. In vitro activity of tigecycline against multidrug-resistant *Enterobacteriaceae* isolates from a Belgian hospital. *Eur J Clin Microbiol Infect Dis*, 2008, Sep 19. [Epub ahead of print] doi 10.1007/s10096-008-0629-9.

[440] Moore IF, Hughes DW, Wright GD. Tigecycline is modified by the flavin-dependent monooxygenase tetX. *Biochemistry*, 2005; 44: 11829-35.

[441] Muralidharan G, Fruncillo RJ, Micalizzi M, Raible DG, Troy SM. Effects of age and sex on single-dose pharmacokinetics of tigecycline in healthy subjects. *Antimicrob. Agents Chemother.*, 2005; 49: 1656-9.

[442] Van Wart SA, Cirincione BB, Ludwig EA, Meagher AK, Korth-Bradley JM, Owen JS. Population pharmacokinetics of tigecycline in healthy volunteers. *J. Clin. Pharmacol.*, 2007; 47: 727-37.

[443] MacGowan AP. Tigecycline pharmacokinetic/pharmacodynamic update. *J. Antimicrob. Chemother.*, 2008; 62(Suppl 1):i11-6.

[444] Tygacil™ [package insert]. Philadelphia, PA: Wyeth Pharmaceuticals Inc., 2005.

[445] Rello J. Pharmacokinetics, pharmacodynamics, safety and tolerability of tigecycline. *J. Chemother.*, 2005; 17(Suppl 1): 12-22.

[446] Rodvold KA, Gotfried MH, Cwik M, Korth-Bradley JM, Dukart G, Ellis-Grosse EJ. Serum, tissue and body fluid concentrations of tigecycline after a single 100 mg dose. *J. Antimicrob. Chemother.*, 2006; 58: 1221-9.

[447] Conte JE, Golden JA, Kelly MG, Zurlinden E. Steady-state serum and intrapulmonary pharmacokinetics and pharmacodynamics of tigecycline. *Int. J. Antimicrob. Agents*, 2005; 25: 523-9.

[448] Meagher AK, Ambrose PG, Grasela TH, Ellis-Grosse EJ. Pharmacokinetic /pharmacodynamic profile for tigecycline: A new glycylcycline antimicrobial agent. *Diagn. Microbiol. Infect. Dis.*, 2005; 52: 165-71.

[449] Hoffmann M, DeMaio W, Jordan RA, Talaat R, Harper D, Speth J, et al. Metabolism, excretion, and pharmacokinetics of [14C] tigecycline, a first-in-class glycylcycline antibiotic, after intravenous infusion to healthy male subjects. *Drug. Metab. Dispos.*, 2007; 35: 1543-53.

[450] Muralidharan G, Micalizzi M, Speth J, Raible DG, Troy SM. Pharmacokinetics of tigecycline after single and multiple doses in healthy subjects. *Antimicrob. Agents Chemother.*, 2005; 49: 220-9.

[451] Passarell JA, Meagher AK, Liolios K, Cirincione BB, Van Wart SA, Babinchak T, et al. Exposure-response analyses of tigecycline efficacy in patients with complicated intra-abdominal infections. *Antimicrob. Agents Chemother.*, 2008; 52: 204-10.

[452] Meagher AK, Passarell JA, Cirincione BB, Van Wart SA, Liolios K, Babinchak T, et al. Exposure-response analyses of tigecycline efficacy in patients with complicated skin and skin-structure infections. *Antimicrob. Agents Chemother.*, 2007, 51: 1939-45.

[453] Agwuh KN, MacGowan A. Pharmacokinetics and pharmacodynamics of the tetracyclines including glycylcyclines. *J. Antimicrob. Chemother.*, 2006; 58: 256-65.

[454] Ellis-Grosse EJ, Babinchak T, Dartois N, Rose G, Loh E. The efficacy and safety of tigecycline in the treatment of skin and skin-structure infections: results of 2 double-blind phase 3 comparison studies with vancomycin-aztreonam. *Clin. Infect. Dis.*, 2005; 41(Suppl 5): S341-53.

[455] Gilson M, Moachon L, Jeanne L, Dumaine V, Eyrolle L, Morand P, et al. Acute pancreatitis related to tigecycline: Case report and review of the literature. *Scand. J. Infect. Dis.*, 2008; 40: 681-3.

[456] Hylands J. Tigecycline: A new antibiotic. *Intensive Crit. Care Nurs.*, 2008; 24: 260-3.

[457] Lentino JR, Narita M, Yu VL. New antimicrobial agents as therapy for resistant gram-positive cocci. *Eur. J. Clin. Microbiol. Infect. Dis.*, 2008; 27: 3-15.

[458] Stein GE. Safety of newer parenteral antibiotics. *Clin. Infect. Dis.*, 2005; 41: S293-302.

[459] Vasilev K, Reshedko G, Orasan R, Sanchez M, Teras J, Babinchak T, et al. A Phase 3, open-label, non-comparative study of tigecycline in the treatment of patients with selected serious infections due to resistant Gram-negative organisms including *Enterobacter* species, *Acinetobacter baumannii* and *Klebsiella pneumoniae*. *J. Antimicrob. Chemother.*, 2008; 62(Suppl. 1): i29-i40.

[460] Tygacyl, Second Periodic Safety Update Report-Preliminary assessment report. Rapporteur: Calvo G. Pharmacovigilance assessors: Macia MA, Martin-Serrano G.

Clinical assessor: Fernandez-Cortizo MJ. Periodcovered by this PSUR: 15 Jun 2006 to 14 December 2006. Date of the assessment report: 17 April 2007.

[461] Tanaseanu C, Bergallo C, Teglia O, Jasovich A, Oliva ME, Dukart G, et al. Integrated results of 2 phase 3 studies comparing tigecycline and levofloxacin in community-acquired pneumonia. *Diagn. Microbiol. Infect. Dis.*, 2008; 61: 329-38.

[462] Karageorgopoulos DE, Kelesidis T, Kelesidis I, Falagas ME. Tigecycline for the treatment of multidrug-resistant (including carbapenem-resistant) *Acinetobacter* infections: a review of the scientific evidence. *J. Antimicrob. Chemother.*, 2008; 62: 45-55.

[463] Reinert RR, Reinert S, van der Linden M, Cil MY, Al-Lahham A, Appelbaum P. Antimicrobial susceptibility of *Streptococcus pneumoniae* in eight european countries from 2001 to 2003. *Antimicrob. Agents Chemother.*, 2005, 49: 2903-13.

[464] Pankuch GA, Lin G, Hoellman DB, Good CE, Jacobs MR, Appelbaum PC. Activity of retapamulin against *Streptococcus pyogenes* and *Staphylococcus aureus* evaluated by agar dilution, microdilution, E-test, and disk diffusion methodologies. *Antimicrob. Agents Chemother.*, 2006; 50: 1727-30.

[465] Parish LC, Jorizzo JL, Breton JJ, Hirman JW, Scangarella NE, Shawar RM, et al. Topical retapamulin ointment (1%, wt/wt) twice daily for 5 days versus oral cephalexin twice daily for 10 days in the treatment of secondarily infected dermatitis: Results of a randomized controlled trial. *J. Am. Acad. Dermatol.*, 2006; 55: 1003-13.

[466] Rittenhouse S, Biswas S, Broskey J, McCloskey L, Moore T, Vasey S, et al. Selection of retapamulin, a novel pleuromutilin for topical use. *Antimicrob. Agents Chemother.* 2006; 50: 3882-5.

[467] Ross JE, Jones RN. Quality control guidelines for susceptibility testing of retapamulin (SB-275833) by reference and standardized methods. *J Clin Microbiol.* 2005; 43: 6212-3.

[468] Davidovich C, Bashan A, Auerbach-Nevo T, Yaggie RD, Gontarek RR, Yonath A. Induced-fit tightens pleuromutilins binding to ribosomes and remote interactions enable their selectivity. *Proc. Natl. Acad. Sci. U S A.*, 2007; 104: 4291-6.

[469] Woodford N, Afzal-Shah M, Warner M, Livermore DM. In vitro activity of retapamulin against *Staphylococcus aureus* isolates resistant to fusidic acid and mupirocin. *J. Antimicrob. Chemother.*, 2008; 62: 766-8.

[470] Gelmetti C. Local antibiotics in dermatology. *Dermatol Ther*, 2008; 21: 187-95.

[471] Goldstein EJ, Citron DM, Merriam CV, Warren YA, Tyrrell KL, Fernandez HT. Comparative in vitro activities of retapamulin (SB-275833) against 141 clinical isolates of *Propionibacterium* spp., including 117 *Propionibacterium acnes* isolates. *Antimicrob. Agents Chemother.*, 2006; 50: 379-81.

[472] Odou MF, Muller C, Calvet, L, Dubreuil L. In vitro activity against anaerobes of retapamulin, a new topical antibiotic for treatment of skin infections. *J. Antimicrob. Chemother.*, 2007; 59: 646-51.

[473] Traczewski MM, Brown SD. Proposed MIC and disk diffusion microbiological cutoffs and spectrum of activity of retapamulin, a novel topical antimicrobial agent. *Antimicrob. Agents Chemother.*, 2008; 52: 3863-7.

[474] Yan K, Madden L, Choudhry AE, Voigt CS, Copeland RA, Gontarek RR. Biochemical characterization of the interactions of the novel pleuromutilin derivative retapamulin with bacterial ribosomes. *Antimicrob. Agents Chemother.*, 2006; 50: 3875-81.

[475] Jones RN, Fritsche TR, Sader HS, Ross JE. Activity of retapamulin (SB-275833), a novel pleuromutilin, against selected resistant gram-positive cocci. *Antimicrob. Agents Chemother.*, 2006; 50: 2583-6.

[476] Oranje AP, Chosidow O, Sacchidanand S, Todd G, Singh K, Scangarella NE, et al. Topical retapamulin ointment, 1%, versus sodium fusidate ointment, 2%, for impetigo: A randomized, observer-blinded, noninferiority study. *Dermatology.* 2007; 215: 331-40.

[477] Altabax™ [package insert]. Research Triangle Park, NC: GlaxoSmithKline, 2007.

[478] Gentry DR, McCloskey L, Gwynn MN, Rittenhouse SF, Scangarella N, Shawar R, et al. Genetic characterization of Vga ABC proteins conferring reduced susceptibility to pleuromutilins in *Staphylococcus aureus. Antimicrob. Agents Chemother.*, 2008; 52: 4507-9.

[479] Altargo®, Prescribing Information by EMEA, 2007 http://www.emea.europa.eu /humandocs /PDFs/EPAR/altargo/H-757-PI-en.pdf

[480] Koning S, van der Wouden JC, Chosidow O, Twynholm M, Singh KP, Scangarella N, et al. Efficacy and safety of retapamulin ointment as treatment of impetigo: randomized double-blind multicentre placebo-controlled trial. *Br. J. Dermatol.*, 2008; 158: 1077-82.

In: Antibiotic Resistance: … ISBN: 978-1-60741-623-4
Editors: Adriel R. Bonilla and Kaden P. Muniz ©2009 Nova Science Publishers, Inc.

Chapter VII

Bacteriophage Therapies and Enzybiotics: Novel Solutions to Antibiotic Resistance

Noémie Manuelle Dorval Courchesne,
Albert Parisien and Christopher Q. Lan[*]
Department of Chemical and Biological Engineering,
University of Ottawa, Ontario, Canada

Abstract

Bacteriophages (phages) and bacterial cell wall hydrolases (BCWHs) have been recognized as promising alternative antibacterials. Phages are bacterial virsuses that kill bacteria by causing bacteriolysis. It is estimated that there are about 10^{31} phages on earth and approximately 5,100 have been identified and reported towards the end of last century, providing a vast pool of candidates for applications such as phage therapy. Phages are highly effective and specific to target bacteria. They have been generally accepted as effective antibacterials that could potentially provide safe and cost effective means for the treatment and prophylaxis of bacterial infections. BCWHs are lytic enzymes that cause bacteriolysis by hydrolyzing the peptidoglycan of bacterial cell wall. BCWHs are also called enzybiotics because they are enzymes that have antibiotic-like antibacterial activities. They are produced by amost all cellular organisms including microorganisms, plants, and animals. Virolysins (also called lysins, endolysins) are a special group of BCWHs encoded by phages but produced naturally by bacteria infected by lytic phages. They are probably the most promising enzybiotics.

Keywords: bacteriophage, virolysin, lysin, antibiotic resistance, enzybiotic

---

[*] Corresponding Author Department of Chemical and Biological Engineering, University of Ottawa, 161 Louis Pasteur St., Ottawa, ON K1N 6N5, Christopher.Lan@uottawa.ca

1. Introduction

For more than half a century, the human society has been relying primarily on antibiotics to treat infectious diseases caused by pathogenic bacteria. However, the emergence of bacterial resistance to antibiotics following widespread clinical, veterinary, and animal agricultural usage [1-3] has made antibiotics less effective. As a result, Gram-positive bacteria have clearly re-emerged as important pathogens world-wide in the past two decades. The hallmark of these Gram-positive pathogens is increasing resistance to available antimicrobial agents. Of particular note is resistance to glycopeptides (Vancomycin), amino glycosides (high-level), and penicillins among the enterococci (especially *E. faecium*), resistance to penicillinase-resistant penicillins (oxacillin and methicillin) and fluoroquinolones (ciprofloxacin and ofloxacin) among staphylococci, and resistance to penicillin, other beta-lactams and macrolides among the pneumococci. The recent detection of decreased susceptibility to Vancomycin among S. *aureus* is also quite disturbing. New antibacterials are clearly needed.

The enormous demand has triggered worldwide efforts in developing novel alternative antibacterials. Bacteriophages (phages), bacterial cell wall hydrolases (especially phage encoded virolysins) are among the most promising candidates. In this chapter, we strive on providing a comprehensive picture outlining current developments regarding these alternative antimicrobials.

2. phages and phage Therapies

Discovered independently by Frederick Twort and Félix d'Hérelle in 1915 and 1917, respectively, phages are bacterial viruses that kill bacteria by causing bacteriolysis. Antibacterial properties of phages were assessed in the pre-biotic era and a few western companies, including French companies Le Laboratoire du Bactériophage and L'Oréal, German company Antipiol and the German phage Society, and American companies Eli-Lilly, Swan-Myers of Abbot Laboratories, Squibb and Sons (now belonging to Brystol-Myers, Squibb Company) and the Parke & Davis Company (now a part of Pfizer), manufactured and/or marketed a variety of different phage preparations to treat various infections including abscesses, suppurating wounds, vaginitis, and infections of the upper respiratory tract [4]. phages were later abandoned in the western countries in favour of the antibiotics because the mechanism was not well defined. Moreover, the exquisite specificity of this treatment limited their use in the ealy days. Consequently, antibiotics whose mechanisms were understood and had a large spectrum of action became popular in western countries. Phage therapy was however extensively used in eastern European countries mainly in the former Soviet Union and in Georgia. Nevertheless, a revitalization of interests on phage therapy has been observed in the last two decades in western countries due to the rise of antibiotic resistant bacterial strains, which is marked by a few excellent recent review works [5-13]. In the USA, although no clinic tests have been reported except the pre-antibiotic era practices， some phages were, however, used for medical studies. For instance, phage ϕX174 was used to monitor humoral immune function in treated ADA-deficient patients [14] and analyze the importance of cell surface-associated molecules in modulating the immune response [15]. In both studies, purified phages were administrated intravenously with consent from volunteers. The interest in phage therapy has grown in western countries in the last two decades due to the rise of antibiotic resistance in bacteria [16, 17].

2.1 Classification of Phages

It is estimated that there are about 10^{31} phages on earth and approximately 5,100 have been identified and reported towards the end of last century [18]. These phages are classified into 13 families according to their morphological characteristics, type of nucleic acid, and presence or absence of envelope or lipid. It was noticed that 4950 out of the 5,100 phages are "tailed phages", which are composed of an icosahedral head and a tail. All those tailed phages have double-stranded DNA as genome and are lytic phages that encode endolysins (endolysin will be referred to as virolysins from here on) [19, 20]. They are classified into three families according to the morphological features of the tail: *Myoviridae* (contractile tail), *Siphoviridae* (long noncontractile tail and *Podoviridae* (extremely short tail). The rest of the phages, constituting only 4% of the total, are classified into ten families. They are cubic, filamentous, or pleomorphic phages containing double-stranded DNA (dsDNA), single-stranded DNA (ssDNA), double-stranded RNA (dsRNA) or single-stranded RNA (ssRNA) as the genome [18].

Phages can also be conventionally classified into two categories according to the strategies they use to escape their hosts [19, 20]: filamentous phages and lytic phages. Filementous phages continuously extrude from their hosts without causing host lysis, whereas all other phages are lytic phages that encode gene products to compromise or destroy the bacterial cell wall. Lytic phages can be further divided into two classes according to their bacteriolytic mechanisms: those encode a virolysin-holin system to hydrolyse host cell wall and those encode a single lytic factor to compromise the strength of cell wall and cause bacteriolysis. About 96% of known phages are lytic phages encoding virolysin-holin system. They are large phages containing dsDNA genome. Only the simplest phages encode single lytic factors for bacteriolysis and they usually contain ssDNA or ssRNA genome. Single lytic factors encoded by small phages causes host lysis by inhibiting cell wall biosynthesis, inducing host autolytic system, or other mechanisms. In the virolysin-holin lysis system, virolysin is a muralytic enzyme that hydrolyses the peptidoglycan in bacterial cell wall and holin is a small peptide that oligomerizes in the membrane to form disruptive membrane lesions, allowing access of virolysin to the cell wall at a programmed timing of the phage's life cycle [21].

2.2 Mode of Action

The most common mode of action of phages is that of lytic phages, i.e., sensitive bacteria are killed by means of bacteriolysis. The lytic life of phages involves several stages including adsorption, injection of nucleic acid, commandeering of host machinery, production of phage components (expression of early and late phage genes), assembly of phage particles, and release of phage particles by cell lysis. Bacteriolysis occurs naturally at the end of the life cycle, in which the peptidoglycan network of bacterial cell wall is disrupted by the action of virolysins. This event is initiated by the formation of holin oligomore pores in cytoplasmic membrane, which allows virolysins to access their substrate [22]. Bacteriolysis could also happen in the adsorption stage if a high multiplication of infection (MOI) is used, in which a substantially large number of phage particles attach to each host cell [23, 24].

Another mode of action involves genetically modified phages, especially filamentous ones, which do not cause cell lysis and cannot be used directly for phage therapy. It has been shown that these phages can be genetically modified in such as way that they lose the ability to extrude from host cells but have the ability to digest the nucleic acid of host (the transportation protein gene is replaced by a restriction enzyme gene) [25, 26]. It has been demonstrated that this type of genetically modified filamentous phages can be used as effective anti-infection agents. Besides, they were shown to have the benefit of reduced release of membrane associated endotoxins, leading to significantly higher survival rates of experimental animals in comparison with therapies using lytic phages [25, 26].

Furthermore, as will be discussed later, phage gene products such as endolysins are also promising alternative antimicriobials that may be ultilized in medical and other applications. These gene products have their unique modes of action.

2.3. Antibacterial Efficacy of Phages

Research in phage therapy in western countries was revived by a series of works on the treatment of *Escherichia coli* infections using experimental mice and calves conducted by Smith and Huggins in late 70s and 80s [27-29]. It was observed that phages multiplied rapidly and profusely after gaining entry to the *E. coli*-infected small intestine of calves, quickly reducing the *E. coli* to numbers that were virtually harmless. It was also demonstrated that a single intramuscular dose of one anti-K1 phage is more effective for treating mice challenged with *E. coli* intramuscularly or intracerebrally than multiple intramuscular doses of tetracycline, ampicillin, chloramphenicol, or trimethoprim plus sulfafurazole.

Since Smith's work, there have been many published reports examining the efficacy of phages against experimental infections by Gram-negative bacteria such as *E. coli*, *Pseudomonas aeruginosa*; *Acinetobacter baumanii*, *Klebsiella pneumoniae*, *Vibrio vulnificus*, *Salmonella* Spp. and Gram-positive bacteria such as *Enterococcus faecium* (vancomycin-resistant strain, VRE) and *Staphylococcus aureus*, mostly in animal models. Nakai et al. succeeded in saving the lives of cultured fish challenged by *Lactococcus garvieae* and *Pseudomonas plecoglossicida*. Phages were also shown to be effective for the elimination of food poisoning pathogens such as *Listeria monocytogenes*, *Campylobacter jejuni* and *Salmonella* Spp. On August 18, 2006, FDA approved the use of phages for the treatment of ready-to-eat meat. A combination of six viruses was designed to be sprayed on ready-to-eat meat to eradicate strains of *Listeria monocytogenes*.

Numerous patents have been filed disclosing methods relating the use of phages for treatment and prophylaxis of bacterial infections [30-37]. There are now evidences that phages can be employed to treat infectious diseases caused by both gram-positive and gram-negative bacteria [38, 39]. For instance, the treatment of *E. coli* infections in experimental mice an calves [40] and recent work in animal models have demonstrated the efficacy of phages against experimental infections by gram-negative and gram-positive bacterial pathogens.

Many of these patents also provide innovative technologies to enhance the efficacy and/or safety of phage therapy. For example, an invention [36] provides *Bacillus* phages to prevent and treat the infection of *Bacillus* bacteria, including *Bacillus anthracis*. Methods and materials to decontaminate a surface or an organism that is contaminated with *Bacillus* bacteria or spores is also provided [36]. Treating acne, which is caused by increased colonization of *Propionibacterium acnes* on human skin, using *P. acnes* phages has also been described [37]. It involves the use of a phage that cannot enter a lysogenic cycle, representing an advantage because the phage cannot lie dormant in the bacterial chromosomal DNA. This way, some of the aforementioned safety concerns such as the lysogenic immunity of pathogenic bacteria and the alternation of bacterial virulence can be avoided. Another innovative approach of phage therapy is the use of lysin-deficient phages [41], which can be generated via targeted mutation or selected by screening through phages that have reduced lysis rates. Without a functional lytic enzyme, phages can infect and kill bacterial cells without causing bacteriolysis, resulting in dead but intact bacterial cells. Therefore, the phage therapies have a reduced immunogenicity and toxicity because cell materials of killed bacteria (e.g. endotoxins) are not released [41, 42]. However, the trade-off of this technology is that phages cannot be propagated if there is no bacteriolysis and a larger dosage of phage would have to be used to eliminate all the bacteria in comparison to therapies involving self-propagating phages.

The extreme specificity of phages renders them ideal candidates for applications designed to increase food safety during the production process as phages can be used for biocontrol of bacteria without interfering with the natural microflora or the cultures in fermented products. They have been shown to be effective against poisoning pathogens such as *Listeria monocytogenes*, *Campylobacter jejuni* and *Salmonella spp.* [43]. Another advantage of phage decontamination is that phage compositions are non-toxic and do not alter color, texture or taste of the food to be decontaminated [43, 44]. In fact, application of phages for food decontamination has been considered to be one of the low-handing fruits since the FDA of the USA and other western authorities have much less rigorous regulations towards food decontamination agents in comparison to human therapeutic agents. As an encouraging notion, FDA approved the use of phages for the treatment of ready-to-eat meat, which is a cocktail of six phages to be sprayed on ready-to-eat meat to eradicate strains of *L. monocytogenes*, in 2006 [45]. *E. coli* 0157:H7 is a leading cause of hemolytic-uremic syndrome (HUS) in the United States and a leading cause of acute renal failure in children. Estimates based on a 1994 outbreak in the Seattle area suggest that more than 20,000 cases occur in the USA each year, and that 250 of them are fatal. This strain of *E. coli* is very dangerous because it can cause disease at very low doses - ingestion of less than 1,000 organisms compared to the more than 10,000,000 needed for *Vibrio cholerae* to cause cholera. Based on continued works, Averback and Gemmell [46] patented *E. coli* phages B1 and B3, which were isolated from raw sewage, and phages 146A and 119U, from a urinary tract infection (UTI) isolate, for the treatment of *E. coli* infections, particularly the enteric diseases caused by the toxin-producing *E. coli 0157:H7* strain [46]. Pasternack and Sulakvelidze [47] patented six *Listeria monocytogenes* phage strains (ATCC Deposit Accession Nos. PTA-5372, PTA-5373, PTA-5374, PTA- 5375, PTA-5376 and PTA-5377), which are capable of controlling the contamination of food products by *L. monocytogenes*. The invention also contemplates the use of these phages, and polynucleotides and polypeptides derived therefrom, for the treatment of host infections or environmental contamination by *L. monocytogenes*.

2.4. Specificity of Phage Therapy

The first essential step of phage infection is the attachment of phage tail to specific receptor on the surface of a bacterial cell. This feature makes phage infection a very specific process. There seem to be some controversies with regard of how specific phage infection really is. While some authors tend to think that phages are generally species-specific [48], it seems to be more accurate to say that phages typically attack bacteria on a strain-specific basis [49]. Nevertheless, there is no doubt that phages are much more specific than antibiotics in therapeutical application. While the high specificity of phages made them less appealing in comparison with broad-spectrum antibiotics in the early days, it is now highly appreciated as a major merit of phage therapy. Because of the high specificity, phage therapies would not affect the microbism of the hosts as antibiotics would normally do.

2.5. Bacterial Resistance to Phages

Bacteria may acquire resistance to phages via at least the following fours mechanisms [11]: 1) integrating a phage into its genome (the lysogenic cycle); 2) losing phage receptor from cell surface; 3) acquiring horizontally a restriction-modification system that degrades the injected phage nucleic acid; and 4) mutating to lose a gene essential for phage replication or assembly. Nevertheless, induced resistance of bacteria to phages is so far not considered a significant obstacle to the clinic applicability of phage therapy. After all, phages mutate at frequencies significantly higher than that of bacteria and there are abudant experimental evidences showing that the co-mutation of phages would be enough to maintain the efficacy of phage therapies (Schuch et al. 2002). However, the dependence on the co-mutation of phages implies that we would have to deal with a constantly mutating phage population for effective phage therapies. This may, even though not necessarily, present a concern in long term application of phage therapy.

2.6. Advantages and Disadvantages of Phage Therapy

Matsuzaki et al. [50] summarized the advantages of phage therapy over antibiotherapy as follows: 1) it is effective against multidrug-resistant pathogenic bacteria as the bacterium-killing mechanism of phage is completely different from that of antibiotics; 2) substituted microbism does not occur because the phages have high specificity to target bacteria; 3) it can respond quickly to the appearance of phage-resistant bacterial mutants because the frequency of phage mutation is significantly higher than that of bacteria; 4) the cost of developing a phage system is cheaper than that of a new antibiotics; 5) the side effects are rare. Nevertheless, there are still some concerns need to be addressed such as: 1) lack of pharmacokinetic data; 2) neutralization of phages by the host immune system may lead to failure of phage therapy; 3) some phages may encode toxins [48]; 4) conversion of lytic phages to lysogenic prophages renders immunity (lysogenic immunity) to the bacteria [51] and may also change the virulence of the bacteria [52, 53]; 5) rapid cell lysis of bacteria may result in the release of large amount of membrane-bound endotoxins of the hosts [54].

Some of the aforementioned concerns have been successfully addressed by different approaches. For instance, the rapid release of endotoxin (e.g. lipopolysaccharide, a component of the outer membrane of Gram-negative bacteria) by phage infection was considered to be a potential problem in phage therapy [25, 54]. Recently, a unique method to minimize the release of endotoxin in phage therapy against *P. aeruginosa* was reported [25, 26, 55, 56]. Hagens et al. [25, 26, 56] constructed a recombinant phage derived from the *P. aeruginosa* filamentous phage. In this phage, the export protein gene was replaced with a restriction endonuclease gene. The mutant phage therefore could not multiply in *P. aeruginosa* cells but the restriction endonuclease encoded by the injected phage DNA digested the host genomic DNA and consequentially killed the bacteria with minimal release of endotoxin in vitro. This modified phage reduced mortality rate to a greater extent than the wildtype in mice challenged with *P. aeruginosa*. However, large dosage than that of wildtype lytic phages would be essential for therapy involving this type of modified phages because they cannot propagate after administration.

In both Gram-positive and Gram-negative bacteria, temperate phage may encode toxins and virulence factors in addition to their essential viral proteins [53, 57, 58]. Examples of phage-associated toxins include the CTX cholera toxin [59-61], botulinum toxin, shiga toxin [62, 63], and diphtheria toxin [57]. Phage-associated conversion of Tox[-] *Streptococcus pyogenes* into Tox[+] bacteria was also confirmed *in vitro* and *in vivo* [52, 53]. We therefore should have rather thorough studies before selecting a canaditate phage for therapeutical applications.

Despite of concerns over phage therapy due to the lack of pharmacological and pharmacokinetic data, possible toxicity of certain phages, and other uncertainties associated with phage therapies, accumulating evidences have shown that phages are effective antibacterial agents that can be employed for clinic treatment or prevention of infectious diseases caused by Gram-positive and Gram-negative bacteria. Facing the threat presented by the rapid emerging of antibiotic resistant pathogenic bacteria, phage therapy is no doubt one of the most promising alternative antibacterial agents. Furthermore, as will be discussed later, phage-encoded gene products such as virolysins, and lytic factors are also promising alternative antibacterials.

3. Enzybiotics: Bacterial Cell Wall Hydrolases (Bcwhs) as Novel Alternatives to Antibiotics

The term "enzybiotics" was first coined for virolysisns, i.e., phage-encoded lytic enzymes, and is now used to describe all bacterial cell wall hydrolases (BCWHs), enzymes that degrade the peptidoglycan, the major component of bacterial cell wall and cause bacteriolysis. The sources of BCWHs include animals, insects, plants, and microbes. Enzymes from different sources, even though may have similar structure and functionalities, do have important differences that may have significant impact on their potential clinic applications. It was proposed to classify BCWHs according to their sources into the following categories [64, 65]: 1) lysozymes, BCWHs of eukaryotic origin; 2) microlysins, BCWHs produced by bacteria and other microorganisms; and 3) virolysins, phage-encoded BCWHs responsible for the lysis of host cells and the release of phage particles at the end of a phage life cycle. The three groups of BCWHs are discussed briefly as follows.

3.1. BCWHs from Different Sources

3.1.1. Lysozymes

Lysozyme is sometimes used as a genric name for BCWHs from different sources. To avoid confusion, it was proposed to explicitly define lysozymes as the BCWHs of eukaryotic origins, e.g., those BCWHs produced by animals and plants. Lysozymes are an important component of the innate defense systems of their hosts and are known to exert antimicrobial activities against a broad spectrum of bacterial, fungal, and viral pathogens [66]. These enzymes, alone or in combinations with other antimicrobials, have found wide applications as food preservatives and pharmaceuticals. A few excellent review works are available on this topic [67-71] , which provide insights regarding the antibacterial properties and mode of action of lysozyme against Gram-positive and Gram-negative bacteria, and the underlying causes of bacterial resistance or sensitivity to lysozyme. The distribution, activity and particularly the number of genes that encode lysozyme vary considerably among species. For instance, it has been reported that in mammals, humans and pigs contain a single lysozyme gene, whereas camels and mice contain 2, and cows, sheep, and deer each contain 10 lysozyme genes [72]. In humans, lysozyme presents in various tissues including skin, and secretions such as saliva, tears, urine, milk, respiratory and cervical secretions [70].

3.1.2 Microlysins

Microlysins can be further classified into two subgroups, autolysins and other microlysins. Most bacterial species contain one or more autolysins, which are usually membrane-bound proteins that have BCWH activities [73-75]. A number of autolysins have been identified and have been shown to be involved in a number of physiological cell functions such as cell wall biosynthesis, cell separation, cell adhesion, and virulence (8, 11, 12, 32, 40, 43, 45, 53, 58, 65, 70, 80, 84, 87, 92, 138). They may also, as the name suggests, cause cell lysis and lead directly to cell death when provoked by various mechanisms [76]. A number of autolysins have been expressed in *E. coli* [77-81]. The concept of activating the autolytic systems of pathogenic bacteria using cationic peptides and other compounds have been investigated with encouraging results [82-87]. Exogenous autolysins such as LytA, an *N*-acetylmuramoyl-L-alanine amidase [88, 89] and the major autolysin of *S. pneumoniae*, which play important roles in the pathogenesis of *S. pneumoniae* [90-92], might be used as vaccines due to its ability to provoke protective responses against streptococci inoculated in the lungs [93, 94].

3.1.3 Virolysins

As aforementioned, virolysins are BCWHs encoded by lytic dsDNA phages and produced in phage-infected bacterial cells toward the end of the lytic cycle. They are capable of degrading peptidoglycan when applied externally (as purified proteins) to the bacterial cell wall, resulting in a rapid lysis of the bacterial cell. The name "virolysin" was first adopted by Rolston et al. in 1950s [95] and was recently suggested to replace the more commonly used but more generic names such as lysozymes, lysins, and lytic enzymes to avoid confusion [64, 65].

The first virolysins was identified as early as in the 1950s [95], however, was reported to be active against dead but not live cells [95]. Then, a second virolysin, PAL (phage-associated virolysin), which lysed dead and live *S. aureus* cells, was identified in the early 1970s [96]. In addition, virolysins from staphylococcal phages Twort [97], 87 [98], phi11 [99], and 80 [100] as well as *Bacillus anthracis* prophage [101], *Listeria monocytogenes* phage and *Clostridium tyrobutyricum* phage, were identified in 1990s. Stimulated by the great potential of virolysins as powerful alternatives to antibiotics, a number of virolysins have been identified and demonstrated to be efficient and safe antimicrobials since 2000 [6, 102-104]. These virolysins have been tested for the control of a variety of pathogens such as *E. faecalis* and *E. faecium*, staphylococci, *B. anthracis*, group A streptococci, *S. pneumoniae*, and Clostridium bacteria [105].

Virolysins possess several important features including a narrow antibacterial spectrum and activity against bacteria regardless of their antibiotic sensitivity. It is also important to notice that there are evidences showing that it is unlikely for sensitive bacteria to develop resstance to virolysins. The results of preclinical studies indicate that the most apparent potential problems associated with phage therapy (e.g., their immunogenicity, the potential toxicity, or the development of resistance) may not be a serious problem to the use of virolysins [10].

3.2. Mode of Action

The primary bactericidal mechanism of BCWHs is the lytic enzymatic activities of these enzymes, which leads to peptidoglycan degradation and consequently bacteriolysis [70].

Bacterial cell wall is a unique structure comprised primary of a peptidoglycan network embedded with other compounds and, in the case of Gram-negative bacteria, surrounded by a lipid-rich outer membrane. The backbone of peptidoglycan is the polymer of the repeat units of two amino sugars, [*N*-acetylglucosamine-*N*-acetylmuramic acid]$_n$. The two amino sugars are linked by a β-1,4 glycoside bond. Tetrapeptides are attached to the D-lactyl moiety of N-acetylmuramic acids. Adjacent tetrapeptide may be cross-linked by an inter-peptide bond (in Gram-positive bacteria) or by an inter-peptide bridge (in Gram-positive bacteria). The tetrapeptides are composed of L-Alanine linked to D-Glutamate, L-lysine and then D-Alanine in the case of gram-positive bacteria. The cross-linked between the two peptide chains connects the L-lysine from one peptide to the D-Alanine of the other. In gram-negative bacteria, such as *E. coli*, L-lysine is replaced by L-diaminopimelic acid (DAP), and this amino acid is cross-linked with the D-Alanine of the other peptide chain. Peptidoglycan forms a closed network around the entire cell that is called the murein sacculus, which defines cellular shape and absorbs cellular turgor pressure [106-110]. Gram-positive bacteria have a thicker peptidoglycan layer (15 to 80nm) than the gram-negative bacteria (10nm) [110]. The peptidolycan is tightly cross-linked on the cytoplamic side and becomes looser for outer layers, and therefore more subject to degradation. Teichoic acid and lipoteichoic acid are two characteristic molecules found in the peptidoglycan layer of gram-positive bacteria. Teichoid acids are chemically bound to peptidoglycan, while lipoteichoic acids are anchored by a fatty acid in the plasma membrane [107]. In the case of gram-negative bacteria, a periplasmic space separates the plasma membrane from a single peptidoglycan layer adjacent to an outer lipopolysaccharide membrane. This outer membrane consists of proteins and lipopolysaccharides, composed of lipid A, the core, and a long repeating O antigen [107].

BCWHs hydrolyse peptidoglycan by attacking specific sites in the peptidolycan network. They can therefore be classified into different groups accordingly: 1) glycosidases, including β-N-acetylmuramidases, attacking the *N*-acetylmuramic acid→*N*-acetylglucosamine β-1-4 glycosidic bond, and β-N-acetylglucosaminidases, hydrolyzing the *N*-acetylglucosamine → *N*-acetylmuramic acid β-1-4 glycosidic bond; 2) transglycosylases, cleaving the same bond that is attacked by β-N-acetylmuramidases but transfering the glycosyl moiety onto the C-6 hydroxyl group of muramic acid; 3) amidases, cleaving the amide bond between the lactyl group of N-acetylmuramic acid and the α-amino group of L-alanine, the first amino acid of the tetrapeptide of peptidoglycan; 4) endopeptidases that cut within the peptide moiety of the peptidoglycan; and 5) other enzymes such as phosphocholine esterase that releases phosphocholine residues from the cell wall teichoic acid (TA) .

The hydrolysis of bacterial cell wall requires two distinct functions of BCWHs: 1) binding to the cell wall leading to the correct positioning of BCWHs as the essential first step; and 2) cleaving specific peptidoglycan bond. These two functions are achieved by two separate domains of BCWHs. It is now clear that most BCWHs have a two-domain modular structure, in which the binding domain is separated from the catalytic domain. For instance, LytA amidase, the major autolysin of pneumococci, has a molecular mass of ~36 kDa and a two-domain modular organization [111]. The C-terminal domain is responsible for the attachment to teichoic or lipoteichoic acid residues on the surface of pneumococci. The N-domain, on the other hand, is responsible for the lytic activity against pneumococcal cell wall. This modular structure is shared by almost all known BCWHs including lysozymes [71, 112-114], autolysins [115-117], and virolysins [101, 118, 119].

A second bactericidal mechanism, the non-lytic mechanism, of BCWHs has also attracted the attention of the research community in recent years [120-122]. The non-lytic mechanism is based on the cationic and amphiphilic properties of BCWH or its peptide derivatives to cause membrane perturbation of its targets through the binding of a certain domains of BCWHs with the bacterial surface or to provoke the autolytic system of bacteria. As will be discussed later, this non-lytic bactericidal mechanism is shared by other antimicrobial peptides.

3.3. Antimicrobial Efficacy of BCHWs

Extensive studies on the antimicrobial efficacy of different groups of BCWHs, mostly of lysozymes [68-71, 123, 124] and virolysins [105, 125, 126], have been carried out in the last two decades.

Lysosomes are a group of broad-spectrum lytic enzymes that exhibit bactericidal activity toward most Gram-positive bacteria [125]. In addition to their bactericidal activities, lysozymes have also been demonstrated to have anti-fungal (e.g. *Fusarium oxysporum, Fusarium solani, Pythium aphanidermatum, Sclerotium rolfsii, and Botrytis cinerea*) [127] and anti-virus (e.g. HIV) [128] activities. Nevertheless, many virulent Gram-positive bacterial pathogens have acquired resistance to lysolyzymes to survive the innate defense of their hosts [66, 129, 130]. It is therefore not surprising to find that the most significant commercial applications of lysozyme are so far in food preservation and processing [131-133]. Lysozyme also found applications in human medicine and veterinary in different ways. For instance, transgenic mice expressing rat lysozyme cDNA in distal respiratory epithelial cells was generated with a significantly enhanced survival rate in comparison with that of wildtype mice when both were challenged with *Pseudomonas aeruginosa* [134]. Lysozymes also have important roles in surveillance of membranes of mammalian cells, enhancement of phagocytic activity of polymorphonuclear leukocytes and macrophages, and stimulation of proliferation and anti-tumor functions of monocytes [121]. It was suggested that lysozymes might be useful as a food additive in the complex treatment of oncological patients for enhancing antineoplastic chemotherapy efficacy [135].

On the other hand, there are abundant evidences showing that endolysins have the capacity of rapidly killing pathogenic Gram-positive bacteria on a generally species-specific basis, *in vitro* or *in vivo*, with effective dosages in the order of milligrams or even micrograms per liter. Nelson *et al.* [104] studied the efficacy of an endolysin encoded by the streptococcal phage C_1, which is specific for groups A, C, and E streptococci with little or no activity against a number of oral streptococci or other commensal organisms tested. Using purified endolysin, Nelson et al. demonstrated that 1,000 units (10 ng) of the enzyme were sufficient to sterilize an *in vitro* culture of about 10^7 group A streptococci within 5 seconds. When a single dose of endolysin (250 units) was first added to the oral cavity of mice, followed by 10^7 live group A streptococci, it provided protection from colonization. Furthermore, when endolysin (500 units) was given orally to 9 heavily colonized mice, no detectable streptococci were observed 2 h after endolysin treatment. Loeffler *et al.* [136] showed that Pal, a purified pneumococcal endolysin, was able to kill 15 common serotypes of pneumococci, including highly penicillin-resistant strains within seconds of contact. The addition of 100 U/ml of endolysin reduced the concentration of bacteria by 4-logs in 30 seconds. *In vivo* experiments showed that mice exposed to a 10^8 CFU of *Streptococcus pneumoniae* did not yield a detectable level of bacteria 5 h after administration of 1400 U of endolysin. This experiment was repeated with 500 U of endolysin resulting in 63 % of the mice being free of bacteria and a significant reduction in the bacterial titer in all the animals. It was also shown that *S. pneumoniae* growing on mucous membranes were sensitive to endolysin; and even though some bacteria reappeared after a certain time, the number was not high enough to cause recolonization of the mucous membrane.

A rapid killing of *Streptococcus pneumoniae* in the nasopharynx of mice has also been reported using other two endolysins, Cpl-1 murein hydrolase and the Pal amidase, in a murine sepsis model. Purified Pal amidase and/or Cpl-1 lysozyme were used alone or in combination. It was concluded that those two endolysins, used separatedly or in combinaition, could protect animals from bacteraemia and death. Moreover, a synergic effect *in vivo* was observed with the combined use of 2.5 µg each of Cpl-1 and Pal [137]. The rapid killing of sensitive bacteria by endolysins at relatively low dosage is not only important in the sense of therapy costs, but could be one of the major reasons whereby the enzymes would avoid being neutralized by the immune response or causing severe allergic responses in hosts [105].

3.4 Bacterial Resistance to BCHWs

In general, Gram-negative bacteria are resistant to exogenous BCWHs due to the protection of their outer membrane. As discussed previously, some successful Gram-positive pathogenic bacteria are also resistant to lysozymes. Several resistant mechanisms have been characterized in pathogens such as *S. aureus*. Those include: 1) O-acetylation of the NAM of peptidoglycan as reported in staphylococci [129, 138, 139]; 2) attachment of other polymers (e.g. polysaccharides) to the cell wall, as described for streptococci [139]; 3) D-Asp (D-aspartic acid) incorporation as discovered in the *Lactococcus lactis* peptidoglycan crossbridge [140]; and 4) some microbes may synthesize lysozyme inhibitors to neutralize the enzymatic activity [141-143]. On the other hand, virolysins apparently have a very different mechanism, which allows specific virolysins to be functional to those Gram-positive bacteria that have acquired resistance to lysozymes.

It is worthy mentioning that studies with a number of pathogenic bacteria, including *S. pneumoniae*, *S. pyogenes* and *B. anthracis* [101], have shown that repeated exposure of those bacteria to sub-lethal doses of corresponding virolysins does not lead to the development of enzyme resistant strains. This observation was tentatively explained by the fact that choline, an essential structural component of many Gram-positive cell wall [144], serves as receptor for binding of virolysins to bacterial cell wall [112, 115, 116, 145, 146].

3.5. Prophylaxis and Pathogen Detection Using BCHWs

Nearly all infections begin at a mucous membrane site and the human mucous membranes are a reservoir for many pathogenic bacteria (e.g., pneumococci, staphylococci, and streptococci) found in the environment [147-149]. This observation, in combination with the fact that induced resistance to virolysins is rarely developed, led to the proposal of a novel method for the control of pathogens by destroying pathogenic bacteria on mucous membranes [104, 136, 150]. Another potential application is in anti-bioterror warfare. Nelson and Fischetti explore the feasibility of exploiting the specific binding and lytic action of virolysins for the rapid detection and killing of *B. anthracis*. PlyG, an virolysin isolated from the γ phage of *B. anthracis* and specifically kills *B. anthracis* and other members of the *B. anthracis* 'cluster' of bacilli, was found satisfactory as a tool for the treatment and detection of *B. anthracis* [151].

4. Virolysins: Promising Enzybiotics

4.1. General Description of Virolysins

As discussed previously, virolysins are phage-encoded BCWHs. They are naturally expressed by phages during their lytic cycle, and aid to the phage release from infected cells [105]. Virolysins are regarded as the most promising enzybiotics among the three groups of BCWHs because of 1) their capacity of rapidly killing sensitive bacteria, even for lysozyme-resistant bacteria; 2) general narrow spectra of sensitive bacteria, minimizing the disturbance to normal microflora; 3) the large diversity of different virolysins from differet lytic phages; and 4) the easily detectable bacteriolytic activity of phages providing a solid basis for rational selection the sources of virolysins [65].

4.2. Antibacterial Efficacy of Virolysins

Virolysins have several known applications, including food decontamination, treatment of bacterial infections in human and animals, prophylaxis, detection of a specific bacterium and diagnostics. All of these uses are possible because of the capacity of virolysin to rapidly kill bacteria and cause bacteriolysis. Extetensive studies have demonstrated that they could represent a realistic alternative to antibiotics. A few virolysins, their target bacteria, and the corresponding health problems are are summarized in Table 1.

4.2.1 Virolysins against Streptococcal Bacteria

Some *Streptococcus* species, such as *Streptococcus pneumonia* (a *Streptococcus* Group A species), can cause respiratory illnesses. A recent patent describes an invention to treat these diseases by administrating a virolysin, Pal that reaches the mucosal lining in the oral or nasal cavity [152]. It has also been demonstrated that amidase Pal and endopeptidase Cpl-1 from the pneumococcal phage Cpl-1 can act synergistically to decrease the occurrence or the severity of local and systemic pneumococcal disease or prevent and eliminate pneumococcal colonization [163]. This virolysin can kill 15 common serotypes of pneumococci, including highly penicillin-resistant strains within seconds of contact [136]. A few virolysins that have bacteriolytic activities to Group A, B and C streptococci have been studied intensively. Group A and C streptococci cause illness such as pharyngitis, toxic shock syndrome, rheumatic fever [153], while group B streptococci are often responsible for neonatal bacterial infections [155]. PlyC virolysin from C1 phage has been found to be an effective antimicrobial agent for group A and C streptococci [164]. *Streptococcus pyogenes,* a Group A *Streptococcus,* can cause diseases such as pharyngitis, rheumatic fever and toxic shock syndrome [153]. The virolysin encoded by the streptococcal phage C1 is also specific for group E streptococci, but has only little or no effect against a number of oral streptococci and other commensal organisms tested [165]. 1,000 units of this enzyme were shown to be sufficient to sterilize *in vitro* culture of about 10^7 Group A streptococci within five seconds, demonstrating the therapeutic efficiency of this virolysin. Its prophylaxis effectiveness has also been verified by administrating first 250 units of virolysin C1 to the oral cavity of mice, followed by 10^7 live Group A streptococci. This prevented colonies to grow [165]. It has also been revealed that *S. pyogenes* is highly sensitive to PlyV12 lysin, a virolysin isolated from the enterococcal phage φ1 [166].

Table 1. Recently discovered virolysins that can be used to treat human or animal bacterial infections

Phage / Lysin	Targeted bacteria	Related health disorders	References
Pal phage / Pal lytic enzyme	Oral streptococci	Pneumonia	[152]
C1 phage / PlyC	Group A or C streptococci bacteria	Pharyngitis, toxic shock syndrome, rheumatic fever [153]	[154]
GBS phage/ PlyGBS	Group B streptococci bacteria	Neonatal infections	[155]
Actinomyces naeslundii phage/Av-1 lysin	*Actinomyces naeslundii*	Periodontal disease (gingivitis) and root surface (cementum) caries	[156]
PlyV12 phage	*Staphylococcus aureus*	Acute dermatitis	[157]
Phage K/LysK	*Staphylococcus aureus* and 8 other species *Staphylococcus*	Abscesses, fatal sepsis, endocarditis, pneumonia, mastitis, phlebitis, meningitis and toxinoses	[158]
B. anthracis γ-phage/PlyG	*Bacillus anthracis*	Anthrax	[159]
PlyV12 phage	*Enterococcus faecalis, Enterococcus faecium, Streptococcus pyogenes*	Nosocomial infections, intraabdominal and pelvic infections	[160]
HL18 phage	*Salmonella typhimurium*	Food-borne illness	[161]
Phage .phi.3626	*Clostridium perfringens*	Necrotic enteritis, gas gangrene, food poisoning	[162]

In the case of Group B streptococci (GBS), the GBS phage NCTC11261 genomic DNA was sequenced and PlyGBS lysin was discovered to be effective against GBS *in vitro* and *in vivo* [167]. Its gene was over 90% identical to several virolysins from various streptococcal species, including GBS phage B30 lysin, *Streptococcus pyogenes* M1 phage-associated lysin, and *Streptococcus equi* phage-associated protein, both at the nucleotide and amino acid level [164].

4.2.2 Virolysins against Cariogenic Bacteria

A bactericide was prepared with an N-acetylmuraminidase, the auto-mutanolysin (Aml) strongly specific to *Streptococcus sobrinus* and *Streptococcus mutans,* two bacteria found in human oral cavity [168]. This preparation could be used to treat dental caries and periodontal disease and easily incorporated into gum, dentifrice or mouthwash. This concept could also possibly be applicable to virolysins. For instance, the virolysin encoded by *Actinomyces naeslundii* phage Av-1 can prevent gingivitis and root surface caries formation [156]. *A. naeslundii* bacteria are resistant to lysozymes but sensitive to virolysins.

4.2.3 Virolysins against Staphylococcus

Phage K, a phage belongs to the Myrovidae phage family, exhibits anti-staphylococcal activity and its virolysin, LysK, has been cloned and expressed in *Lactococcus lactis*. Bioinformatics analysis shows that this enzyme contains two peptidoglycan hydrolase domains at the N- terminus, CHAP and Amidase-2, and a cell wall binding domain at the Cterminus [158]. This virolysin has the advantage of being effective to a wide range of Staphylococci. It was demonstrated that LysK could kill nine species of *Staphylococcus* (*S. aureus, S. epidermidis, S. saprophytics, S. chromogenes, S. captis, S. hominis, S. haemolyticus, S. caprea and S. hyicus*), including some methicillin-resistant *S. aureus* (MRSA) strains that causes serious hospital infections worldwide [169] and the pathogenic *S. aureus* strain associated with bovine mastisis [158]. A patent entitled "Antimicrobial Protein Specific to *Staphylococcus aureus*" also describes a novel virolysin that targets *Staphylococcus aureus* [157]. *S. aureus* is also a bacterial pathogen responsible for nosocomial infections that can be targeted by the PlyV12 virolysin [166]. Methods for controlling the growth and treating the infections of these bacteria using PlyV12 have been patented [160].

4.2.4. Virolysins against Bacilli

A promising approach to treat anthrax involves the isolation of virolysins effective to *B. anthracis* from *B. cereus* phages. *B. cereus* is a bacterium closely related to *B. anthracis* but has a different virulent type. It could be theoretically treated as *B. anthracis* cured of its virulent plasmid [151]. *B. cereus* is related to food poisoning while *B. anthracis* has a recognized potential for biological weapons and mass destruction [151, 170]. The phages of both bacterial species can easily be isolated from top soil [171]. Experiments demonstrated that virolysin PlyG can lyse both spores and vegetative cells of diverse *B. anthracis* strains and no resistance from the bacteria has been developed after several expositions to the enzyme. This lytic enzyme is not blocked by the capsule of many *B. anthracis* strains [151]. A patent entitled "Lytic Enzymes and Spore Surface Antigen for Detection and Treatment of *Bacillus anthracis* Bacteria and Spores" describes the methods of PlyG isolation and the application of the virolysin to treat anthrax [159], a disease caused by highly resistant spore forming bacteria that generally infect animals but can be transmitted to humans under three forms: cutaneous anthrax, gastrointestinal anthrax and inhalation anthrax [172].

A recent patent [160] disclosed the methods, compositions and articles of manufacture useful for the treatment of *B. anthracis* and *B. cereus* bacteria and spores and related conditions. This disclosure further relates to methods for the identification of a virolysin to rapidly and specifically detect and kill *B. anthracis* and other bacteria. Related articles of manufacture, methods of degrading spores and methods of treatment of infections of *B. anthracis* are also provided [173].

4.2.5 Virolysins against Enterococcus Species

Nosocomial infections are caused by *Enterococcus faecalis* and *Enterococcus faecium*, two gram-positive bacteria that normally colonize the lower intestinal track. A PlyV12 phage virolysin has been discovered to have lytic effect on those *enterococcus* species as well as on two vancomycin-resistant *E. faecalis* strains (VRE) and three vancomycin-resistant *E. faecium* strains. Vancomycin is an antibiotic that is considered as the last line of defense against a bacterial pathogen that is already resistant to the other antibiotics [160]. Another patent disclosed a virolysin that is active to various bacteria including both *E. faecalis* and *E. faecium* (including vancomycin resistant strains), as well as other human pathogens [160].

4.2.6. Virolysins against Salmonella

Salmonella is a Gram-negative bacterium. Its cell envelope includes a lipopolysaccharide (LPS) layer (the outer membrane), which can protect it from the lysis caused by lytic enzymes. A novel approach was disclosed pertaining the use of lyases, polysaccharide-degrading enzymes that are normally found on tail spikes of phages and create openings through the outer membrane, to allow the lytic enzymes to access the peptideglycan network of bacterial cell wall [161]. A patent provides HL18 phage virolysins and lyases, enzymatic compositions, and methods of producing and using virolysins and lyases from HL18 phage [161]. It was demonstrated that administration of the purified HL18 phage reduces at least 10-fold the *Salmonella* population in animals. Similarly, by isolating this virolysin gene and producing lyase from *Salmonella* infected cells, a lytic system against several *Salmonella* strains, including multi-drug resistant strains, can be obtained [161]. This bacterium is principally found in contaminated food [174] and in consequence, it was suggested that HL18 lytic enzyme could be preventively added to food products to inactivate *Salmonella*.

4.2.7. Virolysins against Clostridium

Clostridium perfringens, which colonizes intestinal track, can cause diseases such as necrotic enteritis, food poisoning and growth retardation [162]. A virolysin specific to this bacterium was isolated from Clostridium phage phi3626, which was proposed for the treatment of a disorder, disease or condition associated with a Clostridium patho-genic species, in particular, *C. perfringens.*

4.3. Production of Virolysins

Virolysin production cost is one major obstacle associated with this enzybiotic, which can however be resolved by the fast technology development [65]. Two distinct common methods are employed nowadays for virolysin production. The first approach consists in employing high cell density bacterial culture infected with the corresponding phages to allow bacteriolysis to occur. For example, at the end of each phage lytic cycle, using Group C streptococci and C1 phage, the produced virolysins were liberated into the culture medium [175]. Using a similar technique in combination with an alkylating agent, it is possible to obtain a phage-free virolysin preparation at a large scale. *Vibrio harveyi* cultures, isolated from shrimp farms, hatcheries and seawater, were propagated and sodium thiosulphate was added to the cell lysate as alkylating agent. This compound reacts with the phage nucleic acids and deactivates the phage [176]. A more sophisticated and potentially more cost-effective approach involve the cloing and expression of virolysins as recombinant proteins. In the 1970s and 1980s, molecular cloning of DNA fragments via host cells such as E. coli was developed and became a popular technique [102]. At this point of time, virolysins from different phages have started to be expressed and produced in different recombinant bacteria. This consists of the second and more sophisticated approach to produce virolysins, which is more popular and potentially more cost-effective than the infected bacteria strategy. A method was patented in 1985 [103] regarding expression of the lysin gene sequence of phage T7 in E. coli [103]. This was one of the experiments that marked the beginning of high level nontoxic expression of cell wall disrupting proteins and numerous patents have been filed thereafter. In a recent patent [84], a plasmid, pSOFLysK, which contains the gene sequence of virolysin LysK, was constructed and transferred to bacterial strain Lactococcus lactis NZ9800. The recombinant bacterial strain, which was referred to as Lactococcus lactis NZ9800-pSOFLysK and subsequently designated as Lactococcus lactis DPC6132, was claimed to be useful for amplifying large quantities of genetic material providing anti-staphylococcal activity [84]. This technique requires the identification of the potential virolysin using bioinformatics tools and by comparing the homology of the new sequences with those of known virolysins in order to find similar functional domains in the genes. Open reading frame (ORF) analysis can also be carried out, such as in the case of the Clostridium phage phi3626 genome, in which a holing gene was found and permitted to discover a lysin gene encoded downstream of the holin one [162].

5. Conclusion Remarks

A vast number of studies have been carried out on phages and phage-encoded virolysins as promising solutions to antibiotic resistance. Phages, when properly selected, offers the most cost-effective alternative antibacterials. They are also highly specific, effective, and safe for the treatment and prevention of infectious diseases. Virolysins have also been established as promising anternative antibacterials, which are effective to antibiotic resistant strains. In a broader scope, virolysins belong to bacterial cell wall hydrolysases, lytic enzymes produced by animals, plants, and microbes for a diversity of different physiological functionalities. Despite of the well-based optimism, extensive studies are needed to develop these alternative antimicrobials to practical substitutes for antibiotics in term of efficacy, safety, and affordability.

Acknowledgment

Fincial support from the Natural Science and Engineering Research Council of Canada (NSERC) is gratefully acknowledged.

References

[1]   Heuer, O.E., et al., *Human health hazard from antimicrobial-resistant enterococci in animals and food.* Clinical Infectious Diseases, 2006. 43(7): p. 911-916.

[2]   Witte, W., *Selective pressure by antibiotic use in livestock.* International Journal of Antimicrobial Agents, 2000. 16(SUPPL. 1).

[3]   Teuber, M., *Veterinary use and antibiotic resistance.* Current Opinion in Microbiology, 2001. 4(5): p. 493-499.

[4]   Kutateladze, M. and R. Adamia, *Phage therapy experience at the Eliava Institute.* Medecine et Maladies Infectieuses, 2008. 38(8): p. 426-430.

[5]   Brussow, H., *Phage therapy: The E. coli experience.* Microbiology, 2005. 151(7): p. 2133-2140.

[6]   Godany, A., et al., *Phage therapy: Alternative approach to antibiotics.* Biologia - Section Cellular and Molecular Biology, 2003. 58(3): p. 313-320.

[7]   Inal, J.M., *Phage therapy: A reappraisal of bacteriophages as antibiotics.* Archivum Immunologiae et Therapiae Experimentalis, 2003. 51(4): p. 237-244.

[8]   Krylov, V.N., *Phage therapy in terms of bacteriophage genetics: Hopes, perspectives, safety, limitations.* Genetika, 2001. 37(7): p. 869-887.

[9]   Levin, B.R. and J.J. Bull, *Phage therapy revisited: The population biology of a bacterial infection and its treatment with bacteriophage and antibiotics.* American Naturalist, 1996. 147(6): p. 881-898.

[10]   Borysowski, J., et al., *Current status and perspectives of phage therapy.* Advances in Clinical and Experimental Medicine, 2006. 15(4): p. 575-580.

[11]   Skurnik, M. and E. Strauch, *Phage therapy: Facts and fiction.* International Journal of Medical Microbiology, 2006. 296(1): p. 5-14.

[12]   Murthy K, A.B., Roman J-L, Durand S, Fairbrother J, Quessy S, Mandeville R, *Phage therapy: an innovative approach to treat antibiotic-resistant bacterial strains.* Amer. Ass. Swine Vet., 2002: p. 217 -220.

[13]   Mandeville, R., et al., *Diagnostic and Therapeutic Applications of Lytic Phages.* Analytical Letters, 2003. 36(15): p. 3241-3259.

[14]   Ochs, H.D., et al., *Antibody responses to bacteriophage $\phi X174$ in patients with adenosine deaminase deficiency.* Blood, 1992. 80(5): p. 1163-1171.

[15]   Ochs, H.D., et al., *Regulation of antibody responses: The role of complement and adhesion molecules.* Clinical Immunology and Immunopathology, 1993. 67(3 II).

[16]   Brussow, H., *Phage therapy: The E. coli experience.* Microbiology, 2005. 151(7): p. 2133-2140.

[17]   Damasko, C., et al., *Studies of the efficacy of enterocoliticin, a phage-tail like bacteriocin, as antimicrobial agent against Yersinia enterocolitica serotype O3 in a cell culture system and in mice.* Journal of Veterinary Medicine Series B: Infectious Diseases and Veterinary Public Health, 2005. 52(4): p. 171-179.

[18]   Ackermann, H.W., *Frequency of morphological phage descriptions in the year 2000.* Archives of Virology, 2001. 146(5): p. 843-857.

[19]   Young, R., I.N. Wang, and W.D. Roof, *Phages will out: Strategies of host cell lysis.* Trends in Microbiology, 2000. 8(3): p. 120-128.

[20] Bernhardt, T.G., et al., *Breaking free: "Protein antibiotics" and phage lysis.* Research in Microbiology, 2002. 153(8): p. 493-501.

[21] Ugorcakova, J. and G. Bukovska, *Lysins and holins: Tools of phage-induced lysis.* Biologia - Section Cellular and Molecular Biology, 2003. 58(3): p. 327-334.

[22] Wang, I.N., D.L. Smith, and R. Young, *Holins: The protein clocks of bacteriophage infections.* Annual Review of Microbiology, 2000. 54: p. 799-825.

[23] Loeb, M.R., *Bacteriophage T4 mediated release of envelope components from E. coli.* Journal of Virology, 1974. 13(3): p. 631-641.

[24] Tarahovsky, Y.S., G.R. Ivanitsky, and A.A. Khusainov, *Lysis of E. coli cells induced by bacteriophage T4.* FEMS Microbiology Letters, 1994. 122(1-2): p. 195-199.

[25] Hagens, S. and U. Blasi, *Genetically modified filamentous phage as bactericidal agents: A pilot study.* Letters in Applied Microbiology, 2003. 37(4): p. 318-323.

[26] Hagens, S., et al., *Therapy of experimental Pseudomonas infections with a nonreplicating genetically modified phage.* Antimicrobial Agents and Chemotherapy, 2004. 48(10): p. 3817-3822.

[27] Smith, H.W. and M.B. Huggins, *Treatment of experimental E. coli infection in mice with colicine V.* Journal of Medical Microbiology, 1977. 10(4): p. 479-482.

[28] Williams Smith, H. and M.B. Huggins, *Effectiveness of phages in treating experimental E. coli diarhoea in calves, piglets and lambs.* Journal of General Microbiology, 1983. 129(8): p. 2659-2675.

[29] Williams Smith, H., M.B. Huggins, and K.M. Shaw, *Factors influencing the survival and multiplication of bacteriophages in calves and in their environment.* Journal of General Microbiology, 1987. 133(5): p. 1127-1135.

[30] Fischetti, V.A. and J. Loeffler, *App Use Of Synergistic Bacteriophage Lytic Enzymes For Prevention And Treatment Of Bacterial Infections,* In *Patent Cooperation Treaty Application.* 2004.

[31] Rapson, M.E., et al., *Bact Bacteriophages Useful For Therapy And Prophylaxis Of Bacterial Infections,* In *European Patent.* 2005.

[32] Jayasheela, M., B. Sriram, and S. Padmanabhan, *Bact Defined Dose Therapeutic Phage,* In *Patent Cooperation Treaty Application.* 2005.

[33] Piddock, L.J.V. and M.J. Woodward, *Bact Use Of Bacteriophage In Medicaments,* In *Patent Cooperation Treaty Application.* 2006.

[34] Holland, M.A. and N. Lenihan, *Bact Bacteriophage For Lysis Of Methylobacterium And Compositions And Uses Thereof,* In *European Patent Application.* 2006.

[35] Pasternack, G.R., A. Sulakvelidze, and T. Brown, *Bact Method For Vaccination Of Poultry By Bacteriophage Lysate,* In *European Patent Application.* 2006.

[36] Walter, M.H., *Bacteriophages That Infect Bacillus Bacteria (Anthrax),* In *United States Patent And Trademark Office Pre-Grant Publication.* 2008.

[37] West, D., K. Holland, and K. Bojar, *Bact Bacteriophage And Their Uses,* In *Patent Cooperation Treaty Application.* 2007.

[38] Bull, J.J., et al., *Dynamics of success and failure in phage and antibiotic therapy in experimental infections.* BMC microbiology [electronic resource], 2002. 2(1): p. 35.

[39] Stone, R., *Bacteriophage therapy. Stalin's forgotten cure.* Science, 2002. 298(5594): p. 728-731.

[40] Smith, W.H., M.B. Huggins, and K.M. Shaw, *The control of experimental E. coli diarrhoea in calves by means of bacteriophages. Journal of General Microbiology,* 1987. 133(5): p. 1111-1126.

[41] Ramachandran, J., S. Padmanabhan, and B. Sriram, *Lysin-Deficient Bacteriophages Having Reduced Immunogenicity,* In *Patent Cooperation Treaty Application.* 2003.

[42] Ramachandran, J., S. Padmanabhan, and B. Sriram, *Bact Incapacitated Whole-Cell Immunogenic Bacterial Compositions,* In *European Patent.* 2004.

[43] Greer, G.G., *Bacteriophage control of foodborne bacteria. Journal of Food Protection,* 2005. 68(5): p. 1102-1111.

[44] Hagens, S. and M.J. Loessner, *Application of bacteriophages for detection and control of foodborne pathogens. Applied Microbiology and Biotechnology,* 2007. 76(3): p. 513-519.

[45] Macgregor, H.E., *Latest food additive: Viruses,* in *Los Angeles Times.* 2006: Los Angeles. p. F-1.

[46] Averback, P. and J. Gemmell, *BACT Bacteriophage composition useful in treating food products to prevent bacterial contamination,* in *European Patent Application.* 2008.

[47] Pasternack, G.R. and A. Sulakvelidze, *Novel Listeria Monocytogenes Bacteriophage And Uses Thereof,* in *Patent Cooperation Treaty Application.* 2008.

[48] Merril, C.R., D. Scholl, and S.L. Adhya, *The prospect for bacteriophage therapy in Western medicine.* Nature Reviews Drug Discovery, 2003. 2(6): p. 489-497.

[49] Bradbury, J., *"My enemy's enemy is my friend": Using phages to fight bacteria.* Lancet, 2004. 363(9409): p. 624-625.

[50] Matsuzaki, S., et al., *Bacteriophage therapy: A revitalized therapy against bacterial infectious diseases.* Journal of Infection and Chemotherapy, 2005. 11(5): p. 211-219.

[51] Cheng, C.M., et al., *The primary immunity determinant in modulating the lysogenic immunity of the filamentous bacteriophage cf.* Journal of Molecular Biology, 1999. 287(5): p. 867-876.

[52] Broudy, T.B. and V.A. Fischetti, *In vivo lysogenic conversion of Tox- Streptococcus pyogenes to Tox+ with lysogenic streptococci or free phage.* Infection and Immunity, 2003. 71(7): p. 3782-3786.

[53] Dobrindt, U. and J. Reidl, *Pathogenicity islands and phage conversion: Evolutionary aspects of bacterial pathogenesis.* International Journal of Medical Microbiology, 2000. 290(6): p. 519-527.

[54] Chatterjee, S.N. and K. Chaudhuri, *Lipopolysaccharides of Vibrio cholerae: III. Biological functions.* Biochimica et Biophysica Acta - Molecular Basis of Disease, 2006. 1762(1): p. 1-16.

[55] Matsuda, T., et al., *Lysis-deficient bacteriophage therapy decreases endotoxin and inflammatory mediator release and improves survival in a murine peritonitis model.* Surgery, 2005. 137(6): p. 639-646.

[56] Hagens, S., A. Habel, and U. Blasi, *Augmentation of the antimicrobial efficacy of antibiotics by filamentous phage.* Microbial Drug Resistance, 2006. 12(3): p. 164-168.

[57] Brussow, H., C. Canchaya, and W.D. Hardt, *Phages and the evolution of bacterial pathogens: From genomic rearrangements to lysogenic conversion.* Microbiology and Molecular Biology Reviews, 2004. 68(3): p. 560-602.

[58] McGrath, S., G.F. Fitzgerald, and D. Van Sinderen, *The impact of bacteriophage genomics.* Current Opinion in Biotechnology, 2004. 15(2): p. 94-99.

[59] Biswas, B., et al., *Bacteriophage therapy rescues mice bacteremic from a clinical isolate of vancomycin-resistant Enterococcus faecium.* Infection and Immunity, 2002. 70(1): p. 204-210.

[60] Davis, B.M., et al., *CTX prophages in classical biotype Vibrio cholerae: Functional phage genes but dysfunctional phage genomes.* Journal of Bacteriology, 2000. 182(24): p. 6992-6998.

[61] Davis, B.M. and M.K. Waldor, *Filamentous phages linked to virulence of Vibrio cholerae.* Current Opinion in Microbiology, 2003. 6(1): p. 35-42.

[62] Strauch, E., R. Lurz, and L. Beutin, *Characterization of a Shiga toxin-encoding temperate bacteriophage of Shigella sonnei.* Infection and Immunity, 2001. 69(12): p. 7588-7595.

[63] Strauch, E., C. Schaudinn, and L. Beutin, *First-time isolation and characterization of a bacteriophage encoding the Shiga toxin 2c variant, which is globally spread in strains of E. coli O157.* Infection and Immunity, 2004. 72(12): p. 7030-7039.

[64] Parisien, A., et al., *Novel alternatives to antibiotics: Bacteriophages, bacterial cell wall hydrolases, and antimicrobial peptides.* Journal of Applied Microbiology, 2008. 104(1): p. 1-13.

[65] Parisien, A. and C.Q. Lan, *Classification of Bacterial Cell Wall Hydrolysases and Their Potentials as Novel Alternatives to Antibiotics - a response to the letter of Biziulevicius and Kazlauskaite* Journal of Applied Microbiology, 2009. in press.

[66] Abdou, A.M., et al., *Antimicrobial peptides derived from hen egg lysozyme with inhibitory effect against Bacillus species.* Food Control, 2007. 18(2): p. 173-178.

[67] Tenovuo, J., M. Lumikari, and T. Soukka, *Salivary lysozyme, lactoferrin and peroxidases: antibacterial effects on cariogenic bacteria and clinical applications in preventive dentistry.* Proceedings of the Finnish Dental Society. Suomen Hammaslaakariseuran toimituksia, 1991. 87(2): p. 197-208.

[68] Tenovuo, J., *Clinical applications of antimicrobial host proteins lactoperoxidase, lysozyme and lactoferrin in xerostomia: Efficacy and safety.* Oral Diseases, 2002. 8(1): p. 23-29.

[69] Ibrahim, H.R., T. Aoki, and A. Pellegrini, *Strategies for new antimicrobial proteins and peptides: Lysozyme and aprotinin as model molecules.* Current Pharmaceutical Design, 2002. 8(9): p. 671-693.

[70] Masschalck, B. and C.W. Michiels, *Antimicrobial properties of lysozyme in relation to foodborne vegetative bacteria.* Critical Reviews in Microbiology, 2003. 29(3): p. 191-214.

[71] Niyonsaba, F. and H. Ogawa, *Protective roles of the skin against infection: Implication of naturally occurring human antimicrobial agents -defensins, cathelicidin LL-37 and lysozyme.* Journal of Dermatological Science, 2005. 40(3): p. 157-168.

[72] Irwin, D.M., E.M. Prager, and A.C. Wilson, *Evolutionary genetics of ruminant lysozymes.* Animal Genetics, 1992. 23(3): p. 193-202.

[73] Adu-Bobie, J., et al., *GNA33 of Neisseria meningitidis Is A Lipoprotein Required for Cell Separation, Membrane Architecture, and Virulence.* Infection and Immunity, 2004. 72(4): p. 1914-1919.

[74] Blackman, S.A., T.J. Smith, and S.J. Foster, *The role of autolysins during vegetative growth of Bacillus subtilis 168.* Microbiology, 1998. 144(1): p. 73-82.

[75] Garcia, D.L. and J.P. Dillard, *AmiC functions as an N-acetylmuramyl-L-alanine amidase necessary for cell separation and can promote autolysis in Neisseria gonorrhoeae.* Journal of Bacteriology, 2006. 188(20): p. 7211-7221.

[76] Tomasz, A., A. Albino, and E. Zanati, *Multiple antibiotic resistance in a bacterium with suppressed autolytic system.* Nature, 1970. 227(254): p. 138-140.

[77] Beliveau, C., et al., *Cloning, sequencing, and expression in E. coli of a Streptococcus faecalis autolysin.* Journal of Bacteriology, 1991. 173(18): p. 5619-5623.

[78] Vian, A., et al., *Structure of the β-galactosidase gene from Thermus sp. Strain T2: Expression in E. coli and purification in a single step of an active fusion protein.* Applied and Environmental Microbiology, 1998. 64(6): p. 2187-2191.

[79] Croux, C. and J.L. Garcia, *Reconstruction and expression of the autolytic gene from Clostridium acetobutylicum ATCC 824 in E. coli.* FEMS Microbiology Letters, 1992. 95(1): p. 13-20.

[80] Romero, A., R. Lopez, and P. Garcia, *Characterization of the pneumococcal bacteriophage HB-3 amidase: Cloning and expression in E. coli.* Journal of Virology, 1990. 64(1): p. 137-142.

[81] Garcia, E., J.L. Garcia, and C. Ronda, *Cloning and expression of the pneumococcal autolysin gene in E. coli.* Molecular and General Genetics, 1985. 201(2): p. 225-230.

[82] Diaz, E., et al., *The two-step lysis system of pneumococcal bacteriophage EJ-1 is functional in gram-negative bacteria: Triggering of the major pneumococcal autolysin in E. coli.* Molecular Microbiology, 1996. 19(4): p. 667-681.

[83] Biziulevicius, G.A., et al., *Stimulation of microbial autolytic system by tryptic casein hydrolysate.* International Journal of Antimicrobial Agents, 2002. 20(5): p. 361-365.

[84] Wootton, M., et al., *Reduced expression of the atl autolysin gene and susceptibility to autolysis in clinical heterogeneous glycopeptide-intermediate Staphylococcus aureus (hGISA) and GISA strains.* Journal of Antimicrobial Chemotherapy, 2005. 56(5): p. 944-947.

[85] Isturiz, R., J.A. Metcalf, and R.K. Root, *Enhanced killing of penicillin-treated gram-positive cocci by human granulocytes: Role of bacterial autolysins, catalase, and granulocyte oxidative pathways.* Yale Journal of Biology and Medicine, 1985. 58(2): p. 133-143.

[86] Ginsburg, I., *Cationic polyelectrolytes from leukocytes might kill bacteria by activating their autolytic systems: Enigmatically, the relevance of this phenomenon to post-infectious sequelae is disregarded [6].* Intensive Care Medicine, 2002. 28(8): p. 1188.

[87] Ginsburg, I., *Cationic peptides from leukocytes might kill bacteria by activating their autolytic enzymes causing bacteriolysis: Why are publications proposing this concept never acknowledged?* Blood, 2001. 97(8): p. 2530-2531.

[88] Ronda, C., J.L. Garcia, and E. Garcia, *Biological role of the pneumococcal amidase. Cloning of the lytA gene in Streptococcus pneumoniae.* European Journal of Biochemistry, 1987. 164(3): p. 621-624.

[89] Lopez, R., et al., *Structural analysis and biological significance of the cell wall lytic enzymes of Streptococcus pneumoniae and its bacteriophage.* FEMS Microbiology Letters, 1992. 100(1-3): p. 439-447.

[90] Romero, P., R. Lopez, and E. Garcia, *Characterization of LytA-like N-acetylmuramoyl-L-alanine amidases from two new Streptococcus mitis bacteriophages provides insights into the properties of the major pneumococcal autolysin.* Journal of Bacteriology, 2004. 186(24): p. 8229-8239.

[91] Berry, A.M., et al., *Contribution of autolysin to virulence of Streptococcus pneumoniae.* Infection and Immunity, 1989. 57(8): p. 2324-2330.

[92] Sato, K., et al., *Roles of autolysin and pneumolysin in middle ear inflammation caused by a type 3 Streptococcus pneumoniae strain in the chinchilla otitis media model.* Infection and Immunity, 1996. 64(4): p. 1140-1145.

[93] Canvin, J.R., et al., *The role of pneumolysin and autolysin in the pathology of pneumonia and septicemia in mice infected with a type 2 pneumococcus.* Journal of Infectious Diseases, 1995. 172(1): p. 119-123.

[94] Lock, R.A., D. Hansman, and J.C. Paton, *Comparative efficacy of autolysin and pneumolysin as immunogens protecting mice against infection by Streptococcus pneumoniae.* Microbial Pathogenesis, 1992. 12(2): p. 137-143.

[95] Ralston, D.J., et al., *Virolysin: a virus-induced lysin from staphylococcal phage lysates.* Proc. Soc. Exp. Biol. and Med., 1955. 89: p. 502.

[96] Sonstein, S.A., J.M. Hammel, and A. Bondi, *Staphylococcal bacteriophage-associated lysin: a lytic agent active against Staphylococcus aureus.* Journal of Bacteriology, 1971. 107(2): p. 499-504.

[97] Loessner, M.J., et al., *The two-component lysis system of Staphylococcus aureus bacteriophage Twort: A large TTG-start holin and an associated amidase endolysin.* FEMS Microbiology Letters, 1998. 162(2): p. 265-274.

[98] Loessner, M.J., S. Gaeng, and S. Scherer, *Evidence for a holin-like protein gene fully embedded out of frame in the endolysin gene of Staphylococcus aureus bacteriophage 187.* Journal of Bacteriology, 1999. 181(15): p. 4452-4460.

[99] Navarre, W.W., et al., *Multiple enzymatic activities of the murein hydrolase from staphylococcal phage 11: Identification of a D-alanyl-glycine endopeptidase activity.* Journal of Biological Chemistry, 1999. 274(22): p. 15847-15856.

[100] Bon, J., N. Mani, and R.K. Jayaswal, *Molecular analysis of lytic genes of bacteriophage 80 of Staphylococcus aureus.* Canadian Journal of Microbiology, 1997. 43(7): p. 612-616.

[101] Low, L.Y., et al., *Structure and lytic activity of a Bacillus anthracis prophage endolysin.* Journal of Biological Chemistry, 2005. 280(42): p. 35433-35439.

[102] Hermoso, J.A., et al., *Structural basis for selective recognition of pneumococcal cell wall by modular endolysin from phage Cp-1.* Structure, 2003. 11(10): p. 1239-1249.

[103] Monterroso, B., et al., *Unravelling the structure of the pneumococcal autolytic lysozyme.* Biochemical Journal, 2005. 391(1): p. 41-49.

[104] Fischetti, V.A., D. Nelson, and R. Schuch, *Reinventing phage therapy: Are the parts greater than the sum?* Nature Biotechnology, 2006. 24(12): p. 1508-1511.

[105] Fischetti, V.A., *Bacteriophage lytic enzymes: Novel anti-infectives.* Trends in Microbiology, 2005. 13(10): p. 491-496.

[106] Strominger, J.L. and J.M. Ghuysen, *Mechanisms of enzymatic bacteriolysis.* Science, 1967. 156(3772): p. 213-221.

[107] Bower, S. and K.S. Rosenthal, *The bacterial cell wall: The armor, artillery, and Achilles heel.* Infectious Diseases in Clinical Practice, 2006. 14(5): p. 309-317.

[108] Meroueh, S.O., et al., *Three-dimensional structure of the bacterial cell wall peptidoglycan.* Proceedings of the National Academy of Sciences of the United States of America, 2006. 103(12): p. 4404-4409.

[109] Dmitriev, B., F. Toukach, and S. Ehlers, *Towards a comprehensive view of the bacterial cell wall.* Trends in Microbiology, 2005. 13(12): p. 569-574.

[110] Borysowski, J., B. Weber-Dabrowska, and A. Gorski, *Bacteriophage endolysins as a novel class of antibacterial agents.* Experimental Biology and Medicine, 2006. 231(4): p. 366-377.

[111] Garcia, P., et al., *Nucleotide sequence and expression of the pneumococcal autolysin gene from its own promoter in E. coli.* Gene, 1986. 43(3): p. 265-272.

[112] Lopez, R. and E. Garcia, *Recent trends on the molecular biology of pneumococcal capsules, lytic enzymes, and bacteriophage.* FEMS Microbiology Reviews, 2004. 28(5): p. 553-580.

[113] Imoto, T., *Engineering of lysozyme.* EXS, 1996. 75: p. 163-181.

[114] Qian, S.J., et al., *Studies on the engineering of human lysozyme.* Annals of the New York Academy of Sciences, 1995. 750: p. 180-184.

[115] Mesnage, S. and A. Fouet, *Plasmid-encoded autolysin in Bacillus anthracis: Modular structure and catalytic properties.* Journal of Bacteriology, 2002. 184(1): p. 331-334.

[116] Briese, T. and R. Hakenbeck, *Interaction of the pneumococcal amidase with lipoteichoic acid and choline.* European Journal of Biochemistry, 1985. 146(2): p. 417-427.

[117] Lopez, R., et al., *The pneumococcal cell wall degrading enzymes: A modular design to create new lysins?* Microbial Drug Resistance, 1997. 3(2): p. 199-211.

[118] Morita, M., et al., *Functional analysis of antibacterial activity of Bacillus amyloliquefaciens phage endolysin against Gram-negative bacteria.* FEBS Letters, 2001. 500(1-2): p. 56-59.

[119] Cheng, X., et al., *The structure of bacteriophage T7 lysozyme, a zinc amidase and an inhibitor of T7 RNA polymerase.* Proceedings of the National Academy of Sciences of the United States of America, 1994. 91(9): p. 4034-4038.

[120] Masschalck, B., D. Deckers, and C.W. Michiels, *Lytic and nonlytic mechanism of inactivation of gram-positive bacteria by lysozyme under atmospheric and high hydrostatic pressure.* Journal of Food Protection, 2002. 65(12): p. 1916-1923.

[121] Ibrahim, H.R., T. Matsuzaki, and T. Aoki, *Genetic evidence that antibacterial activity of lysozyme is independent of its catalytic function.* FEBS Letters, 2001. 506(1): p. 27-32.

[122] De Vries, J., et al., *The bacteriolytic activity in transgenic potatoes expressing a chimeric T4 lysozyme gene and the effect of T4 lysozyme on soil- and phytopathogenic bacteria.* Systematic and Applied Microbiology, 1999. 22(2): p. 280-286.

[123] Laube, D.M., et al., *Antimicrobial peptides in the airway.* Current topics in microbiology and immunology., 2006. 306: p. 153-182.

[124] Sava, G., *Pharmacological aspects and therapeutic applications of lysozymes.* EXS, 1996. 75: p. 433-449.

[125] Loessner, M.J., *Bacteriophage endolysins - Current state of research and applications.* Current Opinion in Microbiology, 2005. 8(4): p. 480-487.

[126] Bull, J.J. and R.R. Regoes, *Pharmacodynamics of non-replicating viruses, bacteriocins and lysins.* Proceedings of the Royal Society - Biological Sciences (Series B), 2006. 273(1602): p. 2703-2712.

[127] Wang, S., et al., *First report of a novel plant lysozyme with both antifungal and antibacterial activities.* Biochemical and Biophysical Research Communications, 2005. 327(3): p. 820-827.

[128] Lee-Huang, S., et al., *Structural and functional modeling of human lysozyme reveals a unique nonapeptide, HL9, with anti-HIV activity.* Biochemistry, 2005. 44(12): p. 4648-4655.

[129] Bera, A., et al., *Why are pathogenic staphylococci so lysozyme resistant? The peptidoglycan O-acetyltransferase OatA is the major determinant for lysozyme resistance of Staphylococcus aureus.* Molecular Microbiology, 2005. 55(3): p. 778-787.

[130] Solovykh, G.N., et al., *Lysozyme of the mollusk Unio pictorum and the sensitivity of alkanotrophic rhodococci to its effect.* Applied Biochemistry and Microbiology, 2004. 40(5): p. 482-489.

[131] Nattress, F.M., C.K. Yost, and L.P. Baker, *Evaluation of the ability of lysozyme and nisin to control meat spoilage bacteria.* International Journal of Food Microbiology, 2001. 70(1-2): p. 111-119.

[132] Pellegrini, A., S. Schumacher, and R. Stephan, *In-vitro activity of various antimicrobial peptides developed from the bactericidal domains of lysozyme and β-lactoglobulin with respect to Listeria monocytogenes, E. coli O157, Salmonella spp. and Staphylococcus aureus.* Archiv fur Lebensmittelhygiene, 2003. 54(2): p. 34-36.

[133] Cagri, A., Z. Ustunol, and E.T. Ryser, *Antimicrobial edible films and coatings.* Journal of Food Protection, 2004. 67(4): p. 833-848.

[134] Akinbi, H.T., et al., *Bacterial killing is enhanced by expression of lysozyme in the lungs of transgenic mice.* Journal of Immunology, 2000. 165(10): p. 5760-5766.

[135] Shcherbakova, E.G., et al., *Lysozyme effect on the mouse lymphoma growth and antineoplastic activity of cyclophosphamide.* Antibiotiki i Khimioterapiya, 2002. 47(11): p. 3-8.

[136] Loeffler, J.M., D. Nelson, and V.A. Fischetti, *Rapid killing of Streptococcus pneumoniae with a bacteriophage cell wall hydrolase.* Science, 2001. 294(5549): p. 2170-2172.

[137] Jado, I., et al., *Phage lytic enzymes as therapy for antibiotic-resistant Streptococcus pneumoniae infection in a murine sepsis model.* Journal of Antimicrobial Chemotherapy, 2003. 52(6): p. 967-973.

[138] Argueso, P. and M. Sumiyoshi, *Characterization of a carbohydrate epitope defined by the monoclonal antibody H185: Sialic acid O-acetylation on epithelial cell-surface mucins.* Glycobiology, 2006. 16(12): p. 1219-1228.

[139] Fedtke, I., F. Gotz, and A. Peschel, *Bacterial evasion of innate host defenses - The Staphylococcus aureus lesson.* International Journal of Medical Microbiology, 2004. 294(2-3): p. 189-194.

[140] Veiga, P., et al., *Identification of an essential gene responsible for D-Asp incorporation in the Lactococcus lactis peptidoglycan crossbridge.* Molecular Microbiology, 2006. 62(6): p. 1713-1724.

[141] Bukharin, O.V. and A.V. Valyshev, *Microbial inhibitors of lysozyme.* Zhurnal mikrobiologii, epidemiologii, i immunobiologii., 2006(4): p. 8-13.

[142] Nakimbugwe, D., et al., *Inactivation of gram-negative bacteria in milk and banana juice by hen egg white and lambda lysozyme under high hydrostatic pressure.* International Journal of Food Microbiology, 2006. 112(1): p. 19-25.

[143] Callewaert, L., et al., *Purification of Ivy, a lysozyme inhibitor from E. coli, and characterisation of its specificity for various lysozymes.* Enzyme and Microbial Technology, 2005. 37(2): p. 205-211.

[144] Fischer, W., *Phosphocholine of pneumococcal teichoic acids: Role in bacterial physiology and pneumococcal infection.* Research in Microbiology, 2000. 151(6): p. 421-427.

[145] Jedrzejas, M.J., *Pneumococcal Virulence Factors: Structure and Function.* Microbiol. Mol. Biol. Rev., 2001. 65(2): p. 187-207.

[146] Tomasz, A., E. Zanati, and R. Ziegler, *DNA uptake during genetic transformation and the growing zone of the cell envelope.* Proceedings of the National Academy of Sciences of the United States of America, 1971. 68(8): p. 1848-1852.

[147] Coello, R., et al., *Prospective study of infection, colonization and carriage of methicillin-resistant staphylococcus aureus in an outbreak affecting 990 patients.* European Journal of Clinical Microbiology and Infectious Diseases, 1994. 13(1): p. 74-81.

[148] De Lencastre, H., et al., *Carriage of respiratory tract pathogens and molecular epidemiology of Streptococcus pneumoniae colonization in healthy children attending day care centers in Lisbon, Portugal.* Microbial Drug Resistance, 1999. 5(1): p. 19-29.

[149] Von Eiff, C., et al., *Nasal carriage as a source of Staphylococcus aureus bacteremia.* New England Journal of Medicine, 2001. 344(1): p. 11-16.

[150] Fischetti, V.A., *Novel method to control pathogenic bacteria on human mucous membranes.* Annals of the New York Academy of Sciences, 2003. 987: p. 207-214.

[151] Schuch, R., D. Nelson, and V.A. Fischetti, *A bacteriolytic agent that detects and kills Bacillus anthracis.* Nature, 2002. 418(6900): p. 884-889.

[152] Fischetti, V. and L. Loomis, *APP Use of bacterial phage associated lysing enzymes for treating upper respiratory illnesses*, in *United States Patent And Trademark Office Granted Patent.* 2006.

[153] Cunningham, M.W., *Pathogenesis of group a streptococcal infections.* Clinical Microbiology Reviews, 2000. 13(3): p. 470-511.

[154] Nelson, D.C. and V.A. Fischetti, *C1 bacteriophage lytic system*, in *United States Patent And Trademark Office Pre-Grant Publication*. 2002.

[155] Fischetti, V.A. and Q. Cheng, *Ply-Gbs Mutant Lysins*, In *Patent Cooperation Treaty Application*. 2007.

[156] Delisle, A.L., G.J. Barcak, and M. Guo, *Bacteriophage-Encoded Antibacterial Enzyme For The Treatment And Prevention Of Gingivitis And Root Surface Caries*, In *Patent Cooperation Treaty Application*. 2004.

[157] Yoon, S., et al., *App Antimicrobial Protein Specific To Staphylococcus Aureus*, In *Patent Cooperation Treaty Application*. 2008.

[158] Ross, P. and A. Coffey, *App Recombinant Staphylococcal Phage Lysin As An Antibacterial Agent*, In *Patent Cooperation Treaty Application*. 2008.

[159] Fischetti, V.A. and R. Schuch, *Lytic Enzymes And Spore Surface Antigen For Detection And Treatment Of*, In *Patent Cooperation Treaty Application*. 2005.

[160] Yoong, P., Et Al., *Bactiophage Lysins For Enterococcus Faecalis, Enterococcus Faecium And Other Bacteria*, In *United States Patent And Trademark Office Pre-Grant Publication*. 2007.

[161] Harris, D.L. And N. Lee, *App Bacteriophage And Enzymes Lytic To Salmonellae*, In *Patent Cooperation Treaty Application*. 2003.

[162] Zimmer, M., M. Loessner, And A.J. Morgan, *Novel Protein*, In *United States Patent And Trademark Office Pre-Grant Publication*. 2005.

[163] Fischetti, V. And L. Loomis, *App Therapeutic Treatment Of Upper Respiratory Infections Using A Nasal Spray*. United States Patent And Trademark Office Granted Patent, 2005.

[164] Fischetti, V.A., D. Nelson, And R. Schuch, *Nucleic Acids And Polypeptides Of C1 Bacteriophage And Uses Thereof*, In *Patent Cooperation Treaty Application*. 2004.

[165] Nelson, D.C. and V.A. Fischetti, *C1 bacteriophage lytic system*. 2003.

[166] Yoong, P., et al., *Identification of a broadly active phage lytic enzyme with lethal activity against antibiotic-resistant Enterococcus faecalis and Enterococcus faecium*. Journal of Bacteriology, 2004. 186(14): p. 4808-4812.

[167] Nelson, D., L. Loomis, and V.A. Fischetti, *Prevention and elimination of upper respiratory colonization of mice by group A streptococci by using a bacteriophage lytic enzyme*. Proceedings of the National Academy of Sciences of the United States of America, 2001. 98(7): p. 4107-4112.

[168] Yoshimura, G., et al., *Identification and molecular characterization of an N-acetylmuraminidase, Aml, involved in Streptococcus mutans cell separation*. Microbiology and Immunology, 2006. 50(9): p. 729-742.

[169] Hiramatsu, K., et al., *The emergence and evolution of methicillin-resistant Staphylococcus aureus*. Trends in Microbiology, 2001. 9(10): p. 486-493.

[170] Zhong, W., et al., *Differentiation of Bacillus anthracis, B. cereus, and B. thuringiensis by using pulsed-field gel electrophoresis*. Applied and Environmental Microbiology, 2007. 73(10): p. 3446-3449.

[171] Walter, M.H. and D.D. Baker, *Three Bacillus anthracis bacteriophages from topsoil*. Current Microbiology, 2003. 47(1): p. 55-58.

[172] Yoong, P., et al., *App Bactiophage Lysins For Bacillus Anthracis*, In *Patent Cooperation Treaty Application*. 2008.

[173] Fischetti, V.A., R. Schuch, And D. Nelson, *Phage-Associated Lytic Enzymes For Treatment Of Bacillus Anthracis And Related Conditions*, In *United States Patent And Trademark Office Granted Patent*. 2008.

[174] Cetinkaya, F., Et Al., *Shigella And Salmonella Contamination In Various Foodstuffs In Turkey*. Food Control, 2008. 19(11): P. 1059-1063.

[175] Yang, H.-H., S.F. Hiu, And J.L. Harris, *Prod Production Of Phage And Phage-Associated Lysin*, In *United States Patent And Trademark Office Granted Patent*. 1989.

[176] Alday-Sanz, V., I. Karunasagar, And I. Karunasagar, *Prod + App Compositions Comprising Lytic Enzymes Of Bacteriophages For Treating Bacterial Infections*, In *Patent Cooperation Treaty Application*. 2007.

In: Antibiotic Resistance: ...
Editors: Adriel R. Bonilla and Kaden P. Muniz

ISBN: 978-1-60741-623-4
©2009 Nova Science Publishers, Inc.

Chapter VIII

Application of Computational Methods to Study Antibiotic Resistance Mechanisms: Fluoroquinolone Resistance as a Case Study

Sergio Madurga[1], Jordi Vila[2] and Ernest Giralt[3]

[1]Department of Physical Chemistry and IQTCUB, University of Barcelona, Spain
[2]Department of Microbiology, Hospital Clinic, School of Medicine,
University of Barcelona, Spain
[3]Institute for Research in Biomedicine, Barcelona Science Park, Spain; and
Department of Organic Chemistry, University of Barcelona, Spain

Abstract

Antibiotic resistance can occur via three mechanisms: prevention of interaction of the drug with target; decreased uptake due to either an increased efflux or a decreased influx of the antimicrobial agent and enzymatic modification or destruction of the compound. Herein we review the results from computational studies on said mechanisms. For the first mechanism, the bacteria produce mutant versions of antibiotic targets. This process has been studied using several levels of theory, from costly quantum mechanics calculations to classical molecular dynamics calculations. For the decreased uptake mechanisms, since the atomic structure of several influx pores and efflux pumps were resolved recently, homology modelling studies and large molecular dynamics simulations allow us to understand this resistance mechanism at the molecular level. Computational studies with antibiotic molecules (mainly β-lactam compounds) studying the resistance mechanism in which the antibiotic compound is transformed will be also summarized. β-lactamases are bacterial enzymes responsible for most of the resistance against β-lactam antibiotics. These defensive enzymes, prevalent in nearly every pathogenic bacterial strain, hydrolyze the β-lactam ring and release the cleaved, inactive antibiotics. Computational studies on this reaction provided us with knowledge on the molecular mechanism of action of these enzymes. The results may prove valuable in the design of new antibiotic derivatives with improved activity in resistant strains. Finally, a case study on the mechanism of resistance of fluoroquinolones is explained in detail. Extensive use and misuse of fluoroquinolones in human and veterinary medicine has led to the emergence and spread of resistant clones. These have appeared mainly through mutations in the structural genes that encode their intracellular targets (DNA gyrase and topoisomerase IV) as well as via modifications in membrane permeability (e.g. decreased influx and/or increased efflux). We analyzed bacterial resistance to fluoroquinolones that arises from mutations in the DNA gyrase target protein. We studied the binding mode of ciprofloxacin, levofloxacin, and moxifloxacin to DNA gyrase by docking calculations. The binding model obtained enabled us to study, at the atomic level, the resistance mechanism associated with the most common gyrA mutations in *E. coli* fluoroquinolone-resistant strains.

Introduction

Bacterial resistance to antibiotic can occur via three general mechanisms: prevention of interaction of the drug with target; decreased uptake due to either an increased efflux or a decreased influx of the antimicrobial agent; and enzymatic modification or destruction of the compound. These mechanisms have been studied extensively through a variety of techniques, recently including computational tools. Computational simulations of biological systems are now so advanced that they are used to study nearly every experimentally interesting enzymatic system (Garcia et al., 2004; Warshel, 2003; Warshel, 1991; Gao et al., 2002; Benkovic et al., 2003). These simulations complement laboratory experiments by providing important details at the atomic and molecular levels and yielding quantities that are difficult to measure experimentally.

Antibiotic resistance is chiefly simulated at the atomic level through two types of calculations: molecular dynamics (MD) calculations, which use empirical force-field parameters; and quantum mechanics/molecular mechanics (QM/MM) calculations, which use *ab initio* calculations for the most relevant part of the studied protein. Although MD calculations work well for investigating the dynamics and non-covalent binding of biomolecules, they are of limited use in describing enzymatic reactions, since they do not include defined parameters for transition structures in which bonds are partially formed. Albeit MD calculations are fast, they are heavily dependent on the availability of force-field parameters. Moreover, first-principles (*ab initio*) MD calculations are not based on any empirical knowledge, but they can be extremely time consuming when applied to an entire protein. In contrast, QM/MM are more often employed for enzymatic reactions, as they combine accuracy of QM with the speed of MM. QM/MM methodology was introduced by Warshel and coworkers (Warshel et al., 1976) and has been further developed by several groups. In QM/MM, only a small portion of the biomolecule is studied at the quantum level. For instance, the active-site can be treated using high-level QM (the QM region), whereas the more distant parts of the enzyme can be treated using low-cost molecular mechanics (the MM region). The QM region encompasses the reactive species and other moieties that are expected to be involved in the reaction. Although quantum description of the potential for the reactive QM atoms is necessary, a force field approach is often sufficient for describing the MM atoms. The QM/MM approach is a compromise, but numerous studies have demonstrated that it is effective enough for characterising enzymatic reactions (Gao, 1996; Monard et al., 1999; Garcia et al., 2004; Warshel, 2003).

1. Enzymatic Modification or Hydrolysis of the DRUG: β-Lactam Antibiotics

Numerous enzymes confer cells with antibiotic resistance by modifying or destroying the drug (Wright2005). Some enzymes degrade antibiotics via hydrolysis (e.g. β-lactamases, macrolide esterases, and epoxidases), whereas others transfer functional groups on the drug (e.g., acyltransferases and phosphotransferases). Due to the widespread use of β-lactam antibiotics, β-lactamases are among the most important of these enzymes. In this section we discuss several computational studies performed for each class of β-lactamases.

β-lactam antibiotics (e.g., penicillins, cephalosporins and carbapenems) are among the most common drugs prescribed to treat bacterial infections (Demain et al., 1999; Frère et al., 1985). They operate by covalently binding to the active site of D-alanyl-D-alanine carboxy-peptidase/transpeptidase enzymes (also known as penicillin-binding proteins [PBPs]), which are involved in the biosynthesis of bacterial cell wall, to cause cell death (Frère et al., 1985; Waxman et al., 1983; Ghuysen, 1994; Ghuysen, 1997). Resistance to β-lactam antibiotics is principally conferred via β-lactamases, which first bind to the antibiotics analogously to PBPs and then destroy the antibiotics through hydrolysis. The enzymes are regenerated upon hydrolysis of each drug molecule, enabling them to breakdown additional drug molecules (Knott-Hunziker et al., 1982; Frère, 1995; Knox et al., 1996; Pratt, 2002).

Both PBPs and β-lactamases are enzymes that form an acyl-enzyme intermediate with the substrate (Ghuysen, 1991; Ghuysen et al., 1988). Whereas β-lactamases efficiently catalyze hydrolysis of the acyl-enzyme intermediate, PBPs are very poor catalysts of this hydrolysis reaction and therefore, are effectively trapped as the acyl-enzyme intermediate and inactivated. The literature is replete with speculation on the mechanisms by which these acyl-enzyme intermediates are formed (Dubus et al., 1996; Bulychev et al., 1997; Powers et al., 2001; Oefner et al., 1990; Bubus et al., 1994; Lobkovsky et al., 1994, Wilkin et al., 1993; Bernstein et al., 1999). Computational studies are required to characterise the chemistry involved at the atomic level. Once these mechanisms are understood, the main differences between β-lactamases and PBPs can be elucidated, which in turn should facilitate the rational design of new antibiotics that are not susceptible to β-lactamase hydrolysis.

It is widely accepted that β-lactamases evolved from PBPs by acquiring the ability to rapidly hydrolyze the acyl-enzyme species (Knox et al., 1996; Frère et al., 1999; Fisher et al., 2005; Labia, 2004). This led to four distinct β-lactamase classes: A, B, C and D (Fisher et al., 2005; Bush et al., 1995). Like PBPs, classes A, C, D are active-site serine proteases, whereas class B are zinc-dependent proteins. The four classes of β-lactamases inactivate β-lactam antibiotics by hydrolyzing the C-N bond in the lactam ring (Knowles, 1985; Walsh, 2000; Fisher et al., 2005; Page, 1992; Frère, 1995). Understanding β-lactamase function at the molecular level is essential to unravelling the origins of bacterial resistance and to designing novel, effective β-lactamase inhibitors.

In the following subsection, the results of several works that use QM/MM calculations to study the mechanism action of each of the four classes of β-lactamase are presented.

1.1. Class A β-Lactamases

The reaction mechanism of Class A β-lactamases comprises two steps: acylation of Ser70 by the ß-lactam antibiotic (according to the the standard amino acid numbering scheme for β-lactamases of Ambler et al. (Ambler et al., 1991)), followed by hydrolysis of the resulting ester, the acylenzyme intermediate. Lys73 is another catalytically important residue. It forms hydrogen bonds to Ser70, Ser130, Asn132 and Glu166 (Matagne et al., 1998; Lietz et al., 2000; Jelsch et al., 1993). In addition, a special feature of the active site is a structurally-conserved water molecule that is hydrogen bound to Ser70, Glu166 and Asn170. Albeit these residues are likely to be involved in catalysis, the molecular mechanism is unknown. The deacylation mechanism, whereby the conserved water molecule is activated by Glu166 to hydrolyze the acylenzyme intermediate, is widely accepted (Oefner et al., 1990). In contrast, despite the numerous X-ray crystallography structures available (Nukaga et al., 2003; Minasov et al., 2002), the acylation mechanism still remains controversial—chiefly due to the complex ensemble of amino acid residues close to the bound ß-lactam substrate.

There are reviews that summarise the various mechanisms proposed for the acylation reaction (Herzberg et al., 1991; Matagne et al., 1998). These primarily differ by their respective compound which acts as general base and activates Ser70. As laboratory experiments have shown that both Glu166 and Lys73 are essential for efficient acylation (Strynadka et al., 1992; Gibson et al., 1990; Guillaume et al., 1997; Escobar et al., 1991; Adachi et al., 1991; Lietz et al., 2000), the possibility that Lys73 (in neutral state) or Glu166 acting as a base has been studied computationally. Indeed, Glu166-mutants (and Lys73 mutants) are acylated, but at a drastically reduced rate.

In order for Lys73 to be the base, it would have to be in its neutral state, which is rather unusual. However, its neutral state has been suggested to be favoured by the electrostatic environment in the active site and by substrate effects (Swaren et al., 1995; Strynadka et al., 1992). This mechanism in which Lys73 acts as the base was modelled in a QM/MM study by Pitarch et al. (Pitarch et al., 2000). In their study, the acylation step in β-lactamase was explored at the AM1/CHARMM level of theory. The quantum mechanics part of the system was treated with a semiempirical method which is faster—but generally less accurate—than a full *ab initio* method. In contrast, several theoretical and experimental studies have indicated that Lys73 is more likely to be protonated under physiological conditions, and therefore, could not act as the base (Lamotte et al., 1999; Raquet et al., 1997; Damblon et al., 1996). Hermann et al. performed MD simulations which suggest that Lys73 is protonated, by analyzing the stability of the hydrogen-bond network in the active site and RMS deviations of conserved residues (Hermann et al., 2005). Specifically, the conserved water molecule—which is required for deacylation—did not remain in its position in the active site when Lys73 is treated as neutral. Similarly, Díaz et al. concluded from their MD simulations that Lys73 is unlikely to be the base (Díaz et al., 2003).

Using QM/MM calculations on Class A β-lactamase with benzylpenicillin as substrate, Hermann et al. studied the possibility of Glu166 as the base (Hermann et al., 2005), a mechanism supported by previous semiempirical QM/MM calculations (Hermann et al., 2003) and by two X-ray structures of Class A β-lactamases (Minasov et al., 2002; Nukaga et al., 2003). In one of these X-ray structures, in which a transition state analogue is bound to the active site, Glu166 is protonated. The other structure shows Ser70 hydrogen bound to the bridging water molecule. Both structures support a mechanism in which Glu166 acts as the general base.

Hermann et al. (Hermann et al., 2005) showed by QM/MM calculations using AM1/CHARMM22 level with high-level energy corrections (B3LYP/6-31G+(d)//AM1-CHARMM22) that deprotonation of the conserved water molecule by Glu166 is energetically and structurally reasonable, and consistent with experimental data. Hermann et al. chose the high resolution crystal structure of the benzylpenicillin-acylated Glu166Asn mutant TEM1 β-lactamase as the starting geometry to perform QM/MM calculations. First, the Glu166Asn mutation was mutated (*in silico*) back to glutamate to generate a functional (i.e. wild type) active site. The proposed mechanism of Hermann et al. shows that the nucleophile, Ser70, is indirectly activated via deprotonation by Glu166, which abstracts a proton from an intervening water molecule, which in turn deprotonates Ser70. This deprotonation activates the serine for nucleophilic attack of the β-lactam antibiotic.

Analysis of the energy profiles and potential energy surfaces reveals that formation of the tetrahedral intermediate follows a concerted mechanism whereby the two proton transfers (from Ser70 to the water molecule and from the water molecule to the general base, Glu166) are concomitant to nucleophilic attack of the β-lactam carbonyl group by Ser70. Furthermore, the calculations suggest that Asn132, in addition to its attributed role of binding the substrate via interaction with the peptidic side chain of β-lactam compounds, may be crucial to stabilization of the positively charged Lys73.

Finally, Meroueh et al. (Meroueh et al., 2005) studied the serine acylation mechanism for the Class A TEM-1 β-lactamase with penicillanic acid as substrate at a higher level of theory than previous calculations. They concluded that Glu166 and Lys73 both act as base, are compatible and compete (Figure 1.1). Following substrate binding, the pathway starts at a low energy barrier (5 kcal mol^{-1}) and with an energetically favourable proton transfer from Lys73 to Glu166, through the catalytic water molecule and Ser70. This gives deprotonated Lys73 and protonated Glu166. The existence of two routes is fully consistent with experimental data for mutant variants of the TEM β-lactamase.

The results from computational studies suggest routes for modification of β-lactam antibiotics that could increase their stability against Class A β-lactamases. Namely, modifications that impair the deprotonation mechanism of Ser70 could be promising. This activation machinery is different from the actual targets of β-lactams, the PBPs, which lack key residues of the Class A β-lactamase active site, such as the general base Glu166. Therefore, the sensitivity of PBPs to such modified β-lactam antibiotics should not be affected.

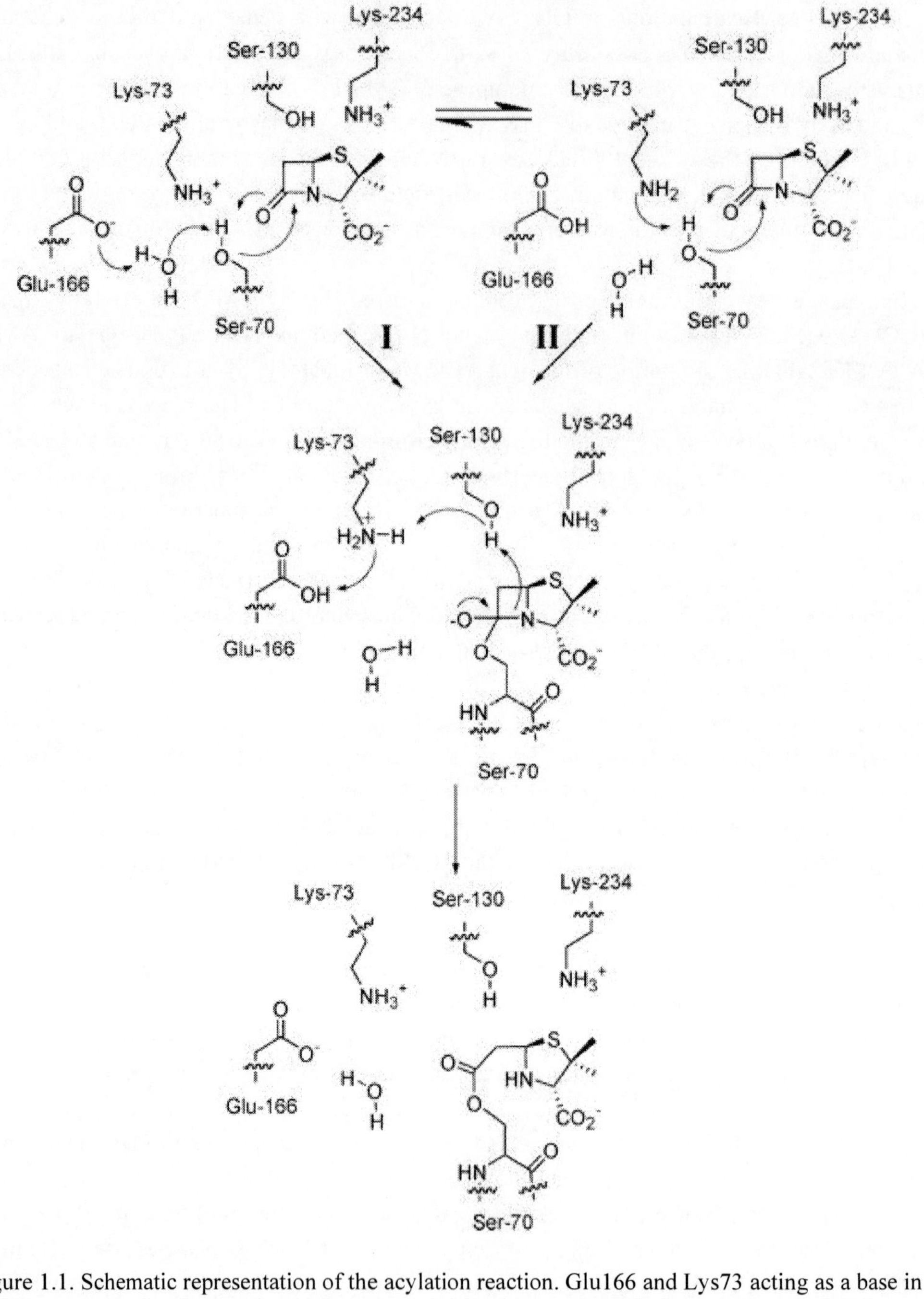

Figure 1.1. Schematic representation of the acylation reaction. Glu166 and Lys73 acting as a base in I) and II), respectively. Figure adapted from the article by Merouerh et al. (Merouerh et al., 2005).

1.2. Class B β-Lactamases

Class B β-lactamases can be further divided into three subclasses: B1, B2 and B3 (Bush, 1998; Galleni et al., 2001). Structural studies have shown that all class B β-lactamases have two potential Zn(II)-binding sites near the bottom of a broad crevasse (Carfi et al., 1995;

Garau et al., 2005; Orellano et al., 1998; Seny et al., 2001): the Zn1 site and the Zn2 site. The Zn1 site comprises three His residues in the B1 and B3 subclasses, and two His and one Asn in the B2 subclass. On the other hand, the Zn2 site consists of an Asp-Cys-His triad in the B1 and B2 subclasses, and an Asp-His-His triad in the B3 subclass.

B1 and B3 ß-lactamases are known to be catalytically active with either one or two zinc cofactors (Paul et al., 1999; Rasia et al., 2002; Wommer et al., 2002). However, B2 enzymes are only active in the monozinc form (Walsh et al., 1996; Valladares et al., 1997). The lactam amide bond is believed to be hydrolyzed by an active site water molecule, which attacks the carbonyl carbon in the lactam ring. The mechanistic details of this reaction are poorly understood.

Some insight into the structure and dynamics of metallo-β-lactamase has been provided by various MD- and QM-based simulations (Díaz et al., 2001; Salsbury et al., 2001; Suárez et al., 2002; Antony et al., 2002; Krauss et al., 2003; Olsen et al., 2004; Peraro et al., 2004; Park et al., 2005a; Park et al., 2005b; Wang et al., 2007; Xu et al., 2006, Oelschlaeger et al., 2003). Xu et al. (Xu et al., 2006) reported a QM/MM study of an apo-subclass B2 metallo-ß-lactamase and its complex with a molecule of the potent ß-lactam antibiotic biapenem. The quantum region in the QM/MM simulations encompasses the Zn(II) ion, the antibiotic molecule, the catalytic water and an active-site His residue. The simulations revealed that the substrate is engaged in direct metal binding through a carboxylate oxygen. The substrate is further anchored by several hydrogen bonds established with active-site residues. Additional molecular dynamics simulations confirmed the stability of the metal-ligand bonds and the hydrogen-bond network of both the apoenzyme and the substrate-enzyme complex. Moreover, the simulations showed that a water molecule resides in a pocket near the lactam carbonyl carbon of the substrate.

For binuclear metallo-ß-lactamases, the molecular basis of substrate specificity was studied using MD calculations on the *Pseudomonas aeruginosa* enzyme IMP-1 and its variant IMP-6 (Oelschlaeger et al., 2003). IMP-6 and IMP-1 differ by a single residue at position 196 (Gly versus Ser, respectively), but have significantly different substrate spectra. To model stability, several MD simulations at 100 K were performed for all enzyme-substrate complexes. Stable structures were further heated to 200 and 300 K. By counting stable structures, the authors derived a stability ranking score which correlated with experimentally determined catalytic efficiency. Interestingly, the authors rationalized the effects of residue 196 on the substrate spectra through a domino effect: upon replacement of Ser with Gly, a hole is created and a stabilizing interaction between Ser196 and Lys33 disappears, rendering the neighboring residues more flexible; this increased flexibility is then transferred to the active site.

1.3. Class C *ß*-Lactamases

Class C ß-lactamases have been computationally modelled to identify their mechanism of action (Castillo et al., 2002; Hata et al., 2000; Fujii et al., 2002; Díaz et al., 2001; Massova et al., 2002). They have a broad spectrum of natural activities and can hydrolyze *ß*-lactamase resistant ß-lactams, such as the third-generation cephalosporins. Moreover, Class C ß-lactamases are not markedly inhibited by clinically used ß-lactamase inhibitors (e.g. clavulanate).

Gherman et al. (Gherman et al., 2004) modelled the deacylation reaction for the ß-lactam antibiotic cephalothin bound to both a PBP (Streptomyces sp. R61 DD-peptidase) and a Class C ß-lactamase (cephalosporinase from *Enterobacter cloacae* P99), using QM/MM calculations. Their computations employ a large QM active site region (150 QM atoms) and a high quality density functional method to compute the structures and energies of the intermediates and transition states. The results of these calculations were in good qualitative—and, in the case of P99, quantitative—agreement with experimental kinetic data for the deacylation rates of the acyl-enzyme intermediates for R61 and P99 with cephalothin (Frère et al., 1975; Dubus et al., 1996). This provided them with confidence that their calculations were sufficiently precise for understanding the crucial differences between the deacylation rates between the PBP and the Class C ß-lactamase.

Powers et al. (Powers et al., 2002) applied several computational studies to the Class C ß-lactamase AmpC. They used X-ray crystal structures of AmpC in complexes with five boronic acid inhibitors and four ß-lactams using three programs (GRID, MCSS and X-SITE) to predict potential binding site hotspots on AmpC. Their results may prove useful for the structure-based design AmpC inhibitors.

1.4. Class D *β*-Lactamases

Class D *β*-lactamases confer high levels of resistance to myriad *β*-lactam antibiotics. The X-ray crystal structures of two Class D lactamases, OXA-10 (Maveyraud et al., 2000) and OXA-1 (Sun et al., 2003, were recently solved. A special characteristic in both of these structures is that Lys-70 is carboxylated, in contrast to the corresponding Lys in the reactive sites of Class A and Class C *β*-lactamases. Carboxylated Lys residues had previously been found in D-ribulose-1,5-bisphosphate carboxylase/oxygenase (Lorimer et al., 1976), urease from *Klebsiella aerogenes* (Jabri et al., 1995), phosphotriesterase from *Pseudomonas diminuta* (Shim et al., 2000), and in a few other proteins (Thoden et al., 2001; Morollo et al., 1999). In these cases the carbamate is stabilized by interactions with metal cations and/or serves a structural role (Jabri et al., 1995; Benning et al., 1995; Shibata et al., 1996).

Studies with $^{14}CO_2$ and $^{13}CO_2$ have shown that carboxylation in OXA-10 is reversible and essential for catalytic activity (Golemi et al., 2001). The fully decarboxylated form is inactive, and the degree of recarboxylation correlates with the degree to which activity is recovered. Independent nuclear magnetic resonance (NMR) experiments with $^{13}CO_2$ confirmed the presence of a carboxylated lysine in the active enzyme (Golemi et al., 2001). The mechanistic role of carboxylated Lys-70 is further supported by the fact that the Lys-70-Ala mutant is entirely inactive.

Li et al. (Li et al., 2005) used QM/MM to study the energetics of the carboxylation of Lys-70 in OXA-10. They and other researchers (Golemi et al., 2003; Birk et al., 2004) have found that understanding the carboxylation/decarboxylation is crucial to understanding the activity of the enzyme. The carboxylated Lys removes a proton from the side chain of the active-site serine of OXA-10, promoting its acylation by the substrate. The same carboxylated Lys activates a water molecule in the second step of the catalytic process, which involves deacylation of the acyl-enzyme species. The carboxylate group of the carboxylated Lys is stabilized by hydrogen bonding interactions with Ser67, by the side chain nitrogen of Trp154 and by a crystallographic water molecule.

2. Efflux of Antibiotics from the Cell

Efflux pumps are transport proteins involved in the extrusion of toxic substrates outside the cell, and are found in the cytoplasmic membranes of all cell types (Bambeke et al., 2000). Pumps may be specific for one substrate or may transport various structurally-dissimilar compounds, including several classes of antibiotics. The latter type of pump is associated with multiple drug resistance (MDR). Bacterial efflux transporters are classified into five major superfamilies (Lomovskaya et al., 2001): major facilitator (MF), multidrug and toxic efflux (MATE), resistance-nodulation-division (RND), small multidrug resistance (SMR) and ATP binding cassette (ABC). These transporters are generally powered by proton transfer (Paulsen et al., 1996), the exception being the ABC family, whose energy source is ATP hydrolysis. MFS dominates in Gram-positive bacteria, whereas the RND family is unique to Gram-negative bacteria.

Multidrug transport proteins extrude structurally-unrelated active molecules. The ability of efflux systems to recognize diverse compounds probably stems from the fact that substrate recognition is based on physicochemical properties (e.g. hydrophobicity, aromaticity and ionizability), rather than on defined chemical properties, as in classical enzyme-substrate or ligand-receptor recognition. Because most antibiotics are amphiphilic they are easily recognized by various efflux pumps.

Reducing efflux-mediated drug resistance will require greater knowledge about two key aspects: firstly, how efflux pumps are able to function with such a broad array of compounds; and secondly, how conformational changes in these pumps are related to transportation of substrates. Here we report on recent advances in understanding the structure and function of drug efflux pumps that have been made possible by computational studies. Once these mechanisms are fully understood the rational design of efflux pump inhibitors could become a reality. This would enable the reutilization of old drugs whose efficacy has been lost due to drug efflux.

Computational studies on bacterial efflux pumps have chiefly focused on two strategies according to the availability of structural data: MD calculations are used when crystal structures are available, whereas homology modelling studies are used when crystal structures are unavailable. However, there is an alternative in the latter case: quantitative structure–activity relationship (QSAR) models could be employed if the affinities of multiple substrates for the same transporter are known.

High-resolution structural data on transport proteins is generally lacking due to two major problems. Firstly, obtaining membrane proteins in the quantities and purity required for crystallization studies is not trivial. And secondly, due to the amphiphilicity of these proteins their crystallization is not straightforward. These proteins feature two types of domains: nucleotide binding domains (NBDs) and transmembrane domains (TMDs). Only a few crystal structures of bacterial transporters with transmembrane domains have been obtained, including those of the ABC transporter Sav1866 from *S. aureus* at 3.0 Å (Dawson et al., 2006; Dawson et al., 2007) and the vitamin B12 transporter BtuCD from *E. coli* (Locher et al., 2002). Several isolated NBDs have also been crystallized (Hung et al., 1998; Diederichs et al., 2000; Gaudet et al., 2001; Yuan et al., 2001; Karpowich et al., 2001; Hopfner et al., 2000; Schmitt et al., 2003).

Among multidrug efflux transporters one of the most relevant to antibiotic resistance is LmrA, an ABC from *Lactococcus lactis* that confers antibiotic resistance to numerous common prescription antibiotics and which has been extensively modelled. Because of the lack of high resolution structural data on the full LmrA transporter, it can be studied using a homology model (i.e. a model based on the structure of a known sequence homolog).

In the following subsection we explain homology modelling of efflux pumps. We then report a recent study of LmrA based on this technique. Finally, we describe several MD calculations for bacterial transport proteins whose crystal structures are known.

2.1. Homology Modelling of Transporters

Homology modelling is useful for modelling transporters whose crystal structure is unavailable. A homology model is generally constructed by extracting structural information from a template protein to generate the three-dimensional structure of a target protein. This requires at least one appropriate and available crystal structure for the template protein, which has to share the same number of transmembrane regions and a high level of either sequence homology or structural homology with the target protein.

There are several algorithms for generating homology models (Bates et al., 2001; Blundell et al., 1988; Contreras et al., 2002; Greer, 1990; Sali et al., 1993, Schwede et al., 2003, Vriend, 1990), including the programs Insight II Homology (Greer, 1990), SYBYL Composer (Blundell et al., 1988) and Modeller (Sali et al., 1993). There are also various online applications such as the WHAT IF server (Vriend, 1990), the Swiss-Model website and server (Schwede et al., 2003) and the 3D-Jigsaw Comparative Modelling Server (Bates et al., 2001, Contreras et al., 2002). Following the analysis of Chang et al., modelling studies applied to transporters follow four steps (Chang et al., 2006): template identification, sequence alignment, model generation, and model optimization and validation.

The first step, template identification, involves the use of sequence similarity search algorithms (e.g. BLAST (Altschul et al., 1990) or PSI-BLAST (Altschul et al., 1997)) or fold recognition algorithms (Godzik, 2003) to search a database of known structures. For transporter proteins the number of available templates is very limited, due to the abovementioned reasons. Consequently, in the selection process the sequence identity is not the most important aspect; rather, what is essential is that the two proteins share the same number of TMD regions and belong to the same superfamily. Different procedures have been developed to select the most appropriate template. One of the most widely used consists in focusing only on isolated parts of the transporter structure, especially the extramembranous domains. This approach has been applied in understanding the functional roles of each specific domain, for example, in studying the structure of the Pho84 phosphate transporter (Lagerstedt et al., 2004).

The second step, sequence alignment, is the most critical step in obtaining a successful homology model. Generally, the sequence alignment of two or more proteins is performed automatically by homology modelling programs. Both sequence alignment and template structure are important factors in the development of a good homology model. Difficulties appear in the generation of the model when there is a structural region present in the target but not in the template (alignment gaps).

In the third step, model generation, a three-dimensional structural model of the target is generated using a given template and an alignment. Three major classes of model generation methods have been proposed (Bakeret al., 2001): fragment assembly, segment matching and satisfaction of spatial restraints. In the fragment assembly method the full model is constructed by assembling several conserved structural fragments from solved structures of related systems. A similar procedure is carried out in the segment matching procedure, but here the target is assembled by using several shorter segments corresponding to different template structures. Finally, the satisfaction of spatial restraints method uses one or more target-template alignments to construct a set of geometrical criteria that are then converted to restraints of C alpha-C alpha distances, main-chain N-O distances, main-chain and side-chain dihedral angles. This method usually employs the program MODELLER (Fiser et al., 2003) in combination with the ModBase database (Pieper et al., 2004).

The final step, model validation, enables us to determine the accuracy of the generated model, and can be based on theoretical and experimental validation. In the case of theoretical validation, different programs that evaluate the three-dimensional structure could be used to verify the quality of the model. In experimental validation the model is compared with biological data. WHAT IF (Vriend, 1990), PROCHECK (Laskowski et al., 1993) and Verify-3D (Bowie et al., 1991, Eisenberg et al., 1997, Luthy et al., 1992) are programs frequently used to perform theoretical validation of homology models. These programs use rules extracted from crystal structures to apply and evaluate the model structure. In general, a significant part of homology modelling studies also involves validating the model by comparing it with experimental data that could be derived from site-directed mutagenesis experiments or low-resolution electron microscopy studies.

In summary, to obtain high-quality models from homology modelling studies these models must be validated and improved with experimental data. Although such models have to be considered provisional until the transporter structure is available, they do provide relevant information in terms of understanding their functional mechanism. Studying the environment of particular amino acids can also be a valuable tool for designing new experiments.

2.2. Homology Modelling of the ABC Multidrug Efflux Transporter LmrA

The ATP binding cassette (ABC) multidrug efflux transporter LmrA from *Lactococcus lactis* confers antibiotic resistance to 17 of the 21 most frequently used antibiotics. This membrane pump, formed by 590 amino acids, was the first ABC transporter to be identified in a prokaryotic organism (Veen et al., 1996). ABC transporters consist of four core domains: two TMDs and two NBDs. The TMDs form a tunnel which allows solutes to pass through the membrane. These transmembrane domains usually have six α-helices that contain the substrate binding sites. The NBDs of ABC transporters are highly conserved and contain the ATP-binding domain of the transporter. Multidrug ABC transporters are responsible for the import and export of a great number of substrates. However, neither the 3D-structure of the binding domain nor the mechanism of transport is well understood at present.

The first X-ray structures of ABC transporters (MsbA from *E. coli* and MsbA from *V. cholera)* became available in 2001 and 2003 (Chang et al., 2001; Chang et al., 2003). In the following years many researchers built homology models of the ABC transporter LmrA using the atomic coordinates of these crystallized MsbA structures (Shilling et al., 2005; Pleban et al., 2004). However, the recently determined crystal structures of the ABC transporter Sav1866 from *S. aureus* at 3.0 Å (Dawson et al., 2006; Dawson et al., 2007) have revealed important inaccuracies in the resolved MsbA structure (Chang et al., 2006). Therefore, only homology modelling studies using the recent Sav1866 structure as a template are able to give reliable details.

In the homology study of Federici et al., a three-dimensional model of the TMD for LmrA was generated (Federici et al., 2007). The alignment was carried out between the primary amino acid sequence of Sav1866 and LmrA. The model was validated using Procheck and Verify3D, and the results showed the model to be of good quality: 94% of residues were in the most favoured region of the Ramachandran plot, 6% in the additionally allowed region, and only two residues out of 590 (0.4%) were in the disallowed region.

From their analysis of this model the authors suggest a structural basis for the role of Glu314 in the transport of protons coupled to a known substrate of LmrA. Although LmrA belongs to an ATP-dependent family of transporters it can also use the proton's electrochemical potential to transport drugs (Venter et al., 2003). Federici et al. suggest a mechanism for the proton conduction pathway using the modelled structural environment of Glu314. In the homology model of LmrA a large tunnel is formed by the TMDs, which is exposed to the exterior of the cell. The interior of the tunnel is positively charged and this charge could explain the observed low affinity of LmrA for hydrophobic cationic drugs.

2.3. Transport Mechanism of Bacterial Transporters by MD Calculations

The transport mechanism of bacterial transporters has been studied by classical MD when the crystal structure of bacterial transport is available. Here we report MD studies of two bacterial proteins: the outer-membrane protein (OMP) TolC and the transporter BtuCD. For Gram-negative bacteria the TolC family of proteins are involved in the secretion of toxins, small peptides and drugs. The transport systems in Gram-negative bacteria are more complex and use a three-protein complex rather than a single transport protein. These complexes enable the translocation of drugs across both the inner and outer membranes. Generally, these transport systems consist of an IMP (inner membrane protein) transporter, a membrane fusion protein (MFP), which is anchored to the inner membrane by either a lipid moiety or a single α-helix, and a porin-like OMP.

Two well-studied examples are the AcrAB/TolC (Nikaido et al., 2001) and MexAB/OprM (Poole, 2001) transport systems that confer multidrug resistance in *E. coli* and *Ps. aeruginosa*, respectively. An MD study of the BtuCD transporter is also discussed below. Although this particular ABC transporter is involved in vitamin B12 uptake, these studies increase our understanding of the structure–function relationship of the NTD and NBDs of ABC transporters.

Vaccaro et al. (Vaccaro et al., 2008) performed classical MD calculations for wild-type TolC and the Tyr362Phe/Arg367Ser mutant. The results of these simulations indicated that the periplasmic gate was involved in the conformational changes of TolC, leading from the closed state that corresponds to the X-ray structure to a proposed open state. The authors suggest that the motions of TolC observed in the simulations facilitate the transport of solutes through the tunnel of the transport system.

As regards BtuCD, a 1110-residue protein found in the inner membrane of various Gram-negative bacteria, Oloo et al. (Oloo et al., 2004) and Ivetac et al. (Ivetac et al., 2007) performed MD calculations of this ABC transporter. In the first paper, Oloo et al. (Oloo et al., 2004) presented extensive MD simulation studies of the ATP binding process in *E. coli* BtuCD. They performed several computer simulations to investigate the hypothesis that the unidirectional transmembrane transport of vitamin B12 is a consequence of important conformational changes produced when passing from the weak to the tight ATP binding state. They simulated the transition of the NBDs of BtuCD from a semi-open state, as observed in the crystal structure, to an MgATP-bound closed state.

The results of these simulations show that in the process of closure of the periplasmic gate and opening of the cytoplasmic gate, the transmembrane domain is affected by conformational changes. Oloo et *al.* suggest that these findings on conformational changes associated with MgATP binding to BtuCD are likely to be representative of bacterial importers in general and may be extrapolated to other ABC transporters.

Recently, Ivetac et al. (Ivetac et al., 2007) performed several MD simulations of the BtuCD and BtuCDF system. BtuCDF is formed by the BtuCD system plus the periplasmic binding protein, which sequesters the solute in the periplasm and delivers it to the TMDs of the BtuCD. The authors used multiple MD simulations to explore the dynamic behaviour of the various components of the BtuCDF import complex, in different configurations. Mechanistic implications were suggested from the conformational dynamics observed in the simulations. They found that the binding of ATP constrains the flexibility of the NBDs. However, it seems that the closure of NBDs can only occur after the binding of BtuF to the complex. This is consistent with observations that solute binding is required to trigger ATP-binding/hydrolysis. The simulations of both Oloo et al. (Oloo et al., 2004) and Ivetac et al. (Ivetac et al., 2007) indicate that closure of the NBDs in BtuCDF is asymmetrical. This behaviour is also referred to in "alternating hydrolysis" models (Veen et al., 2000; Senior et al., 1995) and stoichiometric calculations (Tombline et al., 2005).

3. Preventing the Interaction between Drug and Target: A Case Study Involving Fluoroquinolone Resistance

The antibiotic resistance mechanism for preventing interaction between a drug and its target is achieved by chromosomal mutations in genes that encode the protein targets (Martinez and Baquero, 2000). One of the most representative cases of resistance caused by target alterations is the case of fluoroquinolone antibiotic resistance due to DNA gyrase and/or topoisomerase IV alterations (Fàbrega et al., 2008).

In general, the chromosomal-mediated resistance arises as a result of accumulating mutations. In the case of quinolone resistance the chromosomal mutations may be mainly distributed into mutations in genes (*gyrA, gyrB, parC* and *parE*) encoding the GyrA and GyrB subunits of the protein targets (Vila, 2005). The effect of these mutations in the quinolone resistance phenotype may differ between bacterial species. For example, in *Enterobacteriacea* a single mutation in the *gyrA* gene confers low-level quinolone-resistance (ciprofloxacin MIC of 0.125-0-25 mg/L). The acquisition of a second mutation in *parC* is associated with a moderate level of ciprofloxacin resistance (1–4 mg/L). A third mutation, the second in *gyrA*, is associated with a high level of ciprofloxacin resistance (8–64 mg/L), while a fourth amino acid substitution, the second in *parC*, is associated with the highest level of resistance (128 mg/L) (Vila et al., 1996). In addition, another mechanism of resistance, such as the overexpression of (an) efflux pump(s), may modulate the final MIC (Vila, 2005). Therefore, several mutations are needed to produce a high level of quinolone resistance. The most important mutations leading to a quinolone-resistant phenotype in *E. coli* are in the *gyrA* gene, and they correspond mainly to the amino acids Ser83Leu and Asp87Asn.

Here we report a study that sought to investigate the mechanisms of resistance at the atomic level due to these two mutations in the *gyrA* gene of DNA gyrase. In order to be able to explain the relationship between the observed mutations and their corresponding level of quinolone resistance, we used docking calculations to predict the mode of binding of three characteristic quinolone antibiotics. We begin by explaining the general models of quinolone action described in the literature used to rationalize the experimental data. The molecular basis of quinolone resistance is then studied at the atomic level by means of docking calculations of three fluoroquinolones to DNA gyrase.

3.1. Models Describing the Mode of Action of Quinolone Antibiotics

Quinolone drugs are active against type II topoisomerases (such as DNA gyrase or topoisomerase IV) and act by blocking DNA replication and inhibiting synthesis and cell division (Vila, 2005). The mechanism of quinolone inhibition is known to involve the formation of a ternary cleavage complex with the topoisomerase enzyme and DNA (Hiasa et al., 2000). However, although a lot of experimental work has been carried out to identify the mechanism of action of quinolones, the molecular details of their mode of action remain unclear. Different models have appeared to describe the mode of binding of quinolones to DNA gyrase. In the literature, two models, developed by the groups of Maxwell and Shen, are often used to rationalize experimental data about quinolone action. They differ in their selection of the primary target of quinolones in the ternary complex, this being either DNA gyrase (Maxwell's model) or DNA (Shen's model).

In the model of Shen and coworkers (Shen et al., 1985; Shen et al., 1989a; Shen et al., 1989b; Shen et al., 1989c, Shen et al., 1990) it is postulated that quinolones bind to the single-stranded DNA generated by the action of DNA gyrase; this mechanism is proposed on the basis of the observation that norfloxacin does not bind directly to DNA gyrase but to DNA. In addition, the binding affinity to single-stranded DNA is three to five times higher for this drug. Shen also suggested that in addition to the DNA binding affinity of quinolones, the saturation of the binding site could also be achieved by some quinolones, thereby conferring greater inhibitory activity (Morrissey et al., 1996). The binding mode of saturating quinolones in the binding site was described by a stacking model. This model was supported by the finding that the most potent ofloxacin enantiomer allows the closest stacking between quinolone rings (Hayakawa et al., 1986), and also by the observation of pi-pi stacking interactions of planar quinolone rings in nalidixic acid crystals (Achari et al., 1976; Huber et al., 1980).

The concept of quinolone-DNA binding was revised as a consequence of observations of binding modulation by Mg^{2+} ions. Palù et al. (Palù et al., 1992) showed that norfloxacin binds to plasmid DNA in the presence of an appropriate amount of Mg^{2+}. However, no interaction was found by a fluorescence technique, electrophoretic DNA unwinding, or affinity chromatography techniques in the absence of Mg^{2+} (Palù et al., 1992). These observations led the authors to propose a model for the ternary complex in which the Mg^{2+} ion acts as a bridge between the phosphate groups of nucleic acids and the carbonyl and carboxyl moieties of norfloxacin. In this model it is postulated that quinolones form stacking interactions with the bases in a single-stranded region, in contrast to the initial proposition of the Shen model, where stacking is between quinolone molecules. Molecular details of quinolone–DNA interactions were obtained by Siegmund et al., who solved the structure of a DNA duplex with covalently linked nalidixic acid by NMR and restrained torsion angle MD. The resolved structure showed that nalidixic acid adopts a stacked conformation with nucleotide base pairs (Siegmund et al., 2005).

In contrast to the above the model of Maxwell and co-workers (Reece et al., 1991; Maxwell, 1992; Willmott et al., 1993; Maxwell, 1997; Heddle et al., 2000) proposes that DNA gyrase acts as the primary target of quinolones. This model postulates that both DNA gyrase and DNA are required to bind quinolones in a stable form, and is mainly based on the observation that mutations in DNA gyrase that confer quinolone resistance are clustered principally within a small region (between residues 67 and 106 of GyrA in *E. coli*). This region is often referred to as the quinolone resistance-determining region (QRDR). The most common mutations of the QRDR include the Ser83 and the Asp87 of the *gyrA* gene of *E. coli* (Vila et al., 1994). On the basis of this observation it is thought that these two amino acids directly interact with the quinolone drug in the gyrase-quinolone-DNA ternary complex (Reece et al., 1991; Vila et al., 1994; Lu et al., 1999; Barnard et al., 2001), although the exact quinolone binding site has not been determined. As regards the Topo IV target, mutations in ParC were found in the homologous mutational hotspots (Ser80 and Glu84 in ParC) (Khodursky et al., 1995; Kumagai et al., 1996; Vila et al., 1996; Hiasa, 2002). For both topoisomerase targets these hotspots for quinolone resistance are located close to the active site Tyr, of either the GyrA or ParC subunit. In both cases, binding to the enzyme–DNA complex stabilizes DNA strand breaks created by the two topoisomerases forming ternary complexes. Although a similar inhibitory mechanism is expected for the two quinolone targets, DNA gyrase and Topo IV, they show differential affinity for quinolone drugs (Hooper, 2000; Hooper, 2001; Li 2005).

3.2. Study of the Molecular Mechanism of Quinolone Resistance

We have previously used docking calculations to study (Madurga et al. 2008) the bacterial resistance to fluoroquinolones that arises as a result of the most frequent mutations in the *gyrA* gene of the DNA gyrase target protein. As in the model of Maxwell, we select DNA gyrase as the primary target of quinolones. Thus, the surface of the QRDR of GyrA was used in docking calculations to predict, in terms of atomic details, the mode of binding of ciprofloxacin, levofloxacin, and moxifloxacin fluoroquinolones to DNA gyrase. However, quinolones interact with the DNA-DNA gyrase complex rather than with the enzyme alone, so it is necessary to modify the docking procedure in order to examine the effect of DNA on the binding of fluoroquinolones to DNA gyrase. Therefore, hypotheses derived from the model of Shen were also taken into account to model the contribution of DNA in the ternary complex.

With respect to previous calculations for this target, several docking studies have been conducted with either the ATP binding site of the GyrB subunit (Schulz-Gasch et al., 2003; Boehm et al., 2000) or outside the QRDR region of GyrA (Ostrov et al., 2007). However, this is the first docking study with fluoroquinolones binding to the QRDR region of GyrA, and consequently only this study can provide molecular details of the mechanism of quinolone resistance.

3.2.1. Docking Procedure
In this study, docking calculations were used to determine the binding position of ciprofloxacin, levofloxacin and moxifloxacin quinolones (Figure 3.1) to the QRDR region of DNA gyrase. In general, docking programs provide an automated procedure for predicting the interaction of ligands with biomacromolecular targets. They are designed to predict how small molecules, such as substrates or drug candidates, bind to a receptor of known 3D structure. Here, the software package AutoDock3 (Morris et al., 1998) was used to determine the binding position of ciprofloxacin, levofloxacin and moxifloxacin. The structures of the three fluoroquinolone molecules were obtained by means of ab initio calculations using the density functional method (DFT). To model the target used in docking calculations, the X-ray crystal structure of DNA gyrase (N-terminal portion of E. coli gyrA) was used (1ab4 pdb code). Proper charges and atomic fragmental volumes were assigned by use of the Addsol utility of AutoDock. With the aid of AutoDock Tools, four narrow grids were constructed. The potential grid maps were calculated by use of AutoGrid; these enable a rapid energy evaluation in the docking process by pre-calculating atomic affinity potentials for each atom

type in the substrate molecule. The Autotors utility was used to define the rotatable bonds in the ligand. Ten dockings were performed with the Lamarckian Genetic Algorithm.

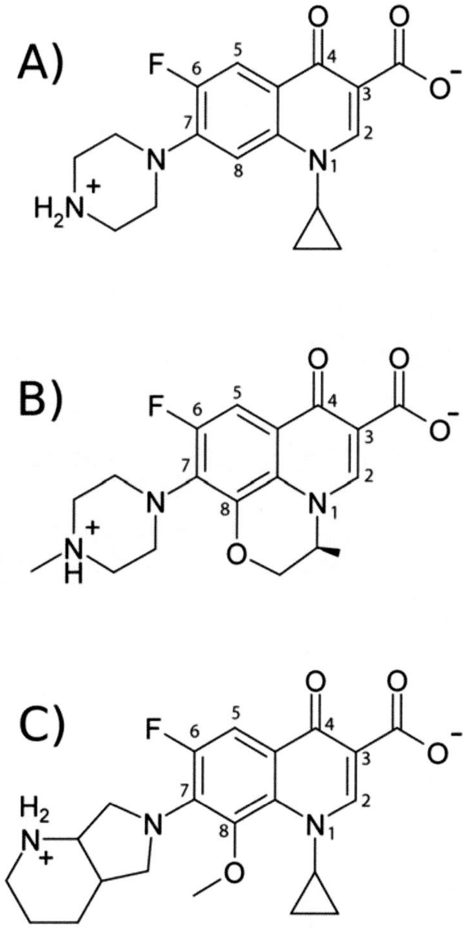

Figure 3.1. Structures of A) ciprofloxacin, B) levofloxacin, and C) moxifloxacin used in docking calculations.

In this docking procedure, the selection of the surface of DNA gyrase, which is proposed to accommodate the ligands, is based on the available information for the residues that are most relevant in achieving the greatest bacterial resistance to fluoroquinolones (Ser83 and Asp87). The potential maps, used to calculate binding free energies to the receptor, are defined in such a way that they contain or are very near these two DNA gyrase residues. In this model the DNA molecule is not present. However, the four overlapping narrow grids used (Figure 3.2) were designed to obtain fluoroquinolone structures oriented perpendicularly to the expected direction of the axes of the DNA. This approach takes into account the effect of DNA in orienting the fluoroquinolones based on the suggested stacking interactions and/or hydrogen bonds with the base pairs of DNA, as referred to in the model of Shen. These docked fluoroquinolones could thus participate in a ternary complex with DNA gyrase and DNA.

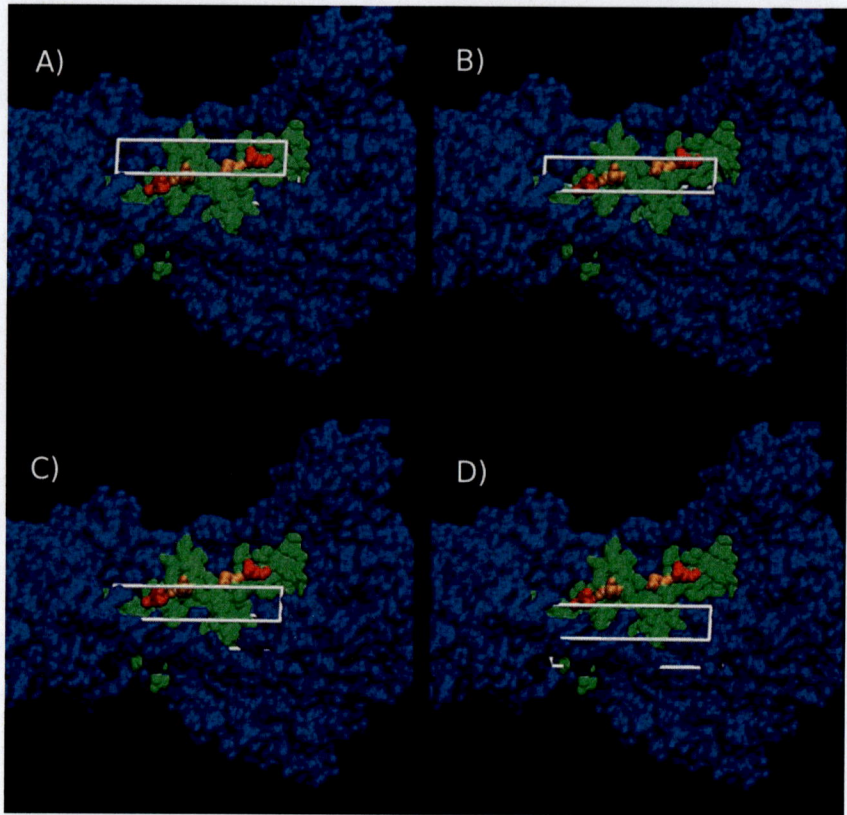

Figure 3.2. The four boxes (A-D) used in the calculations of docking of fluoroquinolones to DNA gyrase. The QRDR of DNA gyrase is represented in green, but Ser83 and Asp87 are shown in orange and red, respectively. Non-QRDR DNA gyrase residues are in blue.

3.2.2. Docking Results

The QRDR region of DNA gyrase was divided into four narrow zones or boxes that could be used in docking calculations to obtain a proposed mode of binding for each one. Thus, the first step of this procedure consists in distinguishing which region of the QRDR is involved in the binding of fluoroquinolones, and then to identify the molecular traits of their mode of action and to explain how point mutations contribute to bacterial resistance to fluoroquinolones.

For each of the four regions of the QRDR a docking calculation was performed with ciprofloxacin, levofloxacin and moxifloxacin. From the analysis of the best interaction docking energy between fluoroquinolones and DNA gyrase, the best structures were obtained for the same box (box C). In addition, similar patterns of binding to DNA gyrase were obtained for the three fluoroquinolones, although slight differences were observed for moxifloxacin (Figure 3.3). The analysis of the interaction pattern for these fluoroquinolones enables us to explain the mechanism associated with the gyrA mutations most commonly found in fluoroquinolone-resistant *E. coli* strains.

A common characteristic observed in the three fluoroquinolones was that their carboxylate group established a salt bridge with the guanidinium group of Arg121. In addition, the positively-charged N atom of the three fluoroquinolones interacted with the carboxylate group of Asp87.

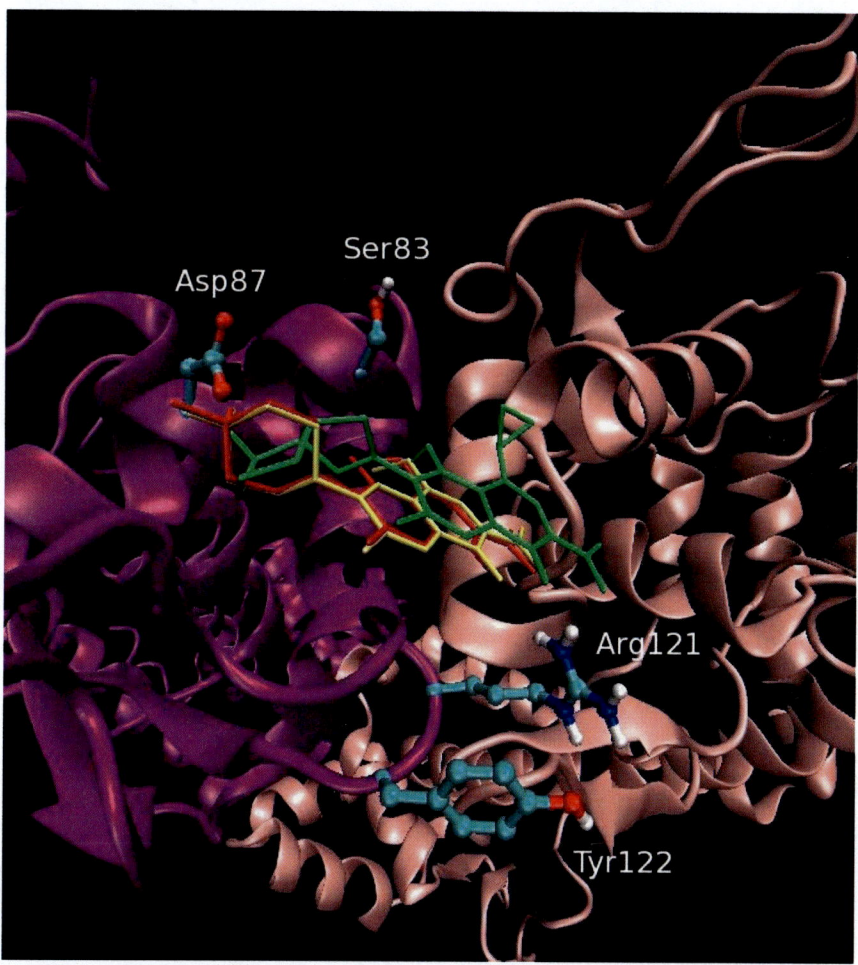

Figure 3.3. The best docked structures for ciprofloxacin (yellow), levofloxacin (red), and moxifloxacin (green) were obtained in Box C. Ser83, Asp87, Arg121, and Tyr122 are also displayed in ball-and-stick representation. The two subunits of DNA gyrase are in ribbon representation.

In contrast, differences were obtained with respect to the interaction with Ser83. For ciprofloxacin and levofloxacin the greatest number of intermolecular contacts was observed for Ser83 with N1 and C8 substituents. For moxifloxacin only a few contacts were observed with these substituents. This difference is due to the fact that the docked structure of moxifloxacin was slightly displaced in relation to the structures of the other two drugs (Fig. 3.3).

3.2.3. Conclusion

From the results of the computational study performed with three representative fluoroquinolones, a binding model for this family of antibiotics to the QRDR of GyrA is proposed. In addition, the analysis of this binding model enables us to understand the resistance mechanism associated with the most commonly found *gyrA* mutations.

In particular, the docking results showed very similar patterns of binding for ciprofloxacin and levofloxacin. It is known that mutation at the amino acid codons for Ser83 and/or Asp87 confers a bacterial resistance mechanism against these two fluoroquinolones. This experimental observation can be attributed to the obtained interactions with Ser83 and Asp87 in the docked structures. First, Asp87 was found to be critical in the binding of these drugs, because it interacts with the positively-charged nitrogen in the fluoroquinolones. Second, Ser83 shows contacts with the N1 and C8 substituents of both quinolones. These contacts can account for the resistance to these fluoroquinolones that is observed when Ser83 is mutated with a residue possessing a side chain which can establish steric hindrance.

For moxifloxacin, the interaction with Asp87 is also critical. However, the Ser83 mutation is tolerated. This tolerance is achieved because this drug can establish better binding to DNA gyrase. Ser83 showed less contact with moxifloxacin than with ciprofloxacin and levofloxacin. Thus, mutation of Ser83 with another residue bearing a larger side chain can produce less steric hindrance with moxifloxacin than with the other two fluoroquinolones.

In addition, the obtained pattern of binding of these fluoroquinolones is also consistent with previous studies which showed that: i) a mutation in the amino acid codon Thr86 (equivalent to Ser83 in E. coli) of GyrA of *Campylobacter jejuni* produces only a slight increase in the minimum inhibitory concentration of moxifloxacin but high increases in resistance to ciprofloxacin and levofloxacin; and ii) a double mutation in the amino acid codons Thr86 and Asp90 (equivalent to Asp87 in E. coli) is required to generate a high level of resistance to moxifloxacin (Ruiz et al., 2005).

Finally, our results show that Arg121 plays a key role in the binding of the antibiotic to GyrA and determines its position in the QRDR of the enzyme. In principle, mutations in the amino acid codon Arg121 could be expected to achieve fluoroquinolone resistance, but this residue has never been found to be mutated. As Arg121 is located next to the active-site tyrosine, we propose that this residue contributes to the activity of DNA gyrase, and consequently Arg121 mutations could be lethal for the microorganism. This hypothesis would explain why this possible escape mechanism suggested by our docking calculations has never been found in nature.

References

Achari, A. and Neidle, S. (1976) Nalidixic acid. *Acta Crystallogr*, B32, 600-602.

Adachi, H., Ohta, T. and Matsuzawa, H. (1991) Site-directed mutants, at position 166, of RTEM-1 beta-lactamase that form a stable acyl-enzyme intermediate with penicillin. *J. Biol. Chem.*, 266, 3186-3191.

Altschul, S.F., Gish, W., Miller, W., Myers, E.W. and Lipman, D.J. (1990) Basic local alignment search tool, *J. Mol. Biol.*, 215, 403-410.

Altschul, S.F., Madden, T.L., Schaffer, A.A., Zhang, J., Zhang, Z., Miller, W. and Lipman, D.J. (1997) Gapped BLAST and PSI-BLAST: a new generation of protein database search programs. *Nucl. Acids Res.*, 25, 3389-3402.

Ambler, R. P., Coulson, A. F. W., Frère, J. M., Ghuysen, J. M., Joris, B., Forsman, M., Levesque, R. C., Tiraby, G. and Waley, S. G. (1991) A standard numbering scheme for the class A beta-lactamases. *Biochem. J.*, 276, 269-272.

Antony, J., Gresh, N., Olsen, L., Hemmingsen, L., Schofield, C. J. and Bauer, R. (2002) Binding of D- and L-captopril inhibitors to metallo-ß-lactamase studied by polarizable molecular mechanics and quantum mechanics. *J. Comput Chem.*, 23, 1281-1296.

Baker, D. and Sali, A. (2001) Protein structure prediction and structural genomics. *Science*, 294, 93-96.

Bambeke, V. F., Balzi, E. and Tulkens, P. M. (2000). Antibiotic efflux pumps. *Biochemical Pharmacol*, 60, 457–70.

Barnard, F.M., and Maxwell, A. (2001) Interaction between DNA Gyrase and Quinolones: Effects of Alanine Mutations at GyrA Subunit Residues Ser83 and Asp87. *Antimicrob. Agents Chemother*, 45, 1994-2000.

Bates, P.A., Kelley, L.A., MacCallum, R.M. and Sternberg, M.J. (2001) Enhancement of protein modeling by human intervention in applying the automatic programs 3D-JIGSAW and 3D-PSSM, *Proteins*, Suppl. 5, 39-46.

Benkovic, S. J. and Hammes-Schiffer, S. (2003) A perspective on enzyme catalysis. *Science*, 301, 1196-1202.

Benning, M.M., Kuo, J.M., Raushel, F.M. and Holden, H.M. (1995) Threedimensional structure of the binuclear metal center of phosphotriesterase. *Biochemistry*, 34, 7973-7978.

Bernstein, N. J. and Pratt, R. F. (1999) On the Importance of a Methyl Group in beta-Lactamase Evolution: Free Energy Profiles and Molecular Modeling. *Biochemistry*, 38, 10499-10510.

Birck, C., Cha, J.Y., Cross, J., Schulze-Briese, C., Meroueh, S.O., Schlegel, H.B., Mobashery, S. and Samama, J.P. (2004) X-ray crystal structure of the acylated beta-lactam sensor domain of BlaR1 from Staphylococcus aureus and the mechanism of receptor activation for signal transduction. *J. Am. Chem. Soc*, 126, 13945-13947.

Blundell, T., Carney, D., Gardner, S., Hayes, F., Howlin, B., Hubbard, T., Overington, J., Singh, D.A., Sibanda, B.L. and Sutcliffe, M. (1988) 18th Sir HansKrebs lecture. Knowledge-based protein modelling and design, *Eur. J. Biochem.*, 172, 513-520.

Boehm, H.J., Boehringer, M., Bur, D., Gmuender, H., Huber, W., Klaus, W., Kostrewa, D., Kuehne, H., Luebbers, T., Meunier-Keller, N. and Mueller, F., (2000) Novel inhibitors of DNA gyrase: 3D structure based biased needle screening, hit validation by biophysical methods, and 3D guided optimization. A promising alternative to random screening, *J. Med. Chem.*, 43, 2664–2674.

Bowie, J.U., Luthy, R. and Eisenberg, D. (1991) A method to identify protein sequences that fold into a known three-dimensional structure. *Science*, 253, 164-170.

Bulychev, A., Massova, I., Miyashita, K. and Mobashery, S. (1997) Nuances of mechanisms and their implications for evolution of the versatile beta-lactamase activity: From biosynthetic enzymes to drug resistance factors. *J. Am. Chem. Soc.*, 119, 7619-7625.

Bush, K. (1998) Metallo-ß-lactamases: a class apart. *Clin. Infect Dis.*, 27, S48-S53.

Bush, K., Jacoby, G. A. and Medeiros, A. A. (1995) A functional classification scheme for ß-lactamases and its correlation with molecular structure. *Antimicrob. Agents Chemother*, 39, 1211-1233.

Carfi, A., Pares, S., Duee, E., Galleni, M., Duez, C., Frère, J.M. and Dideberg, O. (1995) The 3-D structure of a zinc metallo-ß-lactamase from Bacillus cereus reveals a new type of protein fold. *EMBO J.*, 14, 4914-4921.

Castillo, R., Silla, E. and Tuñón, I. (2002) Role of Protein Flexibility in Enzymatic Catalysis: Quantum Mechanical—Molecular Mechanical Study of the Deacylation Reaction in Class A β-Lactamases. *J. Am. Chem. Soc.*, 124, 1809-1816.

Chang, C. and Swaan, P.W. (2006) Computational approaches to modeling drug transporters. *Eur. J. Pharm. Sci.*, 27, 411-424

Chang, G. and Roth, C. B. (2001) RETRACTED: Structure of MsbA from E. coli: A Homolog of the Multidrug Resistance ATP Binding Cassette (ABC) Transporters. *Science*, 293, 1793-1800.

Chang, G. (2003) RETRACTED: Structure of MsbA from Vibrio cholera: A Multidrug Resistance ABC Transporter Homolog in a Closed Conformation. *J. Mol. Biol.*, 330, 419–430.

Chang, G., Roth, C.B., Reyes, C.L. Pornillos, O. and Chen, A.P. (2006) Retraction. *Science*, 314, 1875.

Contreras-Moreira, B. and Bates, P.A. (2002) Domain fishing: a first step in protein comparative modelling. *Bioinformatics*, 18, 1141-1142.

Damblon, C., Raquet, X., Lian, L.Y., Lamotte-Brasseur, J., Fonze, E., Charlier, P., Roberts, G. C. and Frère, J.M. (1996) The catalytic mechanism of beta-lactamases: NMR titration of an active-site lysine residue of the TEM-1 enzyme. *Proc. Natl. Acad. Sci. USA*, 93, 1747-1752.

Dawson, R.J. and Locher, K.P. (2006) Structure of a bacterial multidrug ABC transporter. *Nature*, 443, 180-5.

Dawson, R.J. and Locher, K.P. (2006) Structure of the multidrug ABC transporter Sav1866 from Staphylococcus aureus in complex with AMP-PNP. *FEBS Lett*, 581, 935-8.

de Seny, D., Heinz, U., Wommer, S., Kiefer, J. H., Meyer- Klaucke, W., Galleni, M., Frère, J.M.; Bauer, R. and Adolph, H. W. (2001) Metal ion binding and coordination geometry for wild type and mutants of metallo-ß-lactamase from Bacillus cereus 569/H/9 (BcII). *J. Biol. Chem.*, 276, 45065-45078.

Demain, A. L. and Elander, R. P. (1999) The beta-lactam antibiotics: past, present, and future. *Antonie Van Leeuwenhoek*, 75, 5-19.

Díaz, N., Sordo, T. L., Merz, K. M., Jr. and Suárez, D. (2003) Insights into the acylation mechanism of class A β-Lactamases from molecular dynamics simulations of the TEM-1 enzyme complexed with benzylpenicillin. *J. Am. Chem. Soc*, 125, 672-684.

Díaz, N., Suárez, D. and Merz, K. M., Jr. (2001) Molecular dynamics simulations of the mononuclear zinc-ß-lactamase from Bacillus cereus complexed with benzylpenicillin and a quantum chemical study of the reaction mechanism. *J. Am. Chem. Soc,*. 123, 9867-9879.

Díaz, N., Suárez, D., Sordo, T. L. and Merz, K. M. (2001) Acylation of Class A β-lactamases by Penicillins: A Theoretical Examination of the Role of Serine 130 and the β-lactam Carboxylate Group. *J. Phys. Chem. B*, 105, 11302-11313.

Diederichs, K., Diez, J., Greller, G., Müller, C., Breed, J., Schnell, C., Vonrhein, C., Boos, W. and Welte, W. (2000) Crystal structure of MalK, the ATPase subunit of the trehalose/maltose ABC transporter of the archaeon Thermococcus litoralis. *EMBO J.*, 19, 5951-5961.

Dubus, A., Ledent, P., Lamotte-Brasseur, J. and Frère, J. M. (1996) The roles of residues Tyr150, Glu272, and His314 in class C beta–lactamases. *Proteins: Struct Funct Genet*, 25, 473-485.

Dubus, A., Normark, S., Kania, M. and Page, M. G. P. (1994) The role of tyrosine 150 in catalysis of beta-lactam hydrolysis by AmpC beta-lactamase from Escherichia coli investigated by site-directed mutagenesis. *Biochemistry*, 33, 8577-8586.

Eisenberg, D., Luthy, R. and Bowie, J.U. (1997) VERIFY3D: assessment of protein models with three-dimensional profiles. *Meth. Enzymol.*, 277, 396-404.

Escobar, W. A., Tan, A. K. and Fink, A. L. (1991) Site-directed mutagenesis of beta-lactamase leading to accumulation of a catalytic intermediate. *Biochemistry*, 30, 10783-10787.

Fàbrega, A., Madurga, S., Giralt, E. and Vila, J. (2008) Mechanism of action of and resistance to quinolones. *Microb. Biotech.*, doi:10.1111/j.1751-7915.2008.00063.x.

Federici, L., Woebking, B., Velamakanni, S., Shilling, R.A., Luisi, B. and van Veen, H.W. (2007) New structure model for the ATP-binding cassette multidrug transporter LmrA. *Biochem. Pharmacol.*, 74, 672-678.

Fiser, A. and Sali, A. (2003) Modeller: generation and refinement of homology-based protein structure models. *Methods Enzymol.* 374, 461-91.

Fisher, J. F., Meroueh, S. O. and Mobashery, S. (2005) Bacterial resistance to beta-lactam antibiotics: Compelling opportunism, compelling opportunity. *Chem. Rev.*, 105, 395-424.

Frère, J. M. and Joris, B. (1985) Penicillin-sensitive enzymes in peptidoglycan biosynthesis. *Crit Rev Microbiol*, 11, 299-396.

Frère, J. M. (1995) β-Lactamases and bacterial resistance to antibiotics. *Mol. Microbiol.*, 16, 385-395.

Frère, J. M., Dubus, A., Galleni, M., Matagne, A., Amicosante, G. (1999) Mechanistic diversity of beta-lactamases. *Biochem. Soc. Trans*, 27, 58-63.

Frère, J. M., Ghuysen, J.M. and Iwatsubo, M. (1975) Kinetics of interaction between the exocellular DD-carboxypeptidase-transpeptidase from Streptomyces R61 and beta-lactam antibiotics. A choice of models. *Eur. J. Biochem.*, 57, 343-351.

Fujii, Y., Hata, M., Hoshino, T. and Tsuda, M. (2002) Catalytic Mechanism of Class A β-Lactamase: Role of Lysine 73 and C3-Carboxyl Group of the Substrate Pen G in the Deacylation Step. *J. Phys. Chem. B*, 106, 9687-9695.

Galleni, M., Lamotte-Brasseur, J., Rossolini, G. M., Spencer, J., Dideberg, O. and Frère, J.M. (2001) Standard numbering scheme for class B ß-lactamases. *Antimicrob. Agents Chemother*, 45, 660-663.

Gao, J. and Truhlar, D. G. (2002) Quantum mechanical methods for enzyme kinetics. *Annu Rev. Phys. Chem.*, 53, 467-505.

Gao, J. (1996) Hybrid quantum and molecular mechanical simulations: An alternative avenue to solvent effects in organic chemistry. *Acc. Chem. Res.*, 29, 298-305.

Garau, G., Bebrone, C., Anne, C., Galleni, M., Frère, J.M. and Dideberg, O. (2005) A metallo-ß-lactamase enzyme in action: Crystal structures of the monozinc carbapenemase CphA and its complex with biapenem. *J. Mol. Biol.*, 345, 785-795.

Garcia-Viloca, M., Gao, J., Karplus, M. and Truhlar, D. G. (2004) How enzyme work: Analysis by modern rate theory and computer simulations. *Science*, 303, 186-195.

Gaudet, R. and Wiley, D. C. (2001) Structure of the ABC ATPase domain of human TAP1, the transporter associated with antigen processing. *EMBO J.*, 20, 4964-4972.

Gherman, B.F., Goldberg, S.D., Cornish, V.W. and Friesner, R.A. (2004) Mixed Quantum Mechanical/Molecular Mechanical (QM/MM) Study of the Deacylation Reaction in a Penicillin Binding Protein (PBP) versus in a Class C β-Lactamase. *J. Am. Chem. Soc.*, 126, 7652-7664.

Ghuysen, J.-M. (1991) Serine -lactamases and penicillin-binding proteins. *Annu. Rev. Microbiol.*, 45, 37-67.

Ghuysen, J.-M. (1994) Molecular structures of penicillin-binding proteins and beta-lactamases. *Trends Microbiol*, 2, 372-380.

Ghuysen, J.-M. (1997) Penicillin-binding proteins. Wall peptidoglycan assembly and resistance to penicillin: facts, doubts and hopes. *Int. J. Antimicrob. Agents*, 8, 45-60.

Gibson, R. M., Christensen, H. and Waley, S. G. (1990) Site-directed mutagenesis of beta-lactamase I. Single and double mutants of Glu-166 and Lys-73. *Biochem J.*, 272, 613-619.

Godzik, A. (2003) Structural Bioinformatics: Fold recognition methods (P.E. Bourne and H. Weissig, Editors). Wiley/Liss, Hoboken, NJ.

Golemi, D., Maveyraud, L., Vakulenko, S., Samama, J.P. and Mobashery, S. (2001) Critical involvement of a carbamylated lysine in catalytic function of class D beta-lactamases. *Proc. Natl. Acad. Sci. USA*, 98, 14280-14285.

Golemi-Kotra, D., Cha, J.Y., Meroueh, S.O., Vakulenko, S.B. and Mobashery, S. (2003) Resistance to beta-lactam antibiotics and its mediation by the sensor domain of the transmembrane BlaR signaling pathway in Staphylococcus aureus. *J. Biol. Chem.*, 278,18419-18425.

Greer, J. (1990) Comparative modeling methods: application to the family of the mammalian serine proteases. *Proteins*, 7, 317-334.

Guillaume, G., Vanhove, M., Lamotte-Brasseur, J., Ledent, P., Jamin, M., Joris, B., Frère, J.M. (1997) Site-directed Mutagenesis of Glutamate 166 in Two beta-Lactamases. Kinetic and molecular modeling studies. *J. Biol. Chem.*, 272, 5438-5444.

Hata, M., Fujii, Y., Ishii, M., Hoshino, T. and Tsuda, M. (2000) Catalytic Mechanism of Class A β-lactamase.I. The Role of Glu166 and Ser130 in the Deacylation Reaction. *Chem. Pharm. Bull*, 48, 447-453.

Heddle, J.G., Barnard, F.M., Wentzell, L.M. and Maxwell, A. (2000) The interaction of drugs with DNA gyrase: a model for the molecular basis of quinolone action. *Nucleos Nucleot. Nucl.*, 19, 1249-1264.

Hermann, J. C., Ridder, L., Mulholland, A. J. and Höltje, H.D. (2003) Identification of Glu166 as the General Base in the Acylation Reaction of Class A β-Lactamases through QM/MM Modeling. *J. Am. Chem. Soc*, 125, 9590-9591.

Hermann, J.C., Hensen, C., Ridder, L., Mulholland A. J. and Höe H.D. (2005) Mechanisms of antibiotic resistance: QM/MM modeling of the acylation reaction of a class A ß-lactamase with benzylpenicillin. *J. Am. Chem. Soc*, 127, 4454-4465.

Herzberg, O. and Moult, J. (1991) Penicillin-binding and degrading enzymes. *Curr. Opin. Struct. Biol.*, 1, 946-953.

Hiasa, H. and Shea, M. E. (2000) DNA gyrase-mediated wrapping of the DNA strand is required for the replication fork arrest by the DNA gyrase-quinolone-DNA ternary complex. *J. Biol. Chem.*, 275, 34780–34786.

Hiasa, H. (2002) The Glu-84 of the parC subunit plays critical roles in Both Topoisomerase IV-Quinolone and Topoisomerase IV-DNA interactions. *Biochemistry*, 41, 11779-11785.

Hooper, D.C. (2000) Mechanisms of action and resistance of older and newer fluoroquinolones. *Clin Infect Dis*, 31 (Suppl. 2), S24–8.

Hooper, D.C. (2001) Mechanisms of action of antimicrobials: focus on fluoroquinolones. *Clin. Infect. Dis*, 32 (Suppl. 1), S9–15.

Hopfner, K. P., Karcher, A., Shin, D. S., Craig, L., Arthur, L. M., Carney, J. P. and Tainer, J. A. (2000) Rad50 ATPase: ATP-driven control in DNA double-strand break repair and the ABC-ATPase superfamily. *Cell*, 101,789-800.

Huber, C.P., Gowda, D.S.S. and Acharya, K.R. (1980) Refinement of the structure of nalidixic acid. *Acta Crystallogr*, B36, 497-499.

Hung, L. W., Wang, I. X., Nikaido, K., Liu, P. Q., Ames,G. F. L. and Kim, S. H. (1998) Crystal structure of the ATP-binding subunit of an ABC transporter. *Nature*, 396, 703-707.

Ivetac, A., Campbell, J. D. and Sansom, M. S. P. (2007) Dynamics and function in a bacterial ABC transporter: simulation studies of the BtuCDF system and its components. *Biochemistry*, 46, 2767-2778.

Jabri, E., Carr, M.B., Hausinger, R.P. and Karplus, P.A. (1995) The crystal structure of urease from Klebsiella aerogenes. *Science*, 268, 998-1004.

Jelsch, C., Mourey, L., Masson, J. M. and Samama, J. P. (1993) Crystal structure of Escherichia coli TEM1 beta-lactamase at 1.8 Å. *Proteins*, 16, 364-383.

Joris, B., Ghuysen, J.-M., Dive, G., Renard, A., Dideberg, O., Charlier,P., Frère, J. M., Kelly, J. A., Boyington, J. C., Moews, P. C. and Knox, J. R. (1988) The active-site-serine penicillin-recognizing enzymes as members of the Streptomyces R61 DD-peptidase family. *Biochem J.*, 250, 313-324.

Karpowich, N., Martsinkevich, O., Millen, L., Yuan, Y. R., Dai, P. L., MacVey, K., Thomas, P. J. and Hunt, J. F. (2001) Crystal structures of the MJ1267 ATP binding cassette reveal an induced-fit effect at the ATPase active site of an ABC transporter. *Structure*, 9, 571-586.

Khodursky, A.B., Zechiedrich, E.L. and Cozzarelli, N.R. (1995) Topoisomerase IV is a target of quinolones in Escherichia coli. *Proc. Natl. Acad. Sci. USA*, 92, 11801-11805.

Knott-Hunziker, V., Petursson, S., Waley, S. G., Jaurin, B., Grundstrom, T. (1982) The acyl-enzyme mechanism of beta-lactamase action. The evidence for class C Beta-lactamases. *Biochem. J.*, 207, 315-322.

Knowles, J. R. (1985) Penicillin resistance: The chemistry of ß-lactamase inhibition. *Acc. Chem. Res.*, 18, 97-104.

Knox, J. R., Moews, P. C. and Frère, J. M. (1996) Molecular evolution of bacterial ß-lactam resistance. *Chem. Biol.*, 3, 937-47.

Krauss, M., Gresh, N. and Antony, J. (2003) Binding and hydrolysis of ampicillin in the active site of a zinc lactamase. *J. Phys. Chem. B*, 107, 1215-1229.

Kumagai, Y., Kato, J.I., Hoshino, K., Akasaka, T., Sato, K. and Ikeda, H. (1996) Quinolone-resistant mutants of Escherichia coli DNA Topoisomerase IV parC gene. *Antimicrob. Agents Chemother*, 40, 710-714.

Labia, R. (2004) Plasticity of Class A beta-Lactamases, an Illustration with TEM and SHV Enzymes. Curr Med Chem: *Anti-Infect Agents*, 3, 251-266.

Lagerstedt, J.O., Voss, J.C., Wieslander, A. and Persson, B.L. (2004) Structural modeling of dual-affinity purified Pho84 phosphate transporter. *FEBS Lett.*, 578, 262-268.

Lamotte-Brasseur, J., Wade, R. and Raquet, X. (1999) pKa calculations for class A beta-lactamases: influence of substrate binding. *Protein Sci.*, 8, 404-409.

Laskowski, R.A., MacArthur, M.W., Moss, D.S. and Thornton, J.M. (1993) PROCHECK: a program to check the stereochemical quality of protein structures, *J. Appl. Cryst.*, 26, 283-291.

Li, J., Cross, J.B., Vreven, T., Meroueh, S.O., Mobashery, S. and Schlegel, H. B. (2005) Lysine Carboxylation in Proteins: OXA-10 beta-Lactamase. *Prot. Struct. Funct. Bioinf*, 61, 246-257.

Li, X.Z. (2005) Quinolone resistance in bacteria: emphasis on plasmid-mediated mechanisms. *Int J Antimicrob Agents*, 25, 453–463.

Lietz, E. J., Truher, D. K., Hokenson, M. J. and Fink, A. L. (2000) Lysine-73 is involved in the acylation and deacylation of beta-lactamase. *Biochemistry*, 39, 4971-4981.

Lobkovsky, E., Billings, E. M., Moews, P. C., Rahil, J., Pratt, R. F. and Knox, J. R. (1994) Crystallographic structure of a phosphonate derivate of the enterobacer cloacae P99 cephalosporinase: Mechanistic interpretation of a beta-lactamase transition-state analog. *Biochemistry*, 33, 6762-6772.

Locher, K. P., Lee, A. T. and Rees, D. C. (2002) The E. coli BtuCD Structure: A Framework for ABC Transporter Architecture and Mechanism. *Science*, 296, 1091-1098.

Lomovskaya, O., Warren, M. S., Lee, A., Galazzo, J., Fronko, R., Lee, M., Blais, J., Cho, D., Chamberland, S., Renau, T., Leger, R., Hecker, S., Watkins, W., Hoshino, K., Ishida, H. and Lee, V. J. (2001). Identification and Characterization of Inhibitors of Multidrug Resistance Efflux Pumps in Pseudomonas aeruginosa: Novel Agents for Combination Therapy. *Antimicrob Agents Chemother*, 45, 105-116

Lorimer, G.H., Badger, M.R. and Andrews, J. (1976) Rubisco carboxylation of lysine. *Biochemistry*, 15, 529-536.

Lu, T., Zhao, X. and Drlica, K. (1999) Gatifloxacin activity against quinolone-resistant Gyrase: allele-specific enhancement of bacteriostatic and bactericidal activities by the C-8-methoxy group. *Antimicrob. Agents Chemother*, 43, 2969-2974.

Luthy, R., Bowie, J.U. and Eisenberg, D. (1992) Assessment of protein models with three-dimensional profiles. *Nature*, 356, 83-85.

Madurga, S., Sánchez-Céspedes, J., Belda, I., Vila, J. and Giralt, E. (2008) Binding mechanism of fluoroquinolone to the quinolone resistance-determining region of DNA Gyrase: Towards an understanding of the molecular basis of quinolone resistance. *Chem. Bio. Chem.*, 8, 2081-2086.

Martínez, J. L. and Baquero, F. (2000) Mutation Frequencies and Antibiotic Resistance. *Antimicrob. Agents Chemoth*, 44, 1771–1777.

Massova, I. and Kollman, P. A. (2002) pKa, MM, and QM studies of mechanisms of beta-lactamases and penicillin-binding proteins: acylation step. *J. Comput. Chem*, 23, 1559-1576.

Matagne, A. , Lamotte-Brasseur J. and Frère, J.M. (1998) Catalytic properties of class A beta-lactamases: efficiency and diversity. *Biochem J.*, 330, 581-598.

Maveyraud, L., Golemi, D., Kotra, L.P., Tranier, S., Vakulenko, S., Mobashery, S. and Samama, J.P. (2000) Insights into class D beta-lactamases are revealed by the crystal structure of the OXA10 enzyme from Pseudomonas aeruginosa. *Structure Fold Des*, 8, 1289-1298.

Maxwell, A. (1992) The molecular basis of quinolone action. *J. Antimicrob. Chemother*, 30, 409-414.

Maxwell, A. (1997) DNA gyrase as a drug target. *Trends in Microbiol.*, 5, 102-109.

Meroueh, S. O., Fisher, J. F., Schlegel, H. B. and Mobashery, S. (2005) Ab initio QM/MM study of class A ß-lactamase acylation: Dual participation of Glu166 and Lys73 in a concerted base promotion of Ser70. *J. Am. Chem. Soc.*, 127, 15397-15407.

Minasov, G., Wang, X. and Shoichet, B. K. (2002) An ultrahigh resolution structure of TEM-1 ß-lactamase suggests a role for Glu166 as the general base in acylation. *J. Am. Chem. Soc.*, 124, 5333-40.

Monard, G. and Merz, K. M., Jr. (1999) Combined quantum mechanical/molecular mechanical methodologies applied to biomolecular systems. *Acc. Chem. Res.*, 32, 904-911.

Morollo, A.A., Petsko, G.A. and Ringe, D. (1999) Structure of a Michaelis complex analogue: propionate binds in the substrate carboxylate site of alanine racemase. *Biochemistry*, 38, 3293-3301.

Morris, G., Goodsell, D., Halliday, R., Huey, R., Belew, R. and Olson, A. (1998) Automated docking using a Lamarckian genetic algorithm and an empirical binding free energy function. *J. Comput. Chem.*, 19, 1639-1662.

Morrissey, I., Hoshino, K., Sato, K., Yoshida, A., Hayakawa, I., Bures, M.G. and Shen, L.L. (1996) Mechanism of differential activities of ofloxacin enantiomers. *Antimicrob Agents Chemother*, 40, 1775–1784.

Nikaido, H. and Zgurskaya, H. I. (2001) AcrAB and related multidrug efflux pumps of Escherichia coli. *J. Mol. Microbiol. Biotechnol*, 3, 215–218.

Nukaga, M., Mayama, K., Hujer, A. M., Bonomo, R. A. and Knox, J. R. (2003) Ultrahigh Resolution Structure of a Class A β-Lactamase: On the Mechanism and Specificity of the Extended-spectrum SHV-2 Enzyme. *J. Mol. Biol.*, 328, 289-301.

Oefner, C., D'Arcy, A., Daly, J.J., Gubernator, K., Charnas, R.L., Heinze, I., Hubschwerlen, C. and Winkler, F.K. (1990) Refined crystal structure of beta-lactamase from Citrobacter freundii indicates a mechanism for beta-lactam hydrolysis. *Nature*, 343, 284-288.

Oelschlaeger, P., Schmid, R. D. and Pleiss, J. (2003) Modeling domino effects in enzymes: Molecular basis of the substrate specificity of the bacterial metallo-ß-lactamase IMP-1 and IMP-6. *Biochemistry*, 42, 8945-8956.

Oloo, E.O. and Tieleman, D. P. (2004) Conformational transitions induced by the binding of MgATP to the vitamin B12 ATP-binding cassette (ABC) transporter BtuCD. *J. Biol. Chem.*, 279, 45013-45019.

Olsen, L., Rasmussen, T., Hemmingsen, L. and Ryde, U. (2004) Binding of benzylpenicillin to metallo-ß-lactamase: A QM/MM study. *J. Phys. Chem. B*, 108, 17639-17648.

Orellano, E. G., Girardini, J. E., Cricco, J. A., Ceccarelli, E. A. and Vila, A. J. (1998) Spectroscopic characterization of a binuclear metal site in Bacillus cereus ß-lactamase II. *Biochemistry*, 37, 10173-10180.

Ostrov, D.A., Hernández Prada, J.A., Corsino, P.E., Finton, K.A., Le, N. and Rowe, T. C., (2007) Discovery of Novel DNA Gyrase Inhibitors by High-Throughput Virtual Screening. *Antimicrob Agents Chemother*, 51, 3688–3698.

Page, M. I. (1992) The Chemistry of ß-Lactams; Blackie Academic and Professional: London.

Palù, G., Valisena, S., Ciarrocchi, G., Gatto, B. and Palumbo, M. (1992) Quinolone binding to DNA is mediated by magnesium ions. *Proc. Natl. Acad. Sci. USA*, 89, 9671-9675.

Park, H. and Merz, K. M., Jr. (2005a) Force field design and molecular dynamics simulations of the carbapenem and cephamycinresistant dinuclear zinc metallo-ß-lactamase from Bacteroides fragilis and its complex with a biphenyl tetrazole inhibitor. *J. Med. Chem.*, 48, 1630-1637.

Park, H., Brothers, E. N. and Merz, K. M., Jr. (2005b) Hybrid QM/MM and DFT investigations of the catalytic mechanism and inhibition of the dinuclear zinc metallo-ß-lactamase CcrA from Bacteroides fragilis. *J. Am. Chem. Soc.*, 127, 4232-4241.

Paulsen, I. T., Brown, M. H. and Skurray, R. A. (1996) Proton-dependent multidrug efflux systems. *Microbiol. Reviews*, 60, 575–608.

Paul-Soto, R., Bauer, R., Frère, J.M., Galleni, M., Meyer- Klaucke, W., Nolting, H. F., Rossolini, G. M., de Seny, D., Hernandez-Valladares, M., Zeppenzauer, M. and Adolph, H. W. (1999) Mono- and binuclear Zn2+-ß-lactamase: role of the conserved cysteine in the catalytic mechanism. *J. Biol. Chem.*, 274, 13242-13249.

Peraro, M. D., Vila, A. J. and Carloni, P. (2004) Substrate binding to mononuclear metallo-ß-lactamase from Bacillus cereus. *Proteins*, 54, 412-423.

Pieper, U., Eswar, N., Braberg, H., Madhusudhan, M.S., Davis, F., Stuart, A.C., Mirkovic, N., Rossi, A., Marti-Renom, M.A., Fiser, A., Webb, B., Greenblatt, D., Huang, C., Ferrin, T. and Sali. A. (2004) MODBASE, a database of annotated comparative protein structure models, and associated resources. *Nucleic Acids Res*, 32, D217-D222.

Pitarch, J., Pascual-Ahuir, J.L., Silla, E. and Tuñón, I. J. (2000) A quantum mechanics/molecular mechanics study of the acylation reaction of TEM1 -lactamase and penicillanate. *Chem. Soc., Perkin Trans* 2, 761-767.

Pleban, K., Macchiarulo, A., Costantino, G., Pellicciari, R., Chiba, P. and Ecker, G.F. (2004) Homology model of the multidrug transporter LmrA from Lactococcus lactis. *Bioorg Med. Chem Lett.*, 14, 5823-5826.

Poole, K. (2001) Multidrug efflux pumps and antimicrobial resistance in Pseudomonas aeruginosa and related organisms. *J. Mol. Microbiol. Biotechnol.* 3, 255–264.

Powers, R. A., Caselli, E., Focia, P. J., Prati, F., Shoichet, B. K. (2001) Structures of Ceftazidime and Its Transition-State Analogue in Complex with AmpC β-Lactamase: Implications for Resistance Mutations and Inhibitor Design. *Biochemistry*, 40, 9207-9214.

Powers, R.A. and Shoichet, B. K. (2002) Structure-Based Approach for Binding Site Identification on AmpC β-Lactamase. *J. Med. Chem.*, 45, 3222-3234.

Pratt, R. F. (2002) Functional evolution of the serine-lactamase active site. *J. Chem. Soc-Perkin Trans 2*, 851-861.

Raquet, X., Lounnas, V., Lamotte-Brasseur, J., Frère, J.M. and Wade, R (1997) pKa Calculations for Class A Beta-lactamases: Methodological and Mechanistic Implications. *Biophys. J.*, 73, 2416-2426.

Rasia, R. M. and Vila, A. J. (2002) Exploring the role and the binding affinity of a second zinc equivalent in B. cereus metallo-ß-lactamase. *Biochemistry*, 41, 1853-1860.

Reece, R.J. and Maxwell, A. (1991) DNA gyrase: structure and function. *Crit. Rev. Biochem. Mol. Biol.*, 26, 335-375.

Ruiz, J., Moreno, A., Jimenez de Anta, M. T. and Vila, J. (2005) A double mutation in the gyrA gene is necessary to produce high levels of resistance to moxifloxacin in Campylobacter spp. clinical isolates. *Int. J. Antimicrob Agents*, 25, 542–545.

Sali, A. and Blundell, T.L. (1993) Comparative protein modelling by satisfaction of spatial restraints. *J. Mol. Biol.*, 234, 779-815.

Salsbury, J. F. R., Crowley, M. F. and Brooks, C. L. (2001) III. Modeling of the metallo-ß-lactamase from B.fragilis: Structural and dynamic effects of inhibitor binding. *Proteins*, 44, 448-459.

Schmitt, L., Benabdelhak, H., Blight, M. A., Holland, I.B. and Stubbs, M. T. (2003) Crystal Structure of the Nucleotide-binding Domain of the ABC-transporter Haemolysin B: Identification of a Variable Region Within ABC Helical Domains. *J. Mol. Biol.*, 330, 333-342.

Schulz-Gasch, T. and Stahl, M. (2003) Binding site characteristics in structure-based virtual screening: evaluation of current docking tools. *J. Mol. Model*, 9, 47–57.

Schwede, T., Kopp, J., Guex, N. and Peitsch, M.C. (2003) SWISS-MODEL: an automated protein homology-modeling server. *Nucl. .Acids Res.*, 31, 3381-3385.

Senior, A. E., al-Shawi, M. K. and Urbatsch, I. L. (1995) The catalytic cycle of P-glycoprotein. *FEBS Lett*, 377, 285-9.

Shen, L. L. and Pernet, A. G. (1985) Mechanism of inhibition of DNA gyrase by analogues of nalidixic acid: the target of the drugs is DNA. *Proc. Natl. Acad. Sci. USA*, 82, 307-311.

Shen, L.L., Baranowski, J. and Pernet, A.G. (1989a) Mechanism of inhibition of DNA gyrase by quinolone antibacterials: specificity and cooperativity of drug binding to DNA. *Biochemistry*, 28, 3879-3885.

Shen, L.L., Bures, M.G., Chu, D.T.W. and Plattner, J.J. (1990) Molecular basis of specificity in nucleic acid-drug interactions: Quinolone-DNA interaction: how a small drug molecule acquires high DNA binding affinity and specificity. (B. Pullman ed.). Kluwer Academic Publishers, Dordrecht, The Netherlands.

Shen, L.L., Kohlbrenner, W.E., Weigl, D. and Baranowski, J. (1989b) Mechanism of quinolone inhibition of DNA gyrase. Appearance of unique norfloxacin binding sites in enzyme-DNA complexes. *J. Biol. Chem.*, 264, 2973-2978.

Shen, L.L., Mitscher, L.A., Sharma, P.N., O'Donnell, T.J., Chu, D.W.T., Cooper, C.S., Rosen, T., Pernet, A.G. (1989c) Mechanism of inhibition of DNA gyrase by quinolone antibacterials: a cooperative drug-DNA binding model. *Biochemistry*, 28, 3886-3894.

Shibata, N., Inoue, T., Fukuhara, K., Nagara, Y., Kitagawa, R., Harada, S., Kasai, N., Uemura, K., Kato, K., Yokota, A. and Kai, Y. (1996) Orderly disposition of heterogeneous small subunits in D-ribulose-1,5-bisphosphate carboxylase/oxygenase from spinach. *J. Biol. Chem.*, 271, 26449-26452.

Shilling, R., Federici, L., Walas, F., Venter, H., Velamakanni, S., Woebking, B., Balakrishnan, L., Luisi, B. and van Veen, H.W. (2005) A critical role of a carboxylate in proton conduction by the ATP-binding cassette multidrug transporter LmrA, *FASEB J.*, 19, 1698-1700.

Shim, H. and Raushel, F.M. (2000) Self-assembly of the binuclear metal center of phosphotriesterase. *Biochemistry*, 39,7357-7364.

Siegmund, K., Maheshwary, S., Narayanan, S., Connors, W., Riedrich, M., Printz, M., and Richert. C. (2005) Molecular details of quinolone–DNA interactions: solution structure of an unusually stable DNA duplex with covalently linked nalidixic acid residues and non-covalent complexes derived from it. *Nucleic Acids Res.*, 33, 4838–4848.

Strynadka, N. C. J., Adachi, H., Jensen, S. E., Johns, K., Sielecki, A., Betzel, C., Sutoh, K. and James, M. N. G. (1992) Molecular structure of the acyl-enzyme intermediate in beta-lactam hydrolysis at 1.7 Å resolution. *Nature*, 359, 700-705.

Suárez, D., Díaz, N. and Merz, K. M., Jr. (2002) Molecular dynamics simulations of the dinuclear zinc-ß-lactamase from Bacteroides fragilis complexed with imipenem. *J. Comput .Chem.*, 23, 1587-1600.

Sun, T., Nukaga, M., Mayama, K., Braswell, E.H., Knox, J.R. (2003) Comparison of ß-lactamases of classes A and D: 1.5-Å crystallographic structure of the class D OXA-1 oxacillinase. *Prot. Sci.*, 12, 82-91.

Swarén, P., Maveyraud, L., Guillet, V., Masson, J. M., Mourey, L. and Samama, J. M. (1995) Electrostatic analysis of TEM1 beta-lactamase: effect of substrate binding, steep potential gradients and consequences of site-directed mutations. *Structure*, 3, 603-613.

Thoden, J.B., Phillips, G.N., Jr., Neal, T.M., Raushel, F.M. and Holden, H.M. (2001) Molecular structure of dihydroorotase: a paradigm for catalysis through the use of a binuclear metal center. *Biochemistry*, 40, 6989-6997.

Tombline, G., Muharemagic, A., White, L. B. and Senior, A. E. (2005) Involvement of the "occluded nucleotide conformation" of P-glycoprotein in the catalytic pathway. *Biochemistry*, 44, 12879-12886.

Vaccaro, L., Scott, K.A. and Sansom, M.S.P. (2008) Gating at both ends and breathing in the middle: conformational dynamics of TolC. *Biophys. J. BioFAST*, doi:10.1529/biophysj.108.136028

Valladares, H. M., Felici, A., Weber, G., Adolph, H. W., Zeppezauer, M., Rossolini, G. M., Amicosante, G., Frere, J.M., Galleni, M. (1997) Zn(II) dependence of the Aeromonas hydrophila AE036 metallo-ß-lactamase activity and stability. *Biochemistry*, 36, 11534-11541.

van Veen, H. W., Margolles, A., Muller, M., Higgins, C. F. and Konings, W. N. (2000) The homodimeric ATP-binding cassette transporter LmrA mediates multidrug transport by an alternating two-site (two-cylinder engine) mechanism. *EMBO J.*, 19, 2503-14.

van Veen, H. W., Venema, K., Bolhuis, H., Oussenko, I., Kok, J., Poolman, B., Driessen, A. J. and Konings, W. N. (1996) Multidrug resistance mediated by a bacterial homolog of the human multidrug transporter MDR1. *Proc. Natl. Acad. Sci. USA*, 93, 10668–10672.

Venter, H., Shilling, R. A., Velamakanni, S., Balakrishnan, L., and van Veen, H. W. (2003) An ABC transporter with a secondary-active multidrug translocator domain. *Nature*, 426, 866–870

Vila, J. (2005) Fluoroquinolone Resistance. In Frontiers in Antimicrobial Resístanse: a Tribute to Stuart B. Levy. D.G. White, M.N. Alekshun and P. F. McDermott. (eds). Washington D.C.: ASM Press, 41-52.

Vila, J., Ruiz, J., Goñi, P. and Jiménez de Anta, M.T. (1996) Detection of mutations in parC in quinolone-resistant clinical isolates of Escherichia coli. *Antimicrob. Agents Chemother*, 40, 491-493.

Vila, J., Ruiz, J., Marco, F., Barceló, A., Goñi, P., Giralt, E. and Jiménez de Anta, M.T. (1994) Association between double mutation in gyrA gene of ciprofloxacin-resistant clinical isolates of Escherichia coli and MICs. *Antimicrob. Agents Chemother*, 38, 2477-2479.

Vriend, G. (1990) WHAT IF: a molecular modeling and drug design program. *J. Mol. Graph*, 8, 52-56.

Walsh, C. (2000) Molecular mechanisms that confer antibacterial drug resistance. *Nature*, 406, 775-781.

Walsh, T. R., Gamblin, S. J., Emery, D. C., MacGowan, A. P. and Bennett, B. (1996) Enzyme kinetics and biochemical analysis of ImiS, the metallo-ß-lactamase from Aeromonas sobria 163a. *J. Antimicrob. Chemother*, 37, 423-431.

Wang, C. and Guo, H. (2007) Inhibitor binding by metallo-ß-lactamase IMP-1 from Pseudomonas aeruginosa: quantum mechanical/molecular mechanical simulations. *J. Phys. Chem. B*, 111, 9986-92

Warshel, A. and Levitt, M. (1976) Theoretical Studies of Enzymatic Reactions: Dielectric Electrostatic and Steric Stabilization of the Carbonium Ion in the Reaction of Lysozyme. *J. Mol. Biol.*, 103, 227-249.

Warshel, A. (1991). *Computer Modeling of Chemical Reactions in Enzymes and Solutions*. Wiley: New York.

Warshel, A. (2003) Computer simulations of enzyme catalysis: methods, progress, and insights. *Annu. Rev. Biophys. Biomol. Struct*, 32, 425-443.

Waxman, D. J. and Strominger, J. L. (1983) Penicillin-binding proteins and the mechanism of action of beta-lactam antibiotics. *Annu. Rev. Biochem*, 52, 825-869.

Wilkin, J. M., Jamin, M., Damblon, C., Zhao, G. H., Joris, B., Duez, C. and Frère, J. M. (1993) The mechanism of action of DD-peptidases: the role of tyrosine-159 in the Streptomyces R61 DD-peptidase. *Biochem J.*, 291, 537-544.

Willmott, C.J.R. and Maxwell, A. (1993) A single point mutation in the DNA gyrase A protein greatly reduces binding of fluoroquinolones to the gyrase-DNA complex. *Antimicrob Agents Chemother*, 37, 126-127.

Wommer, S., Rival, S., Heinz, U., Galleni, M., Frère, J.M., Franceschini, N., Amicosante, G., Rasmussen, B. A., Bauer, R. and Adolph, H. W. (2002) Substrate-activated zinc binding of metallo-ß-lactamases. *J. Biol. Chem.*, 277, 24142-24147.

Wright, G.D. (2005) Bacterial resistance to antibiotics: Enzymatic degradation and modification. *Adv. Drug Deliv. Rev.*, 57, 1451-1470.

Xu, D., Xie, D. and Guo, H. (2006) Catalytic mechanism of class B2 metallo-β-lactamase. *J. Bio. Chem.*, 281, 8740-7.

Yuan, Y. R., Blecker, S., Martsinkevich, O., Millen, L., Thomas, P. J. and Hunt, J. F. (2001) The Crystal Structure of the MJ0796 ATP-binding Cassette. Implicatins for the structural consequences of ATP hydrolysis in the active site of an ABC transporter. *J. Biol. Chem.*, 276, 32313-32321.

In: Antibiotic Resistance: …
Editors: Adriel R. Bonilla and Kaden P. Muniz

ISBN: 978-1-60741-623-4
©2009 Nova Science Publishers, Inc.

Chapter IX

"Molecules into systems
To study life, one must take organisms apart and examine their components; to
understand life, one must put the pieces back together. The hallmarks of life are
properties, not of individual molecules but of large organized ensembles; each is a
dynamic pattern deployed in space and time on a scale orders of magnitude above the
molecular. It takes a whole cell to turn nutrients and energy into biological building
blocks, to persist over time, to reproduce, develop and evolve. When they become part of
a cellular system, molecules operate under social control; reactions come to have
location, direction, timing and function. One might describe a cell biologist as a
biochemist who remembers what the question was."

Gleanings of a chemiosmotic eye
Franklin M. Harold BioEssays 23:848±855

Energetics of MDR Microbial Cells

Waché Yves
Laboratoire GPMA,
Université de Bourgogne/AgroSup Dijon, 1, esplanade Erasme, 21000 Dijon, France

Abstract

Multidrug efflux pumps are important in microbial resistance to antibiotics. The energetics of some systems has been characterised in vitro but the impact on whole cell energetics is less studied. In this chapter, after the rapid presentation of the different MDR efflux families, the energetics of some MDR transporters will be described. The impact of these transporters on cell energetics is discussed and the difficulties in studying MDR efflux energetics in whole cell systems will be presented with a description of available techniques. The importance of this field of investigation will be demonstrated with an example of a microbial global strategy to resist to a cationic compound.

Introduction

Comparable to the struggle against water followed in places prone to flooding, cells resist against the invasion of drugs by consolidating their envelope and activating pumps to force drugs out. In conditions of exposure to drugs, the acquisition by cells of an efficient pumping system will confer an advantage by decreasing the intracellular concentration of toxic compounds and thus increasing cell resistance. Many of these pumping systems are unspecific and able to catalyse the transport of a large amount of compounds that are not obviously structurally related. They are called Multi-Drug Efflux Systems/Transporters or Multi-Drug Transporters and they confer to cells a Multi-Drug Resistance (MDR). Many MDR Transporters have been identified both in eukaryotic and prokaryotic cells. They are important to help organisms to resist various chemical stresses but, as a consequence, they enable pathogen or tumor-cells to resist drug therapies. Due to this reason, they are the subject of a fantastic number of studies in the fields of cancer, parasitism and microbial infections. Different classes of MDR Transporters have been identified with a dominant role of ABC-transporters in eukaryotic cells [31] and many secondary transporters in prokaryotic cells (See for instance Paulsen et al [20] or Zgurskaya [37] for reviews) although the role of ATP-dependent transporters in bacteria might be underestimated (16). Some transporters are well conserved between species as, for instance, the P-glycoprotein which is the subject of many studies in tumor cells, in *P. falcyparum* and in *Lactococcus lactis* and is exchangeable between prokaryotic and eukaryotic cells [5]. In all MDR Transporters systems, energy is an important factor and although some efflux mechanisms have been well studied, the impact of the MDR Transporter activity on the global energetic state of cells has been only slightly addressed. The goal of this chapter is to highlight the problems of energy that multi-drug resistant cells can face and show the technical problems that arise when studying this topic.

After a rapid overview of the various families of MDR Transporters, the bases of energetic transport will be given based on some MDR examples which are well documented from an energetic point of view. Then, the energetic perturbation caused by stress resistance and in particular by MDR Efflux will be presented followed by a discussion on the problems related to the evaluation of membrane energetic.

Different Groups of MDR Transporters

Several groups of MDR Transporters have been identified with various mechanisms and energy sources. They have been reviewed many times (see for instance [5, 8, 20, 37] and other reviews cited in the text).

One group, the ATP-Binding Cassette (ABC) superfamily, derives its energy from ATP hydrolysis. These transporters contain four main domains: two transmembrane domains which form a pathway across the membrane for solutes, and two highly conserved nucleotide-binding sites located in the cytoplasmic side. In these domains the ATP hydrolysis, which is coupled to substrate translocation, takes place. ABC transporters play apparently an important role in MDR in eukaryotic cells [31] whereas in bacteria, their role in resistance is usually considered as low (except in *Enterococcus faecalis* [10]). The human

MDR1 has been well characterised and in bacteria, the better characterised example is its lactococcal counterpart, LmrA [35].

The other groups take the energy for transport from the protonmotive force (see figure 1 for the principle). The most studied transporters are from the Major-Facilitator (MF) [12, 15, 27] and the Resistance-Nodulation-cell Division (RND) [19]. Other groups have been characterised such as the small multidrug Resistance family [3], and the newly discovered Multidrug And Toxic Compound Extrusion (MATE) family [14] etc. (see Paulsen et al [20] for the different families). For Gram negative cells, systems often include accessory components enabling drug efflux through the outer membrane (see for instance Andersen et al. [2] and Zgurskaya et al. [39]). These auxiliary proteins belong to the membrane fusion protein (MFP) and outer membrane factor (OMF) families and apparently enable the efflux of drugs across the outer membrane permeability barrier [20].

There are some common features between all known MDR transporters. The first surprising point is the ability of most MDR transporters to transport structurally unrelated substrates. Although some bacterial transporters transport mainly cationic substrates, gram negative transporters can also transport neutral or anionic compounds. Usually, these compounds have in common a hydrophobic domain but some hydrophilic substrates are also transported [37]. The fact that several MDR transport substrates are hydrophobic or possess a delocalised charge and partition therefore in the membrane phase has oriented investigations to the excretion of compounds present in the membrane bilayer. Work with diphenyl hexatriene derivatives (described in the part on energetic evaluation and in Figure 3) have shown for some MDR that substrates of MDR were excreted from the inner leaflet of the membrane (described in Bolhuis et al [4, 5]). However, for other transporters (RND family) the possible substrate binding site might be located in the cytoplasm [37]. The excretion of compounds located in two different compartments is also a possibility as some MDR transporters have at least two drug binding sites (as for instance LmrP, [4] and MsbA [29]). Eventually, the high diversity of compounds that can be transported by MDR can only be explained at a molecular level by structural studies and first results in this field are discussed in Stavrovskaya and Stromskaya [31].

Energy of Transports

As for the evacuation of water in polders in which energy-consuming mills are used, any system favouring the passage of a compound from a lower- to a higher-concentration compartment requires energy. An overview of the possibilities is presented in Figure 1. To give energy to the efflux of a drug against the gradient (A/), transporters can use the energy of a phosphate bond (B/ primary transporters such as ATP Binding Cassette transporters) or the energy of membrane gradients (C/ secondary transporter). In this latter case, the energy comes from a co-catalysed transport of a compound in the way of its gradient. For instance, H^+ can be transported from outside the cell in the way of the proton chemical gradient [1], or a cation can be transported from the outside [2] or an anion from the inside [3], both in the way of the electrical gradient.

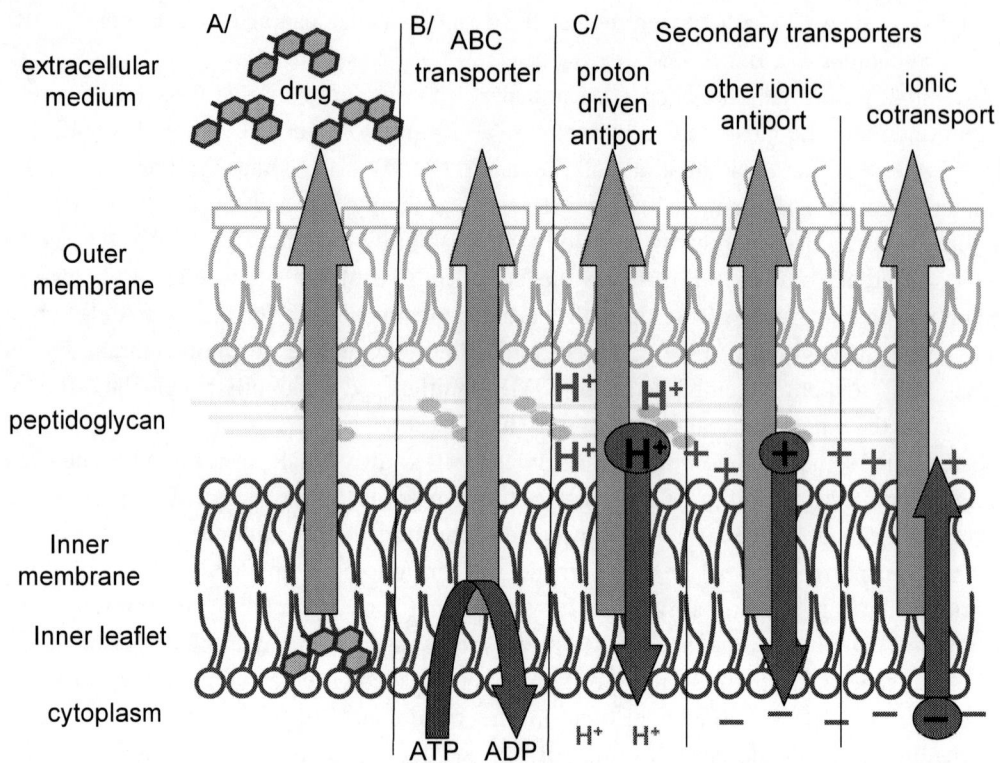

Figure 1. Overview of the possibilities of transport energisation. To give energy to the efflux of a drug against the gradient (A/), transporters can use the energy of a phosphate bond (B/ primary transporters such as ATP Binding Cassette transporters) or the energy of membrane gradients (C/ secondary transporter). In this latter case, the energy comes from a co-catalysed transport of a compound in the way of its gradient. For instance, H^+ can be transported from outside cell in the way of the proton chemical gradient (1), or a cation can be transported from the outside (2) or an anion from the inside (3), both in the way of the electrical gradient.

Some MDR transports have been studied in depth especially in cell free systems. Even in proteoliposomes this investigation is difficult due to the highly lipophilic character of the MDR substrates. They have a high affinity for membranes to such an extent that they go back to the membrane immediately after transport and may even diffuse back across membranes into the origin compartment. To overcome this problem, receptor vesicles can be used. Some secondary transporter mechanisms are presented here from an energetics point of view.

Mechanism of LmrP

The efflux of drug by *Lactococcus lactis* has been studied quite in depth and results are reviewed in Poelarends et al [22]. Actually, investigations have concerned two transporters of this species, the p-glycoprotein primary transporter LmrA and the secondary transporter LmrP, showing a lot of similarities between these two pumps. Experiments have been made with both intact cells and inside-out membrane vesicles. From these results, it has been shown that drug extrusion occurs from the membrane rather than from the cytoplasm [4].

BCECF-AM is excreted from LmrP-producing cells prior to hydrolysis into the fluorescent cellular indicator BCECF by intracellular esterases. Moreover, TMA-DPH is excreted when it is in the inner leaflet of the membrane as shown with the experiment with intact cells and inside out membrane vesicles.

The energetics of transport has also been studied for LmrP and the extrusion of cationic drugs has been shown to be driven by both the membrane potential and the transmembrane proton gradient. The transport of a drug compound involves nH^+ with $n \geq 2$. Without protonmotive force, the protein can also facilitate the diffusion of drugs (in the gradient direction) [17].

Mechanism of AcrAB

As mentioned above, gram negative efflux pumps are usually multicomponents systems that can transport drugs through both membranes thanks to accessory proteins. An interesting work has been carried out on the transport catalysed by AcrAB by using reconstitution of this system in proteoliposomes [38]. Despite the technical problems encountered for investigation, the authors showed that in the presence of a proton chemical gradient, AcrB catalysed the efflux of fluorescent phospholipids however, they could not observe whether non-fluorescent phospholipids were also transported or not, as it has been shown for the mammalian multidrug transporter Mrp1 [11]. Known substrates of AcrAB inhibited this phospholipids transport and it was shown that drug transported by AcrB was accompanied by proton flux.

In proteoliposomes, the kinetic and extent of the efflux depended on ΔpH. The authors showed that the AcrA component of the system was implied in interaction/fusion between membranes and that its localisation depended on ΔpH. With a high proton gradient, AcrA could also cause a slow transport of fluorescent lipids.

Due to the great diversity of compounds that can be transported by AcrAB, a question arises on the effect of the transport on the membrane electrical gradient. These compounds are cationic but also neutral or anionic. Therefore, if the transport involves a proton antiport, it will have a different electrogenic effect depending on the charge of the transported compound.

Na+ Based Multidrug and Toxic Compound Extrusion

Whereas the first families of protonmotive force-based multidrug efflux pumps discovered used the energy of the transport of protons to excrete drugs, the latest secondary transporter MDR family may use the energy of another cation: Na^+. Depending on the medium pH (especially for alkaliphiles [30]) or on the temperature (at high temperature the proton permeation is too high and much higher than the Na^+ permeation), a sodium protonmotive force can be used as cell energy. This way of secondary energisation is particularly used for the MATE family transporters [14].

Energetic Cost (Consequence) of the Transport to Cells

Whatever way transports are energised, they may constitute an important energetic cost for cells. This might not be detectable for energy-rich eukaryotic cells but may play a more significant role for bacteria for which energy is dependent on the level of substrate and addition of glucose in the reaction buffer results in a significant and immediate increase in energy [24]. To give an idea of the relationship between the amount of transported ions and the membrane potential, one can refer to the calculation presented by Schechter [28] in his chapter on ion diffusion and membrane potential. Given a bacterial cell, assimilated to a sphere of one micrometer of radius with an intracellular charge concentration of about 300 mM (the equivalent of 1.2×10^{-10} coulombs). The experimental determination of the membrane potential gives a value of maximum 200 mV which corresponds to a charge amount transferred across the membrane of 2.5×10^{-14} coulombs, which is negligible compared to the initial charge concentration (0.02%). This suggests that only a small perturbation of transport can change in an important way the extent of the membrane potential.

The chemical proton gradient across membranes increases with decreasing pHs (Figure 2). At low pHs, as protons can diffuse across membranes, maintaining a stable intracellular pH is energy consuming for cells. If in addition they have to extrude drugs using the energy of protons coming into the cell, the energetic cost may be too high and the resistance to acidity declines.

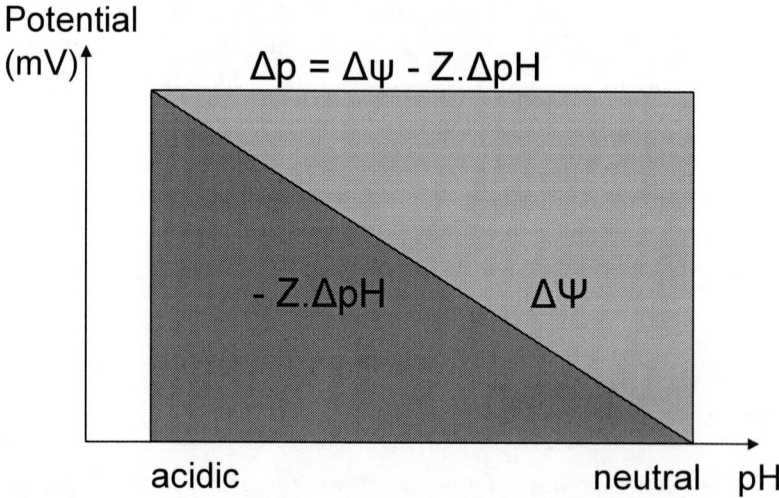

Figure 2. Participation of the electrical potential ($\Delta\psi$) and of the chemical proton gradient (- $Z.\Delta pH^*$) in the global protonmotive force (Δp) depending on the pH for an acidophilic cell. In the physiological range, the global protonmotive force is more or less stable but at acidic pH, the contribution of the difference between the intra- and extra-cellular pH is high whereas, at near neutral pH, when the difference between the intra- and extra-cellular pH is low, the membrane electrical potential is high.*where Z is the conventional factor 2.303 RT/F, which is around 59 at 25°C, when the potentials are expressed in mV.

For instance, the growth of lactococci on lactose is stopped around pH 4.5 due to inhibition by the presence of protons inside cell [36]. This means that, at this pH, the whole cell energy is not sufficient to extrude all the protons diffusing across the membrane. It is therefore very likely that another energy requirement to extrude drug at the expanse of proton entry will cause the energy collapse earlier at a higher pH. However, the membrane proton conductance decreases normally at low pH and this might be stimulated by MDR response but also, this change in proton conductance can be inhibited by the presence of drugs (24). We have observed such a decrease in the acidity resistance for *Escherichia coli* cells expressing an extra MDR system (unpublished data) and this has also been observed by other authors for various bacteria.

Such a phenomenon of hypersensitivity to acidic pH for MDR cells might not be observed for eukaryotic cells which use mainly ATPases and are less subject to de-energisation by sugar depletion. However, the activation of many transporters can result in (and be accompanied by) a perturbation of membrane energetics and ion transports. The group of Roepe has focalised on the relationship between p-glycoprotein MDR expression, drug accumulation and the perturbation of membrane energetics and transport. Although the evaluation of these parameters is not easy (as discussed later), they found that cells overexpressing MDR1 had higher intracellular pH and lower membrane potential and that these perturbation were related to the level of MDR protein expression [25, 32]. Interestingly, they showed that a higher intracellular pH could account for much of the measured drug resistance and that membrane depolarisation could also confer mild drug resistance. They confirmed the relationship between MDR expression and perturbation of energetics and ion transport in a study with huMDR1 expressed in yeast (34) and, together with data obtained on *Plasmodium falcyparum*, this led this group to discuss whether the role of MDR transporters in resistance was not overemphasised and of the importance of ion exchange in this resistance [25]. Beside the modification of diffusion or transport of drugs across the membrane, the intracellular pH of tumor cells is also important for the binding of drugs onto their target which is often based on an acid base interaction. A perturbation of the intracellular pH could thus perturb the distribution of the drug inside the cell, decreasing its efficiency and the more alkaline intracellular compartment of MDR cells could have an impact on drug efficiency [23].

Modification of the Way Energy Is Kept Inside the Cell as a Response to Stress

Beside the fact that the efflux of drug is energy consuming, some cells can adapt the way they keep their energy as a stress response. For instance, *Listeria monocytogenes* responds to acidic stresses through the Acid Tolerance Response (ATR). This response involves several physiological aspects and, interestingly, an energy strategy which is efficient to decrease the sensitivity to the cationic bacteriocin nisin [6]. These authors have observed that ATR+ cells had an intracellular pH lower than ATR- cells and they evaluated their electrical potential as drastically reduced. As a result, ATR+ cells had a very low protonmotive force. However, the overall cell energy was maintained under the form of ATP as the ATP pool was significantly increased for ATR+ cells. Cells could take advantage of this energetic organisation in the presence of antimicrobial cationic compounds. Cationic compounds are attracted by cells possessing a membrane electrical potential (inside negative). After contact, the hydrophobic part of nisin enters membrane forming pores. ATR+ cells that have a decreased membrane potential are thus less sensitive to nisin.

In the case of antibiotics, it has been shown that the presence of MreA, a bifunctional flavokinase/(flavin adenine dinucleotide (FAD) synthetase, which convert riboflavin to flavin mononucleotide (FMN) and FMN to FAD, respectively, results in an increased unspecific resistance to drugs [9]. Although the mechanisms have not yet been elucidated, this resistance could be related to a higher proton transport, giving more energy to the secondary MDR Transporter of the cells and thereby, more efficiency.

Other examples could be given and it is likely that many stress responses involve energetic responses but, as energetic of whole cells is not easy to evaluate, this field of investigation is still rather unexplored.

Energetic Evaluation in Whole Cells

Although the membrane energetic of great size cells can be evaluated through the use of microelectrodes, investigation in small microbial cells requires indirect ways. Many techniques are based on the partition of specific compounds between outside cells and membranes or inside cells. They can bring about interesting data on cells or cell compartments energetic. However, most of them are inadequate for the study of MDR Efflux as the probes used possess an affinity for membranes and, as a result, they are very likely to be themselves the substrate of these pumps. In some cases, the determination of the wanted data is possible but the cross effect is the induction of a cellular response to the presence of drugs (the investigated parameter can only be approached in condition of exposure to drugs), and in other cases, the response modifies the result and we obtain only a bias' response. In this part, the most popular techniques are listed and their use for MDR Efflux studies is discussed. The principles of many techniques mentioned here are described in Cao-Hoang et al [7] and other references are given in the text.

Membrane Physical State

Some physical parameters of the membranes are importantly related to energetic parameters. For instance, the membrane potential depends on the capability of charged compounds to cross the membrane. This diffusion may be related to membrane integrity which depends on membrane structure and fluidity.

Membrane permeability to protons depends on the medium temperature and pH and may be a parameter modified in certain types of multi-drug resistance [24, 33]. It can be evaluated by immerging cells into a liquid rich in protons and monitoring the evolution of their concentration. This technique does utilise only protons as probes and, as it concerns the instantaneous evolution of the proton concentration, it seems adequate for use in the study of MDR Efflux.

Membrane integrity is usually determined by observing the colouration of cells by fluorescent probes such as NPN for the outer membrane and propidium iodide for the inner membrane. If these probes do not cross membranes of living organisms, it is possible that they will not interfere with MDR Transporters, however, as for all fluorescent probes, this point should be checked. However, NPN is known to accumulate more in non-MDR cells [18].

Membrane fluidity can also be evaluated with fluorescent probes that localise inside membranes. There are different types of probes such as fluorochromes of the diphenyl hexatriene (DPH) family for which the fluorescence anisotropy is determined or other probes like laurdan which respond to the fluidity and polarity of the medium by a spectral shift in the emitted fluorescence. Both types of probes are very lipophilic although they may contain a charge. Actually, the presence of a charge let the probe anchored to the polar head part of the membrane phospholipids (Figure 3). However, this polar anchor does not prevent the passage of the probe from the outer to the inner leaflet of the membrane and thus, to the region concerned by the multi-drug efflux. The DPH-related probes have been studied as substrates of the transporters of *Lactococcus lactis*, the ABC-transporter LmrA and the proton motive force-driven LmrP depending on the presence of a charged group [5]. Interestingly, hydrophobic and neutral components of the DPH family (DPH and DMA-DPH) were not extruded by LmrA and LmrP whereas amphiphilic compounds were extruded if they were positively charged (TMA(P)-DPH).

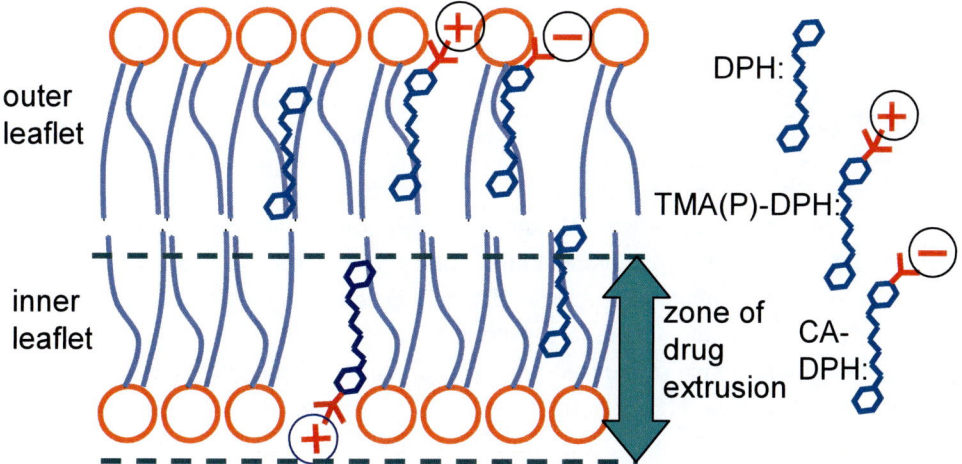

Figure 3. Localisation of DPH-derived compounds in the membrane and extrusion by LmrA and LmrP. Only the compounds located in the inner leaflet « zone of drug extrusion » are transported but not DPH, which is more in the hydrophobic core of the membrane, or probes located in the outer leaflet of the membrane. Polar parts are represented in red and apolar in blue.

The negatively charged amphiphilic CA–DPH was not extruded. These observations were used to understand how LmrA and LmrP work but they have also brought about interesting results on the localisation of DPH related compounds in the membrane. Kaiser and

London [13] and Pebay-Peroula et al. [21] have already studied the location of these compounds in a model membrane, observing that the presence of a charged group anchoring the compound to the polar head layer of the membrane modified only slightly the position of the diphenyl hexatriene part in the membrane, with DPH being slightly more in the hydrophobic core of the membrane.

However, the study by Bolhuis et al. [4] brings indirectly information on the localisation in regard to the inner or outer leaflet of the membrane. Cationic DPH derived compounds were extruded by these MDR Transporters whereas the anionic CA-DPH was not. The authors suggest that the negative charge could prevent this compound from a localisation in the inner leaflet of the membrane in presence of a membrane potential (interior negative). From these results with a cationic probe being anchored in both leaflets of the membrane and being extruded by LmrA and P and likely by other MDR Transporters, and an anionic probe in the outer leaflet and not extruded, it is possible to choose the latter probe accounting only for the outer leaflet fluidity and thus not being extruded (at least by LmrA and P) and DPH, giving information for a deeper localisation in the membrane and not being extruded by this system. Other techniques may be used for the study of membrane fluidity for instance, by introducing spin-labelled nitroxide radicals in the membrane (ESR) [28]. Some bias can avoid MDR Efflux problems by extracting membranes constituents and evaluating membrane fluidity by the fluorescence techniques mentioned above or by Fourier Transformed Infra Red spectroscopy. Eventually, other techniques for the determination of diffusion of a compound in a membrane can be used like FRAP (Fluorescence Recovery After Photobleaching) and FCS (Fluorescence Correlation Spectroscopy), but once again, the use of probes having an affinity for membranes suggest that these compounds are very likely substrates of MDR Efflux.

Membrane Energetical State

Determination of Intracellular pH

In an environment of known pH, the determination of the intracellular pH enables investigators to calculate the membrane proton gradient. The classical method is based on the use of weak acids for which the protonated form can diffuse freely across the membrane while the ionised form is membrane impermeant. From the knowledge of the initial and final concentrations and of the pH of the medium, it is possible to deduce the intracellular pH. The final concentration can both be determined by using labelled acids or specific electrodes. However, weak acids are usually quite different from classical drugs and they give an evaluation of the intracellular pH but they are also effectors of the multiple antibiotic resistance (Mar) system [1, 26]. It is also possible to evaluate the intracellular pH using fluorescent pH-sensitive probes. The first probes developed were derived from fluorescein. The efflux of some of these probes by MDR Transporters has been observed [4]. As the determination of the intracellular pH is based on a dual measurement at a pH-dependent wavelength and at a concentration dependent wavelength, it is possible even despite probe extrusion. However, the value obtained account only for pH in the condition of the presence of drug. Other pH-sensitive fluorescent probes might be of interest, such as the green fluorescent protein but genetic modification and GFP production in bacteria has to be based on a MDR-free selection system.

Determination of the Membrane Potential

This electrical component of the protonmotive force is probably the biggest source of problem for investigation of the MDR cells energetic. For small cells, electrodes cannot be employed and the determination of the membrane potential depends indirectly on the behaviour of probes. These compounds have an affinity for cell membranes depending on the membrane potential: they are charged with a charge opposite from the one of the intracellular charge. They are commonly cationic for membrane potential with a negative charge inside. However, beside this charge, these compounds possess a hydrophobic part (and the charge is delocalised on the compound) to favour affinity for membranes. Such a description of a hydrophobic compound possessing a positive charge corresponds to many antimicrobial drugs and probes of the membrane potential are therefore good substrates of MDR Transporters, such as the widely used tetraphenylphosphonium (TPP+). The concentration of this compound is usually evaluated through labelled TPP+ or with specific electrodes (24). Fluorescent probes possessing similar physicochemical properties can also be used as long as their accumulation on membranes can be estimated through a spectral shift. Many carbocyanin derivatives are used for this purpose.

Another type of fluorescent probe may be used to indicate the absence of membrane potential. These probes are also hydrophobic with one charge but in this case, they are negatively charged. As they are very hydrophobic, they have an important affinity for membranes and lipid rich domains of the cells but, with the same charge as the inside part of the membrane, they cannot enter cells unless cells have a depolarised membrane. As for the DPH derivatives, it is likely that cationic probes are transported by MDR transporters whereas anionic ones are not. If these fluorochromes can give a graduate response depending on membrane potential, they might be a solution to the evaluation problem.

Conclusion

The use of MDR efflux pumps by microorganisms is energy consuming and could result, in very unfavourable conditions, to a loss of activity. This is particularly true for prokaryotic cells using mainly secondary transporters but energetic perturbation are also observable for eukaryotic microorganisms for which the efflux relies more on ABC transporters. The understanding of this energetic counterpart of MDR could result in new strategies to deal with resistant cells. However, such an issue is not easy to investigate due to difficulties to evaluate these parameters. From the number of fluorescent probes investigated in the frame of MDR, it is however possible to choose experimental conditions, probes and MDR substrates competing with them that can enable investigators to approach cell energetics parameters.

References

[1]   Alekshun, M. N., and S. B. Levy. 1997. Regulation of chromosomally mediated multiple antibiotic resistance: the mar regulon. *Antimicrob. Agents Chemother.* 41:2067-75.

[2]   Andersen, C., C. Hughes, and V. Koronakis. 2001. Protein export and drug efflux through bacterial channel-tunnels. *Curr. Opin. Cell Biol.* 13:412-6.

[3]   Bay, D. C., K. L. Rommens, and R. J. Turner. 2008. Small multidrug resistance proteins: a multidrug transporter family that continues to grow. *Biochim. Biophys. Acta* 1778:1814-38.

[4]   Bolhuis, H., H. W. van Veen, J. R. Brands, M. Putman, B. Poolman, A. J. Driessen, and W. N. Konings. 1996. Energetics and mechanism of drug transport mediated by the lactococcal multidrug transporter LmrP. *J. Biol. Chem.* 271:24123-8.

[5]   Bolhuis, H., H. W. van Veen, B. Poolman, A. J. Driessen, and W. N. Konings. 1997. Mechanisms of multidrug transporters. *FEMS Microbiol. Rev.* 21:55-84.

[6]   Bonnet, M., M. M. Rafi, M. L. Chikindas, and T. J. Montville. 2006. Bioenergetic mechanism for nisin resistance, induced by the acid tolerance response of *Listeria monocytogenes*. *Appl. Environ. Microbiol.* 72:2556-2553.

[7]   Cao-Hoang, L., P. A. Marechal, M. Le-Thanh, P. Gervais, and Y. Waché. 2008. Fluorescent probes to evaluate the physiological state and activity of microbial biocatalysts: a guide for prokaryotic and eukaryotic investigation. *Biotechnol. J.* 3:890-903.

[8]   Cattoir, V. 2004. [Efflux-mediated antibiotics resistance in bacteria]. *Pathol. Biol.* (Paris) 52:607-16.

[9]   Clarebout, G., C. Villers, and R. Leclercq. 2001. Macrolide resistance gene mreA of Streptococcus agalactiae encodes a flavokinase. *Antimicrob. Agents Chemother* 45:2280-6.

[10] Davis, D. R., J. B. McAlpine, C. J. Pazoles, M. K. Talbot, E. A. Alder, C. White, B. M. Jonas, B. E. Murray, G. M. Weinstock, and B. L. Rogers. 2001. Enterococcus faecalis multi-drug resistance transporters: application for antibiotic discovery. *J. Mol. Microbiol. Biotechnol.* 3:179-84.

[11] Dekkers, D. W., P. Comfurius, A. J. Schroit, E. M. Bevers, and R. F. Zwaal. 1998. Transbilayer movement of NBD-labeled phospholipids in red blood cell membranes: outward-directed transport by the multidrug resistance protein 1 (MRP1). *Biochemistry* 37:14833-7.

[12] Fluman, N., and E. Bibi. 2008. Bacterial multidrug transport through the lens of the major facilitator superfamily. *Biochim. Biophys Acta.*

[13] Kaiser, R. D., and E. London. 1998. Location of diphenylhexatriene (DPH) and its derivatives within membranes: comparison of different fluorescence quenching analyses of membrane depth. *Biochemistry* 37:8180-90.

[14] Kuroda, T., and T. Tsuchiya. 2008. Multidrug efflux transporters in the MATE family. *Biochim. Biophys. Acta.*

[15] Law, C. J., P. C. Maloney, and D. N. Wang. 2008. Ins and outs of major facilitator superfamily antiporters. *Annu. Rev. Microbiol.* 62:289-305.

[16] Lubelski, J., W. N. Konings, and A. J. Driessen. 2007. Distribution and physiology of ABC-type transporters contributing to multidrug resistance in bacteria. *Microbiol. Mol. Biol Rev* 71:463-76.

[17] Mazurkiewicz, P., A. J. Driessen, and W. N. Konings. 2004. Energetics of wild-type and mutant multidrug resistance secondary transporter LmrP of Lactococcus lactis. *Biochim. Biophys. Acta 1658*:252-61.

[18] Nikaido, H. 1996. Multidrug efflux pumps of gram-negative bacteria. *J. Bacteriol.* 178:5853-9.

[19] Nikaido, H., and Y. Takatsuka. 2008. Mechanisms of RND multidrug efflux pumps. *Biochim. Biophys. Acta.*

[20] Paulsen, I. T., M. H. Brown, and R. A. Skurray. 1996. Proton-dependent multidrug efflux systems. *Microbiol. Rev.* 60:575-608.

[21] Pebay-Peyroula, E., E. J. Dufourc, and A. G. Szabo. 1994. Location of diphenyl-hexatriene and trimethylammonium-diphenyl-hexatriene in dipalmitoylphosphatidyl choline bilayers by neutron diffraction. *Biophys. Chem.* 53:45-56.

[22] Poelarends, G. J., P. Mazurkiewicz, and W. N. Konings. 2002. Multidrug transporters and antibiotic resistance in Lactococcus lactis. *Biochim. Biophys. Acta* 1555:1-7.

[23] Rajae Belhoussine, H. M. S. S. D. P. M. M. 1999. Characterization of intracellular pH gradients in human multidrug-resistant tumor cells by means of scanning microspectrofluorometry and dual-emission-ratio probes. *Int. J. Cancer* 81:81-89.

[24] Riondet, C., R. Cachon, Y. Waché, G. Alcaraz, and C. Diviès. 1999. Changes in the proton-motive force in Escherichia coli in response to external oxidoreduction potential. *Eur. J. Biochem.* 262:595-9.

[25] Roepe, P. D., L. Y. Wei, J. Cruz, and D. Carlson. 1993. Lower electrical membrane potential and altered pHi homeostasis in multidrug-resistant (MDR) cells: further characterization of a series of MDR cell lines expressing different levels of P-glycoprotein. *Biochemistry* 32:11042-56.

[26] Rosner, J. L., and J. L. Slonczewski. 1994. Dual regulation of inaA by the multiple antibiotic resistance (mar) and superoxide (soxRS) stress response systems of Escherichia coli. *J. Bacteriol.* 176:6262-9.

[27] Saier, M. H., Jr., J. T. Beatty, A. Goffeau, K. T. Harley, W. H. Heijne, S. C. Huang, D. L. Jack, P. S. Jahn, K. Lew, J. Liu, S. S. Pao, I. T. Paulsen, T. T. Tseng, and P. S. Virk. 1999. The major facilitator superfamily. *J. Mol. Microbiol. Biotechnol.* 1:257-79.

[28] Schechter, E. 2000. Biochimie et biophysique des membranes, aspects structuraux et fonctionnels, p. pp370-374, 2nd ed. Dunod, Paris.

[29] Siarheyeva, A., and F. J. Sharom. 2009. The ABC transporter MsbA interacts with lipid A and amphipathic drugs at different sites. *Biochem. J.*

[30] Skulachev, V. P. 1999. Bacterial energetics at high pH: what happens to the H+ cycle when the extracellular H+ concentration decreases? *Novartis Found Symp.* 221:200-13; discussion 213-7.

[31] Stavrovskaya, A. A., and T. P. Stromskaya. 2008. Transport proteins of the ABC family and multidrug resistance of tumor cells. *Biochemistry* (Mosc) 73:592-604.

[32] Touhami, A., B. Hoffmann, A. Vasella, F. A. Denis, and Y. F. Dufrene. 2003. Aggregation of yeast cells: direct measurement of discrete lectin-carbohydrate interactions. *Microbiology* 149:2873-8.

[33] van de Vossenberg, J. L. C. M., A. J. M. Driessen, M. S. da Costa, and W. N. Konings. 1999. Homeostasis of the membrane proton permeability in Bacillus subtilis grown at different temperatures. *Biochim. Biophys. Acta (BBA) - Biomembranes* 1419:97-104.

[34] van Helvoort, A., A. J. Smith, H. Sprong, I. Fritzsche, A. H. Schinkel, P. Borst, and G. Van Meer. 1996. MDR1 P-glycoprotein is a lipid translocase of broad specificity, while MDR3 P-glycoprotein specifically translocates phosphatidylcholine. *Cell* 87:507-517.

[35] van Veen, H. W., A. Margolles, M. Muller, C. F. Higgins, and W. N. Konings. 2000. The homodimeric ATP-binding cassette transporter LmrA mediates multidrug transport by an alternating two-site (two-cylinder engine) mechanism. *Embo. J.* 19:2503-14.

[36] Waché, Y., C. Riondet, C. Diviès, and R. Cachon. 2002. Effect of reducing agents on the acidification capacity and the proton motive force of *Lactococcus lactis* ssp *cremoris* resting cells. *Bioelectrochem.* 57:113-118.

[37] Zgurskaya, H. I. 2002. Molecular analysis of efflux pump-based antibiotic resistance. Int *J. Med. Microbiol.* 292:95-105.

[38] Zgurskaya, H. I., and H. Nikaido. 1999. Bypassing the periplasm: reconstitution of the AcrAB multidrug efflux pump of Escherichia coli. *Proc. Natl. Acad. Sci. USA* 96:7190-5.

[39] Zgurskaya, H. I., Y. Yamada, E. B. Tikhonova, Q. Ge, and G. Krishnamoorthy. 2008. Structural and functional diversity of bacterial membrane fusion proteins. *Biochim. Biophys. Acta.*

In: Antibiotic Resistance: …   ISBN: 978-1-60741-623-4
Editors: Adriel R. Bonilla and Kaden P. Muniz   ©2009 Nova Science Publishers, Inc.

Chapter X

Low Impact of OmpC and OmpF on Susceptibility to Antibiotics in Clinical Isolates of *Escherichia coli* Producers of Extended-Spectrum Beta-Lactamases

A. Sorlózano[a], A. Salmerón[b], F. Martínez-Checa[a], E. Villegas[a], J. D. Luna[c] and J. Gutiérrez[a]*

[a]Department of Microbiology, University of Granada, Spain
[b]Pharmacy Service, San Cecilio University Hospital. Granada, Spain
[c]Department of Biostatistics, University of Granada, Spain

Abstract

The activity of 12 antibiotics in Mueller-Hinton (MH) broth and Nutrient-Broth (NB) was assessed by microdilution in 50 clinical isolates of *Escherichia coli* producers of extended-spectrum beta-lactamases (ESBLs). In addition, the expression pattern of OmpC and OmpF porins was analyzed after culture of isolates in the two media. Three porin expression patterns were obtained: 13 isolates expressed both porins in both media, 8 expressed one porin in both media, and 29 expressed both porins in NB and one in MH. Analysis of the relationship between modification of porin expression and MIC values of the different antibiotics tested was unable to demonstrate, using this methodology, that porin loss was responsible for clinically relevant changes in the MIC of these clinical isolates.

* Correspondence: Dr. José Gutiérrez, Departamento de Microbiología, Facultad de Medicina, Avda. de Madrid 11. E-18012 Granada, Spain. Tfn: 34-958 24 20 71; Fax: 34-958 24 61 19; E-mail: josegf@ugr.es

Introduction

Porins are outer membrane proteins (OMPs) that form water filled channels that permit diffusion of small hydrophilic solutes, e.g., antibiotics, across the membrane. This process, which does not require energy, is directly proportional to the antibiotic concentration in the extrabacterial medium [1].

In *Escherichia coli*, several studies have associated loss of OmpC and OmpF porins with resistance to various antibiotic groups [2]. Porin loss in an isolate may increase the MIC value of an antibiotic, although not necessarily high enough to be detected as clinically relevant [3]. However, the effect of a decrease in permeability may be increased by the presence in the same isolate of other resistance mechanisms, e.g., enzymatic inactivation or active efflux of the antibiotic. In *E. coli*, effects on the MIC of the production of extended spectrum beta-lactamases (ESBLs) and a decrease in porin expression have been simultaneously studied. Thus, Reguera et al. [4] found that a decrease in the expression of OmpC and OmpF had no major effect on the activity of beta-lactams, whereas a marked increase in MICs was observed in presence of beta-lactamase. In addition, the lack of both OmpC and OmpF showed a greater increase in MICs than did the absence of OmpF alone [4].

In *E. coli*, levels of the two major OMPs, OmpC and OmpF, are regulated in response to various environmental parameters, and numerous factors have been shown to influence porin synthesis [5]. Their expression may be regulated by the pH, osmolarity, or O_2 concentration at the colonization or growth site, among other factors [6], which must all be considered in the study of susceptibility in any culture medium.

With this background, the aim of this study was to determine porin expression in clinical isolates of ESBL-producing *E. coli* after culture in two media with different osmolarities, and to relate possible porin expression phenotypes in the media to changes in susceptibility of the isolates.

Material and Methods

Bacterial Isolates

A study was conducted in 50 randomly selected ESBL-producing *E. coli* from a previous study on clinical isolates of this species obtained at the San Cecilio University Hospital in Granada. Following phenotypic confirmation, determination of beta-lactamase and clonality was carried out by means of biochemical (determination of the isoelectric point) and molecular (PCR, PFGE) studies, following the procedures described elsewhere by our group [7]. CTX-M9 enzymes were produced by 33 of these isolates and SHV by 17.

Susceptibility Study

Activity of 12 antibiotics was determined in the 50 isolates (table 1) by a microdilution method in Mueller-Hinton broth (MH) and Nutrient-Broth (NB) (Becton Dickinson, Spain), following CLSI recommendations [8]. Each antibiotic was dissolved according to the manufacturers' recommendations. Only the MIC value was determined, not the clinical category, because NB is not an accepted medium for *in vitro* susceptibility studies.

Table 1. MIC range (in μg/ml), of the studied antibiotic for the three porin expression patterns

Antibiotics	2 in NB and 2 in MH (n=13)		1 in NB and 1 in MH (n=8)		2 in NB and 1 in MH (n=29)	
	NB	MH	NB	MH	NB	MH
Amoxicillin-clavulanic acid	2-16	2-32	8-32	4-32	4-32	4-32
Piperacillin-tazobactam	0.5-4	≤0.25-32	1-32	1-32	1-32	≤0.25-64
Cefoxitin	1-8	1-32	4-16	8-32	2-16	2-32
Ceftazidime	≤0.25-64	≤0.25-64	1-32	0.5-32	0.5-128	≤0.25->256
Cefepime	≤0.25-32	≤0.25-16	2-32	1-32	0.5-64	0.5-64
Imipenem	≤0.008-0.016	0.03-2	≤0.008-0.016	0.125-0.25	≤0.008-0.03	0.06-0.25
Meropenem	≤0.008-0.03	≤0.008-0.25	≤0.008-0.125	≤0.008-1	0.016-0.03	≤0.008-0.03
Ertapenem	0.016-0.06	≤0.008-0.125	0.03-0.125	≤0.008-0.5	0.016-0.125	≤0.008-0.25
Amikacin	≤0.25-0.5	0.5-4	≤0.25-0.5	1-8	≤0.25-0.5	0.5-4
Tobramycin	≤0.125-0.25	≤0.125-4	≤0.125-32	0.25-128	≤0.125-1	≤0.125-16
Ciprofloxacin	≤0.125-64	≤0.125-32	2-128	8-128	≤0.125-64	≤0.125-128
Levofloxacin	≤0.125-32	≤0.125-16	1-32	4-16	≤0.125-32	≤0.125-32

Porin Expression Analysis

All isolates were cultured in parallel in MH and NB. Cells from overnight cultures were recovered by centrifugation, washed with 10 mM Tris-HCl and lysed by sonication (UP 200s Ultraschallprozessor, Germany). Unbroken cells were removed by centrifugation at 3000 g for 10 min, and cell envelopes were recovered at 100000 g for 45 min. After solubilization in 10 mM Tris-HCl, 2% sodium lauroyl sarcosinate for 30 min at room temperature, insoluble OMPs were recovered at 100000 g. The OMP profile was analyzed by polyacrylamide gel electrophoresis (12% acrylamide-0.4% bisacrylamide, 6M urea, 0.1% SDS). Gels were visualized by staining with Coomassie blue (Bio-Rad, Spain) [9].

In order to establish the porin pattern of each isolate, *E. coli* K-12 (strain JF568) was included in each gel (supplied by Sebastian Alberti of the Universitat de les Illes Balears, Palma de Mallorca, Spain). This strain expresses the structural protein OmpA, non-specific porins OmpF and OmpC and, in media with maltose or derivatives, the specific porin LamB [10, 11].

Statistical Analysis

A regression analysis with interval-censored data was performed in order to determine, for each antibiotic, any variations in MIC values among isolates presenting different porin expression patterns in each medium [12].

In order to determine whether differences in MIC values between media were related to distinct porin expression or characteristics of the media, a test of interaction between porin expression pattern and medium was first applied. When the result was significant, paired comparisons were performed between each porin expression group and each medium using Bonferroni´s correction. When the interaction test was not significant, marginal means of porin expression pattern and medium were separately compared [13]. $p < 0.05$ was considered significant in all analyses.

Results

Figure 1 depicts porin expression patterns in NB (figure 1A) and MH (figure 1B). In NB medium, both porins (OmpC and OmpF) were expressed by 84% (42/50) of isolates and one porin by 16% (8/50), without being able to determine whether it was OmpC or OmpF. In MH medium, both porins were expressed by 26% (13/50) of isolates and one porin by 74% (37/50), with OmpC expressed by 29 of these and with an OMP that could not be determined (OmpC or OmpF) in the remaining 8, the same 8 isolates that showed this result in NB. Simultaneous loss of OmpF and OmpC was not observed in any isolate.

Therefore, three patterns could be observed. The most frequent pattern (29 isolates, 58%), was characterized by expression of both porins in NB and one in MH (group A). The other two patterns were characterized by expression of the same number of porins (group B), with 26% expressing both porins in both media and 16% expressing one porin in both media. All isolates expressed an OMP compatible with OmpA of *E. coli* JF568 in both MH and NB.

Table 1 shows the MIC range (in µg/ml) obtained for each antibiotic in each porin expression group and medium. A wide variability of MIC values was observed for each antibiotic in all porin expression patterns, regardless of the culture medium. In the NB medium, comparison of MIC values showed that cefoxitin, cefepime, ertapenem, tobramycin, ciprofloxacin, and levofloxacin were significantly more active against the isolates expressing both porins (n=42) than against those expressing only one (n=8) (*p<0.001, p=0.012, p=0.017, p<0.001, p=0.009, p=0.026*, respectively). This comparison revealed no significant differences in the MICs of amoxicillin-clavulanic acid, piperacillin-tazobactam, ceftazidime, imipenem, meropenem, or amikacin as a function of porin loss.

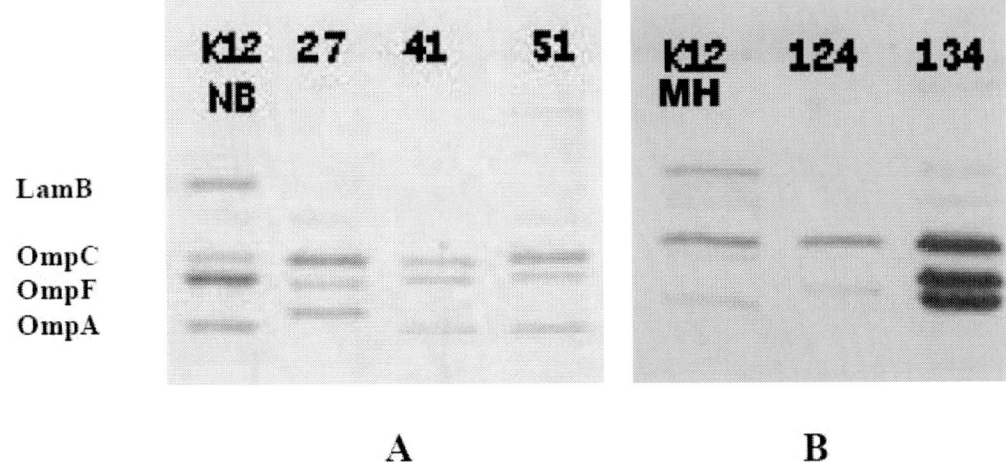

Figure 1A. Expression of porins OmpC and OmpF in K12 strain and isolates 27, 41 and 51 after culture in NB. Figure 1B. Expression of porin OmpC in K12 strain and isolate 124, and of OmpC and OmpF in isolate 134, after culture in MH. Porin OmpA is expressed in all isolates in both media.

In the MH medium, cefoxitin was significantly more active in isolates expressing both porins (n=13) than in those expressing only one (n=37) ($p=0.007$), with no difference in the activity of the other antibiotics as a function of porin loss.

Table 2 shows the results of comparing mean MIC values (adjusted by the statistical test) in each culture medium between group A (expressing both porins in NB and one porin in MH) and group B (expressing same type of porin in each medium) isolates. The aim of these comparisons was to determine whether mean MIC values differed between media and whether any differences detected were associated or not with the modification in porins between the media. For amoxicillin-clavulanic acid, ceftazidime, cefepime, meropenem, and ertapenem, the interaction was not significant ($p=0.372$, $p=0.170$, $p=0.441$, $p=0.175$, $p=0.302$, respectively), i.e., there was no association between porin pattern and medium. Porin pattern and medium had no significant effect on MIC values for any of these antibiotics ($p=0.727$, $p=0.257$, $p=0.897$, $p=0.485$, $p=0.076$, respectively), i.e., mean MIC values did not significantly differ between groups A and B in either medium. Therefore, the activity of these antibiotics was not affected by either the number of porins or the culture medium.

No significant interaction was found for piperacillin-tazobactam, cefoxitin, imipenem, amikacin, tobramycin, or levofloxacin, ($p=0.634$, $p=0.988$, $p=0.574$, $p=0.563$, $p=0.535$, $p=1.000$, respectively), i.e., there was no association between porin pattern and medium. Analysis of the effects of porin pattern and medium on MIC values showed a significant effect only for the medium ($p=0.013$, $p<0.001$, $p<0.001$, $p<0.001$, $p<0.001$, $p=0.013$, respectively), with lower mean MIC values in NB versus MH for both groups (A and B) with the exception of piperacillin-tazobactam, which showed the opposite result. Therefore, in both groups, isolates were more susceptible in NB than in MH to cefoxitin, imipenem, amikacin, tobramycin and levofloxacin but were more resistant to piperacillin-tazobactam.

A. Sorlózano, A. Salmerón, F. Martínez-Checa et al.

Table 2. Mean and standard deviation of MIC values (adjusted by statistical test) of the 50 isolates by group and culture medium

Antibiotic	Medium	Values adjusted by statistical test	Group A (n=29)	Group B (n=21)
Amoxicillin-clavulanic acid	NB	Mean	2.59	2.52
		SD	0.1655	0.2151
	MH	Mean	2.50	2.57
		SD	0.1595	0.2168
Piperacillin-tazobactam	NB	Mean	1.30	0.88
		SD	0.2736	0.3320
	MH	Mean	0.82	0.50
		SD	0.2734	0.3318
Cefoxitin	NB	Mean	1.57	1.58
		SD	0.2037	0.2423
	MH	Mean	2.06	2.07
		SD	0.2037	0.2420
Ceftazidime	NB	Mean	0.19	1.55
		SD	0.4810	0.4982
	MH	Mean	0.59	1.55
		SD	0.4814	0.4982
Cefepime	NB	Mean	2.14	2.07
		SD	0.4507	0.4041
	MH	Mean	2.18	1.98
		SD	0.4504	0.4040
Imipenem	NB	Mean	-6.95	-7.21
		SD	0.1397	0.1646
	MH	Mean	-3.40	-3.49
		SD	0.1399	0.1632
Meropenem	NB	Mean	-6.19	-6.26
		SD	0.1773	0.2080
	MH	Mean	-6.26	-5.92
		SD	0.1773	0.2074
Ertapenem	NB	Mean	-5.09	-4.88
		SD	0.2202	0.2588
	MH	Mean	-5.26	-5.45
		SD	0.2200	0.2583
Amikacin	NB	Mean	-2.36	-2.21
		SD	0.1333	0.1563
	MH	Mean	0.05	0.03
		SD	0.1316	0.1546
Tobramycin	NB	Mean	-3.23	-2.45
		SD	0.3642	0.4324
	MH	Mean	-0.74	-0.26
		SD	0.3641	0.4323

Antibiotic	Medium	Values adjusted by statistical test	Group A (n=29)	Group B (n=21)
Ciprofloxacin	NB	Mean	1.00	1.46
		SD	0.3902	0.5665
	MH	Mean	1.90	2.13
		SD	0.3901	0.5667
Levofloxacin	NB	Mean	1.06	0.74
		SD	0.3972	0.5324
	MH	Mean	1.55	1.12
		SD	0.3971	0.5325

NB: Nutrient-Broth; MH: Mueller-Hinton broth; SD: Standard deviation.
Group A: Isolates with different number of porins in each medium (2 in NB and 1 in MH).
Group B: Isolates with same number of porins in each medium (1 in NB and MH, 2 in NB and MH).

Finally, a significant interaction was found for ciprofloxacin ($p=0.036$), indicating a relationship between porin pattern and the medium. Consequently, the effects of the medium were compared in each group, finding a significant difference in each group (group A, $p<0.001$; group B, $p=0.024$), with a lower mean MIC in NB than in MH. Since the interaction was significant, this trend was more important in group A. It can be concluded that the isolates were more susceptible to ciprofloxacin in NB because they expressed both porins in this medium.

Discussion

The present study assessed the activity of various antibiotics in clinical isolates of ESBL-producing *E. coli* in two culture media with different osmolarities [14] and porin expressions. Porin expression differed between these media, and in MH, a high osmolarity medium, there was a significant loss of porin OmpF [15,16]. Independent analyses of the activity of each antibiotic in each culture medium demonstrated a relationship between porin loss and a decrease in the activity of some antibiotics, especially cefoxitin. Cefoxitin was the only antibiotic tested that showed a significant decrease in activity as a consequence of porin loss in both NB and MH. Various authors also reported this direct relationship between cefoxitin activity and porin loss in both *K. pneumoniae* and *E. coli* [17].

Various studies have investigated the activity of different antibiotics in relation to porin loss in these bacterial species [18,19]. However, authors considered only one culture medium, usually Mueller-Hinton broth, which best reproduces physiological concentrations of the different ions. Further research is required into the effect on antibiotic activity of the medium, since it has been reported that high-osmolarity media not only reduce expression of porins but can also increase expression of active expulsion pumps, which contributes to a reduced activity of some antibiotics [16].

The present study demonstrated that the osmolarity of the medium had a greater effect on the activity of piperacillin-tazobactam, cefoxitin, imipenem, amikacin, tobramycin, and levofloxacin than did porin loss, likely due to mechanisms other than reduction of porin expression [16]. However, the activity against *E. coli* isolates of amoxicillin-clavulanic acid, ceftazidime, cefepime, meropenem, and ertapenem was not affected by the type of culture medium (MH or NB) or number of porins. The only decrease in activity was observed for ciprofloxacin in MH, as a consequence of the lower porin expression in this medium. Some authors consider that the presence of suprainhibitory concentrations of fluoroquinolones may also reduce OmpF expression [16].

In both culture media, the MIC values of the beta-lactams, especially ceftazidime and cefepime, showed a high variability in each of three porin expression patterns studied. This is explained by hydrolysis due to the presence of ESBL enzymes. Thus, isolates with a CTX-M9 enzyme showed high resistance to cefepime but virtually no increase in the MIC of ceftazidime, while isolates with a SHV enzyme were more resistant to ceftazidime. This suggests that the action of the beta-lactamase itself plays a greater role than porin loss in the resistance of ESBL-producing *E. coli* to beta-lactam antibiotics. The variability of fluoroquinolones MIC values can also be explained by the presence in some isolates but not others of *gyrA*, *parC* and *parE* mutations, previously reported in the same ESBLs-producing isolates [20].

Separation of *E. coli* porins by electrophoresis is difficult because of their similar molecular weight (OmpC, 38.284 kDa; OmpF, 37.061 kDa). Their differentiation was facilitated in this study by using urea in the SDS polyacrylamide gel, which causes OmpC to migrate more slowly due its slightly higher weight [9]. Nevertheless, the porin expressed by eight of the isolates could not be identified. In this context, although some authors have used a complementary methodology with Western-Blot to identify porins, this was not considered appropriate for the present study because it has been reported that some porins may not be detected. We therefore propose the inclusion of extract of *E. coli* JF568 in each gel, since the porin expression of this reference strain is well characterized [9].

In conclusion, it was not possible to demonstrate, using this methodology, that loss of porin expression is responsible for clinically relevant changes in the MIC of clinical isolates of ESBL-producing *E. coli*.

References

[1]   Nikaido H. Molecular basis of bacterial outer membrane permeability revisited. *Microbiol. Mol. Biol. Rev.*, 2003; 67: 593-656.

[2]   Harder KJ, Nikaido H, Matsuhashi M. Mutants of *Escherichia coli* that are resistant to certain beta-lactam compounds lack the ompF porin. *Antimicrob. Agents Chemother.*, 1981; 20: 549-52.

[3]   Nikaido H. Outer membrane barrier as a mechanism of antimicrobial resistance. *Antimicrob. Agents Chemother.*, 1989; 33: 1831-6.

[4]   Reguera JA, Baquero F, Pérez-Díaz JC, Martínez JL. Factors determining resistance to beta-lactam combined with beta-lactamase inhibitors in *Escherichia coli. J. Antimicrob. Chemother.*, 1991; 27: 569-75.

[5]   Pratt LA, Hsing W, Gibson KE, Silhavy T. From acids to osmZ: multiple factors influence synthesis of OmpF and OmpC porins in *Escherichia coli. Mol. Microbiol.*, 1996; 20: 911-7.

[6]   Pages JM. Bacterial porin and antibiotic susceptibility. *Med. Sci. (Paris)*, 2004; 20: 346-51.

[7]   Sorlozano A, Gutierrez J, De Luna JD, Oteo J, Liebana J, Soto MJ, et al. High presence of extended-spectrum β-lactamases and resistance to quinolones in clinical isolates of *Escherichia coli. Microbiol. Res.*, 2007; 162: 347-54.

[8]   Clinical and Laboratory Standards Institute. Methods for dilution antimicrobial susceptibility tests for bacteria that grow aerobically, 7th ed., M7-A7. Clinical and Laboratory Standards Institute, Wayne, PA. 2006.

[9]   Hernandez-Alles S, Alberti S, Alvarez D, Domenech-Sanchez A, Martinez-Martinez L, Gil J, et al. Porin expression in clinical isolates of *Klebsiella pneumoniae. Microbiology*, 1999, 145: 673-9.

[10]   Foulds J, Chai TJ. New major outer membrane protein found in an *Escherichia coli* tolF mutant resistant to bacteriophage Tulb. *J. Bacteriol.*, 1978; 133: 1478-83.

[11]   Gibbs KA, Isaac DD, Xu J, Hendrix RW, Silhavy TJ, Theriot JA. Complex spatial distribution and dynamics of an abundant *Escherichia coli* outer membrane protein, LamB. *Mol. Microbiol.*, 2004; 53: 1771-83.

[12]   Long JS, Freese J. Regression models for categorical and limited dependent variables using Stata. College Station TX: Stata Press. 2006.

[13]   Long JS. Regression models for categorical and limited dependent variables. Thousands Oaks CA: Sage. 1997.

[14]   Beggs WH, Andrews FA. Role of ionic strength in salt antagonism of aminoglycoside action on *Escherichia coli* and *Pseudomonas aeruginosa. J. Infect. Dis.*, 1976; 134:500-4.

[15]   Yoshida T, Qin L, Egger LA, Inouye M. Transcription regulation of OmpF and OmpC by a single transcription factor, OmpR. *J. Biol. Chem.*, 2006; 281:17114-23.

[16]   Giuliodori AM, Gualerzi CO, Soto S, Vila J, Tavío MM. Review on bacterial stress topics. *Ann. NY Acad. Sci.*, 2007; 1113: 95-104.

[17]   Ananthan S, Subha A. Cefoxitin resistance mediated by loss of a porin in clinical strains of *Klebsiella pneumoniae* and *Escherichia coli. Indian J. Med. Microbiol.*, 2005, 23: 20-3.

[18]   Hancock RE, Farmer SW, Li ZS, Poole K. Interaction of aminoglycosides with the outer membranes and purified lipopolysaccharide and OmpF porin of *Escherichia coli. Antimicrob. Agents Chemother.*, 1991; 35:1309-14.

[19]   Hernandez-Alles S, Conejo MC, Pascual A, Tomas JM, Benedi VJ, Martinez-Martinez L. Relationship between outer membrane alterations and susceptibility to antimicrobial agents in isogenic strains of *Klebsiella pneumoniae. J. Antimicrob. Chemother.*, 2000; 46: 273-7.

[20]   Sorlozano A, Gutierrez J, Jimenez A, De Luna JD, Martinez JL. Contribution of a new mutation in *parE* to quinolone resistance in extended-spectrum beta-lactamase-producing *Escherichia coli* isolates. *J. Clin. Microbiol.*, 2007; 45: 2740-2.

In: Antibiotic Resistance: …
Editors: Adriel R. Bonilla and Kaden P. Muniz

ISBN: 978-1-60741-623-4
©2009 Nova Science Publishers, Inc.

Chapter XI

Antibiotic Resistance in Mariculture Environments of China

Jingyi Zhao and Hongyue Dang

Centre for Bioengineering and Biotechnology, China University of Petroleum
(East China), Qingdao 266555, China

Abstract

China has become the largest mariculture country of the world. The extensive and intense use of antibiotics in mariculture for the prevention and treatment of microbial infections of the farmed marine animals exerts a selective pressure on environmental bacteria. The mariculture environment may have become a reservoir and dissemination source of antibiotic resistance. The prevalence of antibiotic resistance may undermine the effectiveness of various antibiotics, alter the natural microbiota, disturb the ecological equilibria, and create a potential threat to human health and welfare. The emergence of antibiotic resistant bacteria in mariculture and related environments has become a great concern of environmental and human health. There is an urgent need to develop a monitoring platform to investigate the antibiotic resistant bacteria and their resistance mechanisms in mariculture environments, for effective prevention and control of the spread and evolution of harmful antibiotic resistant bacteria and their resistance determinants. Certain research effort has been made to evaluate the abundance and diversity of the antibiotic-resistant microbes and their resistance genes in China mariculture environments. A preliminary review on this issue is provided in this paper. As the biggest mariculture country, China will take the responsibility and resolution for the control and elimination of antibiotic resistance in mariculture environment.

Introduction

A large number of marine animals, such as sea cucumbers, sea urchins, abalones, clams, oysters, shrimps and fishes, have been successfully cultured along the 18,400 km coast of

China, making China one of the largest producers and consumers of mariculture products all over the world. But the old-fashioned and unscientific management may result in a great threat to the healthy and sustainable development of the Chinese mariculture industry, especially due to the overuse of antibiotics and the resultant antibiotic-resistance issues. Cultured marine animals are frequently subjected to infectious diseases (Wang et al., 2004; Zhang et al., 2004), which lead to great losses every year by almost 1.5 billion dollars. Bacteria are the causative agents for most of the infections, such as septicopyaemia, pustule and fester disease (Ma et al., 1996; Ye et al., 1997; Li et al., 1998). Various antibiotics, such as oxytetracycline, penicillin and streptomycin, are used for the prevention and treatment of infections in mariculture. The extensive and intense use of antibiotics creates a selective pressure for bacteria, making the mariculture environment become a reservoir and dissemination source of antibiotic resistance. However, only very limited information about antibiotic resistance in aquacultural and related natural environments is available in China (Li et al., 1999).

The antibiotic resistance has been recognized as not only a serious public health issue, but also an important ecological problem. The prevalence of antibiotic resistant bacteria in mariculture and related natural environments has become a great concern of environmental and human health. Without accurate monitoring and prompt action, resistant bacteria in mariculture environments might become a harmful reservoir for both marine animals and human beings.

Oxytetracycline and chloramphenicol were once widely used in aquaculture of China. Although chloramphenicol was banned since 1999, oxytetracycline is still used as the major prophylactic reagent. Bacteria resistant to these antibiotics were screened to gain a basic understanding of antibiotic resistance in China mariculture environments. Studies indicate that the China maricultural environments are populated with antibiotic resistant microorganisms.

Abundance of Antibiotic-Resistant Bacteria in China Mariculture Environments

Dang et al. have investigated the multidrug-resistant bacteria from four rearing water samples in a maricultural farm in Dalian of China, for the cultivation of sea cucumbers, sea urchins, turbots and abalones, respectively (Dang et al., 2006a, 2006b, 2007). The 2216 marine agar were used for the count measurement of culturable bacteria, and the tryptic soy agar with 3% NaCl and screening antibiotic, oxytetracycline or chloramphenicol, were used for the isolation of antibiotic resistant bacteria. High incidence of antibiotic resistant bacteria occurred in the water samples (Table 1).

For chloramphenicol- and oxytetracycline-resistance, the most serious contamination situation took place in the sea cucumber rearing water, where the chloramphenicol- and oxytetracycline-resistant bacteria accounted for 36.2% and 32.2% of the total culturable microbes respectively (Dang et al., 2006a, 2006b).

Table 1. Comparison of antibiotic-resistant bacterial isolates and their chloramphenicol- and oxytetracycline-resistance genes from four different rearing water sources in a mariculture farm of China

	Abalone		Sea cucumber		Sea urchin		Turbot	
	CP[a]	OTC[b]	CP[a]	OTC[b]	CP[a]	OTC[b]	CP[a]	OTC[b]
Total cultural bacterial counts (cells ml^{-1})	$(1.40\pm0.25) \times 10^5$		$(1.82\pm0.14) \times 10^5$		$(4.74\pm0.35) \times 10^5$		$(1.91\pm0.13) \times 10^5$	
Antibiotic resistant bacteria counts (cells ml^{-1})	$(1.19\pm0.03) \times 10^4$	$(5.13\pm0.42) \times 10^3$	$(6.60\pm1.15) \times 10^4$	$(5.87\pm0.97) \times 10^4$	$(7.17\pm0.76) \times 10^4$	$(2.67\pm0.29) \times 10^4$	$(2.73\pm0.12) \times 10^4$	$(1.90\pm0.44) \times 10^4$
Multidrug Resistance[c]	8.5%	3.7%	36.2%	32.2%	15.1%	5.6%	14.3%	9.9%
Strains								
Vibrio splendidus	*cat* II, *floR*, *tet*(B), *tet*(D), *tet*(E), *tet*(M)	*cat* II, *floR*, *tet*(A), *tet*(B), *tet*(D), *tet*(M)	*cat* II, *cat* IV, *floR*, *tet*(D), *tet*(E), *tet*(M)	*cat* II, *cat* IV, *floR*, *tet*(B), *tet*(D), *tet*(M)	*cat* II, *floR*, *tet*(B), *tet*(D), *tet*(E), *tet*(M)	*floR*, *tet*(A), *tet*(B), *tet*(D), *tet*(M)	*cat* II	*cat* II, *floR*, *tet*(A), *tet*(B), *tet*(D), *tet*(M)
V. tasmaniensis	*cat* II, *cat* IV, *floR*, *tet*(B), *tet*(D), *tet*(M)	*cat* II, *tet*(D)	*cat* II, *cat* IV, *floR*, *tet*(A), *tet*(B), *tet*(D), *tet*(M)	*cat* II, *cat* IV, *floR*, *tet*(B), *tet*(D), *tet*(M)	*cat* II, *tet*(D)		*cat* II, *cat* IV, *floR*, *tet*(B), *tet*(D), *tet*(E), *tet*(M)	*cat* II, *floR*, *tet*(A), *tet*(B), *tet*(D), *tet*(M)
Listonella (*Vibrio*) *pelagius*						*cat* IV, *tet*(B), *tet*(M)		
other vibrio							*cat* II	

Table 1. (Continued)

	Abalone		Sea cucumber		Sea urchin		Turbot	
	CP[a]	OTC[b]	CP[a]	OTC[b]	CP[a]	OTC[b]	CP[a]	OTC[b]
Pseudoalteromonas atlantica			*cat* IV, *tet*(B), *tet*(D), *tet*(M)		*floR*	*cat* IV, *floR*, *tet*(B), *tet*(D), *tet*(E)	*cat* II, *floR*, *tet*(D)	*floR*
P. haloplanktis					*floR*	*floR*		*floR*
P. marina		*cat* II, *floR*, *tet*(M)						
P. mariniglutinosa		*floR*						*floR*
P. carrageenovora						*cat* IV, *tet*(M)		
Alteromonas marina		*floR*						
References	Dang et al., 2009	Dang et al., 2007	Dang et al., 2006a; Chen and Dang, 2008	Dang et al., 2006b; Zhang et al., 2007	Dang et al., 2006a; Chen and Dang, 2008	Dang et al., 2006b; Zhang et al., 2007	Dang et al., 2009	Dang et al., 2007

[a] CP, chloramphenicol was used as the initial antibiotic for multidrug-resistant bacteria isolation;

[b] OTC, oxytetracycline was used as the initial antibiotic for multidrug-resistant bacteria isolation;

[c] Multidrug resistance was calculated as the percentage of strains that were resistant to at least two different types of antibiotics tested to the total culturable bacterial count.

The abalone rearing water showed the lowest level of antibiotic resistance contamination, with about 8.5% and 3.7% of the total culturable microbes being identified as chloramphenicol- and oxytetracycline-resistant (Dang et al., 2007). Less than 9% of the total bacteria were found to be florfenicol-resistant in water samples collected from two Chilean salmon farms (Miranda and Rojas, 2007). About 4.8% of the culturable bacteria on average proved to be oxytetracycline resistant in four fish farms situated in western Denmark (Schmidt et al., 2000). Studies on seawater samples in Jiaozhou Bay on the China coast showed that respectively 0.15%-6.70% and lower than 0.6% of the culturable microbes could be classified as chloramphenicol- and oxytetracycline-resistant (Dang et al., 2008a, 2008b). The more severe contamination of antibiotic resistance in China mariculture environments indicates that more research efforts should be invested.

All the screened oxytetracycline- or chloramphenicol-resistant isolates from the studied water samples can be resistant to at least two types of antibiotics. And 4.1% of the resistant isolates (3/74) in the sea cucumber farm could be resistant to all the antibiotics tested, including ampicillin, chloramphenicol, erythromycin, nalidixic acid, oxytetracycline and streptomycin (Dang et al., 2006b). The most common resistance phenotype of the isolates was the simultaneous resistance to oxytetracycline, chloramphenicol and ampicillin. Prevalence of multidrug resistant bacteria in aquaculture was common all over the world. The majority of the *Aeromonas* spp. isolated from South African aquaculture environments displayed resistance to the β-lactams, tetracycline and nalidixic acid, and showed decreased susceptibility to erythromycin (Jacobs and Chenia, 2007). The multidrug-resistant isolates from Chilean salmon farms showed high percentages of resistance to erythromycin, ampicillin, furazolidone and cotrimoxazole (Miranda and Rojas, 2007).

The incidence and widespread of the multidrug resistance may create great threat to the development of mariculture industry. Once the infectious diseases broke out, the effectiveness of these antibiotics or their derivatives may be undermined.

Diversity of Antibiotic-Resistant Bacteria in China Mariculture Environments

Based on the 16S rRNA gene sequences of the respective isolates and the phylogenetic tree constructed, most oxytetracycline- or chloramphenicol-resistant isolates belonged to *Vibrio* or *Pseudoalteromonas* bacteria for the studied mariculture environments of China (Dang et al., 2006a, 2006b, 2007). The bacteria closely related to *Vibrio* were the predominant resistant strains, accounting for 70%-100% of the determined isolates. *V. tasmaniensis* and *V. splendidus* were the predominant antibiotic resistant *Vibrio* strains. But the florfenicol-resistant bacteria in Chilean salmon farms mainly belonged to *Pseudomonas* genus, and the predominant species were *P. putida*, *P. viridilivida*, and *P. fluorescens* (Miranda and Rojas, 2007). *Bacillus* and *Vibrio* were the common antibiotic resistant species in shrimp faming of Vietnam (Le et al., 2005). The differences of antibiotic resistant microbial species may be due to the different species of cultured marine animals. Some *V. splendidus* strains were found to be pathogenic to some cultured mollusks, crustaceans and fishes (Prayitno and Latchford, 1995; Miranda and Rojas, 1996; Balebona et al., 1998;

Sugumar et al., 1998; Gay et al., 2004; Gomez-Leon et al., 2005). The prevalence of these potentially pathogenic multidrug-resistant bacteria may result in catastrophic losses to the mariculture ponds when the infectious diseases broke out. In Jiaozhou Bay, more diverse chloramphenicol- and oxytetracycline-resistant bacteria were found (Dang et al., 2008a, 2008b), including *Aeromonas, Shewanella, Pseudoalteromonas, Klebsiella, Escherichia, Proteus, Vibrio, Pseudomonas, Psychrobacter, Roseobacter, Micrococcus, Arthrobacter, Kocuria, Bacillus, Raoultella, Photobacterium, Acinetobacter, Halomonas, Formosa* and *Citrobacter*. The less diverse antibiotic resistant bacteria species in China mariculture environments may be caused by the intense use of various antibiotic compounds. The combination of the use of various antibiotics with high dose may eliminate most of the bacteria having low and narrow-spectra of resistance.

Diversity of Antibiotic Resistance Determinants in China Mariculture Environments

Various antibiotic resistance determinants were detected in the mariculture environments of China (Dang et al., 2006a, 2006b, 2007). The common oxytetracycline resistance genes in aquatic bacteria could be divided into two types: the genes encoding the active efflux pumps, such as *tet*(A)-*tet*(E), *tet*(G) and *tet*(Y) (Furushita ct al., 2003; Jun ct al., 2004; Akinbowale et al., 2007; Jacobs and Chenia, 2007; Heepngoen et al., 2008), and the genes encoding the ribosomal protection proteins like *tet*(M) and *tet*(S) (Kim et al., 2004; Akinbowale et al., 2007). The gene segments of *tet*(A), *tet*(B), *tet*(D), *tet*(E) and *tet*(M) could be identified in all rearing water samples in the studied China mariculture environments (Dang et al., 2006a, 2006b, 2007). *Tet*(A) is always combined with other *tet* genes, in patterns of *tet*(A) and *tet*(D), *tet*(A) and *tet*(B), *tet*(A), *tet*(B) and *tet*(D), and *tet*(A), *tet*(B) and *tet*(M). The other four *tet* genes could be detected in single pattern, or combined ones, such as *tet*(B) and *tet*(D), *tet*(D) and *tet*(E), *tet*(B) and *tet*(M), and *tet*(B), *tet*(D) and *tet*(M).

The predominant *tet* genes in vibrio isolates from the China mariculture farm were *tet*(A), *tet*(B) and *tet*(D). However, studies in Jiaozhou Bay indicated that the *tet*(A), *tet*(B) and *tet*(G) were the most predominant gene determinants, with the vibrio harboring *tet*(B), occasionally *tet*(A) or *tet*(G) (Dang et al., 2008b). As previously reported results, the *tet* gene carried on R plasmids from fish pathogen *V. anguillarum* isolated from 1973 to 1977 in Japan was *tet*(B), from 1980-1983 was *tet*(G), and from 1989 to 1991 was *tet*(D) (Aoki, 2000). The *tet* gene carried on R plasmids from fish pathogen *Edwardsiella tarda* in Korea was *tet*(A) and *tet*(D), and *tet*(B) and *tet*(G) were detected on nonmobile nucleic acid (Jun et al., 2004). The prevalence of similar *tet* genes in Korea and China in recent years to the originally detected *tet* genes in Japan decades ago may indicate the origin and spread of some antibiotic resistance factors in the three neighboring countries.

The chloramphenicol resistance genes carried by the marine bacteria are usually the genes encoding chloramphenicol acetyltransferases to cause the antibiotic inactivation, mainly *cat*I-IV (Yoo et al., 2003). The resistance gene *floR* was also found to be responsible for some of the resistance to chloramphenicol. The *cat*II, *cat*IV and *floR* could be detected in most of the mariculture environments of China so far studied (Dang et al., 2006a, 2006b,

2007). The *cat*II and *cat*IV were always separately identified, but coexisted in some of the vibrio strains. Some strains carried simultaneous *cat*II and *floR,* and a vibrio strain harbored simultaneously the above three resistance genes. The prevalence of *cat*II and *cat*IV in China maricultural environments showed similar *cat* gene profiles from the aquaculture environments of Japan (Aoki, 2000) and Korea (Yoo et al., 2003) with a progressive timeline, in contrary to *cat*I and *cat*III predominant gene profiles in Jiaozhou Bay (Dang et al., 2008a).

It is also proven that comparative studies with different antibiotics as the first screening reagents could be helpful to detect a wider diversity of the resistance genes. When chloramphenicol was used as the screening antibiotic, *cat*II, *cat*IV, *floR*, *tet*(B), *tet*(D), *tet*(E) and *tet*(M) could be detected in the turbot rearing water sample, but only *cat*II and *floR*, *tet*(A), *tet*(B), *tet*(D) and *tet*(M) can be identified in the same sample when oxytetracycline was used as the screening antibiotic (Dang et al., 2007).

Reasons for Prevalence of Antibiotic Resistance in the Mariculture Environments

Marine vibrios have been recognized as reservoirs and vehicles of antibiotic resistance. Their abundance and diversity in marine environments and the capacity of developing and acquiring resistance determinants help antibiotic resistance spread by horizontal gene transfer (Thompson et al., 2004, 2005). Epidemics of pathogens in marine environments could rapidly spread due to their potential for long-term survival outside the host and the lack of barriers to dispersal (McCallum et al., 2003).

In agreement with the presumption, vibrio, the predominant antibiotic resistant bacteria in the microbiota of China mariculture environments so far studied, may play an important role in the prevalence of antibiotic resistance in marine environments.

The chloramphenicol resistant bacteria could persist in mariculture environments even after the drug use has been banned. Cross-resistance and co-resistance might be the mechanisms involved (Alonso et al., 2001; Courvalin and Trieu-Cuot, 2001; Schwarz et al., 2004). Besides the chloramphenicol acetyltransferases, multidrug transporters (Poole, 2005) may provide the cross-resistance in marine environments.

For the mechanisms of co-resistance, the usage of one kind of antibiotic may increase level of resistance to another specific drug, even with different active modes (Kummerer, 2004). Based on our study, it is predicted that co-selection by oxytetracycline might be the molecular mechanism for the maintenance of the *cat* genes in marine environments (Dang et al., 2006b). Besides antibiotics, heavy metal and other contamination may also contribute to the cross-selection and co-selection of antibiotic resistance (Schwarz et al., 2004; Baker-Austin et al., 2006). Plasmids with resistance to heavy metal and antibiotics have been found in *E. coli* (Johnson et al., 2005) and marine *Pseudomonas* (Rajini Rani and Mahadevan, 1992).

Conclusion

Extensive use and misuse of antibiotic in mariculture result in global serious issue for public health and environmental management. Due to lack of studies on pharmacokinetics and pharmacodynamics of antibiotics used in mariculture, misuse of antibiotics stimulates the propagation of multidrug resistant bacteria in aquatic water. The resistant microbes and their resistance determinants may pass from the aquatic environment to the terrestrial environment through food chain and human activities, creating a great threat to human health and welfare. Previous studies indicated that more and more resistance bacteria were identified from coastal (Herwig et al., 1997) and aquacultural environments, due to increasing antibiotic selective pressure. The mariculture environments may become the reservoir and dissemination source of antibiotic resistance. The joint FAO/OIE/WHO recommended that "*Measures should be developed and implemented at national and international levels to prevent development and spread of antimicrobial resistance in aquaculture*" (WHO, 2006). However, the studies of this issue have just started recently in China. The lack of systematic research on antibiotic resistance in mariculture environments in China imparts a hindrance to the healthy development of mariculture and management of marine environments. Basic investigations on the abundance, diversity, distribution and source of antibiotic resistant bacteria and their resistance determinants in China mariculture farms and Jiaozhou Bay have been taken for gaining the necessary basic understanding and for eventually effective prevention and control of environmental antibiotic resistance.

Nevertheless, studies on antibiotic resistance on a global scale encountered lots of problems. Due to the lack of required data and the extreme diversity and complexity of mariculture, it is difficult to develop some consensus standardization for evaluation and interpretation of the antibiotic resistance in mariculture for international communications (Smith, 2008). Because of the laboratory variations on the data collection and interpretation, the presumptions in various published studies may be misleading and erroneous. The development and validation of the model of resistance gene flow and gene ecology is urgently needed to design optimal risk management strategies, making the antibiotic use more efficacious and reducing the emergence of antibiotic resistance (Smith, 2008).

More professional supervision should be taken in the amounts and varieties of antibiotics in mariculture to help the effective use of antibiotics in mariculture. The use of antibiotics in mariculture as the prophylactic and therapeutic agents must be strictly monitored and well regulated, and public awareness of the terrible consequences of antibiotic resistance has to be raised. Experience gained in Norway shows that development of effective vaccines based on the detailed investigation on immunology of cultured animals will help to reduce the use of antibiotics in mariculture (Markestad and Grave, 1997).

Certain mobile genetic elements, such as plasmids, transposons and integrons, could facilitate the transfer of antibiotic resistance (Olsen, 1999; White and McDermott 2001). The *intI1* and *intI2* integrase genes and the *dfr* and *aadA* gene cassettes were identified from the resistant isolates in Jiaozhou Bay (Wang et al., 2008). Some investigations on molecular characterization of more resistance determinants in antibiotic resistant strains, likelihood of gene transfer and evolution origin of these determinants among the terrestrial and marine environments should be carried out to clarify the mechanisms of resistance gene flow. The assessment of co-resistance mechanism between antibiotic and other contamination factors also needs further consideration and investigation.

Antibiotic resistant bacteria can be recognized as bioindicators of the environmental quality and potential biotracers of contaminations. The biological, environmental and anthropogenic factors and their interaction that may contribute to the antibiotic resistance issue are an important research direction for Chinese microbiologists. There is also an urgent need to develop a monitoring platform for further investigation on the antibiotic resistant bacteria and their resistance mechanisms in other mariculture environments of China.

As the biggest mariculture country, China scientists would take a more active part in the global effort on monitoring and surveillance of the use of antibiotics in mariculture, and of the consequences of its use for the control and elimination of antibiotic resistance in mariculture environments.

References

[1]   Akinbowale, O.L.; Peng, H.; Barton, M.D. *J. Appl. Microbiol.* 2007, 103, 2016-2022.

[2]   Alonso, A.; Sanchez, P.; Martinez, J.L. *Environ. Microbiol.* 2001, 3, 1-9.

[3]   Aoki, T. *Use of chemicals in aquaculture in Asia*; Transferable drug resistance plasmids in fish-pathogenic bacteria; SEAFDEC Aquaculture Department: Tigbauan, Iloilo, PH, 2000; pp 31-33.

[4]   Baker-Austin, C.; Wright, M.S.; Stepanauskas, R.; McArthur, J.V. *Trends Microbiol.* 2006, 14, 176-182.

[5]   Balebona, M.C.; Zorilla, I.; Morinigo, M.A.; Borrego, J.J. *Aquaculture* 1998, 166, 19-35.

[6]   Chen, M.N.; Dang, H.Y. *Mar. Sci.* 2008, 32, 13-18.

[7]   Courvalin, P.; Trieu-Cuot, P. *Clin. Infect. Dis.* 2001, 33, S138-S146.

[8]   Dang, H.; Ren, J.; Song, L.; Sun, S.; An, L. *World J. Micribiol. Biotechnol.* 2008a, 24, 209-217.

[9]   Dang, H.; Ren, J.; Song, L.; Sun, S.; An, L. *Microb. Ecol.* 2008b, 55, 237-246.

[10]   Dang, H.; Song, L.; Chen, M.; Chang, Y. *Microb. Ecol.* 2006a, 52, 634-643.

[11]   Dang, H.; Zhang, X.; Song, L.; Chang, Y.; Yang, G. *Mar. Pollut. Bull.* 2006b, 52, 1494-1503.

[12]   Dang, H.; Zhang, X.; Song, L.; Chang, Y.; Yang, G. *J. Appl. Microbiol.* 2007, 103, 2580-2592.

[13]   Dang, H.; Zhao, J.; Song, L.; Chen, M.; Chang, Y. *Mar. Pollut. Bull.* 2009, 58, 987-994.

[14]   Furushita, M.; Shiba, T.; Maeda, T.; Yahata, M.; Kaneoka, A.; Takahashi, Y.; Torii, K.; Hasegawa, T.; Ohta, M. *Appl. Environ. Microbiol.* 2003, 69, 5336-5342.

[15]   Gay, M.; Renault, T.; Pons, A.M.; Le Roux, F. *Dis. Aquat. Organ.* 2004, 62, 65-74.

[16]   Gomez-Leon, J.; Villamil, L.; Lemos, M.L.; Novoa, B.; Figueras, A. *Appl. Environ. Microbiol.* 2005, 71, 98-104.

[17] Heepngoen, P.; Sajjaphan, K.; Ferguson, J.A.; Sadowsky, M.J. *J. Microbiol. Biotechnol.* 2008, 18, 199-206.

[18] Herwig, R.P.; Gray, J.P.; Weston, D.P. *Aquaculture* 1997, 149, 263-283.

[19] Jacobs, L.; Chenia, H.Y. *Int. J. Food Microbiol.* 2007, 114, 295-306.

[20] Johnson, T.J.; Siek, K.E.; Johnson, S.J.; Nolan, L.K. *Antimicrob. Agents Chemother.* 2005, 49, 4681-4688.

[21] Jun, L.J.; Jeong J.B.; Huh, M.D.; Chung, J.K.; Choi, D.L.; Lee, C.H.; Jeong, H.D. *Aquaculture* 2004, 240, 89-100.

[22] Kim S.R.; Nonaka, L.; Suzuki, S. *FEMS Microbiol. Lett.* 2004, 237, 147-156.

[23] Kummerer, K. *J. Antimicrob. Chemother.* 2004, 54, 311-320.

[24] Le, T.X.; Munekage, Y.; Kato, S. *Sci. Total Environ.* 2005, 349, 95-105.

[25] Li, J.; Yie, J.; Foo, R.W.T.; Ling, J.M.L.; Xu, H.S.; Woo, N.Y.S. *Mar. Pollut. Bull.* 1999, 39, 245-249.

[26] Li, T.W.; Ding, M.J.; Zhang, J.; Xiang, J.H.; Liu, R.Y. *J. Shellfish Res.* 1998, 17, 707-711.

[27] Ma, J.M.; Wang, Q.; Ma, F.H.; Liu, M.Q. *J. Fishery China* 1996, 20, 332-336.

[28] Markestad, A.; Grave, K. *Fish Vaccinol.* 1997, 90, 365-369.

[29] McCallum, H.; Harvell, D.; Dobson, A. *Ecol. Lett.* 2003, 6, 1062-1067.

[30] Miranda, C.D.; Rojas, R. *Rev. Biol. Mar.* 1996, 31, 1-9.

[31] Miranda, C.D.; Rojas, R. *Aquaculture* 2007, 266, 39-46.

[32] Olsen, J.E. *Acta Vet. Scand. Supp.* 1999, 92, 15-22.

[33] Poole, K. *J. Antimicrob. Chemoth.* 2005, 56, 20-51.

[34] Prayitno, S.B.; Latchford, J.W. *Aquaculture* 1995, 132, 105-112.

[35] Rajini Rani, D.B.; Mahadevan, A. *BioMetals* 1992, 5, 73-80.

[36] Schmidt, A.S.; Bruun, M.S.; Dalsgaard, I.; Pedersen, K.; Larsen, J.L. *Appl. Environ. Microbiol.* 2000, 66, 4908-4915.

[37] Schwarz, S.; Kehrenberg, C.; Doublet, B.; Cloeckaert, A. *FEMS Microbiol. Rev.* 2004, 28, 519-542.

[38] Smith P. *Rev. Sci. Tech.* 2008, 27, 243-264.

[39] Sugumar, G.; Nakai, T.; Hirata, Y.; Matsubara, D.; Muroga, K. *Dis. Aquat. Organ.* 1998, 33, 111-118.

[40] Thompson, F.L.; Iida, T.; Swings, J. *Microbiol. Mol. Biol. Rev.* 2004, 68, 3403-3431.

[41] Thompson, J.R.; Pacocha, S.; Pharino, C.; Klepac-Ceraj, V.; Hunt, D.E.; Benoit, J.; Sarma-Rupavtarm, R.; Distel, D.L.; Polz, M.F. *Science* 2005, 307, 1311-1313.

[42] Wang, C.; Dang, H.; Ding, Y. *World J. Microbiol. Biotechnol.* 2008, 24, 2889-2896.

[43] Wang, Y.G.; Zhang, Z.; Qin, L.; Shi, C.Y.; Chen, J.J.; Yang, S.L.; Ma, A.J. *Mar. Fisheries Res.* 2004, 25, 61-68.

[44] White, D.G.; McDermott, P.F. *Curr. Opin. Microbiol.* 2001, 4, 313-317.

[45] WHO. (2006). Report of a joint FAO/OIE/WHO expert consultation on antimicrobial use in aquaculture and antimicrobial resistance. http://www.who.int/topics/foodborne_diseases/aquaculture_rep_13_16june2006%20.pdf

[46] Ye, L.; Yu, K.K.; Wang, R.C.; Liu, L.Y.; Zou, F.G.; Liang, Y.J.; Chen, G. *J. Fishery Sci. China* 1997, 4, 43-48.

[47] Yoo, M.H.; Huh, M.D.; Kim, E.H.; Lee, H.H.; Jeong, H.D. *Aquaculture* 2003, 217, 11-21.

[48] Zhang, G.F.; Que, H.Y.; Liu, X.; Xu, H.S. *J. shellfish Res.* 2004, 23, 947-950.

[49] Zhang, X.X.; Dang, H.Y.; Yang, G.P. *Period. Ocean Univ. China* 2007, 37, 86-90.

In: Antibiotic Resistance...   ISBN 978-1-60741-623-4
Editors: A. R. Bonilla and K. P. Muniz   © 2009 Nova Science Publishers, Inc.

Chapter XII

Antibiotic Resistance as a Method for Determining Sources of Fecal Pollution in Water

Alexandria K. Graves[*,1] *and Charles Hagedorn*[2]
[1]Department of Soil Science, North Carolina State University,
Raleigh, NC, USA
[2]Department of Crop and Soil Environmental Sciences
401 Price Hall, Virginia Tech, Blacksburg, VA, USA

Abstract

Understanding the origin of fecal pollution is essential in assessing potential health risks as well as for determining the actions necessary to remediate the problem of waters contaminated by fecal matter. As a result, microbial source tracking (MST) methods aimed at determining sources of fecal pollution have evolved over the past decade. Antibiotic resistance analysis (ARA) has emerged as one MST tool that has proven useful for determining the sources of fecal pollution in environmental waters.

Antibiotic resistance analysis is a simple, rapid, and inexpensive method for performing MST. It is a published method that has been independently validated by a variety of tests designed to improve library-based methods, and is currently being used in laboratories across the United States as well as internationally.

The ARA method is based on the rationale that antibiotics exert selective pressure on the fecal flora of the animals that ingest antibiotics. Different types of animals receive differential exposure to antibiotics and as a result, different animals will have bacteria with at least reasonably source-specific patterns of antibiotic resistance. The ARA procedure involves the isolation and culturing of a target organism, (usually *Escherichia coli* or *Enterococcus sp.*), then replica plating the isolates on media containing various antibiotics at pre-selected concentrations. After the plates are incubated, the organisms are scored according to their resistance to the antibiotics to generate an antibiotic

* Corresponding author: Phone: 919.513.0635; Fax: 919.515.2167; Email: Alexandria_Graves@ncsu.edu

resistance profile (phenotypic fingerprint). These fingerprints are then evaluated by a multivariate statistical method such as discriminate analysis (DA).

Discriminant analysis classifies the bacteria based on shared patterns of antibiotic resistance, and the results are pooled to form a "known source database" (or library) of antibiotic resistance patterns from different fecal sources. The known source database is summarized in the form of a classification table. The average rate of correct classification is the average rate that known source isolates are correctly classified, and is used to measure the reliability of the library. Additional method performance criteria to ensure the reliability of the database are also used, including library decloning, construction of larger libraries representing more diverse host populations, and realistic tests of method accuracy, such as incorporating independently collected proficiency isolates and samples. Isolates recovered from water samples are compared to the known source database to identify an isolate as being either human or animal derived.

Antibiotic resistance analysis is an MST tool that is most appropriate for small, relatively simple rural watersheds. The application of ARA to large-scale complex systems is more problematic as the wider genetic variability present in target organism populations impacts the phenotypic expression of antibiotic resistance. The potential of this genetic diversity occurring in many different host sources leads to the concern of not being able to fully capture that diversity in a known source library, with subsequent reductions in classification accuracy of water isolates (unknown sources). This is particularly relevant when multiple sources of pollution are contributing to watershed contamination at comparatively similar levels. However, the method performance issues that must be addressed with ARA (and are described in this chapter) are identical for any library-based approach and can also be modified to evaluate library-independent MST methods as well.

This chapter describes the advantages and disadvantages of ARA, presents case studies where the method has been used in a variety of different environmental situations, responds to criticisms of ARA, and details six method performance criteria that should be applied to every MST method. Such evaluations are long overdue in the rapidly developing field of MST.

Introduction

Two major classes of MST methods have been developed and widely used in water quality projects around the world. Known as library-dependent and library-independent approaches, each currently possesses both strengths and weaknesses for source identifications. Library-dependent methods rely on the construction of a host-origin database, or library, of isolates from known fecal sources. Bacterial isolates collected from these known fecal sources are assayed to provide a collection of possible 'fingerprint' patterns that allow for a direct comparison with the fingerprints of isolates of unknown origin (water isolates) using statistical classification algorithms. The rate at which host-origin isolates within the library are correctly classified, using the models generated from those same isolates, is referred to as the rate of correct classification (RCC) for a single category, and the average rate of correct classification (ARCC) for the entire library.

Antibiotic Resistance and MST

MST methods employing antibiotic resistance were some of the earliest developed, and have been deployed in a variety of different watershed environments (Wiggins, 1996; Hagedorn et al., 1999; Parveen et al., 1997; Harwood et al., 2000). The basis of antibiotic resistance analysis (ARA), multiple antibiotic resistance (MAR) and the Kirby-Bauer (KB) disk diffusion methods is that enteric bacterial strains from different host organisms have acquired and retain unique patterns of antibiotic resistance as selected for by the differential exposure of their host-animal to antibiotics or other xenobiotic compounds. Growth of these bacterial isolates in the presence of varying antibiotics and/or concentrations will produce a 'fingerprint' pattern unique to a specific, or group of, host animals. Use of different panels of antibiotics in humans and domestic animals, as well as antibiotics added to many types of animal feeds has likely selected for resistant strains, and resistance is also seen in strains from wild animals as well, but typically at greatly reduced levels (Butaye et al., 2001; Sayah et al., 2005). Following early work by Kaspar et al., 1990, studies have confirmed the existence of quantifiable and consistent differences in the antibiotic resistance patterns of streptococci isolated from the feces of a variety of host organisms (Wiggins 1996; Wiggins et al., 1999). While enterococci have received the most application in antibiotic resistance studies, both *E. coli* and fecal coliforms (FCs) have been employed as well (Hagedorn et al., 1999; Harwood et al., 2000; Whitlock et al., 2002).

All current antibiotic resistance methods are culture-based, requiring the physical isolation of the organism, followed by inoculation onto a variety of antibiotics and/or antibiotic concentrations. Individual isolates are assessed as to their resistance/susceptibility to different antibiotics at pre-selected concentrations. Although typically scored by hand, at least one study has attempted to develop an automated version (Ebdon et al., 2004) using the PhenePlate™ system plate reader (PhPlate AB, Stockholm, Sweden). Following evaluations of growth patterns among isolates, results are generally converted to binary data (1 or 0) representing growth or no growth, respectively. Data are characterized using a statistical algorithm, typically discriminate analysis (DA) to generate a model that identifies the fingerprint patterns of isolates of unknown origin collected from environmental water samples (Wiggins, 1996). Several protocol variations employing antibiotic resistance have been evaluated as MST tools.

Antibiotic Resistance Method Variations

ARA has been the most commonly used library-dependent MST method and has undergone widespread field application. In ARA, isolates are cultured in microtiter plates and then replica plated onto between 20 and 40 media plates (typically trypticase soy agar) containing different antibiotics and concentrations, allowing for the simultaneous evaluation of up to 48 isolates. ARA has consistently demonstrated effectiveness in small watersheds (Hagedorn et al., 1999; Graves et al., 2002; Booth et al., 2003) and on modest budgets (Crozier et al., 2002), and has shown success in moderately-sized and/or mixed-used watersheds, especially those with just one dominant source (Burnes, 2003; Carroll et al.,

2005; Dickerson et al., 2007b, Graves et al., 2007). However, questions concerning the ability of the method to discriminate between sources in large, urban watersheds have been raised (Moore et al., 2005).

In one of the first field applications, Hagedorn et al., 1999 assembled a known-source library of 7,058 fecal streptococci (FS) isolates from known human, livestock, and wildlife sources in Montgomery County, VA, achieving an average rate of correct classification (ARCC) of 87% for the three-way classification split. Application of this library to Page Brook in Clarke Co., VA identified cattle with unrestricted stream access as the dominant contributing source. An average reduction of 94% in FS counts was achieved by fencing streams and installing watering stations within pastures.

In additional Virginia studies, Graves et al., 2002 identified the appearance of enterococci of human origin in Spout Run, a small Virginia stream, as it passed through the non-sewered community of Millwood; with the human signature fading in the stream with increasing distance from the town. Booth et al., 2003, using a library of 1,451 enterococci isolates, employed ARA as a means to identify livestock as the dominant fecal source in the Blackwater River, in Virginia as part of a Total Maximum Daily Load (TMDL) project. Within the coastal region of Virginia, Dickerson et al., 2007b used ARA with DA and logistic regression to identify human fecal pollution at two Virginia beaches, and monitor successful remediation efforts over two consecutive summers.

Within the tropical waters of Florida, Harwood et al., 2000 used ARA to classify fecal pollution from a variety of animal sources in coastal waters using libraries with ARCCs of 63.9% and 62.3% for FC and enterococci, respectively. A study in Stevenson Creek in Clearwater, FL by Whitlock et al., 2002, using an ARA library of 2398 FCs, identified wildlife as the dominant fecal source when coliform counts were high and human when counts were low.

In mixed-use watersheds, Burnes 2003 used six antibiotics and a library of 1125 FCs isolates to identify chickens and livestock as the major contributors to fecal contamination in a mixed-use Georgia watershed. Choi et al., 2003 used ARA to identify birds as the dominant fecal source (vs urban runoff sources) in at Huntington Beach, CA, achieving a library ARCC above 80%.

Internationally, Carroll et al., 2005 used eight different antibiotics to generate fingerprints for a library of 717 *E. coli* isolates from humans, wildlife, domestic animals, and livestock in the Gold Coast region, Queensland State, Australia. Results indicated that sources in rural areas were dominantly non-human, while isolates classified as human in origin increased dramatically in urban areas where septic tanks predominated. Edge and Hill, 2005 identified birds as a primary fecal contributor to the waters of Bayfront Park in Hamilton, Ontario using an *E. coli* library with an ARCC of 68% for bird and wastewater sources.

In multiple antibiotic resistance (MAR), isolates are replica plated on multiple plates, each containing a single concentration of an antibiotic and results are based on the highest level of resistance for each isolate. Early in method development, Parveen et al., 1997, using 10 different antibiotics, concluded that *E. coli* MAR profiles were capable of discriminating between point and nonpoint sources of pollution in isolates collected from Apalachicola Bay, FL. Kelsey et al., 2003 used MAR analyses of *E. coli* isolates to determine that the fecal pollution in a South Carolina estuary was not human in origin, even in areas surrounded by clusters of active septic tanks.

In another South Carolina study, Webster et al., 2004 used MAR to successfully differentiate human- and wildlife-derived *E. coli*. Vantarakis et al., 2006 used MAR with cluster and DA to separate 128 *E. coli* isolates collected from humans and animals in southwestern Greece, achieving an ARCC of 99.2%. In a recent study employing multiple MST methods, *E. coli* MAR was used in conjunction with human-specific molecular markers for *Bacteroides* and *Enterococcus faceium* at two Lake Erie beaches in Ohio. Results among all methods were consistent in determining that mixed bird and wastewater fecal sources were the likely contributors to the fecal impairment of beach waters (Francy et al., 2006).

Use of the Kirby-Bauer (KB) tests, where antibiotic susceptibility is assessed by zones of clearing around antibiotic impregnated disks on a plate inoculated with a specific bacterial strain, has only been reported in a method comparison study (Harwood et al., 2003). Initial results found this method poorly identified fecal sources in blind water samples, and further testing was suspended.

Current Status of Antibiotic Resistance and MST

The widespread application of antibiotic resistance patterns in field studies can be contributed largely to the relative simplicity with which each isolates can be fingerprinted, the suitability of the method for different fecal indicator bacteria (FIB), the lack of specialized equipment required, and the ability to rapidly fingerprint a large number of isolates. All of these factors are desirable as researchers discovered the diversity of FIB populations present even within small watersheds (Stewart et al., 2003), and recognized the need to collect large numbers of isolates and samples to achieve a representative population, avoiding errors generated by under sampling (Choi et al. 2003). However, the need to collect and maintain a large host-origin library is also a major disadvantage for all library-based MST methods.

In two attempts to assess the temporal stability of fingerprint patterns used for library construction, Wiggins et al., 2003 and Dickerson et al., 2007b, used a variety of procedures with ARA to prove the stability of patterns for at least a one- and two-year period, respectively (See section on Persistence of Antibiotic Resistance).

Questions of method effectiveness have been raised in method comparison (MC) studies, as well as individual reports. Unfortunately, most negative reports based conclusions on results obtained from a relatively small collection of isolates. Guan et al., 2002 created MAR profiles of 319 *E. coli* isolates, and found that only 46% of the livestock isolates, 95% of the wildlife isolates, and 55% of livestock isolates were correctly classified. Samadpour et al., 2005 determined ARA was less successful at discriminating between sources that ribotyping based on a collection of 120 *E. coli* isolates.

In addition, the reproducibility and stability of antibiotic resistance patterns has been questioned (Parveen et al., 1999), but remains unconfirmed. Moore et al., 2005 found problems repeating ARA patterns in a subset of isolates fingerprinted over several days, a problem also encountered in most library-based methods, as well as ARA (Stoeckel et al., 2004).

Method Comparison Studies

Three multi-laboratory, independently-evaluated method comparison (MC) studies have been conducted to date. The first, sponsored by the Southern California Coastal Water Research Project (SCCRWP) encompassed a wide variety of both library-dependent and – independent methods, attempting to identify fecal sources from southern California (Griffith et al., 2003). The second study, sponsored by the United States Geological Survey (USGS), involved only library-dependent methods, and used *E. coli* isolates collected from West Virginia (Stoeckel, et al., 2004). The final MC study was conducted in Europe focusing solely in library-independent methods (will not be considered further in this chapter) and attempted identification of human and farm wastewaters from Spain, France, Sweden, Cyprus, and the U.K. (Blanch et al., 2006).

The SCCWRP MC Study

The primary goal of the SCCRWP MC study was the evaluation of numerous MST protocols for the detection, or identification of fecal sources present in laboratory-created, blind water samples. With 11 total sponsors, including public health and sanitation districts, a primary focus for all methods involved was the ability to correctly identify the presence, or absence, of human fecal pollution. The additional identification of the dominant fecal material within samples, and ability to detect all sources present in a sample, were applied to largely library-dependent methods, as well as selected library-independent methods with protocols capable of distinguishing between a greater variety of sources. Results of this study were published in a series of seven papers (Field et al., 2003, Griffith et al., 2003, Harwood et al, 2003, Myoda et al., 2003, Noble et al, 2003, Ritter et al., 2003, Stewart et al., 2003).

Of the three MC studies, the SCCRWP study tested the widest variety of protocols, selecting 22 different researchers to analyze blind water samples using 12 different MST methods, often with several variations on each. Source-tracking methods involved in the study included both phenotypic and genotypic library-dependent methods, as well a variety of library-independent methods. The SCCRWP study was only MC study to examine the ability of library-independent methods to identify the host origins of fecal pollution. Just the library-dependent results are described here as the other methods are outside the scope of this chapter.

All methods tested used water matrix samples (fresh, salt, and brackish) created in a laboratory to contain fecal material from a single, or combination of animal sources. These samples were constructed using feces directly from humans, birds, cattle, dogs or sewage influent collected in Southern California. Only the methods detecting *Escherichia coli* toxin-genes, adenovirus, and the library-based pulsed-field gel electrophoresis (PFGE) were not tested by at least two separate laboratories. However within the study the use of identical methods at different labs could not be considered replicates, as the protocols and data analysis were not standardized and varied between laboratories.

Results of the phenotypic and genotypic library-based methods were published in separate papers (Harwood et al., 2003; Myoda et al., 2003). A negative aspect of this approach was the reporting of data in different forms and with different procedural variations applied in the final data analyses. This oversight makes the direct comparison across the method categories difficult.

The phenotypic methods investigated (Harwood et al., 2003) include four ARA protocols each selecting a different set or subset of indicator organisms, including enterococci, *E. coli*, fecal coliforms, and fecal streptococci. Similar in protocols, the concentrations and antibiotics selected varied for each ARA method, as did the researcher's criteria for considering bacterial growth as positive or negative. Two carbon source utilization methods using *E. coli* and fecal streptococci were also included, as were the MAR and Kirby-Bauer antibiotic susceptibility tests, both with *E. coli*.

The genotypic portion of the study (Myoda et al., 2003) selected six researchers to employ one or more of three MST methods. The popular rep-PCR was performed by three researchers all using the fecal indicator *E. coli* and BOXA1R primers. Ribotyping was also selected for use by three investigators; with two using the restriction endonuclease *Eco*RI on *E. coli* and the third using *Pst*I for enterococci. The final genotypic method selected was PFGE, in which the sole researcher elected to use the enzyme *XBa*I on isolates of *E. coli*. Although procedures were often similar, variations existed in the similarity thresholds (none were used in phenotypic study) required for a positive identification (e.g. 80% matches) as well as both the selection and analyses of banding patterns produced.

The average accuracy for all known source isolates was high for the majority of the methods, ranging from 78% to 100%, with only the Kirby-Bauer test falling below this range, correctly identifying less than 50% of sources present. However, for all methods the percentage of false-positives was high. A later attempt to improve results in the data analysis phase was the application of a minimum detectable percentage (MDP), or a minimum percentage of isolates which must be classified within a source category for that source to be considered relevant. A MDP of 5% showed a slight decrease in false positives, while the application of a 15% cut-off level decreased false positives substantially for most of the methods.

Within the genotypic study, in general, the false negatives were low, however, this was due mainly to the abundance of false positives reported. Although no matrix sample contained fecal material from all four potential sources, collectively, the genotypic methods indicated all four sources were present in 37% of the samples analyzed. Overall two of the ribotyping methods and PFGE produced the lowest numbers of false positives and the highest number of true negatives (both used 100% similarity thresholds), and the lowest number of isolates that could not be classified.

In evaluations based strictly for the ability to correctly identify the dominant source in a water sample (unreported in the phenotypic study), most genotypic methods performed reasonably well, correctly identifying the dominant source in greater than two-thirds of the total water samples. When the identified secondary source was included, dominant source identification of five of the seven methods increased by 10% or more.

Conclusions of the SCCWRP MC study were (1) optimize existing MST methods, (2) improve quality control techniques in laboratories, (3) evaluate library size issues, and (4) consider the effects of geographic variability. The SCCWRP authors recommended the use of multiple methods when attempting to perform MST in natural waters. The SCCWRP study did result in a major change in MST. Realization of the difficulty in establishing adequate libraries even for small watersheds focused the attention of the MST community on the need for accurate library-independent methods.

The USGS MC Study

The goal of the USGS MC study was an evaluation of the ability of seven library-based MST protocols to correctly identify *E. coli* isolates of unknown origin using identical known-source libraries (Stoeckel et al., 2004). Method effectiveness was determined by the correct source classification of pre-selected individual isolates, as opposed to the general source category identification of randomly selected isolates from a laboratory inoculated water sample, as was the case in the SCCWRP study. The success of a given protocol was assessed through the ability to correctly classify three categories of blind isolates: those already present within the library (REPLICATE), those not present but from a source animal represented in the library (ACCURACY), and those from a source animal not present in the library (RINGER).

One MST researcher was selected for each method to perform the necessary protocols for ARA, carbon source utilization, ribotyping (with *Hin*dIII or *Eco*RI), PFGE, BOX-PCR, and rep-PCR. Known-source libraries were constructed from fecal samples collected within Berkeley County, WV, where scat was collected and *E. coli* isolates were obtained centrally for distribution to individual laboratories. Libraries of 900 identical isolates were constructed from nine sources (human, beef cattle, dairy cattle, chickens, swine, white-tailed deer, horses, dogs, and Canada geese). However, researchers using carbon sources, ribotyping-*Hin*dIII, and rep-PCR elected to use a smaller subset of 630 isolates drawn from the 900 (due to costs).

Focusing strictly on the ability of a method to correctly classify blind isolates, three distinct collections of isolates (REPLICATE, ACCURACY, and RINGER), and three source-level splits (2-way, human and non-human; 3-way, human, livestock and wildlife; and 8-way, human cattle, chickens, swine, deer, horses, dogs, and geese) were used to assess method effectiveness. Identical sets of blind isolates, collected post-library construction were provided to researchers for source identification. REPLICATE and ACCURACY results will be discussed as these included evaluations of antibiotic resistance analysis data.

The REPLICATE set should have allowed for the correct identification of the majority of isolates tested (although ARCCs were not reported), as all 26 isolates were present within the libraries of each method. However, the results were extremely varied and the percentage of correctly identified isolates using the 8-level split ranged from 13% (Ribotyping-*Hin*dIII) to 100% (PFGE). ARA had a percent correct classification rate of 23%.

A total of 150 isolates, composing the ACCURACY test, were provided to researchers to evaluate method classification of non-library isolates. Only the ARA, CUP, RT-*Hin*dIII, and BOX-PCR attempted to classify all isolates provided. The ARA procedure produced the highest classification rate of only 27% for the 8-way split. Of those methods employing thresholds, Ribotyping-*Eco*I only attempted 5% of isolates provided, but correctly classified 90%.

Classification rates increased for all methods using the 3 source-level split. The highest averages of those attempting to classify all isolates was BOX-PCR at 48%, and of those not attempting all isolates, RT-*Eco*I successful classifying 100% of the 6% of isolates attempted. ARA correctly classified 39% of the isolates. Classification based on 2 source-levels again increased classification rates. The highest average of those attempting to classify all isolates was REP-PCR at 77% and ARA had a correct classification rate of 55%, while of the methods not attempting the classification all isolates, RT-*Eco*I again, correctly identified 100% of the 6% of isolates attempted.

Library sizes, although greatly increased in size from the SCCWRP study, were still deemed too small to accurately represent an entire county watershed, with scats samples from only 20 host organisms used per source category. As the diversity of *E. coli* genotypes and phenotypes present in the scat of warm-blooded animals currently remains poorly understood, the standardization of isolates used in the library and challenge sets of this study allowed for increased confidence in contrasting results. Issues in quality assurance/quality control (QA/QC) described in the SCCRWP study should have prompted the enlistment of at least one replicate lab for each protocol tested. The employment of replicate protocols would have provided information in method reproducibility beyond the results of the REPLICATE test. Temporal strain variability, as acknowledged by researchers, may have also played a role in the low number isolates correctly identified from the ACCURACY set, which was collected nine months after samples used in library construction.

The single most significant result of the USGS study revealed the lack of knowledge among the MST community concerning known-source library construction. As pointed out in the study recommendations, better host species representation was needed in the libraries. An additional recommendation was the development of better methods, although in light of the library representativeness problems, a retesting of some library-dependent methods may be warranted once greater understanding of how to best build a known-source library has been established.

Lessons from both the SCCWRP and USGS MC studies should be taken with an understanding that the source-tracking community did not understand the diversity of bacteria or abundance of viruses and chemical markers likely to be present in host organisms and/or natural waters. This is still unresolved. Questions relating to MST that must be addressed in the future include issues of fecal abundance and source-specificity of tracers. For those engaged specifically in bacterial source tracking, issues of host and environmental strain prevalence, library-size, as well as temporal, seasonal, geographic, and within-host variability of fecal indicator communities must also be addressed.

Limitations and Unanswered Questions in MST

Strain Variability

After more than a decade of research into MST methods and applications, the most effective means to construct a known-source library (such as those developed in ARA), or collect isolates to test a suspected library-independent method, still remains largely unknown. Although certain aspects have received minor attention, library-based methods have relied on untested assumptions, and generally ignored research that does not support the current direction of source-tracking. The sole purpose of a known-source library is to provide a collection of 'fingerprints' in which to reference environmental isolates of unidentified origin. Isolates of known-origin are most commonly obtained through the collection of fecal scat, sewage, or septage samples; however questions remain concerning how, when, and where isolates should be obtained for library construction or library-independent marker testing (Table 1).

Known-Source Collection

Only a few publications report the number of isolates obtained from each scat/sewage sample, although this should be reported in every source tracking paper, including those based on library independent methods. The studies that report these numbers typically used from 1 to 5 isolates per sample (Dombek et al., 2000; Albert et al., 2003; Hagedorn et al., 2003; McLellan et al., 2003; Johnson, et al., 2004; Moore et al., 2005; Dickerson et al., 2007b) although some have used numbers as high as 20 to 32 (Graves et al., 2002; Ahmed et al., 2005). It has been suggested that a dominant *E. coli* strain exists in individuals (McLellan et al., 2003), however the results of the SCWWRP study seemed to indicate that five isolates from each fecal samples is probably inadequate to account for the variability within one host organism. Classification rates were generally low among all methods when attempting to identify additional isolates collected from the library-building scat samples. The single exception was the success of classifying isolates of human origin, an anomaly with several possible explanations. One possibility is the imbalance of the libraries, as isolates of human origin were represented by twice as many isolates as any other single category, and represented 40% of the total library, which can tend to bias classifications (Ritter and Robinson, 2004). Another plausible explanation is that the use of 60 isolates from a single untreated sewage sample was sufficient to account for the variability within that one sample.

Studies using PFGE have shown that only an average of 12 distinct patterns exists within a single sewage sample of less than 1 L (Simmons et al., 2002; O'Brien et al., 2005). A single sewage influent sample likely consists of fecal material from a relatively small number of individuals; however no studies have been conducted to determine the diversity of isolates in sewage samples collected over regular hourly, daily, or seasonal intervals from a single sewage treatment plant. The USGS study, also using 5 isolates from each fecal sample, suffered from similar poor classification rates among all methods involved. Although challenge set isolates were obtained from different scat/fecal samples than those used for library construction, the considerably larger (than the SCCWRP library) 630- or 900-isolate library still proved insufficient.

Several studies have reported higher than expected diversity in *E. coli* isolated from farm animals. In a sample of 481 isolates, 240 different ribotype patterns were observed in two herds of cattle (Jenkins et al., 2003). Isolates collected from cattle, swine, chicken and horses in Georgia and Idaho, displayed 213 ribotypes in a collection of 568 *E. coli* isolates (Hartel et al., 2002). A sampling of *E. coli* diversity from pigs found an average of 2.4 phenotypes per 9.5 strains tested from an individual (Katouli et al., 1995). Using rep-PCR, Lu et al., 2005, predicted that approximately 60 different genotypes may be present in single herd of swine or dairy cattle on a given day. Analysis of two collections taken from manure holding tanks on these swine or cattle farms yielded estimates that between 70-158 genotypes were likely present (Lu et al., 2005). Using PCR-based methods, a required 32 isolates per individual was deemed sufficient for fecal characterization of sewage, horse, cow, gull, and dog fecal samples (Seurinck et al., 2005).

These studies indicate that a larger sampling of isolates per fecal sample may be necessary for account for the variability within a single individual, with size likely dependent on the MST method employed. The possibility of such variability within a single host raises questions concerning how much of the reported geographic variability is a result of actual differences in the individuals from different areas, and how much is by pure chance, as studies generally collected far less than 32 isolates per individual for analyses. Although largely uninvestigated, the possibility of dominant strains within an individual may still prove to be geographically dependent as seen in one library-independent method (Hamilton et al., 2006). However, once outside of the host animals, some strains may come to dominate in an environmental setting such as a septic system (Gordon, 2001) or irrigation water (Lu et al., 2004), and the once dominant intra-host strain may display an increasing die-off rate relative to less prevalent strains under environmental conditions.

One suggestion to help increase library diversity is the collection of both fresh and dry manure from livestock (Weaver et al., 2005). Dry manure is generally more abundant on farms, and *E. coli* and fecal streptococcus populations showed a decrease in numbers over time in scat from horse, sheep and cattle populations. Thus, the collection of both dried and fresh scat may increase library diversity and yield information about the differential survival of strains outside the host organism. However, in a different study by Graves et al., 2007 used the Biolog™ system to identify enterococci at the species level in both dry and fresh livestock manure. No significant differences were detected in species survival rates within the environment. The conclusion was made that, the frequency of enterococci species likely to enter waterways would be consistent with those found in collected manure samples and used for the construction of known-source libraries. However, the possibility exists that differences in strain survival are present, but undetectable using the Biolog™ system and by only looking at the species level (Table 1).

Strain Overlap

Further compounding source identification is the possibility of genetic and phenotypic strain overlap between host-sources (Table 1). Using rep-PCR, shared banding patterns have been observed between gulls and sewage samples (McLellan et al., 2003) and overlapping phenotypic profiles were observed for human and livestock in the European MC study (Blanch et al., 2006). The potential acquisition of new strains from external sources also requires the consideration of source-tracking researchers. Although a study from Kenya isolated distinct strains of *E. coli* from children living in close proximity to chickens (Kariuki et al., 1999), other publications point to the possibility of acquiring and incorporating environmentally persistent strains into an individual's intestinal flora. Gulls have been shown to contain an incredible diversity of strains (Fogarty et al., 2003), possibly resulting from the feeding habits of these birds that frequent areas of polluted rivers, water treatment facilities or areas containing human trash, such as landfills. New strains may also be obtained from ingested food and water. Further supporting the idea of this acquired diversity is a study that found the range of genotypes present in a single mouse increased as the age increased (Gordon, 1997), suggesting the acquisition of long-term enteric residents over time. Additionally, *E. coli* from an isolated subset of a litter of pigs found more similarity among *E. coli* from the isolated litter than other members of the same litter that had mixed with other pigs (Katouli et al, 1995).

Geographic Variability

Issues of geographic variability in fecal indicator strains isolated from identical host species have been a major concern of ARA and other library–dependent methods, and a largely untested aspect of library-independent methods (Table 1). A study of 568 *E. coli* isolates from Idaho and Georgia (3 locations) from cattle, swine, chicken and horses found that similarity in strains decreased with increasing geographic distance for cattle and horses (although not for swine and chickens; Hartel et al., 2002). Additional difficulties have also been encountered in attempts to distinguish between farm animals in Florida over a large region (Scott et al., 2003). Using isolates collected from mice inhabiting two geographically isolated farms, some *E. coli* genotypes that were dominant at one farm proved to be very rare at the other, thus demonstrating localized geographic variability (Gordon, 1997). It has been widely assumed that geographic variability could be circumvented with library-independent approaches, and field applications continue to be reported with these methods even though this assumption remains largely unproven. One recent study demonstrated that sets of *E. coli*-based library-independent markers found in waterfowl were geographically limited, although it is not known if this reported regional specificity will apply to other sources or other organisms (Hamilton et al., 2006).

Seasonal/Temporal Variability

Additional questions still remain concerning when to collect known-source samples for library construction when using ARA, as well as other library dependent methods. Issues of seasonal or temporal variability have received only minor attention, and application of these principles has generally not been reported within the literature. Inadvertently, the USGS MC study raised the concern for seasonal variability of enteric communities within host organisms. The nine-month separation between the collection of library isolates and the collection of what would be the challenge set of isolates was suggested as a possibility for the poor performance of those methods tested. A study of sewage-isolated *E. coli* saw significant changes in strain prevalence over four months (Pupo and Richardson, 1995), although sample sizes were generally small. Similar results were seen in populations of mice over a period of 6 months (Gordon, 1997). In addition, dietary changes have been shown to shift enteric populations in rats, pigs, cattle and humans (Silvi et al., 1999; Leser et al., 2000; Russell et al., 2000; McDonald et al., 2001). Katouli et al., 1995, tested isolates obtained from individual pigs through their life and concluded that *E. coli* populations changed over the lifetime of the pigs. A dietary influence on *E. coli* populations was found in deer, with the nutritionally diverse wild deer displaying a greater variety of genotypes than those in captivity (Hartel et al., 2003).

More diversity was seen in dairy cattle or swine manure holding tanks than from individuals on the farm, and may represent a temporal variability as enteric populations shift, and tanks receive additional input throughout the year (Lu et al., 2005). For known-source collections assuming that, as the seasonal food supply of wildlife changes, enteric populations undergo a shift as well, may warrant the simultaneous collections of both water and scat samples (Table 1).

Environmental Persistence

Further compounding the efforts of an MST researcher to collect isolates representative of the fecal pollution in an area may be bacterial survival in soils, sediments or on vegetation. Both *E. coli* and enterococci have been found to survive at least 19 weeks from cow manure in soil at temps from 9-21°C (Lau and Ingham, 2001). The pathogenic *E. coli* O157:H7, following land application, was recoverable from up to 6 weeks post-application on vegetation (Avery et al., 2005) and 15 weeks in soil (Ogden et al., 2002). Cow manure is believed to provide a substantial *E. coli* contribution for overland runoff for periods greater than 30 days (Muirhead et al., 2005). Such increased persistence in the soil and potential to enter natural waters in surface runoff may require MST researchers to begin collecting source samples in a watershed several months before collecting water samples, the opposite approach for what may be necessary to account for season/temporal variability (preceding section and Table 1).

Within streambed sediments, *E. coli* has been reported to remain viable for up to 6 weeks (Jamieson et al., 2005), lending further support to the idea of early known-source collections. Survival of *E. coli* in filtered irrigation water was found to exceed 8 weeks, however survival rates differed between strains, with one of the three strains tested increasing in relative percentage over the 8 week period (Lu et al., 2004). The survival of *E. coli* for greater than 28 days in coastal sediments has been observed (Craig et al., 2004) noting that survival is improved at lower temperatures. Resuspension of sediments and release of bacteria into the water column is considered to be primarily the result of wave action (LeFevre and Lewis, 2003). This may require researchers to begin library collecting known-source samples even earlier in colder areas or in field projects spanning primarily winter months.

Differences have been observed between *E. coli* strain persistence in freshwater (Anderson et al., 2005) with these differences in modeled systems failing to represent the true fecal inputs into a water body (Barnes and Gordon, 2004). However, as the relative risk of a water body is currently determined for fecal pollution strictly based on the prevalence of indicator organisms (USEPA, 1986), source tracking protocols employing the recommended fecal indicators should provide a means to lower bacterial counts nevertheless.

Library Representativeness

The use of average rate of correct classification (ARCC) and average frequency of misclassification (AFM) to assess predictive abilities has resulted in the construction and application of potentially undersized and non-representative known-source libraries. Although few studies have been conducted to date, results have shown that small libraries tend to have better internal classification rates than larger libraries (Dickerson et al., 2007a), but are generally less capable of correctly identifying non-library isolates than their larger counterparts (Wiggins, et. al., 2003).

In the post-MC field of source-tracking, all testing or field applications of MST methods should now report an assessment of method/library competence using a validation set of known-source isolates (Harwood et al., 2003; Stoeckel et al., 2004: Moore et al., 2005; Dickerson et al., 2007b). However, since the publication of the final U.S.-based MC study in 2004, the willingness to employ a validation set in library-based applications has been largely ignored.

Application has been sporadic, ranging from collection of isolates specifically for validation (Moore et al., 2005), to use of a holdout set of library isolates (Wiggins et al., 2003; Carroll et al., 2005), to the failure to apply a validation set of any kind (e.g. Ahmed et al., 2005; Edge and Hill, 2005; Shehane et al., 2005).

The optimal size of a known-source library for a given watershed is likely dependent on the MST method(s) selected. Any future attempts to determine library size should also be accompanied by a validation set. Moore et al., 2005 used a set of 97 *E. coli* and 99 *Enterococcus* isolates to assess the capabilities of ribotype library consisting of 997 *E. coli* isolates, as well as two ARA libraries of 3657 *Enterococcus* and 3477 *E. coli* isolates. Using ARCC as the desired level of proficiency, only the *Enterococcus* ARA library was able to correctly classify both internal and external validation sets equally well, although ARCC was generally low for the library itself (44%).

The recommendation of validation set application in this chapter is consistent with the recommendations from both MC studies. Using a hold-out sample of isolates from an ARA library, Wiggins et al., 2003 reported that only the largest library, of 2931 isolates, was able to reach acceptable ARCC levels. Using a smaller, 717 isolate *E. coli* ARA library with a high correct classification rate (89.2%) and a human/non-human split, a hold-out, cross-validation ARCC of 93.2% was achieved (Carroll et al., 2005), however fecal samples were obtained from a potentially undersized sampling of fecal sources.

Based primarily on reasons discussed in previous sections, some general guidelines should be applied to validation set applications. The potential for environmental persistence indicates that known-source fecal acquisition should begin prior to the collection of initial water samples. Efforts to avoid potential seasonal variability warrants the collection of all validation set isolates simultaneously with both the library and water sample isolates.

None of the validation set isolates should be obtained from the same fecal scat sample used to construct the library. Multiple isolates from the same sample may possess identical genotypes or phenotypes, and a potential biasing of challenge set isolates may occur. Use of the internal classification ability (ARCC and AFM) as seen in Moore et al., 2005, should serve as the desired external classification standard for assessing library representativeness.

Source Tracking Issues with ARA and Potential Solutions

Persistence of Antibiotic Resistance

Early in the development of MST protocols, a criticism of ARA was introduced that was based on antibiotic resistance patterns being less stabile for library construction than genotypic patterns (Parveen et al., 1999), and thus represented an inferior long-term source-tracking tool. However, since that time evidence has not emerged supporting the temporal instability of antibiotic resistance patterns, nor has evidence been reported to advocate the stability over time of genotypic patterns in MST applications. The only MST publications to assess temporal stability concluded that the antibiotic resistance patterns used for known-source library construction were stable over periods of one and two years (Wiggins et al., 2003; Dickerson et al., 2007b). In the short-term, antibiotic resistance was found to persist in enteric bacteria isolated from swine manure lagoons (Graves, pers. comm.). Although still debated within the MST community, the long-term stability of antibiotic resistant enteric bacteria has been clearly demonstrated by medical and public health researchers.

One such study has shown that antibiotic resistance is prevalent within some (unexposed) wild animal populations, concluding that a discontinuity in the supply of antibiotics to animals harboring resistant strains is unlikely to decrease populations of resistant microbes (Gilliver et al., 1999). Antibiotic resistant genes are considered stable even in the absence of obvious antibiotic selections pressures (Salyers and Amábile-Cuevas, 1997), making them difficult to eliminate from enteric populations.

In a comparative study of oral streptococci obtained from healthy Mexican and Cuban volunteers, researchers found that in Mexico, where antibiotics are freely available (and used in agriculture), multi-drug resistance was high. Streptococci isolates from Cuba, where antibiotics have been tightly controlled since 1990 (having very limited availability and no agricultural application), displayed similar resistance profiles to those found in Mexico, implying retention of resistance genes over more than a decade (Díaz-Mejía et al., 2002).

Genes encoding resistance to the antibiotic chloramphenicol were found in poultry broiler litter despite its discontinued use for greater than 15 years (Lu et al., 2003). Recent evidence has refuted claims that the retention of resistance genes reduces bacterial fitness (Björkman et al., 2000). In the environment, antibiotic resistance genes have been found to provide a selective advantage in systems polluted with heavy metals (McArthur et al., 2000) or organic solvents (Li et al., 1998). Thus, the antibiotic resistance would seem to provide suitable stability (although possibly geographically restrictive) for MST employment over extended periods of time. Genotypic libraries have shown geographic limitations, however, strain variability and limited sample sizes may have unfairly skewed these results; larger libraries will be required to fully test this contention.

Method Reproducibility

Reproducibility has proven to be problematic for both genotypic and phenotypic library-based methods. Poor method reproduction was seen in six of the seven protocols used in the USGS study (Stoeckel et al., 2004). Of the limited studies addressing the duplication of results, problems were found in both ARA and ribotyping methods when performed in the same lab over multiple days (Moore et al., 2005). Only limited research, however, has been conducted to assess the variability of identical protocols in generating fingerprint patterns across independent laboratories (Lefrense et al., 2004). The relative complexity of genotypic methods, as compared to most phenotypic methods requires increasing quality control and expertise, and may limit application to only select laboratories. As widespread application to water quality issues is a major goal of source-tracking, reproducibility across labs is becoming increasingly important. State regulatory agencies closely regulate and certify labs that conduct water quality monitoring where the results could be used for regulatory purposes, and such agencies will expect the same levels of quality control and reproducibility from source tracking labs (Table 1).

Method Costs and Related Issues

Using any MST method also involves dealing with the cost per isolate of performing the analyses (factoring in the price of equipment, materials, and trained staff). These costs need to be considered for watershed analysis when evaluating appropriate library and sample size concerns. Pulsed-field gel electrophoresis, although considered by both MC studies to be one of the most accurate options, also features a high per isolate cost and a very slow turnaround time (Hager, 2001a), potentially limiting construction of a representative library and analyses of a sufficient number of isolates per sample. With varying degrees of severity, these fiscal and temporal problems exist for numerous genotypic methods. One source-tracking researcher using ribotyping has received criticism for using only two to three isolates per water sample (Hager, 2001b).

Phenotypic methods, such as ARA, have seen increased application for field studies as the method requires only basic laboratory equipment, minimal personal training, and a turn-around time of about one week (Hager, 2001a). In addition, ARA is suitable for inexpensive testing of the large number of isolates required for simultaneous library building and water samples analyses. The ability of phenotypic methods to produce rapid and high-volume results can allow for the simultaneous construction of a known-source library with a field application; a limiting factor in the usage of many genotypic methods. While library-independent methods may offer a less expensive alternative to the analyses of thousands of isolates, these methods still have problems with rates of false-negatives, due to scarcity of the target bacteria or viruses in open waters, from host sources (Soule et al., 2006), or outside of a geographic range (Hamilton et al., 2006). Additionally, means of quantification (Field et al., 2003) and correlation to fecal indicators has yet to be established (Jiang et al., 2001). However, in their current forms these methods still make desirable methods (when applicable) for validation of results (Table 1).

Performance Criteria

Stoeckel and Harwood (2007) recently proposed a standardized approach to implementing MST projects that included performance criteria plus recommendations for field study design. The goal of performance criteria is to be able to evaluate any particular source tracking method (biological or chemical) in such a way that a decision can be made regarding its performance, and then the method either retained as an option (with its strengths and weaknesses quantified), or discarded as ineffective. We propose that every method should be evaluated against the following six performance criteria, largely mirroring those suggested for microbial-based methods (USEPA 2007). The first two criteria are focused on whether any single method is inherently appropriate, while the latter four describe criteria for measuring and assessing the method.

i. Specificity

Specificity is best described in terms of false positive and false negative rates. The false positive approach determines if the method is significantly more likely or less likely to detect non-target organisms or other sample constituents that could be reported as the target organism when compared to the reference method. To assess whether the false positive rates are significant, replicates known to contain non-target organisms that could be falsely identified as the target organism should be analyzed. The determination that the samples do not contain the target organism should be based on a third independent test. For example, if the target organism is cultured *E. coli*, the test should be used against at least other enterobacteria and, depending on what the test is, potentially gram positive organisms as well. If the test is for genetic material, then the primers and probes should be tested against Genbank to look for potential false positives from non-*E. coli* species with the same sequences.

Specificity also includes the false negative issue that deals with whether the new method is significantly more likely or less likely to exhibit non-detections for samples containing the target organism or to exhibit results that are biased low when compared to the reference method. To assess whether the false negative rates are significantly different between methods, replicates known to contain target organisms should be analyzed. As in false positive studies, the determination that the samples do not contain the target organism should be based on a third independent test. For example, if the target organism is genetic material from *E. coli*, then a method for culturable *E. coli* can be used. If the culture method is able to detect *E. coli*, then the genetic method should, in general, also detect *E. coli*.

Estimates of false positive and negative rates as percentages can be calculated as follows:

- false positive rate = # false positives / (# of true negatives + false positives) multiplied by 100%
- false negative rate = # false negatives / (# true positives + false negatives) multiplied by 100%

ii. Temporal, Geographic, and Matrix Applicability

The range of applicability deals with the issue of whether or not a method is reliable on a nationwide basis (e.g. does it work equally well in temperate and tropical climes, in the Great Lakes and other inland waters, etc.), in the presence of inhibitors (e.g., turbidity, alkalinity, organics [humic acids]), and in a variety of matrices (e.g., sewage, septic tanks, urban runoff, agricultural waste, known animal sources), and over what time period. In general, the range of applicability does not apply to matrices other than the one for which the test was designed - i.e., a recreational water method should not be expected to perform equally well in sewage sludge. Like robustness, this is not a measurable attribute but must be considered and applied for overall method performance.

The best methods should produce a comparable signal across a large geographic range (and not lose the signal over time), although such applicability can be affected by varying local situations. For example, antibiotic use differs substantially among countries and methods such as ARA may not perform as well in locations where there is less antibiotic use. The presence of a chosen indicator should also not be seasonal, or seasonality of its presence should be understood so that the results can be interpreted in context of those patterns.

Many waters that are tested for microbiological quality are saline, turbid, or have a high organic content, all of which have the potential to interfere with the selected MST method. For example, tannic and humic acids from decaying plant material can interfere with certain methods, as can low levels of residual chlorine from waste treatment facilities. Methods that require filtration are also susceptible to interference from high suspended solid loads. Matrix-related issues have yet to be examined for most MST methods.

iii. Sensitivity and Accuracy

Sensitivity and accuracy are measurement corollaries to indicator specificity. Indicators that are specific to a source must have accompanying methods that allow their detection with easy to collect sample volumes. It is always possible to measure lower concentrations of indicators through use of high volume collection strategies, but it is typically preferable for indicators to be present at high enough density to be easily detected in sample volumes that are convenient to collect and transport to a laboratory for analysis.

The sensitivity of a test is the analytical detection limit of the test (the smallest amount detectable using the method). For microbial methods, sensitivity is the limit of detection of a particular method. In general, methods are not used at this level since confidence around that level is lower and more subject to user error. For chemical methods, the sensitivity may be defined as the minimum amount of a particular component that can be determined by a single measurement with a stated confidence level. Generally, these refer to instrument analysis, and thus, it is the lowest quantity of a substance that can be distinguished from the absence of that substance (a blank).

Accuracy measures the degree to which the method identifies its target. It is defined as the degree of agreement between an observed value and an accepted reference value. Accuracy includes random error (precision) and systematic error (recovery) that are caused by sampling and analysis.

iv. Repeatability

Repeatability is often referred to as precision and can be expressed both on an absolute scale (i.e., standard deviation) and on a relative scale [i.e., relative standard deviation (RSD)]. The RSD (also referred to as coefficient of variation) is calculated as the standard deviation divided by the mean, expressed as a percent. For the purpose of summarizing data, both standard deviations and RSDs should be calculated. Generally, RSDs are most appropriate for summarizing precision when variability increases as concentration increases. To give an indication of the effect of multiple matrices on precision, standard deviations should be calculated separately for each matrix as well as for the method over all matrices. In addition to within and among matrix/matrices for repeatability, it is important to test intra (within lab) and interlaboratory (among labs) repeatability to insure consistency. Preferred methods will also measure indicator concentrations precisely, which is particularly important when decisions must be made on a limited number of samples. Method precision includes not only repeatability within a laboratory, but variability across labs. Generally, greater precision is better, but in particular the precision must meet the needs for the decision process.

v. Practicality

Practicality for any given method can be subdivided into capital costs, training costs, per sample costs, and additional sampling requirements. Capital costs include the up-front costs such as equipment purchase and the actual space required for the test. For example, when performing genetic testing, aside from the equipment needed (e.g. platform [specific machine], laminar flow hoods, dedicated pipettors), space is needed, optimally in separate rooms, for reagent preparation (material not containing any genetic materials) and for the two types of sample preparation (those containing high target sequence DNA concentrations such as DNA standards and calibrator samples) and those containing expected low target sequence DNA concentrations (e.g., filter blanks and water samples), which should also be in separate laminar flow hoods.

Training costs are those incurred prior to routine testing so that the user can perform the test within the performance criteria of the test; these may include going to a workshop for hands-on experience or completing a training module. The other two issues regard routine use of the test. A high per sample cost may become an issue if a large volume of tests need to be completed on a routine basis. Some labs do not object to capital or training costs, but find issue with a high per sample cost or with additional sampling requirements. Logistical feasibility will often govern the method of choice. Cost concerns can be important when large numbers of samples are needed for screening purposes, but may be less important when the consequences to be addressed have major impacts on human health risk, such as the risk of an outbreak or a high burden of disease related to the exposure. Simpler methods with proven field utility and small volume requirements may be preferred when applications are implemented on-site using less well-trained personnel.

vi. Robustness and Time Constraints

The robustness of a test is the degree to which the method can perform in the presence of incorrect inputs or stressed conditions. More simply put, how poorly can a method perform and still produce useful results. For example, does the method perform as intended in the hands of a semi-novice user (e.g. qPCR method in the hands of a user having knowledge of molecular methods, but having done only PCR methods rather than quantitative PCR)? If the test is for cultured organisms, can it detect stressed organisms in ambient waters (e.g. the EPA *E. coli* methods have a 2 hour resuscitation step at a lower temperature for stressed organisms)? Robustness is not a measurable attribute but must be considered and applied for overall method performance.

Speed of the analytical or detection method is also an important characteristic, particularly when warning decisions are involved and potential human exposure might occur during the laboratory analysis period.

We have attempted to further develop and better describe six evaluation criteria and we propose that ARA as well as all other microbe and chemical based MST methods be subjected to these same criteria (USEPA, 2007). Only with consistent evaluation against specific performance criteria can decisions be made to deem any particular method as either suitable or unsuitable. Such evaluations are long overdue in the rapidly developing field of MST.

The Future of Source Tracking

In the future, MST will likely move away from library-dependent methods in exchange for the less expensive and more rapid library-independent means of assessing and identifying fecal pollution in waterways (if such can be found). Currently, however, most library-independent methods are restricted by the undeveloped protocols for multiple potential sources, inadequate sensitivity (leading to high false-negatives), inability to quantify source contributions (Field et al., 2003, Noble et al., 2003), and possible geographic limitations (Hamilton et al., 2006). Questions still remain as to how the detection of a bacterial species, viruses, chemicals, or gene-specific markers can be quantitatively related to the FIB used by state agencies. In addition, the major supporters of MST research, the European Union, USEPA, USGS, and SCCWRP are at present working independently. Failure of these agencies to collaboratively set goals and objectives in the future will continue to the fragment the field of MST and hinder advances in the development of consistent, reproducible and widely accessible methods.

Library-independent methods do not require the collection and fingerprinting of known-source isolates, offering a distinct advantage in terms of time and overall expense to perform MST in a watershed. However, few if any current methods have proven to be consistently unique to a specific species, detectable in significant quantities in environmental waters, and/or geographical stable in different regions of the United States or Europe.

The possibility exists that as methods improve, public health standards for fecal indicators as set by USEPA, 2002 may be redefined in terms of percentage of animal contributions. However, the current TMDL projects continue to use quantifications of animal fecal inputs, a required input which continues to remain beyond the scope of the available library-independent methods. Current options still involve the use multiple methods (both library-dependent and independent) as recommend by Stewart et al., 2003 and applied by McDonald et al., 2006 and Dickerson et al., 2007b for cross-validation and increased confidence in results.

Table 1. Topic to be addressed for different MST approaches and issues to be considered for each.

Topic:	Applicable to:*	Issues to be considered:
Known Source (Host-Origin) Collection and Strain Variability	Primarily LD and LICD, less to LCI	Adequate time period for collection of representative fecal samples. Age and condition of samples collected. Location of samples in the target environment and numbers of fecal samples to be collected. Number of isolates selected per sample for analysis
Strain Overlap	All approaches	Degree of overlap of phenotypic and/or genotypic characteristics (LD and LICD) or DNA markers (LCI) among different sources.
Geographic Variability	All approaches	Geographic limitations or range of phenotypic and/or genotypic characteristics or DNA markers.
Seasonal/Temporal Variability	All approaches	Stability of phenotypic and/or genotypic characteristics or DNA markers over time. Appearance of new strains or characteristics and/or disappearance of older strains or characteristics over time.

Table 1. (Continued)

Environmental Persistence	All approaches, especially LCI	Survival/persistence of phenotypic and/or genotypic characteristics or DNA markers in different media (e.g. soil and sediments). May require additional sampling. Survival/persistence of phenotypic and/or genotypic characteristics or DNA markers when fecal indicator bacteria (FIB) are below standard, and relationship of the MST approach to the FIB in general.
Library Representativeness	LD only	Related to first topic (above), but including number of source categories included and number of isolates per source category (balanced or not, and library size). Inclusion of a validation set to assess representativeness. Uniqueness of each isolate in the library and degree of overlap among source categories.
Method Reproducibility	All approaches	Variability of identical protocols in different independent labs, and also within the same lab over time.
Method Costs and Related Issues	All approaches	Costs of whatever analytical equipment is needed and trained personnel dedicated to the equipment. Level of difficulty of the procedure and ease of performance in the analytical lab. Ability of the analytical lab to perform hundreds (or thousands) of analyses in large watershed projects. Obtaining results in a timely manner - schedule of the analytical lab.

* The three MST approaches are library-dependent (LD), library-independent but culture dependent (LICD), and library and culture independent (LCI).

References

Ahmed, W., R. Neller, and M. Katouli. 2005. Host species-specific metabolic fingerprint database for enterococci and *Escherichia coli* and its application to identify sources of fecal contamination in surface waters. *Appl. Environ. Microbiol.* 71:4461-4468.

Albert, J.M., J. Munkata-Marr, L. Tenorio, and R.L. Siegrist. 2003. Statistical evaluation of bacterial source tracking data obtained by rep-PCR DNA fingerprinting of *Escherichia coli*. *Environ. Sci. Technol.* 37:4554-4560.

Anderson, K.L., J.E., Whitlock, and V.J. Harwood. 2005. Persistence and differential survival of fecal indicator bacteria in subtropical waters and sediments. *Appl. Environ. Microbiol.* 71:3041-3047.

Avery, L.M., K. Killham, and D.L. Jones. 2005. Survival of *E. coli* O157:H7 in organic wastes destined for land application. *J. Appl. Microbiol.* 98:814-822.

Barnes, B. and D.M. Gordon. 2004. Coliform dynamics and the implications for source tracking. *Environ. Microbiol.* 6:501-509.

Björkman, J., I. Nagaev, O.G. Berg, D. Hughes, and D.I. Anderson. 2000. Effects of environment on compensatory mutations to ameliorate costs of antibiotic resistance. *Science.* 287: 479-1482.

Blanch, A.R., L. Belanche-Munoz, X. Bonjoch, J. Ebdon, C. Gantzer, F. Lucena, J. Ottoson, C. Kourtis, A. Iverson, I. Kuhn, L. Moce, M. Muniesa, J. Schwartzbrod, S. Skraber, G.T. Papageorgiou, H. Taylor, J. Wallis, and J. Jofre. 2006. Integrated analysis of established and novel microbial and chemical methods for microbial source tracking. *Appl. Environ. Microbiol.* 72:5915-5926.

Booth, A.M., C. Hagedorn, A. K. Graves, S.C. Hagedorn, and K.H. Mentz. 2003. Sources of fecal pollution in Virginia's Blackwater River. *J. Environ. Eng.* 6:547-552.

Burnes, B.S. 2003. Antibiotic resistance analysis of fecal coliforms to determine fecal pollution sources in a mixed-use watershed. *Environ. Mon. Assess.* 85:87–98.

Butaye, P., L.A. Devriese, and F. Haesebrouck, 2001. Differences in antibiotic resistance patterns of *Enterococcus faecalis* and *Enterococcus faecium* strains isolated from farm and pet animals. *Antimicrob Agents Chemother.* 45:1374-1378.

Carroll, S., M. Hargreaves, and A. Goonetilleke. 2005. Sourcing faecal pollution from onsite wastewater treatment systems in surface waters using antibiotic resistance analysis. *J. Appl. Microbiol.* 99:471-482.

Choi, S., W. Chu, J. Brown, S.J. Becker, V.J. Harwood, and S.C. Jiang. 2003. Application of *Enterococci* antibiotic resistance patterns for contamination source identification at Huntington Beach, California, *Marine Pollution Bulletin* 46: 748–755.

Craig, D.L., H.J. Fallowfield, and N.J. Cromar. 2004. Use of microcosms to determine persistence of *Escherichia coli* in recreational coastal water and sediment and validation with *in situ* measurements. *J. Appl. Microbiol.* 96:922-930.

Crozier, J.B., B, Clark, and H. Weber. 2002. Identifying sources of fecal pollution in the Roanoke River, Roanoke County, Virginia. *Va. J. Sci.* 53:157-166.

Díaz-Mejía, J.J., A. Carbajal-Saucedo, and C.F. Amábile-Cuevas. 2002. Antibiotic resistance in oral commensal streptococci from healthy Mexicans and Cubans: resistance prevalence does not mirror antibiotic usage. *FEMS Microbiol.* L. 217:173-176.

Dickerson, J.W. Jr, J. B. Crozier, C. Hagedorn, and A. Hassall. 2007a. Assessment of the 16S-23S rDNA intergenic spacer region in *Enterococcus spp.* for microbial source tracking. *Journal of Environmental Quality* 36:1661-1669.

Dickerson, J. W. Jr., C. Hagedorn, and A. Hassall. 2007b. Detection and remediation of human-origin pollution at two public beaches in Virginia using multiple source tracking methods. *Water Res. Water Research* 41:3758-3770.

Dombek, P.E., L.K., Johnson, S.T, Zimmerley, and M.J. Sadowsky. 2000. Use of repetitive DNA sequences and PCR to differentiate *Escherichia coli* isolates from human and animal sources. *Appl. Environ. Microbiol.* 66:2572-2577.

Ebdon, J.E., J.L. Wallis, and H.D. Taylor. 2004. A simplified low-cost approach to antibiotic resistance profiling for faecal source tracking. *Water Sci. Tech.* 1:185-191.

Edge, T. A., and S. Hill. 2005. Occurrence of antibiotic resistance in *Escherichia coli* from surface waters and fecal pollution sources near Hamilton, Ontario. *Can. J. Microbiol.* 51:501-505.

Field, K.G., E.C. Chern, L.K. Dick, J. Fuhrman, J. Griffith, P.A. Holden, M.G. LaMontagne, J. Le, B. Olson, and M.T. Simonich. 2003. A comparative study of culture-independent genotypic methods of fecal source tracking. *J. Wat. Health* 1: 181-194.

Fogarty, L.R., S.K. Haack, M J. Wolcott, and R.L. Whitman. 2003. Abundance and characteristics of the recreational water quality indicator bacteria *Escherichia coli* and enterococci in gull feces. *J. App. Microbiol.* 94:865-878.

Francy, D.S., E.E. Bertke, D.P. Finnegan, C.M. Kephart, R.A. Sheets, J. Rhoades, and L. Stumpe. 2006. Use of spatial sampling and microbial source-tracking tools for understanding fecal contamination at two Lake Erie beaches, U.S. Geological Survey *Scientific Investigations Report* 2006-5298, 29 p.

Gilliver, M.A., M. Bennett, M. Begon, S.M. Hazel, and C.A. Hart. 1999. Antibiotic resistance found in wild rodents. *Nature.* 401:233-234.

Gordon, D.M. 1997. The genetic structure of *Escherichia coli* populations in feral house mice. *Microbiology.* 143:2039-2046.

Gordon, D. M. 2001. Geographical structure and host specificity in bacteria and the implications for tracing the source of coliform contamination. *Microbiol.* 147: 1079-1085.

Graves, A. K., C. Hagedorn, A. Teetor, M. Mahal, A. M. Booth, and R. B. Reneau, Jr. 2002. Antibiotic resistance profiles to determine sources of fecal contamination in water for a rural Virginia watershed. *J. Environ. Qual.* 31:1300-1308.

Graves, A.K., C. Hagedorn, A. Brooks, R.L. Hagedorn, and E. Martin. 2007. Microbial source tracking in a rural watershed dominated by cattle. *Water Research* 41:3729-3739.

Griffith, J. F., S.B. Weisberg, and C.D. McGee. 2003. Evaluation of microbial source tracking methods using mixed fecal sources in aqueous test samples. *J. Wat. Health* 1:141-151.

Guan, S., R. Xu, S. Chen, J. Odumeru, and C. Gyles. 2002. Development of a procedure for discriminating among *Escherichia coli* isolates from animal and human sources. *Appl. Environ. Microbiol.* 68:2690-2698.

Hagedorn, C., S.L. Robinson, J.R. Filtz, S.M. Grubbs, T.A. Angier, and Reneneau, R.B. 1999. Determining sources of fecal pollution in a rural Virginia watershed with antibiotic resistance patterns in fecal streptococci. *Appl. Environ. Microbiol.* 65:5522-5531.

Hagedorn, C., J.B. Crozier, K.A. Mentz, A.M. Booth, A.K. Graves, N.J. Nelson, and R.B. Reneau Jr. 2003. Carbon source utilization profiles as a method to identify sources of faecal pollution in water. *Appl. Environ. Microbiol.* 94:792-799.

Hager, M.C. Detecting bacteria in coastal waters. 2001a. Part 1, *The Journal for Surface Water Quality Professionals* 2(3), pp. 16–25.

Hager, M.C. Detecting bacteria in coastal waters. 2001b. Part 2, *The Journal for Surface Water Quality Professionals* 2 (2001) (4).

Hamilton, M.J., T. Yan, and M.J. Sadowsky. 2006. Development of goose- and duck-specific DNA markers to determine sources of *Escherichia coli* in waterways. *Appl. Environ. Microbiol.* 72: 4012-4019.

Hartel, P. G., J. D. Summer, J. L. Hill, J. V. Collins, J. A. Entry, and W. I. Segers. 2002. Geographic variability of *Escherichia coli* ribotypes from animals in Idaho and Georgia. *J. Environ. Qual.* 31:1273–1278.

Hartel, P.G., J.D. Summer, and W.I. Segars. 2003. Deer diet affects ribotype diversity of *Escherichia coli* for bacterial source tracking. *Wat. Res.* 37:3263-3268.

Harwood, V.J., J. Whitlock, and V. Withington. 2000. Classification of antibiotic resistance patterns of indicator bacteria by discriminant analysis: use in predicting the source of fecal contamination in subtropical waters. *Appl. Environ. Microbiol.* 66:3698-3704.

Harwood, V.J., B. Wiggins, C. Hagedorn, R.D. Ellender, J. Gooch, J. Kern, M. Samadpour, A.C.H. Chapman, and B.J. Robinson. 2003. Phenotypic library-based microbial source tracking methods: efficacy in the California collaborative study. *J. Wat. Health* 1:153-166.

Jamieson, R.C., D.M. Joy, H. Lee, R. Kostachik, and R.J. Gordon. 2005. Resuspension of sediment-associated *Escherichia coli* in a natural stream. *J. Environ. Qual.* 34:581-589.

Jenkins, M.B., P.G. Hartel, T.J. Olexa, and J.A. Stuedemann. 2003. Putative temporal variability of *Escherichia coli* ribotypes from yearling steers. *J. Environ. Qual.* 32:305-309.

Jiang, S. C., R. T. Noble, and W. Chu. 2001. Human adenoviruses and coliphage in urban runoff-impacted coastal waters of southern California. *Appl. Environ. Microbiol.* 67:179-184.

Johnson, L.K., M.B. Brown, E.A. Carruthers, J.A. Ferguson, P.E. Dombeck, and M.J. Sadowsky. 2004. Sample size, library composition, and genotypic diversity among natural populations of *Escherichia coli* from different animals influence accuracy pf determining sources of fecal pollution. *Appl. Environ. Microbiol.* 70: 4478-4485.

Kariuki, S., C. Gilks, J. Kimari, A. Obanda, J. Muyodi, P. Waiyaki, and C.A. Hart. 1999. Genotype analysis of *Escherichia coli* strains isolated from chickens and children living in close contact. *Appl. Environ. Microbiol.* 65:472-476.

Kaspar, C. W., J. L. Burgess, I. T. Knight, and R. R. Colwell. 1990. Antibiotic resistance indexing of *Escherichia coli* to identify sources of fecal contamination in water. *Can. J. Microbiol.* 36:**891-894**.

Katouli, M., A. Lund, P. Wallgren, I. Kühn, O. Söderlind, and R. Möllby. 1995. Phenotypic characterization of intestinal *Escherichia coli* of pigs during suckling, postweaning, and fattening periods. *Appl. Environ. Microbiol.* 61:778–783.

Kelsey, R.H., G.I. Scott, D.E., Porter, B. Thompson, and L. Webster. 2003. Using multiple antibiotic characteristics to determine sources of fecal coliform bacterial pollution. *Environ. Mon. Assess.* 81: 337–348.

Lau, M.M. and S.C. Ingham. 2001. Survival of faecal indicator bacteria in bovine manure incorporated into soil. L. *Appl. Microbiol.* 33:131-136.

LeFevre, N.M. and G.D. Lewis. 2003. The role of resuspension in enterococci distribution in water at an urban beach. *Wat. Sci. Technol.* 47:205-210.

Lefresne, G., E. Latrille, F. Irlinger, and P. A. D. Grimont. 2004. Repeatability and reproducibility of ribotyping and its computer interpretation. *Res. Microbiol.* 155:154-161

Leser, T.D., R.H. Lindecrona, T.K. Jensen, B.B. Jensen, and K. Moller. 2000. Changes in bacterial community structure in the colon of pigs fed different experimental diets and after infection with *Brachyspira hyodysenteriae*. *Appl. Environ. Microbiol.* 66:3290-3296.

Li, X.-Z., L. Zhang, and K. Poole. 1998. Role of the multidrug efflux systems of *Pseudomonas aeruginosa* in organic solvent tolerance. *J. Bacteriol.* 180:2987-2991.

Lu, J., S. Sanchez, C. Hofacre, J.J. Maurer, B.G. Harmon, and M.D. Lee. 2003. Evaluation of broiler litter with reference to the microbial composition as assessed by using 16S rRNA and functional gene markers. *Appl. Environ. Microbiol.* 69:901-908.

Lu, L., M.E. Hume, K.L. Sternes, and S.D. Pillai. 2004. Genetic diversity of *Escherichia coli* isolates in irrigation water associated sediments: implications for source tracking. *Wat. Res.* 38:3899-3908.

Lu, Z., D. Lapen, A. Scott, A. Dang, and E. Topp. 2005. Identifying host sources of fecal pollution: diversity of *Escherichia coli* in confined dairy and swine production systems. *Appl. Environ. Microbiol.* 71:5992-5998.

McArthur, J.V. and R.C. Tuckfield. 2000. Spatial patterns in antibiotic resistance among stream bacteria: effects of industrial pollution. *Appl. Environ. Microbiol.* 66:3722-3726.

McDonald, D.E., D.W. Pethick, B.P. Mullan, and D.J. Hampson. 2001. Increasing viscosity of the intestinal contents alters small intestinal structure and intestinal growth, and stimulates proliferation of enterotoxigenic *Escherichia coli* in newly-weaned pigs. *Br. J. Nutr.* 86:487–498.

McDonald, J.L., P.G. Hartel, L.C. Gentit, C.N. Belcher, K.W. Gates, K. Rodgers, J. A.Fisher, K.A. Smith, and K.A. Payne. 2006. Identifying sources of fecal contamination inexpensively with targeted sampling and bacterial source tracking. *J. Environ. Qual.* 35:889-897.

McLellan, S. L., A. D. Daniels, and A. K. Salmore. 2003. Genetic characterization of *Escherichia coli* populations from host sources of fecal pollution by using DNA fingerprinting. *Appl. Environ. Microbiol.* 69:2587-2594.

Moore, D. F., V. J. Harwood, D.M. Ferguson, J. Lukasik, P. Hannah, M. Geitrich, and M. Brownell. 2005. Evaluation of antibiotic resistance analysis and ribotyping for identification of faecal pollution sources in urban watershed. *J. Appl. Microbiol.* 99:618-628.

Muirhead, R.W., R.P. Collins, and P.J. Bremer. 2005. Erosion and subsequent transport state of *Escherichia coli* from cowpats. *Appl. Environ. Microbiol.* 71:2875-2879.

Myoda, S. P., C. A. Carson, J. J. Fuhrmann, B.K. Hahm, P.G. Hartel, H. Yampara-Iquise, L. Johnson, R.L. Kuntz, C.H. Nakatsu, M.J. Sadowsky, and M. Samadpour. 2003. Comparison of genotypic-based microbial source tracking methods requiring a host origin database. *J. Wat. Health* 1:167-180.

Noble, R.T., S.M. Allen, A.D. Blackwood, W. Chu, S.C. Jiang, G.L. Lovelace, M.D. Sobsey, J.R. Stewart, and D.A. Wait. 2003. Use of viral pathogens and indicators to differentiate between human and non-human fecal contamination in a microbial source tracking comparison study. *J. Wat. Health* 1:195-207.

O'Brien, T.L., D. Bailey, A. Gill, and P. Station. 2005. Considerations for using sewage versus direct human samples to generate a bacterial source tracking database. *ASM Poster* Q-416.

Ogden, I.D., N.F. Hepburn, M. MacRae, N.J.C. Strachan, D.R. Fenlon, S.M. Rusbridge, and T.H. Pennington. 2002. Long-term survival of *Escherichia coli* O157 on pasture following an outbreak associated with sheep at a scout camp. L. *Appl. Microbiol.* 38:100-104.

Parveen, S., R.L. Murphree, L. Edminston, C.W. Kaspar, K.M. Portier, and M.L. Tamplin. 1997. Association of multiple-antibiotic resistance profiles with point and non-point sources of *Escherichia coli* in Apalachicola Bay. *Appl. Environ. Microbiol.* 63:2607-2612.

Parveen, S., K.M. Portier, K. Robinson, L. Edminston, and M.L. Tamplin. 1999. Discriminant analysis of ribotype profiles of Escherichia coli for differentiating human and nonhuman sources of fecal pollution. *Appl. Environ Microbiol* 65, 3142–3147.

Pupo, G.M. and B.J. Richardson. 1995. Biochemical genetics of a natural population of *Escherichia coli*: season changes in alleles and haplotypes. *Microbiol.* 141:1037-1044.

Ritter, K.J., Carruthers, C., Carson, C.A., Ellender, R.D., Harwood, V.J., Kingsley, K., Nakatsu, C., Sadowsky, M., Shear, B., West, B., Whitlock, J.E., Wiggins, B.A. and Wilbur, J.D. 2003. Assessment of statistical methods using in library-based approaches to microbial source tracking. *J. Wat. Health* 1:209-223.

Ritter K. and B. Robinson. 2004. Statistical appraisal of disproportional versus proportional libraries. Presentation, presentation given during the Gulf of Mexico Bacterial Source Tracking workshop in Biloxi, MS, Nov 11-13, 2004. Moderator: R.D. Ellender, University of Southern Mississippi, Hattisburg, MS.

Russell, J. B., F. Diez-Gonzalez, and G.N. Jarvis. 2000. Symposium: Farm Health and Safety. Invited Review: Effects of Diet Shifts on *Escherichia coli* in Cattle. *J. Dairy Sci.* 83:863–873.

Salyers, A.A. and C.F. Amábile-Cuevas. 1997. Why are antibiotic resistance genes so resistant to elimination? *Antimicrobial Agents and Chemotherapy.* 41:2321-2325.

Samadpour, M., M.C. Roberts, C. Kitts, W. Mulugeta, and D. Alfi. 2005. The use of ribotyping and antibiotic resistance patterns for identification of host sources of *Escherichia coli* strains. *Letters in Applied Microbiology* 40, 63-68.

Sayah, R.S., J. B. Kaneene, Y. Johnson, and R. Miller. 2005. Patterns of antimicrobial resistance observed in *Escherichia coli* isolates obtained from domestic- and wild-animal fecal samples, human septage, and surface water. *Appl. Environ. Microbiol.* 71:1394-1404.

Scott, T.M., S. Parveen, K.M. Portier, J.B. Rose, M.L. Tamplin, S.R. Farrah, A. Koo, and J. Lukasik. 2003. Geographical variation in ribotype profiles of *Escherichia coli* isolates from human, swine, poultry, beef, and dairy cattle in Florida. *Appl. Environ. Microbiol.* 69:1089-1092.

Seurinck, S., W. Verstraete, and S.D. Siciliano. 2005. Microbial source tracking for identification of fecal pollution. *Rev. Environ. Sci. Bio/Technol.* 4:19-37.

Shehane, S.D., V.J. Harwood, J.E. Whitlock, and J. B . Rose. 2005. The influence of rainfall on the incidence of microbial faecal indicators and the dominant sources of faecal pollution in a Florida river. *J. Appl. Microbiol.* 98:1127-1136.

Silvi, S., C.J. Rumney, A. Cresci, and I.R. Rowland. 1999. Resistant starch modifies gut microflora and microbial metabolism in human flora-associated rats inoculated with faeces from Italian and UK donors. *J. Appl. Microbiol.* 86, 521–530.

Simmons, G.M., D.F. Waye, S. Herbein, S. Myers, and E. Walker 2002. Estimating nonpoint fecal coliform sources in Northern Virginia's Four Mile Run watershed, p. 143-167. In Younos, T. (ed.), *Advances in Water Monitoring Research*. Water Resources Publications, LLC.

Soule, M., E. Kuhn, F. Loge, J. Gay, and D. R. Call. 2006. Using DNA microarrays to identify library-independent markers for bacterial source tracking. *Appl. Environ. Microbiol.* 72:1843-1851.

Stewart, J.R., R.D. Ellender, J.A. Gooch, S. Jiang, S.P. Myoda, and S. B. Weisberg. 2003. Recommendations for microbial source tracking: lessons learned from a methods comparison study. *J. Water Health* 1:225-231.

Stoeckel, D.M., M.V. Mathes, K.E. Hyer, C. Hagedorn, H. Kator, J. Lukasik, T.L. O'Brien, T.W. Fenger, M. Samadpour, K.M. Strickler, and B.A. Wiggins. 2004. Comparison of seven protocols to identify fecal contamination sources using *Escherichia coli*. *Environ. Sci. Technol.* 38:6109-6117.

Stoeckel, D. M., and V. J. Harwood. 2007. Performance, design, and analysis in microbial source tracking studies. *Appl. Environ. Microbiol.* 73:2405-2415.

USEPA. 1986. Ambient Water Quality Criteria for Bacteria - 1986. U.S. Environmental Protection Agency, Office of Water, Washington, D.C. EPA-440/5-84-002.

USEPA. 2002. Implementation Guidance for Ambient Water Quality Criteria for Bacteria. U.S. Environmental Protection Agency, Washington, D.C. May 2002 Draft.

USEPA. 2007. Experts Scientific Workshop on Critical Research Needs for the Development of New or Revised Recreational Water Quality Criteria. EPA-OW-823-R-07-006. (http://www.epa.gov/waterscience/criteria/recreation/experts/index.html).

Vantarakis, A., D. Venieri, G. Komninou, and M. Papapetropoulou. 2006. Differentiation of faecal *Escherichia coli* from humans and animals by multiple antibiotic resistance analysis. L. *Appl. Microbiol.* 42:71-77.

Weaver, R.W., J.A. Entry, and A. Graves. 2005. Numbers of fecal streptococci and *Escherichia coli* in fresh and dry cattle, horse, and sheep manure. *Can. J. Microbiol.* 51:847-851.

Webster, L.F., B.C. Thompson, M.H. Fulton, D.E. Chestnut, R.F. Van Dolah, A.K. Leight, and G.I. Scott. 2004. Identification of sources of *Escherichia coli* in South Carolina estuaries using antibiotic resistance analysis. *J. Exper. Mar. Biol. Ecol.* 298:179-195.

Whitlock, J.E., D.T. Jones, and V.J. Harwood. 2002. Identification of the sources of fecal coliforms in an urban watershed using antibiotic resistance analysis. *Wat. Res.* 36:4273-4282.

Wiggins, B. A. 1996. Discriminant analysis of antibiotic resistance patterns in fecal streptococci, a method to differentiate human and animal sources of fecal pollution in natural waters. *Appl. Environ. Microbiol.* 62:3997-4002.

Wiggins, B. A., R. W. Andrews, R. A. Conway, C. L. Corr, E. J. Dobratz, D. P. Dougherty, J. R. Eppard, S. R. Knupp, M. C. Limjoco, J. M. Mettenburg, J. M. Rinehardt, J. Sonsino, R. L. Torrijos, and M. E. Zimmerman. 1999. Identification of sources of fecal pollution using discriminant analysis: Supporting evidence from large datasets. *Appl. Environ. Microbiol.* 65:3483-3486.

Wiggins, B.A., P.W. Cash, W.S. Creamer, S.E. Dart, P.P. Garcia, T.M. Gerecke, J. Han, B.L. Henry, K.B. Hoover, E.L. Johnson, K.C. Jones, J.G. McCarthy, J.A. McDonough, S.A. Mercer, M.J. Noto, H. Park, M.S. Phillips, S.M. Purner, B.M. Smith, E.N. Stevens, and A.K. Varner. 2003. Use of antibiotic resistance analysis for representativeness testing of multiwatershed libraries. *Appl. Environ. Microbiol.* 69:3399-3405.

In: Antibiotic Resistance…   ISBN 978-1-60741-623-4
Editors: A. R. Bonilla and K. P. Muniz   © 2009 Nova Science Publishers, Inc.

Chapter XIII

Genetic Regulation, Physiology, Assessment and Inhibition of Efflux Pumps Responsible for Multi-Drug Resistant Phenotypes of Bacterial Pathogens

L. Amaral[*,1,2,3], *S. Fanning* [3,4], *G. Spengler* [1,2], *L. Rodrigues* [1,2], *C. Iversen* [4], *M. Martins* [1,2], *A. Martins* [1,2], *M. Viveiros* [1,3] and *I. Couto*[1,5]

[1]Unit of Mycobacteriology and [2] UPMM, Instituto de Higiene e Medicina Tropical, Universidade Nova de Lisboa (IHMT/UNL), Rua da Junqueira 96, 1349-008 Lisboa, Portugal
[3]COST ACTION BM0701 (ATENS) of the European Commission/ European Science Foundation
[4]Centres for Food Safety and Food-borne Zoonomics, UCD Veterinary Sciences Centre, University College Dublin, Belfield, Dublin 4, Ireland
[5]Centro de Recursos Microbiológicos (CREM), Faculdade de Ciências e Tecnologia, Universidade Nova de Lisboa, 2829-516 Caparica, Portugal

Abstract

The response of bacteria to a given antibiotic or other toxic agent that does not immediately kill them results in an adaptive response that secures their survival. This response may involve a number of distinct mechanisms, among which is the activation of genes that promote the appearance of transporters that extrude the agent prior to its reaching its target. These transporters extrude a large variety of chemically unrelated

---

[*] Corresponding author: Leonard Amaral, Unit of Mycobacteriology, Instituto de Higiene e Medicina Tropical, Universidade Nova de Lisboa (IHMT/UNL). Rua da Junqueira, 96, 1349-008 Lisboa, Portugal. Tel: +351 21 365 2600, Fax: +351 21 363 2105. E-mail: lamaral@ihmt.unl.pt.

compounds and hence they bestow on the bacterium a multi-drug resistant (MDR) phenotype. The appearance of this MDR phenotype during therapy makes therapy problematic. Understanding the genetic and physiological properties of MDR efflux pumps is an absolute requirement if MDR bacterial infections are to be successfully managed. There is much to learn and methods that afford the needed understanding will eventually pave the way for the successful management of an MDR bacterial infection. Therefore, the application of recently developed methods that assess the MDR bacterium at its genetic and physiological levels is the focus of this chapter. The material presented in this chapter is only the beginning for the evaluation and assessment of MDR efflux pumps.

Introduction

Multi-drug resistance of bacterial clinical isolates to representative antibiotics from two or more unrelated classes, is now accepted to be due to over-expressed efflux pumps which extrude the antibiotics prior to their reaching their intended targets [1-5]. Although the manner by which multi-drug resistance develops during infection is still not precisely demonstrated, prolonged *in vitro* exposure of reference bacterial strains to increasing concentrations of given antibiotics results in the appearance of a multi-drug resistant (MDR) phenotype. In this manner, prolonged exposure of *Staphylococcus aureus*, *Escherichia coli*, and *Mycobacterium tuberculosis*, to increasing concentrations of oxacillin [6] tetracycline [7, 8] and isoniazid [9], respectively, renders the respective organism resistant to the antibiotic to which it has been exposed, as well as to other classes of antibiotics. MDR phenotypes can also result from prolonged exposure to increasing concentrations of ethidium bromide (EB) [10], thereby reminding us that as far as the organism is "concerned", the response is due to exposure to a noxious agent, be it an antibiotic or other toxic substances. The response to prolonged exposure to a noxious agent may be considered to be one of "adaptation" inasmuch as when the organism is transferred to drug-free medium, restoration of initial susceptibility to the antibiotic takes place, albeit, over a lengthy number of replications in drug-free medium [8, 9]. Because agents that are known to inhibit efflux pump activity [11, 12] can also render the MDR bacterium susceptible to the antibiotics to which it had been induced to high-level resistance [6-10], the demonstration of reversal of resistance by a given agent constitutes *prima facia* evidence that the agent inhibits the efflux pump system of the MDR bacterium, provided that the resistance has been demonstrated to be due to efflux [1]. To this extent, thousands of compounds have been studied for their effects on over-expressed efflux pumps of MDR bacteria [13, 14] and as of this writing, although many agents have been shown to be effective efflux pump inhibitors (EPIs) [15-19], they have little clinical relevance since they are toxic. Phenothiazines and their derivatives have been shown to have inhibitory activity against many types of over-expressed multi-drug resistance mediating efflux pump systems [6, 8-12, 20-23] and because many have been used for the therapy of non-infectious pathology and produce few serious side effects [24-28], it is this class of compounds which will eventually yield an effective adjuvant for the therapy of MDR bacterial infections. It is therefore the intent of this chapter to discuss these compounds and the mechanism by which they affect efflux pumps of important MDR bacterial pathogens.

Efflux Pumps of MDR Bacteria:
The Major Facilitator Superfamily

The Major Facilitator Superfamily (MFS) of transporters is a diverse superfamily that consists of more than a thousand aminoacid sequenced members. They catalyze the exchange of monovalent cations H^+ or Na^+ for unrelated and structurally different antibiotics. Most are of 400-600 aminoacid residues in length and possess either 12, 14 or 24 putative transmembrane α-helical spanning domains although with respect to Gram-negative bacteria, most MFS transporters are of a 12-domain type. The energy that drives the pump and therefore expels the antibiotic from the region immediately medial to the outer component of the cytoplasmic membrane is the proton motive force (PMF). In Gram-positive bacteria, efflux of antibiotics is mainly mediated by MFS-type transporter proteins. About 10% of the total transport proteins of Gram-positive bacteria are putative MFS-type multi-drug efflux pumps which when over-expressed are solely responsible for the MDR phenotype (29 and see also www.membranetransport.org). Examples of this type of pump is the *S. aureus* NorA, which when over-expressed renders the organism resistant to fluoroquinolones [10, 29-31] and the Qac system of efflux, which makes the organism extremely resistant to biocides [32-34]; and, the PmrA efflux pump of *Streptococcus pneumoniae* that when over-expressed results in resistance to fluoroquinolones (FQs) (35). Examples of inhibitors of the MFS-type efflux pump are: an ofloxacin-based EPI that is a potent inhibitor of NorA [36]; phenothiazines [11, 12], reserpine [11, 12, 35], citral derived amides [37], pyrazine derivatives [38] and N-caffeoylphenalkylamide derivatives [39]. Omeprazole derivatives have also been recently shown to inhibit the NorA efflux pump [40].

The NorA Efflux Pump of *Staphylococcus Aureus*

Susceptibility of wild-type *S. aureus* to FQs is dependent upon the permeability of the cell envelop and to the presence of intrinsic efflux pump systems, most commonly NorA, that extrudes the antibiotic, albeit, weakly [41]. Increased resistance to FQs is due to mutations that result in lower affinity of the gyrases GrlA and GyrA for FQs [41, 42]. In *S. aureus* most of these mutations occur in *grlA*. Greater than 97% of all clinical isolates that show resistance to norfloxacin, enoxacin, ciprofloxacin, fleroxacin, sparfloxacin and levofloxacin possess mutations in *grlA* and *gyrA*. Double mutations in both loci result in high-level resistance to these and newer FQs [42]. Examples of single mutations found in the GrlA and which produce intermediate to high-level resistance to ciprofloxacin are: Ser-80-->Phe or Tyr or Glu-84-->Lys or Ala-116-->Glu or Pro or a combination of Ser-80>Phe and Glu-84>Val. When these aminoacid substitutions are combined with alterations in GyrA, namely, Ser-84>Leu or Lys or Glu-88>Lys or Val, high-level resistance results [43].

Although the above mutations account for the vast majority of resistance to FQs, resistance has also been shown to involve the over-expression of the NorA efflux pump [41]. Although mutations of the promoter region of *norA* can lead to the over-expression of NorA [44], over-expression has been shown for some isolates to be independent of changes within the promoter region [45]. Over-expression has been reported in the absence of any mutation within the *norA* promoter region [46, 31].

Efflux mediated resistance to FQs can be induced in *S. aureus* by exposure to substrates recognized by the NorA efflux pump system (47). Among these substrates is EB, which when present in ever-increasing concentration, over-time, promotes the development of extreme resistance of wild-type *S. aureus* to the agent [minimum inhibitory concentration (MIC) increases from 5 to over 150 mg/L] [10]. Accompanying this increased resistance is resistance to FQs which can be reversed upon exposure to reserpine, and a more pronounced effect is seen with phenothiazines chlorpromazine and thioridazine [10]. Evaluation of the activity of *norA* and other efflux pump-encoding genes, active efflux of EB, along with the sequencing of the *norA* gene, yielded a 35-fold increase in the activity of *norA*, no change in the activity of other genes that encode other efflux pumps, a 4-fold increase in the efflux of EB and no mutations within *norA*. However, a 70 bp deletion was noted within the *norA* promoter region [10]. The precise genetic mechanism by which an efflux pump substrate of NorA that has no structural relationship to FQs can initiate the above, remains to be elucidated. These observations are not surprising inasmuch as the mechanism, by which efflux-mediated resistance is normally brought about in FQs resistant clinical isolates, is yet to be defined.

Other Intrinsic Efflux Pumps of Gram-Positive Bacteria

Intrinsic MFS-type efflux pumps of bacteria have not been readily studied due to the lack of sensitivity of the systems employed. However, the main intrinsic MFS-type efflux pump of the Gram-positive *Enterococcus faecalis* is the EmeA pump which has been characterized by Lee et al. [48], and as is the case for all MFS-type pumps, derives the energy needed for its activity from the PMF (48). We have studied the efflux of EB by the *E. faecalis* ATCC29212 reference strain under conditions which are more physiological than those usually employed. These studies were undertaken in the presence of a source of metabolic energy, at different medium pHs [ranging from 5 to 8] and an incubation temperature of 37°C [49] using a semi-automated method that utilizes the common efflux pump substrate EB [50]. At pH 5, metabolic energy is not required for efflux of EB; in contrast at pH 8 catabolism of glucose is required to energise efflux. These physiological conditions are summarized in Figure 1 showing an increase in EB accumulation at pH 8, with the concomitant increase in slope of the line at this pH, as efflux decreased. In contrast, at pH 5, EPIs such as thioridazine, verapamil and reserpine and the uncoupler of the PMF, carbonyl cyanide m-chlorophenylhydrazone (CCCP) have no effect on the efflux of EB. In the presence of these EPIs, at pH 8 efflux is completely eliminated (as shown for CCCP in Figure 2). These results suggest that at pH 5 the PMF is capable of energizing efflux as a result of the potential difference across the membrane, due to the high concentrations of protons. At pH 8, the PMF is somewhat dissipated and hence the concentration of CCCP that had no affect on efflux at pH 5 completely inhibited efflux at pH 8 by collapsing the proton gradient. If the PMF was to be the only source required to energise this MFS-type efflux, then EPIs which are known to inhibit the hydrolysis of ATP, such as thioridazine, should have no affect on efflux. A similar scenario would be expected to occur in the absence of a source of metabolic energy. Thus, whereas an MFS-type efflux pump readily derives energy from protons at pH 5, when the availability of those protons is reduced as would be the case at pH 8, energy must be provided through the hydrolysis of ATP. Moreover, unlike other Gram-positive bacteria, *E. faecalis* has another efflux system, namely the EfrAB that can extrude antibiotics. This pump is a member of the ATP-Binding Cassette (ABC) superfamily [51] and derives its energy from the hydrolysis of ATP [52], by ATPase enzymes that are inhibited by phenothiazines at pH 8 and not at pH 5 [53].

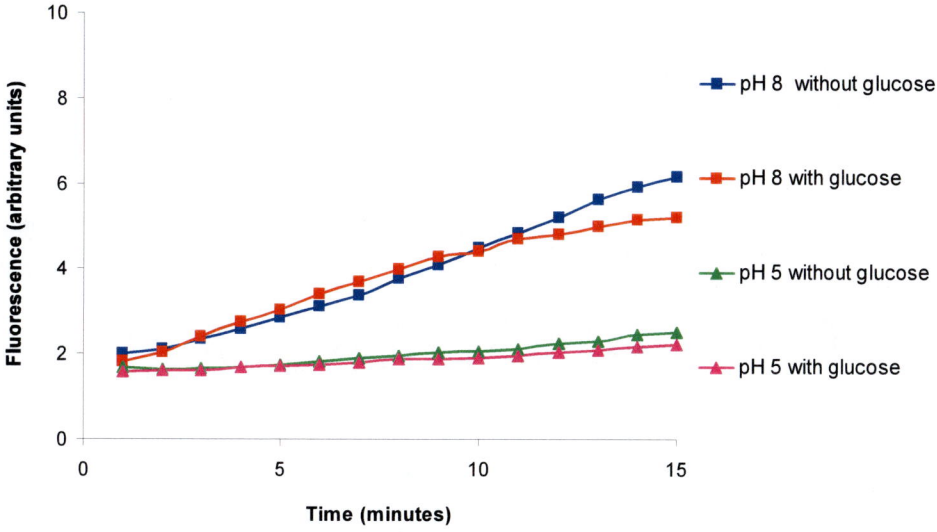

Figure 1. Accumulation of EB at 0.5 mg/L by E. faecalis ATCC29212 at pH 8 and 5 in the presence and absence of glucose 0.6%.

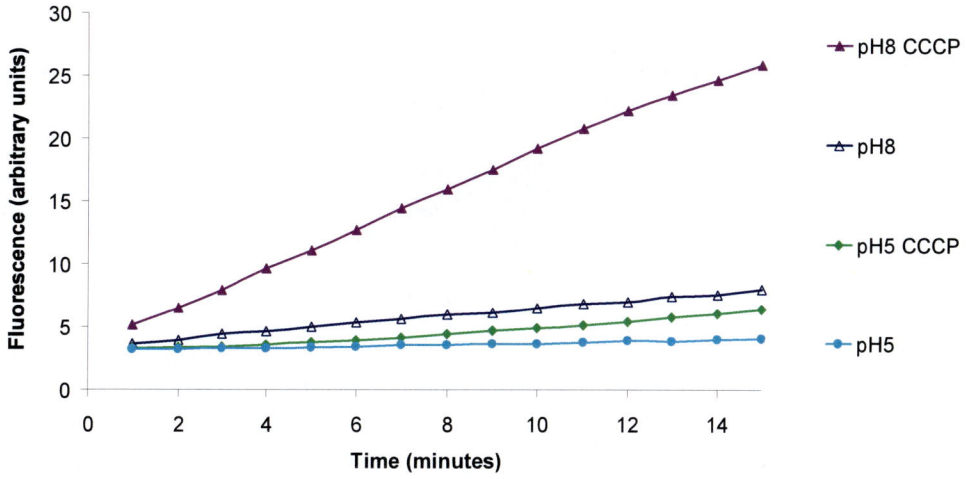

Figure 2. Effect of CCCP 100 μM (½ MIC) on accumulation of EB at 0.5 mg/L by *E. faecalis* ATCC29212 at pH 8 and 5 in the presence of glucose 0.6%.

Efflux Pumps of Gram-Negative Bacteria: The Resistance Nodulation Division (RND) Family

The efflux pumps of Gram-negative bacteria that promote an MDR phenotype when over-expressed, are part of the Resistance Nodulation Division (RND) family of transporters, and consist of tripartite units that span the plasma membrane from the outer membrane to the inner membrane being closely associated with the interstitial periplasm. These tripartite pumps comprise an outer-membrane channel, TolC, which connects to the transporter located in the inner-membrane and which transduces the electrochemical energy of proton gradients. A fusion protein then links the transmembrane component in the periplasm with TolC [54-56]. Although more than two dozen structures of the inner-membrane transporter protein AcrB have been determined for various ligand (substrate) bound states [57, 58], the actual structure as it exists in the cell envelope remains for now as a conjecture. Nevertheless, a variety of models have been presented to represent the relationship of the transporter component to TolC along with its anchorage to the cytoplasmic side of the inner membrane [59-61]. Figure 3 presents such a model (62) which in the opinion of the authors, seems to be supported by the studies of others.

THE RND EFFLUX PUMP

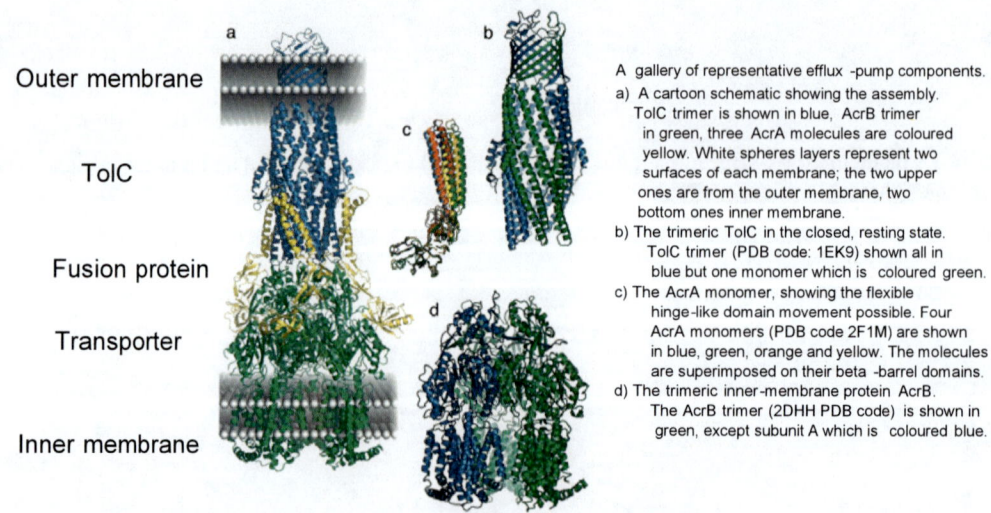

Outer membrane

TolC

Fusion protein

Transporter

Inner membrane

A gallery of representative efflux -pump components.
a) A cartoon schematic showing the assembly.
   TolC trimer is shown in blue, AcrB trimer
   in green, three AcrA molecules are coloured
   yellow. White spheres layers represent two
   surfaces of each membrane; the two upper
   ones are from the outer membrane, two
   bottom ones inner membrane.
b) The trimeric TolC in the closed, resting state.
   TolC trimer (PDB code: 1EK9) shown all in
   blue but one monomer which is coloured green.
c) The AcrA monomer, showing the flexible
   hinge-like domain movement possible. Four
   AcrA monomers (PDB code 2F1M) are shown
   in blue, green, orange and yellow. The molecules
   are superimposed on their beta -barrel domains.
d) The trimeric inner-membrane protein AcrB.
   The AcrB trimer (2DHH PDB code) is shown in
   green, except subunit A which is coloured blue.

Courtesy of Ben Luisi-Cambridge Univ

Figure 3. Model representing the assembly of TolC, the transporter protein AcrB and the fusion protein AcrA. Adapted from Pietras Z. et al. (63).

The mechanism by which unrelated antibiotics are extruded by this tripartite efflux pump of Gram-negative MDR bacteria is thought to involve the transport of a proton from the surface of the cell where the proton gradient is strongest through the TolC channel and finally, through the transporter itself. The passage of the proton energises the transporter component to expell the antibiotic from the region of the inner membrane to the TolC where it makes its way to the outside of the cell. The physical chemistry behind this process is beyond the scope of this review and the reader is encouraged to refer to an excellent review by Ben Luisi et al. [62].

Genetic Regulation of Efflux Pumps of Gram-Negative Bacteria (ex. *Escherichia coli*)

E. coli has at least eight tripartite efflux pumps that, when over-expressed, contribute to the MDR phenotype of the organism [7]. Over-expression of these RND efflux pumps results when the organism is exposed to increasing concentrations of an antibiotic, such as tetracycline [7, 8]. The over-expression of these efflux pumps renders the bacterium increasingly resistant to tetracycline along with other antibiotics [7]. At the onset of exposure to tetracycline, the stress regulator genes *soxS* and *rob* are immediately increased. Soon thereafter, the first regulatory gene showing an increased expression is *marB* which is soon followed by *marA*. After the regulatory genes are activated, the expression of the stress genes begins to decrease and the expression of genes that code for the transporters of the main efflux pumps of *E. coli*, namely, *acrB*, *acrF* and *yhiV* are progressively increased with each increase in tetracycline concentration to which the bacterium is exposed.

Figure 4 summarises these findings. Following transfer of the tetracycline induced resistant strain (AG100$_{TET}$) to drug-free media (and hence the removal of the transient selective pressure) initial susceptibility to tetracycline, as well as to the other antibiotics that constituted this MDR phenotype, is restored [7]. Therefore, under these conditions, the genetic response to exposure to increasing concentrations of the antibiotic may be considered as one of adaptation. However, if the tetracycline induced strain is serially passed in medium containing a constant concentration of tetracycline such as 10 mg/L, the organism becomes increasingly resistant, reaching levels of resistance greater than 120 mg/L of tetracycline even though it had never been exposed to a concentration of the agent above 10 mg/L. The expression of genes that encode the global regulators of efflux pumps such as *marA, marB,* stress genes such as *soxR* and *soxS,* and genes that encode the transporters *acrB* and *acrF* of this high-level tetracycline induced resistant strain is now similar to that of the parental wild-type.

To determine whether any broader pleiotrophic effects could be recognized, these strains were investigated using a phenotypic microarray. The complete panel of reactions was analysed and when compared to the isogenic wild-type strain *E. coli* AG100, demonstrated a large number of potential genetic targets whose activities had been altered (data not shown). Moreover, because this strain did not revert to initial susceptibility [to tetracycline (MIC of 2 mg/L)] after greater than 50 serial passages in 500 mL of drug-free medium, the existence of one or more mutations cannot be ruled out. The possibility that such mutations had taken place as a consequence of a master mutator gene, as described by Chopra et al. [63], may represent a reasonable hypothesis.

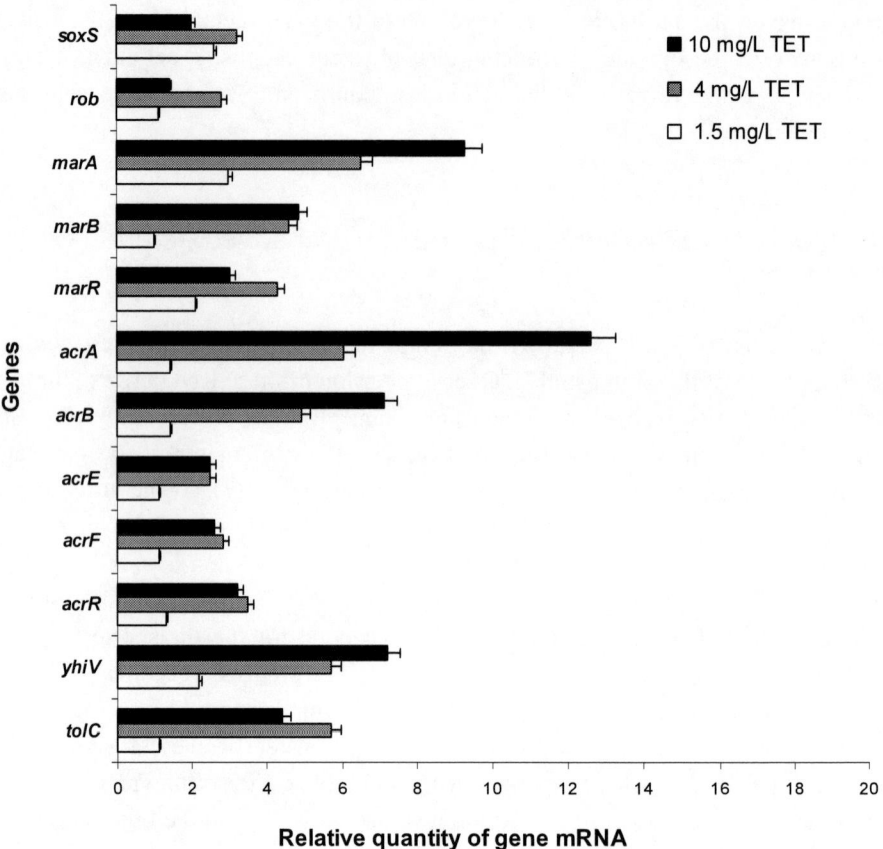

Figure 4. Relative expression of regulators and inner membrane transporter genes of *E. coli* AG100 gradually exposed to 1.5 mg/L, 4 and 10 mg/L of tetracycline (TET) compared to its parental non-induced strain.

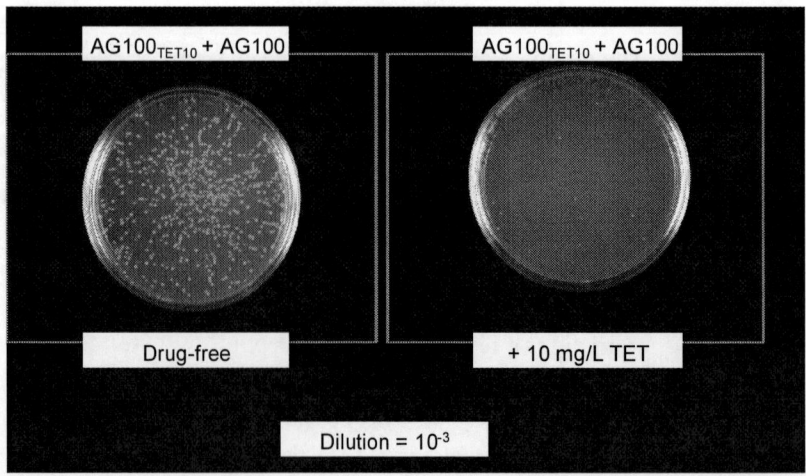

Figure 5. Survival fitness of AG100$_{TET10}$, that has been serially exposed to 10 mg/L of tetracycline. Plate on left is drug free and on right place contains 10 mg/L of tetracycline.

The question of whether the development of an extreme, non-reversible resistance phenotype to tetracycline caused a decrease of fitness was studied by inoculating 500 mL drug-free medium with equal numbers of the wild-type isogenic reference strain (AG100) and the strain that was now resistant to 120 mg/L of tetracycline (AG100$_{TET10}$), incubated at 37°C, and determination of cell number expressed as colony forming units (CFU) from both drug-free and tetracycline (10 mg/L) containing agar plates. As is shown by Figure 5, very few colonies detected on drug-free agar were of the highly tetracycline resistant strain. Indeed, the AG100$_{TET10}$ appears to pay a high fitness cost when it "decides" to reduce the available energy required to maintain a high efflux activity and embark on a rapid evolutionary pathway.

Evaluation of Intrinsic and Over-Expressed Efflux Pumps of Gram-Negative Bacteria

The recently developed semi-automated method that utilizes the common efflux pump fluorochrome substrate EB, affords the sensitivity for the characterization and assessment of the intrinsic efflux pump system of *E. coli* wild-type reference strain, as well as those that express an MDR phenotype [50, 64]. Laboratory methods used to evaluate an efflux pump system are best conducted as close to physiologically relevant conditions as possible, namely, conditions provided by the *in vivo* environment during infection of the human. Such conditions usually involve a temperature of 37°C, the presence of a metabolic energy source in the event that such a source is needed and suitable ionic conditions similar to the interstitial fluids of the infected host. EB must be at a concentration in the medium that does not yield a fluorescence signal, and yet, if and when it begins to be accumulated within the periplasmic space of the bacterium, the relative concentration much reach detectable levels that can be measured by an instrument on a real-time basis. Accumulation of EB is considered to be due to a concentration of EB that exceeds the efflux capacity of the pump or to the presence of an agent that inhibits the pump [50, 64]. As an example of the method, the *E. coli* tetracycline induced strain AG100$_{TET}$ is incubated at 37°C in a saline phosphate solution that is buffered at varying pH, containing glucose and increasing concentrations of EB. As shown by Figure 6, accumulation of EB by this over-expressing efflux pumps strain is minimal at low pH (5 to 7) compared to the accumulation observable at the higher pH of 8.

Efflux of EB and the physiological conditions that influence it are demonstrated by the following: cells are pre-loaded with EB under conditions that minimize efflux (temperature of 25°C; no energy source; presence of an EPI) and the accumulation of EB is followed on a real-time basis. When sufficient EB has accumulated in the presence of an EPI, the medium is replaced with EB-free medium at pH 7 containing an energy source (glucose) and efflux is followed at 37°C. As shown by Figure 7, efflux of EB by a strain of *E. coli* that over-expresses its efflux pump (AG100$_{TET}$) can be inhibited by the phenothiazine chlorpromazine in a concentration dependent manner. The phenothiazine thioridazine is less effective.

The activity of an over-expressed efflux pump system is readily demonstrated by the method. Employing a *Salmonella* Enteritidis, that has been selected and made resistant to ciprofloxacin (*Salmonella* 5408$_{cip}$) and which over-expresses *acrAB* some 6-fold over that of its parent *Salmonella* 5408, one can readily see that the *Salmonella* 5408$_{cip}$ strain begins to accumulate EB at a concentration of EB (5 mg/L) and above (Figure 8a) compared to its isogenic parent wherein accumulation of EB begins at lower concentrations (1 mg/L) (Figure 8b).

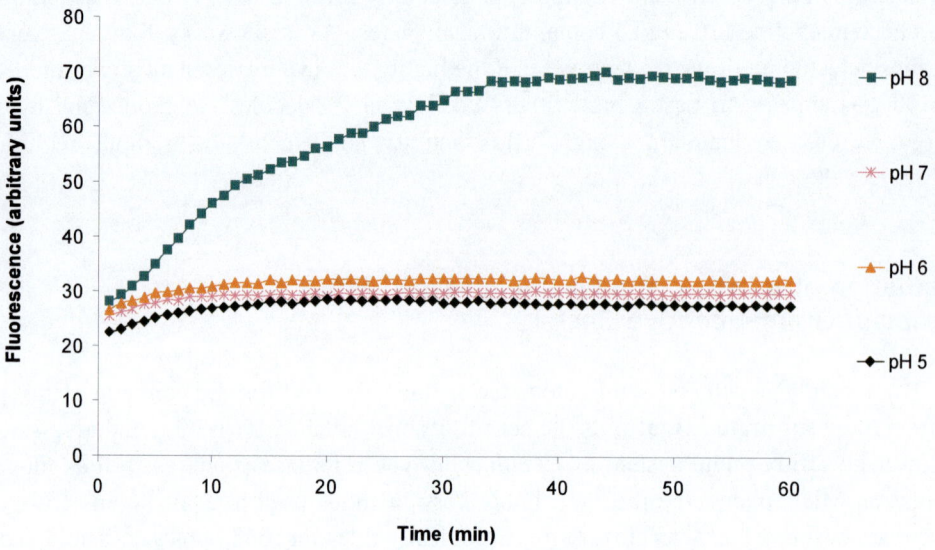

Figure 6. The effect of pH on the accumulation of EB used at 5 mg/L by *E. coli* AG100$_{TET}$ that over-expresses its AcrAB efflux pump.

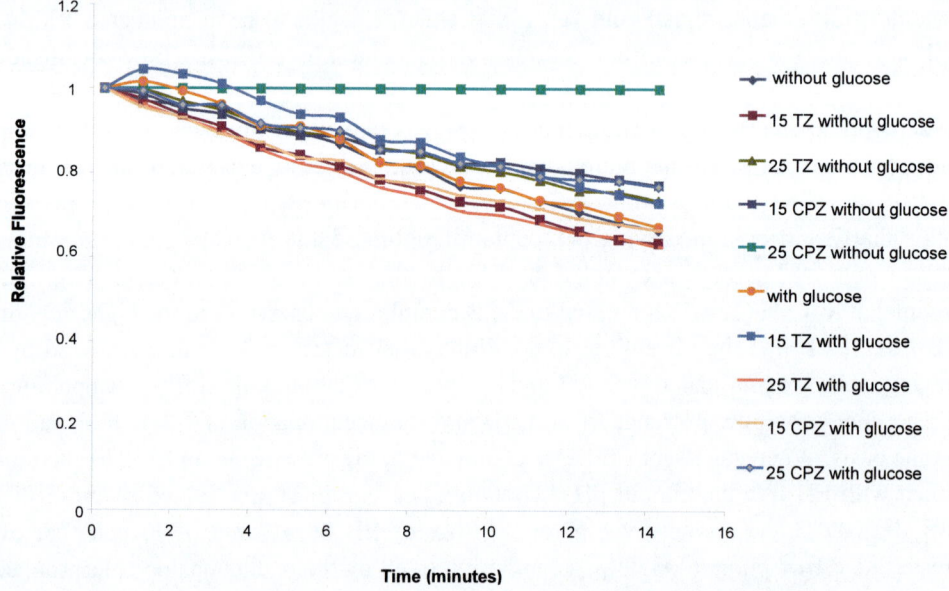

Figure 7. Demonstration of efflux of EB by *E. coli* AG100$_{TET}$ in the presence or absence of glucose at 0.4%.

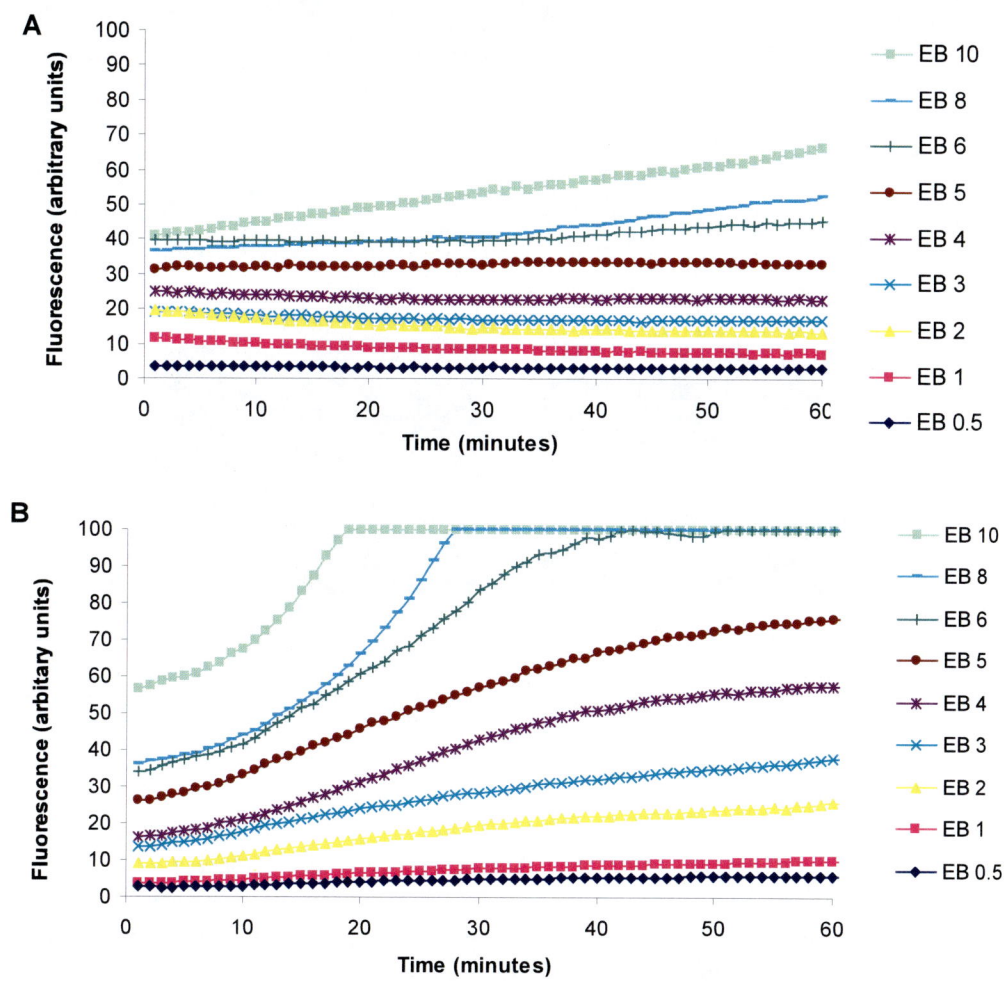

Figure 8. Determination of the highest concentration of EB that can be handled by Salmonella 5408cip (A) and Salmonella 5408 (B). The lines represent increasing concentrations of EB in mg/L.

These results are comparable to those obtained by the EB-agar cartwheel method [64, 65], which show that whereas 1.0 mg/L of EB causes the colonies of the *Salmonella* 5408 strain to fluoresce, the *Salmonella* 5408$_{cip}$ does not fluoresce even with a concentration of EB of 2.5 mg/L (Figure 9).

The accumulation of EB by Gram-negative and Gram-positive bacteria, as previously discussed, is affected by pH; at low pH accumulation is minimal, at higher pH it is far greater. This observation can be reproduced using the EB-agar cartwheel method as shown by Figure 10. Note that at pH 5 the concentration that produces fluorescence of the colonies is always much higher than at pH 8. Also, at pH 8, a concentration of EB as high as 3 mg/L does not produce fluorescence of the *Salmonella* 5408$_{cip}$.

The permeability of *Salmonella* to antibiotics and other noxious agents and the bacterium response to these differs from that of *E. coli*.

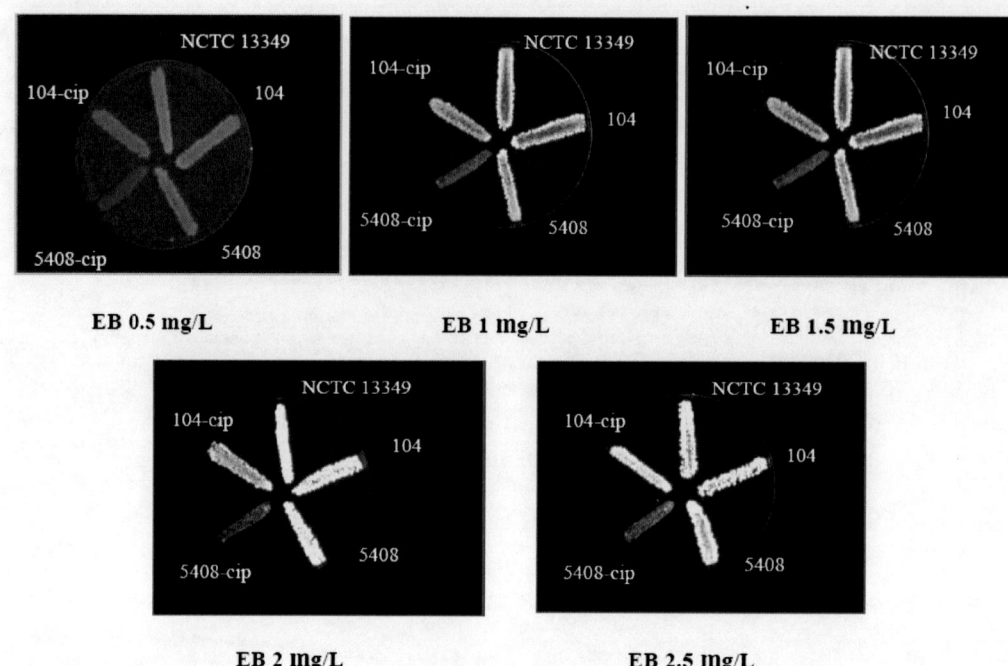

Figure 9. The EB-agar cartwheel method applied to a set of five Salmonella strains at pH 7. Salmonella 5408cip.

The major differences include: i) the regulation of the main efflux pump of *Salmonella* *acrAB* which although very similar to that of *E. coli* [66] is also influenced by *ramA* a gene that is absent in *E. coli* [67, 68] ii) the regulation of permeability in *Salmonella* takes place as a consequence of the activation of *pmrA* by its cognate sensor kinase PmrB when the organism is cultured in medium at pH 5 [69] and the subsequent increase in the lipopolysaccharide deposition by the organism through the over-expression of genes that collectively result in the increased synthesis of Lipid A [70, 71]. That the pH of the medium is a major regulator of the permeability of *Salmonella* to an efflux pump substrate such as EB is clearly demonstrated by Figure 10.

The selection of the highest concentration at each pH that does not produce accumulation affords the opportunity to study additional conditions that may affect the concentrations of EB accumulated, such as the modulation of permeability to EB promoted by an EPI. As shown by Figure 11, the accumulation of EB by a *Salmonella* strain, in this case *Salmonella* 104, at pH 8 in the presence of 50 mg/L of the phenothiazine promotes rapid and substantial accumulation of EB. This step accumulation is soon followed by efflux. Because thioridazine inhibits ATPases and kinases [72-74], a metabolic source of protons would be required for activation of the efflux pump. Considering that *Salmonella* is primed for the activation of genes that are involved in the synthesis of Lipid A and increased deposition of the lipopolysaccharide layer [72-74], we considered the possibility that the source of energy that afforded the extrusion of EB as a consequence of exposure to thioridazine came from the metabolism of fatty acids. In *Salmonella* Enteritidis 104$_{cip}$, the *lpxC* gene is up-regulated (data not shown), resulting increased lipopolysaccharide synthesis. As shown by Figure 11, the addition of palmitic acid reduces thioridazine promoted accumulation of EB.

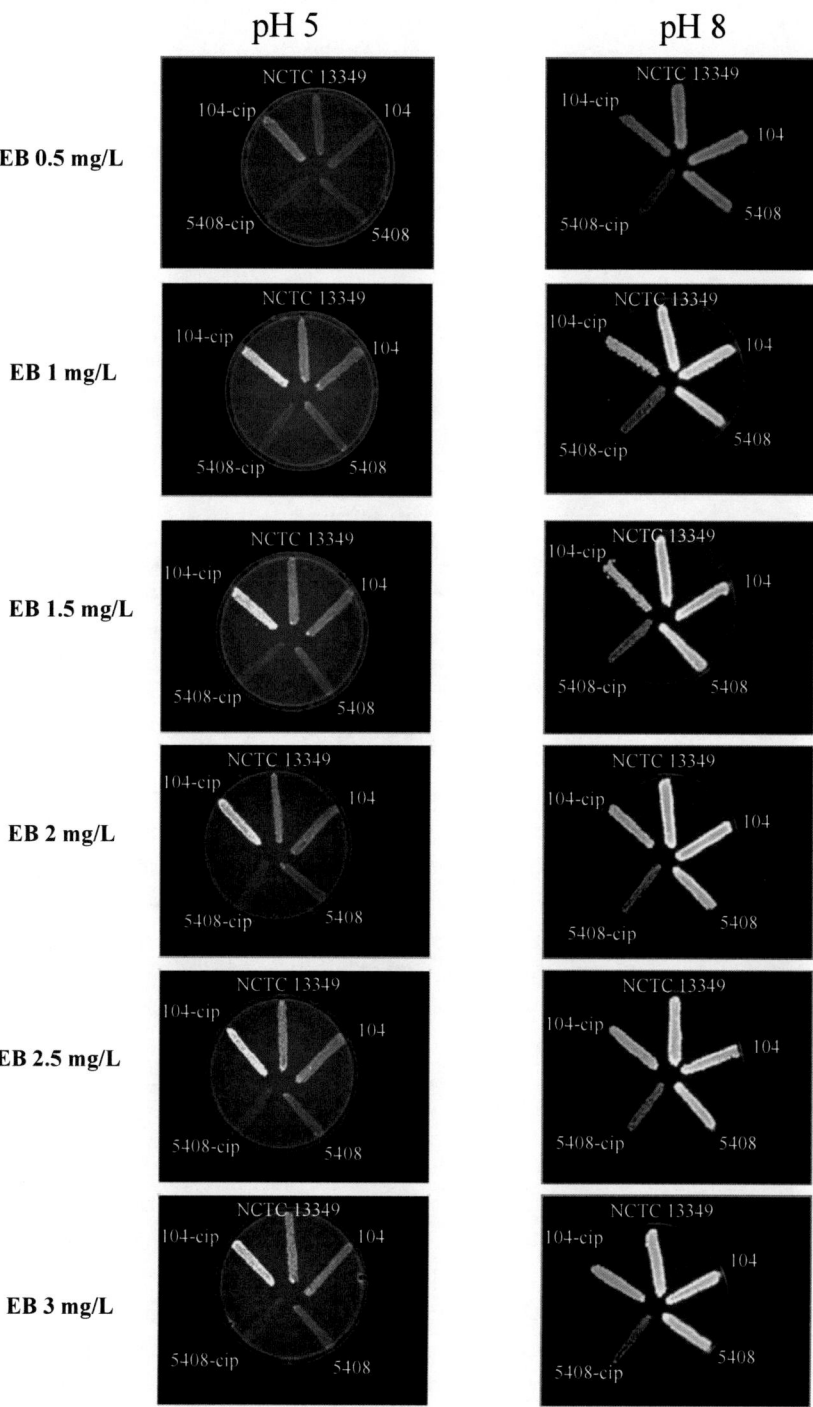

Figure 10. The EB-agar cartwheel method applied to a set of five *Salmonella* strains at pH 5 and 8. Note that at pH 5 the concentration of EB that produces fluorescence of the strains is higher than at pH 8. Moreover, even at pH 8, a concentration of EB as high as 3 mg/L does not produce fluorescence of the *Salmonella* 5408$_{cip}$.

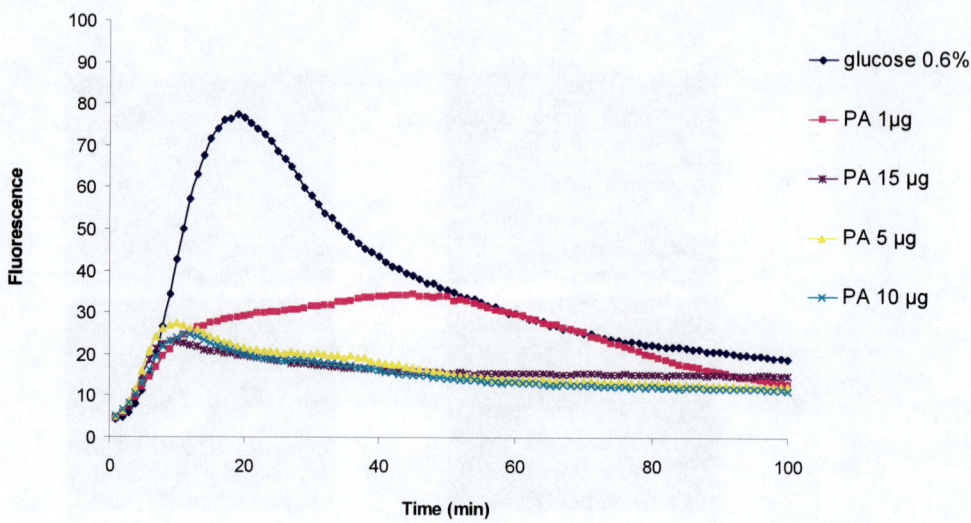

Figure 11. Accumulation of EB at 1 mg/L in the presence of thioridazine (TZ) at 50 mg/L by *Salmonella* 104 at pH 8. The addition of palmitic acid (PA) reduces the accumulation of EB.

Although far from being understood, the above experiments demonstrate that for *Salmonella*, the status of permeability to a noxious agent such as EB involves a pH dependent efflux pump system which is supplemented in its activity by metabolic energy when conditions of the environment does not support the source of protons needed to drive the pump. It is important to note that although hydrolysis of ATP is increased at high pH due to the F_1F_o ATP synthase [72], because the oxyreductase II as well as the F_1F_o ATP synthase are inhibited by phenothiazines [73, 74] the source of protons needed to drive the efflux pump is removed. Because this organism is already primed by its PmrA/kinase PmrB to respond to a noxious agent by up-regulation of its lipopolysaccharide and Lipid A content, the source of protons needed to drive the efflux pump at pH 8 is assured.

Summary and Perspectives

The response of bacteria to a given antibiotic or other toxic agent that does not immediately kill them results in an adaptive response that secures their survival. This response may involve a number of distinct mechanisms, among which is the activation of genes that promote the appearance of transporters that extrude the agent prior to its reaching its target. These transporters extrude a large variety of chemically unrelated compounds and hence they bestow on the bacterium a MDR phenotype. The appearance of this MDR phenotype during therapy makes therapy problematic. Understanding the genetic and physiological properties of MDR efflux pumps is an absolute requirement if MDR bacterial infections are to be successfully managed. The material presented in this chapter is only the beginning for the evaluation and assessment of MDR efflux pumps. There is much to learn and methods that afford the needed understanding will eventually pave the way for the successful management of an MDR bacterial infection.

References

[1]   Martins M., Dastidar S.G., Fanning S., Kristiansen J.E., Molnar J., Pagès J.M., Schelz Z., Spengler G., Viveiros M., Amaral L. (2008) Potential role of non-antibiotics (helper compounds) in the treatment of multidrug-resistant Gram-negative infections: mechanisms for their direct and indirect activities. *Int. J. Antimicrob. Agents* 31: 198-208.

[2]   Poole K. (2007) Efflux pumps as antimicrobial resistance mechanisms. *Ann. Med.* 39: 162-176.

[3]   Mahamoud A., Chevalier J., Davin-Regli A., Barbe J., Pagès J.M. (2006) Quinoline derivatives as promising inhibitors of antibiotic efflux pump in multidrug resistant *Enterobacter aerogenes* isolates. *Curr. Drug Targets* 7: 843-847.

[4]   Piddock L.J. (2006). Clinically relevant chromosomally encoded multidrug resistance efflux pumps in bacteria. *Clin. Microbiol. Rev.* 19: 382-402.

[5]   Pagès JM, Masi M, Barbe J. (2005) Inhibitors of efflux pumps in Gram-negative bacteria. *Trends Mol. Med.* 11: 382-389.

[6]   Martins A., Couto I., Aagaard L., Martins M., Viveiros M., Kristiansen J.E., Amaral L. (2007) Prolonged exposure of methicillin-resistant *Staphylococcus aureus* (MRSA) COL strain to increasing concentrations of oxacillin results in a multidrug-resistant phenotype. *Int. J. Antimicrob. Agents* 29: 302-305.

[7]   Viveiros M., Dupont M., Rodrigues L., Couto I., Davin-Regli A., Martins M., Pagès J.M., Amaral L. (2007) Antibiotic stress, genetic response and altered permeability of *E. coli*. *PLoS ONE* 2: e365.

[8]   Viveiros M., Jesus A., Brito M., Leandro C., Martins M., Ordway D., Molnar A.M., Molnar J., Amaral L. (2005) Inducement and reversal of tetracycline resistance in *Escherichia coli* K-12 and expression of proton gradient-dependent multidrug efflux pump genes. *Antimicrob. Agents Chemother.* 49: 3578-3582.

[9]   Viveiros M., Portugal I., Bettencourt R., Victor T.C., Jordaan A.M., Leandro C., Ordway D., Amaral L. (2002) Isoniazid-induced transient high-level resistance in *Mycobacterium tuberculosis*. *Antimicrob. Agents Chemother.* 46: 2804-2810.

[10] Couto I., Costa S.S., Viveiros M., Martins M., Amaral L. (2008) Efflux-mediated response of *Staphylococcus aureus* exposed to ethidium bromide. *J. Antimicrob. Chemother.* 62: 504-513.

[11] Kristiansen M.M., Leandro C., Ordway D., Martins M. Viveiros M., Pacheco T., Kristiansen J.E. and Amaral L. (2005) Thioridazine Reduces Resistance Of Methicillin Resistant *Staphylococcus aureus* By Inhibiting A Reserpine Sensitive Efflux Pump. *In Vivo* 20: 361-366.

[12] Kaatz G.W., Moudgal V.V., Seo S.M., Kristiansen J.E. (2003) Phenothiazines and thioxanthenes inhibit multidrug efflux pump activity in *Staphylococcus aureus*. *Antimicrob. Agents Chemother.* 47: 719-726.

[13] Lomovskaya O., Bostian K.A. (2006) Practical applications and feasibility of efflux pump inhibitors in the clinic – a vision for applied use. *Biochem. Pharmacol.* 71:910-918.

[14] Lomovskaya O., Watkins W.J. (2001) Efflux pumps: their role in antibacterial drug discovery. *Curr. Med. Chem.* 8:1699-1711.

[15] Kamicker B.J., Sweeney M.T., Kaczmarek F., Dib-Hajj F., Shang W., Crimin K., Duignan J. , Gootz T.D. (2008) Bacterial efflux pump inhibitors. *Methods Mol. Med.* 142: 187-204.

[16] German N., Kaatz G.W., Kerns R.J. (2008) Synthesis and evaluation of PSSRI-based inhibitors of *Staphylococcus aureus* multidrug efflux pumps. *Bioorg. Med. Chem. Lett.* 18: 1368-1373.

[17] Robertson G.T., Doyle T.B., Du Q., Duncan L., Mdluli K.E., Lynch A.S. (2007) A Novel indole compound that inhibits *Pseudomonas aeruginosa* growth by targeting MreB is a substrate for MexAB-OprM. *J. Bacteriol.* 189: 6870-6881.

[18] Ball A.R., Casadei G., Samosorn S., Bremner J.B., Ausubel F.M., Moy T.I., Lewis K. (2006) Conjugating berberine to a multidrug efflux pump inhibitor creates an effective antimicrobial. *A.C.S Chem. Biol.* 1:594-600.

[19] Pannek S., Higgins P.G., Steinke P., Jonas D., Akova M., Bohnert J.A., Seifert H., Kern W.V. (2006) Multidrug efflux inhibition in *Acinetobacter baumannii*: comparison between 1-(1-naphthylmethyl)-piperazine and phenyl-arginine-beta-naphthylamide. *J. Antimicrob. Chemother.* 57:970-974.

[20] Ramón-García S., Martín C., Aínsa J.A., De Rossi E. (2006) Characterization of tetracycline resistance mediated by the efflux pump Tap from *Mycobacterium fortuitum. J. Antimicrob. Chemother.* 57:252-259.

[21] Marquez B. (2005) Bacterial efflux systems and efflux pumps inhibitors. *Biochimie* 87: 1137-1147.

[22] Hendricks O., Butterworth T.S., Kristiansen J.E. (2003) The in-vitro antimicrobial effect of non-antibiotics and putative inhibitors of efflux pumps on *Pseudomonas aeruginosa* and *Staphylococcus aureus*. *Int. J. Antimicrob. Agents* 22: 262-264.

[23] Molnár J., Hevér A., Fakla I., Fischer J., Ocsovski I., Aszalós A. (1997) Inhibition of the transport function of membrane proteins by some substituted phenothiazines in *E. coli* and multidrug resistant tumor cells. *Anticancer Res.* 17: 481-486.

[24] Amaral L., Viveiros M., Kristiansen J.E. (2006) "Non-Antibiotics": alternative therapy for the management of MDRTB and MRSA in economically disadvantaged countries. *Curr. Drug Targets* 7: 887-891.

[25] Amaral L., Viveiros M., Molnar J. (2004) Antimicrobial activity of phenothiazines. *In Vivo* 18: 725-731.

[26] Amaral L., Viveiros M., Kristiansen J.E. (2001) Phenothiazines: potential alternatives for the management of antibiotic resistant infections of tuberculosis and malaria in developing countries. *Trop. Med. Int. Health* 6: 1016-1022.

[27] Amaral L., Kristiansen J.E., Viveiros M., Atouguia J. (2001) Activity of phenothiazines against antibiotic-resistant *Mycobacterium tuberculosis*: a review supporting further studies that may elucidate the potential use of thioridazine as anti-tuberculosis therapy. *J. Antimicrob. Chemother.* 47: 505-511.

[28] Amaral L., Kristiansen J.E. (2000) Phenothiazines: an alternative to conventional therapy for the initial management of suspected multidrug resistant tuberculosis. A call for studies. *Int. J. Antimicrob. Agents* 14: 173-176.

[29] Lorca G.L., Barabote R.D., Zlotopolski V., Tran C., Winnen B., Hvorup R.N., Stonestrom A.J., Nguyen E., Huang L.W., Kim D.S., Saier M.H. Jr. (2007) Transport capabilities of eleven gram-positive bacteria: comparative genomic analyses. *Biochim. Biophys. Acta* 1768: 1342-1366.

[30] Piddock L.J., Jin Y.F. (1999) Antimicrobial activity and accumulation of moxifloxacin in quinolone-susceptible bacteria. *J. Antimicrob. Chemother.* 43: 39-42.

[31] Muñoz-Bellido J.L., Alonzo Manzanares M., Martínez Andrés J.A., Guttiérrez Zufiaurre M.N., Ortiz G., Segovia Hernández M., García-Rodríguez JA. (1999) Efflux pump-mediated quinolone resistance in *Staphylococcus aureus* strains wild type for *gyrA*, *gyrB*, *grlA*, and *norA*. *Antimicrob. Agents Chemother.* 43: 354-356.

[32] Jia B., Zhou T.Q., Huang A.L., Huang W.X. (2008) Role of TMS5: staphylococcal multidrug-efflux protein QacA. *Chin. Med. J. (Engl).* 121: 409-413.

[33] Smith K., Gemmell C.G., Hunter I.S. (2008) The association between biocide tolerance and the presence or absence of *qac* genes among hospital-acquired and community-acquired MRSA isolates. *J. Antimicrob. Chemother.* 61: 78-84.

[34] Sekiguchi J., Hama T., Fujino T., Araake M., Irie A., Saruta K., Konosaki H., Nishimura H., Kawano A., Kudo K., Kondo T., Sasazuki T., Kuratsuji T., Yoshikura H., Kirikae T. (2004) Detection of the antiseptic- and disinfectant-resistance genes *qacA*, *qacB*, and *qacC* in methicillin-resistant *Staphylococcus aureus* isolated in a Tokyo hospital. *Jpn. J. Infect. Dis.* 57: 288-291.

[35] Piddock L.J., Johnson M.M., Simjee S., Pumbwe L. (2002) Expression of efflux pump gene *pmrA* in fluoroquinolone-resistant and –susceptible clinical isolates of *Streptococcus pneumoniae. Antimicrob. Agents Chemother.* 46: 808-812.

[36] German N, Wei P, Kaatz GW, Kerns RJ. (2008) Synthesis and evaluation of fluoroquinolone derivatives as substrate-based inhibitors of bacterial efflux pumps. *Eur. J. Med. Chem.* 43: 2453-2463.

[37] Thota N., Koul S., Reddy M.V., Sangwan P.L., Khan I.A., Kumar A., Raja A.F., Andotra S.S., Qazi G.N. (2008) Citral derived amides as potent bacterial NorA efflux pump inhibitors. *Bioorg. Med. Chem.* 16: 6535-6543.

[38] Vidaillac C., Guillon J., Moreau S., Arpin C., Lagardère A., Larrouture S., Dallemagne P., Caignard D.H., Quentin C., Jarry C. (2007) Synthesis of new 4-[2-(alkylamino) ethylthio]pyrrolo[1,2-a]quinoxaline and 5-[2-(alkylamino) ethylthio]pyrrolo[1,2-a]thieno[3,2-e]pyrazine derivatives, as potential bacterial multidrug resistance pump inhibitors. *J. Enzyme. Inhib. Med. Chem.* 22: 620-631.

[39] Michalet S., Cartier G., David B., Mariotte A.M., Dijoux-franca M.G., Kaatz G.W., Stavri M., Gibbons S. (2007) N-caffeoylphenalkylamide derivatives as bacterial efflux pump inhibitors. *Bioorg. Med. Chem. Lett.* 17: 1755-1758.

[40] Vidaillac C., Guillon J., Arpin C., Forfar-Bares I., Ba B.B., Grellet J., Moreau S., Caignard D.H., Jarry C., Quentin C. (2007) Synthesis of omeprazole analogues and evaluation of these as potential inhibitors of the multidrug efflux pump NorA of *Staphylococcus aureus. Antimicrob. Agents Chemother.* 51: 831-838.

[41] Kaatz G.W., Seo S.M., Barriere S.L., Albrecht L.M., Rybak M.J. (1991) Development of resistance to fleroxacin during therapy of experimental methicillin-susceptible *Staphylococcus aureus* endocarditis. *Antimicrob. Agents Chemother.* 35: 1547-1550.

[42] Noguchi N., Okihara T., Namiki Y., Kumaki Y., Yamanaka Y., Koyama M., Wakasugi K., Sasatsu M. (2005) Susceptibility and resistance genes to fluoroquinolones in methicillin-resistant *Staphylococcus aureus* isolated in 2002. *Int. J. Antimicrob. Agents* 25: 374-379.

[43] Schmitz F.J., Fluit A.C., Brisse S., Verhoef J., Köhrer K., Milatovic D. (1999) Molecular epidemiology of quinolone resistance and comparative in vitro activities of new quinolones against European *Staphylococcus aureus* isolates. *FEMS Immunol. Med. Microbiol.* 26: 281-287.

[44] Ng E.Y., Trucksis M., Hooper D.C. (1994) Quinolone resistance mediated by *norA*: physiologic characterization and relationship to *flqB*, a quinolone resistance locus on the *Staphylococcus aureus* chromosome. *Antimicrob. Agents Chemother.* 38: 1345-1355.

[45] Kaatz G.W., Seo S.M. (1997) Mechanisms of fluoroquinolone resistance in genetically related strains of *Staphylococcus aureus*. *Antimicrob. Agents Chemother.* 41: 2733-2737.

[46] Muñoz Bellido J.L., Alonso Manzanares M.A., Yagüe Guirao G., Gutiérrez Zufiaurre M.N., Toldos M.C., Segovia Hernández M., Garcia-Rodríguez J.A. (1999) In vitro activities of 13 fluoroquinolones against *Staphylococcus aureus* isolates with characterized mutations in *gyrA*, *gyrB*, *grlA*, and *norA* and against wild-type isolates. *Antimicrob. Agents Chemother.* 43: 966-968.

[47] Kaatz G.W., Seo S.M. (1995) Inducible NorA-mediated multidrug resistance in *Staphylococcus aureus*. *Antimicrob. Agents Chemother.* 39: 2650-2655.

[48] Lee E.W., Chen J., Huda M.N., Kuroda T., Mizushima T., Tsuchiya T. (2003) Functional cloning and expression of *emeA*, and characterization of EmeA, a multidrug efflux pump from *Enterococcus faecalis*. *Biol. Pharm. Bull.* 26: 266-270.

[49] Spengler G., Martins A., Schelz Z., Rodrigues L., Aagaard L., Martins M., Costa S.S., Couto I., Viveiros M., Kristiansen J.E., Fanning S., Molnar J. and Amaral L. Characterisation of intrinsic efflux activity of *Enterococcus faecalis* ATCC29212 by a semi-automated ethidium bromide method. Accepted by *In Vivo*.

[50] Viveiros M., Martins A., Paixão L., Rodrigues L., Martins M., Couto I., Fähnrich E., Kern W.V., Amaral L. (2008) Demonstration of intrinsic efflux activity of *Escherichia coli* K-12 AG100 by an automated ethidium bromide method. *Int. J. Antimicrob. Agents* 31: 458-462.

[51] Lee E.W., Huda M.N., Kuroda T., Mizushima T., Tsuchiya T. (2003) EfrAB, an ABC multidrug efflux pump in *Enterococcus faecalis*. *Antimicrob. Agents Chemother.* 47: 3733-3738.

[52] Davidson A.L., Dassa E., Orelle C., Chen J. (2008) Structure, function, and evolution of bacterial ATP-binding cassette systems. *Microbiol. Mol. Biol. Rev.* 72: 317-364.

[53] Zakharov S.D., Li X., Red'ko T.P., Dilley R.A. (1996) Calcium binding to the subunit c of *E. coli* ATP-synthase and possible functional implications in energy coupling. *J. Bioenerg. Biomembr.* 28: 483-494.

[54] Thanassi D.G. and Hultgren S.J. (2000) Multiple pathways allow protein secretion across the bacterial outer membrane. *Curr. Opin. Cell Biol.* 12: 420-430.

[55] Borges-Walmsley M.I., McKeegan K.S., Walmsley A.R. (2003) Structure and function of efflux pumps that confer resistance to drugs. *Biochem. J.* 376: 313-338.

[56] Delepelaire P. (2004) Type I secretion in gram-negative bacteria. *Biochim. Biophys. Acta*; 1694: 149-161.

[57] Murakami S., Nakashima R., Yamashita E., Matsumoto T. and Yamaguchi A. (2006) Crystal structures of a multidrug transporter reveal a functionally rotating mechanism. *Nature* 443: 173-179.

[58] Akama H., Matsuura T., Kashiwagi S., Yoneyama H., Narita S., Tsukihara T., Nakagawa A. and Nakae T. (2004) Crystal structure of the membrane fusion protein, MexA, of the multidrug transporter in *Pseudomonas aeruginosa*. *J. Biol. Chem.* 279: 25939-25942.

[59] Higgins M.K., Bokma E., Koronakis E., Hughes C., Koronakis V. (2004) Structure of the periplasmic component of a bacterial drug efflux pump. *Proc. Natl. Acad. Sci. U.S.A.* 101: 9994-9999.

[60] Fernandez-Recio J., Walas F., Federici L., Venkatesh Pratap J., Bavro V.N., Miguel R.N., Mizuguchi K. and Luisi B. (2004) A model of a transmembrane drug-efflux pump from Gram-negative bacteria. *FEBS Lett.* 578: 5-9.

[61] Lobedanz S., Bokma E., Symmons M.F., Koronakis E., Hughes C. and Koronakis V. (2007) A periplasmic coiled-coil interface underlying TolC recruitment and the assembly of bacterial drug efflux pumps. *Proc. Natl. Acad. Sci. U.S.A.* 104: 4612-4617.

[62] Pietras Z., Bavro V.N., Furnham N., Pellegrini-Calace M., Milner-White E.J. and Luisi B.F. (2008) Structure and mechanism of drug efflux machinery in Gram negative bacteria. *Curr. Drug Targets* 9: 719-728.

[63] Chopra I., O'Neill A.J., Miller K. (2003) The role of mutators in the emergence of antibiotic-resistant bacteria. *Drug Resist. Updat.* 6: 137-145.

[64] Viveiros M., Martins M., Martins A., Rodrigues L., Couto I., Fanning S. and Amaral L. (2008) New methods for the identification of efflux mediated MDR bacteria, genetic assessment of regulators and efflux pump constituents, characterization of efflux systems and screening for inhibitors of efflux pumps. *Curr. Drug Targets* 9: 760-778.

[65] Martins M., Santos B., Couto I., Viveiros M., Pages J.M., Molnar M., Cruz A. and Amaral L. (2006) Instrument free method for the demonstration and assessment of efflux pumps that cause bacterial resistance. *In Vivo* 20: 657-664.

[66] Mahamoud A., Chevalier J., Alibert-Franco S., Kern W.V., Pagès J.M. (2007) Antibiotic efflux pumps in Gram-negative bacteria: the inhibitor response strategy. *J. Antimicrob. Chemother.* 59: 1223-1229.

[67] Nikaido E., Yamaguchi A., Nishino K. (2008) AcrAB multidrug efflux pump regulation in *Salmonella enterica* serovar Typhimurium by RamA in response to environmental signals. *J. Biol. Chem.* 283: 24245-24253.

[68] Dowd S.E., Killinger-Mann K., Brashears M., Fralick J. (2008) Evaluation of gene expression in a single antibiotic exposure-derived isolate of *Salmonella enterica* typhimurium 14028 possessing resistance to multiple antibiotics. *Foodborne Pathog. Dis.* 5: 205-221.

[69] Perez J.C., Groisman E.A. (2007) Acid pH activation of the PmrA/PmrB two-component regulatory system of *Salmonella enterica*. *Mol. Microbiol.* 63: 283-293.

[70] Murata T., Tseng W., Guina T., Miller S.I., Nikaido H. (2007) PhoPQ-mediated regulation produces a more robust permeability barrier in the outer membrane of *Salmonella enterica* serovar typhimurium. *J. Bacteriol.* 189: 7213-7222.

[71] Gunn J.S. (2008) The Salmonella PmrAB regulon: lipopolysaccharide modifications, antimicrobial peptide resistance and more. *Trends Microbiol.* 16: 284-290.

[72] see: http://www.rpi.edu/dept/bcbp/molbiochem/MBWeb/mb1/part2/f1fo.htm for complete review of scheme.

[73] Teh J.S., Yano T., Rubin H. (2007) Type II NADH: menaquinone oxidoreductase of *Mycobacterium tuberculosis*. *Infect. Disord. Drug Targets* 7: 169-181.

[74] Tran S.L., Cook G.M. (2005) The F1Fo-ATP synthase of *Mycobacterium smegmatis* is essential for growth. *J. Bacteriol.* 187: 5023-5028.

In: Antibiotic Resistance…

Editors: A. R. Bonilla and K. P. Muniz

ISBN 978-1-60741-623-4

© 2009 Nova Science Publishers, Inc.

Chapter XIV

Genetic and Phenotypic Characterization of Drug-Resistant *Mycobacterium Tuberculosis* Isolates

Maysaa El Sayed Zaki[*]

Professor of Clinical Pathology, Faculty of Medicine,
Mansoura University, Egypt

Abstract

The reemergence of Mycobacterium tuberculosis with increasing numbers of multi-drug resistant (MDR) strains has increased the need for rapid diagnostic methods.

Molecular bases of drug resistance have been identified for all of the main antituberculous drugs, and drug resistance results from changes in several target genes, some of which are still undefined. Drug resistance in M. tuberculosis is due to the acquisition of mutations in chromosomally encoded genes and the generation of multidrug resistance is a consequence of serial accumulation of mutations primarily due to inadequate therapy. Several studies have shown that resistance to isoniazid (INTI) is due to mutaions in kat G gene. The rpo B gene, which encodes the subunit of RNA polymerase, harbors a mutation in an 81 bp region in about 95% of rifampicin (RIF) reistant M. tuberculosis strains recovered globally. Streptomycin (STR) resistance is due to mutations in rrs and rpsl genes which encodes 16S SrRNA and ribosomal protein S12 respectively. Approximately 65% of clinical isolates resistant to ethambutol have a mutation in the embB gene.

Several susceptibility phenotypes methods have been developed. Among them were radiometric systems such as the BACTEC460 TB system reduces the test time considerably, but they still labor intensive, expensive and require manipulation of radioactive substances.

Rapid promising approach to determine drug resistant strains especially for rifampicin (RIF) is the use of mycobacteriophage. A number of low-cost colorimetric

---

[*] e-mail:may_s65@hotmail.com. Mail : Egypt-Mansoura University-Faculty of Medicine-Clinical Pathology

AST assays, such as the 3-(4,5-dimethylthiazol- 2-yl)-2,5-diphenyl tetrazolium bromide (MTT) assay, the Alamar blue assay, and an assay based on microscopic detection of cord-like growth by *M. tuberculosis*, have been described. However, these tests have limitations; mycobacteria other than *M. tuberculosis* can produce cord factor, and INH can interfere with the formazan production in the MTT assay and give rise to false resistant results. Moreover, the use of a liquid medium in a microtiter plate format in these tests may be disadvantageous not only as a biohazard but also due to possible Contamination between wells.

The goal of the present study is to characterize 100 drug-resistant Mycobacterium tuberculosis (MTB) isolates with respect to their drug susceptibility phenotypes to four common anti-tuberculosis drugs (rifampicin, ethambutol, isoniazid andstreptomycin) and the relationship between such phenotypes and the patterns of genetic mutations in the corresponding resistance genes (rpoB, embB, katG, Rpsl) METHODS: The MIC values of the aforementioned anti-tuberculosis drugs were determined for each of the 100 drug-resistant MTB clinical isolates by the absolute concentration method and by BACTEC460). Genetic mutations in the corresponding resistance genes in these MTB isolates were identified by PCR-single-stranded conformation polymorphism/multiplex PCR amplimer conformation analysis (SSCP/MPAC).

Phenotypic resistance was found in all isolates. All isolates were resistant to ethambutol, 70% isolates were resistant to isoniazid, 50% isolates were resistant to streptomycin and 20% of the isolates were resistant to rifampicin. Genotypic mutations in the studied resistance to rifampicin, isoniazid, streptomycin and ethambutol were 20%, 70%, 80%, and 100% respectively.

These findings expand the spectrum of potential resistance-related mutations in MTB clinical isolates and help consolidate the framework for the development of molecular methods for delineating the drug susceptibility profiles of MTB isolates in clinical laboratories.

Key words: Mycobacterium tuberculosis, Molecular study of Drug resistance.

Introduction

The wide spread emergence of isolates of Mycobacterium tuberculosis(M. tuberculosis) resistant to one or more antituberculous drugs represents one of the most alarming corollaries of AIDS related tuberculosis during recent years. Delayed detection, identification, and susceptibility testing of drug resistant isolates and failure to appropriately isolate contagious patients and to begin adequate chemotherapy have all been identified as predisposing factors of transmission of drug resistant M. tuberculosis [1].

Radiometric systems such as the BACTEC460 TB system reduce the test time considerably, but they still labor intensive, expensive and carries the hazards of use of radioactive materials [2].

A method has been developed for the detection of mycobacteria by using modified Middle brook 7H9 broth which contains silicon rubber impregnated with ruthenium metal complex as a fluorescence quenching-based oxygen sensor. It is called Mycobacteria growth indicator tube (MGIT). It is read either manually or by BACTEC 9500. Manual reading require only a UV lamp and has been reported as a sensitive and rapid method for the growth and detection of mycobacteria from clinical specimens [3]. Studies have reported that MGIT can also be used for antituberculous susceptibility testing either using the primary cultured M. tuberculosis strains on Middlebrook media or by direct sensitivity testing of the decontaminated samples on antituberculous containing MGIT [4, 5].

Rapid promising approach to determine drug resistant strains especially for rifampicin (RIF) is the use of mycobacteriophage. It is based on using bacteriophage D29 to detect viable M. tuberculosis after RIF blocked productive infection in sensitive but not resistant strains. Aphagicidal agent was used to neutralize extracellular viruses and infected M. tuberculosis cells were demonstrated by the production of plaques on a rapidly grown lawn of Mycobacterium smegmatis [6]. Current evidence is largely restricted to the use of phage assays for the detection of RIF resistance in culture isolates. When used on culture isolates, these assays appear to have high sensitivity, but variable and slightly lower specificity. In contrast, evidence is lacking on the accuracy of these assays when they are directly applied to sputum specimens [7].

A number of low-cost colorimetric AST assays, such as the 3-(4,5-dimethylthiazol- 2-yl)-2,5-diphenyl tetrazolium bromide (MTT) assay [8,9] the Alamar blue assay [10] and an assay based on microscopic detection of cord-like growth by M. tuberculosis, [10] have been described. However, these tests have limitations; mycobacteria other than M. tuberculosis can produce cord factor, and INH can interfere with the formazan production in the MTT assay and give rise to false resistant results.10 Moreover, the use of a liquid medium in a microtiter plate format in these tests may be disadvantageous not only as a biohazard but also due to possible contamination between wells.

Recently, an AST for M. tuberculosis based on a nitrate reductase assay performed in nitrate-containing Lowenstein–Jensen (LJ) solid medium was described. The test was comparable to the BACTEC 460TB system in detecting INH and RIF resistance, and the AST results were available in 10 days for 87% of the strains tested [11].

The nitrate reductase-based test was adapted for use as a colorimetric nitrate reductase-based antibiotic susceptibility (CONRAS) test for M. tuberculosis in Middlebrook 7H9 broth cultures. The method is based on the ability of M. tuberculosis to reduce nitrate to nitrite by using the nitrate reductase enzyme [12]. Most a pathogenic mycobacteria lack this enzyme. The presence of nitrite is detected by a color change to pink upon the addition of specific reagents. The reduction of nitrate to nitrite was detected visually and, on a subset of samples, also by spectrophotometry. The performance of the CONRAS test was proved to be rapid and sensitive against two commercial liquid-based systems, the radiometric BACTEC 460TB and the manual MGIT, for determining the susceptibilities of 74 M. tuberculosis strains to INH and RIF [13].

Molecular bases of drug resistance have been identified for all of the main antituberculous drugs, and drug resistance results from changes in several target genes, some of which are still undefined [14,15]. These factors highlights the need to implement the rapid detection of drug resistance, for better management of patients as well as for control of the outbreaks and prevention of future nosocomial drug- resistant tuberculosis transmission [16].

Drug resistance in M. tuberculosis is due to the acquisition of mutations in chromosomally encoded genes and the generation of multidrug resistance is a consequence of serial accumulation of mutations primarily due to inadequate therapy [17, 18].

Several studies have shown that resistance to isoniazid (INH) is due to mutaions in *kat G* gene. The *rpoB* gene, which encodes te subunit of RNA polymerase, harbors a mutation in an 81 bp region in about 95% of rifampicin (RIF) reistant M. tuberculosis strains recovered globally [18,19]. Streptomycin (STR) resistance is due to mutations in rrs and rpsl genes which encodes 16S SrRNA and ribosomal protein S12 respectively [18,20]. Approximately 65% of clinical isolates resistant to ethambutol have a mutation in the embB gene [21, 22]. Owing to the advent of molecular detection techniques, it is envisaged that a more thorough understanding of the genetic basis of drug resistance shall facilitate the development of rapid methods for assessing the antibiotic susceptibility phenotypes of clinical MTB isolates, thereby allowing more effective drug usage and treatment of the disease, and hence reduction in resistance development

The goal of the present study is to characterize 100 drug-resistant Mycobacterium tuberculosis (MTB) isolates with respect to their drug susceptibility phenotypes to four common anti-tuberculosis drugs (rifampicin, ethambutol, isoniazid andstreptomycin) and the relationship between such phenotypes and the patterns of genetic mutations in the corresponding resistance genes (*rpoB, embB, katG, Rpsl*)

Clinical *M. tuberculosis* isolates from 100 respiratory samples (sputum, induced sputum and bronchoalveolar lavage fluid) were collected from January 2005 until September 2008 from Mansoura, Egypt. All the isolates chosen were resistant to at least one drug of the first line antituberculous drugs (rifampicin, isoniazid, streptomycin and ethambutol).

Detection of mycobacteria was performed by use of acid – fast analysis, then isolation and identification for MTB was performed by BACTEC460 (Becton Dickinson, Sparks, MD) radiometric system and Lowenstein-Jenseen media. The isolation was followed by antimicrobial phenotypic drug susceptibility testing (AST).

Isolated colonies were subjected to AST using both agar proportion method and BACTEC 460 TB system.

Agar Proportion Method

We followed the modified agar proportion method using Middlebrook 7H10 agar plates to determine the susceptibility of MTB isolates [23]. Briefly, antibiotic stock solutions were diluted and added to Middlebrook 7H10 agar containing 10% oleic acid–albumin–dextrose to give the following critical concentrations in quadrant plates: INH, 0.2 mg/mL; RIF, 1 mg/mL; ethambutol (EMB), 5.0 mg/mL; and streptomycin (SM), 2.0 mg/mL. One hundred-microliter aliquots of diluted bacterial samples was inoculated to quadrants of drug-containing or drug-free media. Drug resistance in 7H10 method of proportion was defined as 1% or more growth of colonies on the drug-containing agar quadrant compared to growth on the drug-free quadrant. Results were recorded at 21 days after inoculation.

Bactec 460 Tb System

We used the recommendation of the manufacturer for sensitivity testing. The modified critical concentrations of provided drugs (SIRE, Becton Dickinson Microbiology System) were adopted:

SM, 2 mg/mL; INH, 0.1 mg/mL; RIF, 2.0 mg/mL; and EMB, 2.5 mg/mL.

Polymerase Chain Reaction (PCR)

Material collected from BACTEC cultures (growth index 30) was prepared for PCR by rapid purification method, including digestion with protease K (QIA mp, Qiagen, Hilden, Germany). The SSCP/MPAC analysis was performed as described [23] to elucidate the genetic profiles of the five resistance genes. These included the region containing hot-spot mutations in the *rpoB* gene and those in the *embB*, *katG*, *Rpsl* genes. Information regarding primer sequences is listed in Table S1. The drug susceptibility phenotypes of MTB isolates in the specimens were predicted on the basis of the SSCP/MPAC patterns generated. Wild-type and known mutation controls were included in the analysis to facilitate the identification of SSCP/MPAC or SSCP types of specimens. The primers used and the PCR conditions for each of the target regions were derived from published sequences [2, 10, 24, 25, 26, 27] (table 1).

Table 1. Conditions for PCR mutational analysis of target regions analyzed for drug resistance in patients with tuberculosis.

Drug	Gene	Concentration of primers	Ength of amplicon	Sequences
Rifampicin	Rpo B	0.1μM	157	5′ - TGCACGTCGCGGACCTCCA-′3 5′-TCGCCGCGCGATCAAGGAGT - ′3
Isoniazid	Kat G	0.2 μM	422	5′- TGGCACGCTGCCGGCACCTA-′3 5′—-AATGTCGACCGCCGCCGCGGCCA-′3
Streptomcin	Rpsl	0.1 μM	306	5′- CCCACCATTCAGCAGCTGGT -′3 5′-GTCGAGCGAACCGCGAATGA- ′3
Ethambutol	EmbB	0.5μM	399	5′-ACAGACTGGCGTCGCTGACA - ′3 5′-ACGCTGAAACTGCTGGCGAT-′3

The study comprised MTB isolates, each of which exhibited resistance to one or more of the following anti-tuberculosis agents: rifampicin, isoniazid, ethambutol and streptomycine. Detailed analysis of the resistance phenotypes of these isolates revealed that all isolates were resistant to ethambutol.

Resistance to rifampicin was found in 20% of the isolates, whereas 70%of the isolates were resistant to isoniazid, 50% of the isolates were resistant to streptomycine and all (Table 2).

Table 2. Analysis of drug resistant Mycobacterium tuberculosis isolates for mutations conferring resistance to rifampicin, isoniazid, streptomycin and ethambutol.

Drug	Phenotype pattern		Genotype pattern		Concordance	
	No.	%	No.	%	No.	%
Rifampicin	20	20%	20	20%	20	20%
Isoniazid	70	70%	70	70%	60	60%
Streptomycin	50	50%	80	80%	50	50%
Ethambutol	100	100%	100	100%	100	100%

All 20 strains with phenotypic resistance displayed mutations within the rpo B gene. No mutations in rpoB were observed in susceptible isolates.

For study of genotypic study of resistance to isoniazid, sixty strains with phenotypic resistance to isoniazid displayed mutation in *katG* sequence. Ten strains with phenotypic susceptible pattern had mutations in *katG* sequence

For resistance to streptomycin, all phenotypic resistant strains had mutations in rpsl sequence. Thirty strains with susceptible phenotype pattern had mutations in rpsl sequence.

For resistance to ethambutol, all strains resistant to ethambutol had mutations in embB sequence.

Sensitivity, specificity and predictive values of mutational analysis: For rifampicin, the sensitivity, specificity, positive and negative predictive values of PCR were 100%. For isoniazid, these values were 85.7%, 66.7% 85.7% and 66.7%. For streptomycin, the values were 100%, 40%, 100%, 40%. For ethambutol, these values were 100% (Table 3).

Table 3. Sensitivity, specificity, positive predictive value and negative predictive value of genotyping of resistant strains

	Sensitivity	Specificity	PPV	NPV
Rifampicin	100%	100%	100%	100%
Isoniazid	85.7%	66.7	85.7%	66.7
Streptomycin	100%	40%	100%	40%
Ethambutol	100%	-	100%	-

Drug resistance of MTB is generally believed to be caused by point mutations in several key resistance genes within the MTB genome. Although hot-spot mutations have been identified in these resistance genes, few studies have managed to reveal the range of phenotypic and mutational profiles that may be recovered in clinical MTB isolates. Our data suggested that the majority of these isolates displayed multiple drug resistance phenotypes that involved two or more drugs.

It should be noted that, to our knowledge, the majority of the 100 strains in this study were isolated from patients who had previously received anti-tuberculosis treatment. Although we lack the precise data on the relative proportion of isolates obtained from the first-time or re-treated patients, our finding that co-resistance to the first-line drugs, rifampicin and isoniazid, accounted for an overwhelming majority of all resistance phenotypes, tends to suggest that resistance in clinical MTB isolates is essentially 'multiple' in nature once it develops. It also appears that resistance to the other drugs develops on the basis of resistance to the first-line drugs of ethambutol and isoniazid. This phenomenon is probably related to the consecutive use of different anti-tuberculosis drugs for treatment, as well as to dissemination of the MDR strains. Whether this phenomenon is related to the differential pattern of drug prescription among the patients from whom the isolates were collected remains to be investigated. It should also be noted that our approach of drug susceptibility testing in this study, in which only a small number of susceptibility levels were tested, did not allow us to examine whether there were any enhancement effects on specific resistance phenotypes that could be attributable to accumulation of mutations in different resistance genes.

The results of the present study revealed a high level of correspondence between in vitro resistance to isoniazid and rifampicin and the presence of genotypic mutations. Hence it is likely that there are additive effects on multiple drug resistance as a result of accumulation of multiple gene mutations. Our results are online with previous reports that demonstrated some correlation between specific mutation types and resistance phenotypes [28.29].

As in previous observations, rpoB testing is confirmed to be highly sensitive and specific for rifampicin [18].

Sixty strains with phenotypic resistance to isoniazid were found to be associated with mutation in Kat G gene. However, 10 isolates with phenotypic resistance failed to detect the presence of such mutations. A previous report detected these mutations in 21% of isoniazid – resistant isolates with a high specificity [30].

Such findings prompted us to consider the need to investigate the direct effect of such hot-spot mutations on the basic structures and functional mechanisms concerning mycobacterial growth and survival. In fact, it is entirely possible that an identical mutation may be associated with different phenotypic characteristics of two bacterial strains if they simultaneously harboured different types of compensatory mutations,[31,32] although mutations that lead to a reversal of resistance phenotypes have not been documented.

However, a better selection of target regions seems to be crucial to enable rapid recognition of resistance to isoniazid, considering that the sequencing of a region of 72000 bp of the KatG gene involves an excessive delay. In our experience, the selection of genetic region of kat G codone 463 allowed detection of 60/70 of isoniazid – resistant isolates in < 72h.

In contrast to rifampicin, genotypic testing for resistance to INH presents obvious difficulties. First, alterations in at least three genes kat G, inh A, and alpC, are associated with INH resistance. Second, mutations may occur at multiple sites in Kat G, in the regulatory regions of inh A [33] or alpc [34] or much more rarely in the inh A structural genes [35] third, some mutations in kat G are associated with high level resistance e.g deletions or (S315T), where as others may not confer resistance to clinically significant concentrations of INH [36]. Despite these potential limitations, in the strategy of confining the analysis to kat G most frequently involved in resistance to INH provided satisfactory results in our study

Mutations in rpsl were found in all strains resistant to streptomycin. In line with other study that about two thirds of strepomycin resistant strains of M. tuberculosis have detectable mutations associated with resisance to this antimicrobial agent [31]. However, it seems that mutations in this sequence may be not always associated with phenotypic resistance.

PCR analysis for detection of resistance to ethambutol in all of isolates included in the study confirmed the strong association between genotypic alteration in the embB gene and phenotypic resistance to this drug, which has already been verified in other populations [16]

Although the data in the literature as well as those gathered in this study suggested that the mutational and phenotypic patterns for multidrug resistance in MTB vary geographically, it is still possible that a significant proportion of multidrug resistance cases were due to clonal spread of certain types of resistant isolates, rather than intrinsic resistance development that involves spontaneous mutation and selection during the course of treatment. It remains to be seen whether clonal spread of resistant mutants accounts for the higher rate of multidrug resistance among re-treated cases, when compared with that of primary infections. This hypothesis may be tested through investigation of the epidemiological profiles of our collection of resistant isolates. Since high rates of acquired MDR-TB have also been reported in various parts of the world including Nepal (48.0%), Gujarat, India (33.8%), New York City, USA (30.1%), Bolivia (15.3%) and Korea (14.5%),[37] future research should focus on analyzing factors that determine dissemination of known resistant isolates.

Conclusion

It would be advisable that the molecular tests for drugs susceptible pattern include rpoB, embB, katG, Rpsl genes as there is extremely good correlation between the presence of mutations in these genes and resistance phenotypes. Positive detection of mutations in one or more of these genes would infer a very high possibility of the presence of a multidrug resistance phenotype. A positive result should therefore be followed by either sequencing analysis of all known resistance genes or routine susceptibility testing, so as to reveal the entire drug susceptibility spectrum of the potentially multidrug-resistant isolate. On the other hand, we believe that a lack of mutations in all the test genes infers that the test isolate is susceptible to all anti-tuberculosis drugs and that no further standard susceptibility tests need to be performed. In addition, the molecular test should be carried out with smear-positive sputum specimens so as to speed up the susceptibility testing process. As a concluding note, we wish to stress that rapid and reliable identification of MDR-TB and their drug susceptibility phenotypes is instrumental in facilitating more effective treatment as well as control of spread of diseases involving this notorious pathogen. It is envisaged that such a goal may be attained through the development of new-generation molecular methods for MTB susceptibility testing.

References

[1] Fieden TR, Sherman LF, Maw KL, et al. (1996). A multi-institutional outbreak of highly drug – resistant tuberculosis. *JAMA*. 276:1229-35.

[2] Palaci M, Ueki SYM, Sato DN. Evaluation of mycobacterium growth indicator tube for recovery and drug susceptibility testing of Mycobacterium tuberculosis isolates from respiratory specimens. *J Clin Microb* 1996;34(3):762.

[3] Gerdes SR, Dmehi C, Nardi G. Multicenter evaluation of mycobacteria growth indicator tube for testing susceptibility of Mycobacterium tuberculosis to first line drugs. *J Clin Microb* 1999;37(1):45–9.

[4] Suzuki KK, Tsuyuguchi H, Matsumoto A. Evaluation of mycobacterium Growth indicator tube (MGIT) for drug susceptibility testing of Mycobacterium tuberculosis isolates. *Kekkkaku* 1997;72:187–90.

[5] Gloubeva V, Lecocq M, Lassowsky P, et al. Evaluation of Mycobacterium growth indicator tube for direct and indirect drug susceptibility of Mycobacterium tuberculosis from respiratory specimens in a Siberian prison hospital. *J Clin Microb* 2001;39(4):1501–6.

[6] Marei AM, El-Behedy EM, Mhtady HA. Evaluation of a rapid bacteriophage—based method for the detection of Mycobacterium tuberculosis in clinical sample. *J Med Microb* 2003;52(4):331–5.

[7] Pai M, Kalantri S, Pascopella L, Riley LW, Reingold AL. Bacteriophage-based assays for the rapid detection of rifampicin resistance in Mycobacterium tuberculosis: a meta-analysis. *J Infect* 2005;51(3):175–87.

[8] Caviedes L, Delgado J, Gilman RH. Tetrazolium microplate assay as a rapid and inexpensive colorimetric method for determination of antibiotic susceptibility of Mycobacterium tuberculosis. J Clin Microbiol 2002;40:1873–4.

[9] Caviedes L, Lee T, Gilman RH, Sheen P, Spellman E, Lee EH, The Tuberculosis Working Group in Peru., et al. Rapid, efficient detection and drug susceptibility testing of Mycobacterium tuberculosis in sputum by microscopic observation of broth cultures. *J Clin Microbiol* 2000;38:1203–8.

[10] Mshana RN, Tadesse G, Abate G, Miørner H. Use of 3-(4,5-dimethylthiazol-2-yl)-2,5-diphenyl tetrazolium bromide for rapid detection of rifampin-resistant Mycobacterium tuberculosis. *J Clin Microbiol* 1998;6:1214–9.

[11] A¨ ngeby KAK, Klintz L, Hoffner SE. Rapid and inexpensive drug susceptibility testing of Mycobacterium tuberculosis with a nitrate reductase assay. *J Clin Microbiol* 2002;40:553–5.

[12] Master RN. Identification tests for mycobacteria, part 3.122. In: Isenberg HO, editor. Clinical microbiology procedures handbook, vol. 1. Washington, DC: *American Society for Microbiology;* 1992. p. 1–29.

[13] Syre H, Phyu S, Sandven P, Bjorvatn B, Grewal HMS. Rapid colorimetric method for testing susceptibility of Mycobacterium tuberculosis to isoniazid and Rifampin in Liquid Cultures. *Clin Microbiol* 2003;41(11):5173–7.

[14] Zhang Y, Heym B, Allen B, Young D, Cole ST. (1992). The catalase – peroxidase gene and isoniazid resistace of Mycobacterium tuberculosis. *Nature*:358:591-3.

[15] Mdluli K, Slayden RA, Zhu Y, et al. (1998). Inhibition of a Mycobbacterium tuberculosis ketoacyl ACP synthase by isoniazid. *Science*. 280:1607-10.

[16] Cingolani A, Antinori A, Sanguinetti M, et al. (1999). Application of molecular methods for detection and transmission analysis of Mycobacterium tuberculosis drug resistance in patients attending a reference hospital, Italy. *J Infect dis*.179:1025-9.

[17] Marttila H J, Soini, H, Eerola, E, Vyshnevskaya E , Vyshnevskiy B I, Otten TF, Vasilyef AV & Viljanen, M K (1998). A Ser315Thr substitution in KatG is predominant in genetically heterogeneous multidrug- resistant Mycobacterium tuberculosis isolates originating from the Petersburg area in Russia. *Antimicrob Agents Chemother*. 42, 2443-2445.

[18] Ramaswamy S and Musser JM (1998). Molecular genetic basis of antimicrobial agent resistance in Mycobacterium tuberculosis, 1998 update. *Tuber. Lung Dis* . 9:3-29.

[19] Telenti A, Imboden P, Marchesi P,Marchesi nF, Schmidheinin T, Bodmer T. (1993). Direct, automated detection of rifampicin – resistant Mycobacterhun tuberculosis by polmerase chin reaction and single – strand conformation polymorphism analysis. *Antimicrob Agets Chemother*.37:2054-8.

[20] Sreevatsan S, Pan X, Stockbauer K E, Williams, D L, Kreiswirth, B N, Musser JM. (1996). Characterization of rpsL and rrs mutations in streptomycin-resisant Mycobacterium tuberculosis isolates from diverse geographic localities. *Antimicrob Agents Chemothe*. 40/1024-1026.

[21] Ramswamy S V, Amin A G, Ksel G S, Stager C E, et al. (2000).Molecular genetic analysis if Mycobacterium tuberculosis. *Antimicrob Agents Chemother* .44/ 326-336.

[22] Telenti, A., Philipp, W.J., Sreevatsan, S., Bernasan. S., Bernansconi, C, et al. (1997). The emb operon, a gene cluster of Mycobacterium tuberculosis involved in resistance to ethambutol. *Nat Med.* 3/567-570.

[23] INDERLIED, K.A. 1996. Antimycobacterial Agents: *In Vitro Susceptibility Testing, Spectra of Activity, Mechanisms of Action and Resistance, and Assays for Activity in Biologic Fluids*, 4th Ed., Williams & Wilkins, Baltimore, MD.

[24] Banerjee A, Dubnau E, Quemaid A, et al.(1994). Inh A, a gene encoding a target for isoniazid and ethionamide in Mycobacterium tuberculosis. *Science*. 263/227-30

[25] Wilson TM, collins D. Ahp C (1996). A gene involved in isoniazid resistance of the M. tuberculosis complex. *Mol Microbiol*. 19/1025-34.

[26] Telenti, A., Imboden P., Marchesi, F., Lowrie D, Cole S, Colston, M J, Matter L, Schopfer K, Bodmer T. (1993). Detection of rifampicin – resistance mutation in Mycobacterium tuberculosis. *Lancet*. 31/ 647-650

[27] Honore N. and Cole ST (1994). Streptomycin resistance in mycobacteria. *Antmicrob Agents Chemother*. 38/238-42

[28] Siddiqi N, Shamim M, Hussain S, et al. (2002) Molecular characterization of multidrug-resistant isolates of *Mycobacterium tuberculosis* from patients in North India. *Antimicrob Agents Chemother* 46:443–50.

[29] Taniguchi H, Aramaki HH, Nikaido Y, et al. (1996) Rifampicin resistance and mutation of the *rpoB* gene in *Mycobacterium tuberculosis*. *FEMS Microbiol Lett* 144:103–8.

[30] Musser JM (1995) Antimicrobial Agent Resistance in Mycobacteria: Molecular Genetic Insight. *Clin Microbiol Rev*. 8 (4)/ 496-514.

[31]   Bottger EC, Springer B, Pletschette M, et al. (1998) Fitness of antibiotic-resistant microorganisms and compensatory mutations. *Nat Med* 4:1343–4.

[32]   Levin BR, Perrot V, Walker N. (2000) Compensatory mutations, antibiotic resistance and the population genetics of adaptive evolution in bacteria. *Genetics* 154:985–97.

[33]   Kapur VL, Ling-ling MR., Hamrick BB, et al. (1995). Rapid Mycobacterium species assignment and unambiguous identification of mutations associated with antimicrobial resistance in Mycobacterium tuberculosis by automated DNA sequencing. *Arch Pathol Lab Med.*119/138-40.

[34]   Wilson TM, collins D. Ahp C (1996). A gene involved in isoniazid resistance of the M. tuberculosis complex. *Mol Microbiol.* 19/1025-34.

[35]   Ristow M M, Moehling M, Rifai H, et al. (1995). New isoniazid/ethionamide resistance gene mutations and screening for multi-drug resistant Mycobacterium tuberculosis strains. *Lancet.* 346:502-3.

[36]   Heym B, Alzari PM, Honore N and ColesT (1995). Missense mutations in the catalase – peroxidase gene, kat G, are associated with isoniazid resistance in tuberculosis in Mycobacterium tuberculosis. *Mol Microbiol.* 15/235-245.

[37]   Cohn DL, Bustreo F, Raviglione MC. (1997) Drug-resistant tuberculosis: review of the worldwide situation and the WHO/IUATLD Global Surveillance Project. International Union Against Tuberculosis and Lung Disease. *Clin Infect Dis* 24:Suppl. 1, S121–30.

In: Antibiotic Resistance…
Editors: A. R. Bonilla and K. P. Muniz

ISBN 978-1-60741-623-4
© 2009 Nova Science Publishers, Inc.

Chapter XV

Tracking Down a New Putative Drug Target for Osteoporosis: Structure of an Essential Region of the Proton Translocation Channel of H^+-V_O-ATPase

*Afonso M. S. Duarte** and *Marcus A. Hemminga*

Laboratory of Biophysics,
Wageningen University, The Netherlands

Abstract

In the last decades, osteoporosis has become a major subject in the field of drug discovery and design. One of the proteins recently considered relevant to use as a drug target is the membrane-bound enzyme H^+-V_O-ATPase. This proton pump is located in the osteoclast cells, which are positioned at the bone surface. In these cells the enzyme controls the proton flux to the bone and consequently bone resorption. One major task on drug design is the knowledge of the secondary and tertiary structure of the enzyme involved. The topology of the V-ATPase protein complex has been largely established, however, the three-dimensional structure is only known for some individual subunits. This chapter reviews our recently published work on the secondary and tertiary structure of the proton translocation channel located in subunit *a* of the V-ATPase complex. For this purpose, we designed two peptides consisting of 25 and 37 amino acid residues, representing the seventh transmembrane segment of subunit *a*, which encompass the proton translocation channel as well as the region of interest for interaction with possible inhibitors. Using a combination of NMR (nuclear magnetic resonance) and CD (circular dichroism) spectroscopy the structure of these V-ATPase peptides was studied in different membrane-mimicking environments. The results indicate that a primordial transmembrane segment of this protein region adopts an α-helical conformation and is

---

* Current address: Cellular Protein Chemistry, Utrecht University, The Netherlands.

longer than proposed by topological studies. Moreover, this segment exhibits a hinge region located near the cytoplasmic end of the channel. It is proposed that the presence of this hinge allows the opening and closing of the proton translocation channel and provides flexibility for the channel to act as a binding pocket for inhibitors. These findings can be used as tools in the design of new drugs that can control the activity of V-ATPase in osteoclast cells, helping in this way the fight against osteoporosis.

Introduction

Proton Vacuolar ATPase

As life expectancy increases, the frequency of fractures originated by bone illnesses like osteoporosis is increasing throughout the world. According to the World Health Organization (WHO), between six and seven percent of people in the world are affected by this disease (WHO, 2007). Approximately one in three women and one in seven men over the age of 50 years will at some stage suffer a bone fracture as a result of osteoporosis. This particular disease is therefore regarded by the WHO as one of the world's most important health problems.

Osteoporosis leads to a decrease of the skeletal mass to the point of structural bone instability and makes the patient susceptible to spontaneous bone fracture. As adult osteoporosis is always associated with enhanced bone resorption, advances in understanding and treating this type of diseases require the study of osteoclast biology. Osteoclasts, the bone-resorbing cells, and osteoblasts, the bone-forming cells, play a central role in the formation of the skeleton and regulation of its mass. A difference in activity of osteoclast and osteoblast bone cells can trigger the appearance of osteoporosis. During the bone-resorbing activity the extracellular proton concentration is regulated via vacuolar proton V-ATPases (see Figure 1).

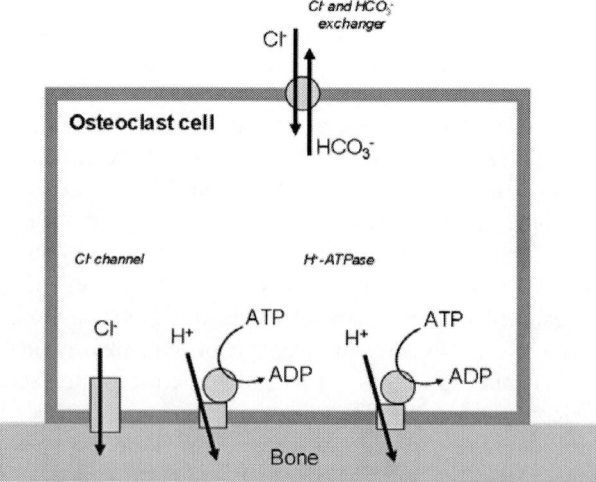

Figure 1. Schematic illustration of the location of the H^+-V-ATPase proton pumps in the cell membranes of osteoclast cells.

The first evidences of the existence of V-ATPases in eukaryotic cells date from studies of about 30-40 years ago (Bashford et al., 1975; Njus and Radda, 1979; Kirshner, 1962; Mellman et al., 1986). These early studies demonstrated that catecholamine uptake is driven by proton pumping generated by an ATP-dependent proton pump, later named V-ATPase. Following these studies, V-ATPase was found to be present in the intracellular and plasma membranes of all eukaryotic cells, playing an important role in endocytosis, intracellular targeting, protein processing and degradation (Finbow and Harrison, 1997; Stevens and Forgac, 1997; Forgac, 1998; Forgac, 1999; Nishi and Forgac, 2002; Kane, 2006). When located in the plasma membrane the protein is involved in renal acidification, pH homeostasis, and bone resorption (Wieczorek et al., 1999). One of the possible deregulations identified for osteoporosis is due to an over-function of the V-ATPase, which makes the bone tissue more acidic, leading to its demineralization (Finbow and Harrison, 1997; Arata et al., 2002). In this respect, V-ATPase inhibitors are thought to have a potential to act as agents to fight against many common lytic bone disorders, e.g., osteoporosis. The drugs available at the moment to reduce bone loss only have a temporary effect, so new therapies with a higher specificity and longer time of action are needed. However, the discovery of new inhibitors for V-ATPase has been hampered by the absence of a high-resolution structure of the entire V-ATPase system. This information together with studies of the dynamics of the system would help to identify possible target points to control the function of V-ATPase in human osteoclast cells. Along with the recent advances in the biophysics of structure determination of membrane proteins, the structure of the V-ATPase has been intensively studied during the past few years.

The topology and arrangement of the different subunits of the V-ATPase from *Saccharomyces cerevisiae* are shown in Figure 2 (Manolson et al., 1992; Kawasaki-Nishi and Forgac, 2003). V-ATPase is formed by two domains: the catalytic cytoplasmic domain V_1 that is connected via a stalk to the proton translocation transmembrane domain V_O. In Table 1 a list of the V-ATPase subunits is presented, including the subunit name, molecular mass, corresponding gene in *Saccharomyces cerevisiae* and function. The V_1 domain is composed of eight subunits with stoichiometry $A_3B_3CDEFG_2H_{1-2}$ and has a total molecular weight of 640 kDa. Because of the relatively high sequence identity between the catalytic subunits α and β of the F-ATPase and subunits A and B of the V-ATPase, the V_1 domain is assumed to use ATP to drive proton translocation across the membrane.

The rotary catalytic mechanism of ATP hydrolysis and proton transportation (Abrahams et al., 1994; Boyer, 1997) is thought to be very similar among the two classes of enzymes, but the different subunit stoichiometry and architectural appearance in electron micrographs suggests that V-type ATPases are more complex (Boekema et al., 1999; Wilkens et al., 1999). The transmembrane V_O domain has a molecular weight of 260 kDa and is composed of five subunits (a, d, c, c', c) with stoichiometry adc'c'c. During proton translocation, the subunits c, c' and c, driven by the ATP hydrolysis in subunits A and B, rotate in the membrane about the central stalk subunit D. Therefore the c subunits are called "rotor" subunits and subunit a is called the "stator" subunit. Subunit a from V-ATPase is composed of nine putative transmembrane sections and a 400-residue cytoplasmic section (Table 1 and Figure 2). Arginine residue R735 of the seventh transmembrane section (TM7) is fundamental to proton translocation, since its mutation blocks the enzyme (Kawasaki-Nishi and Forgac, 2003).

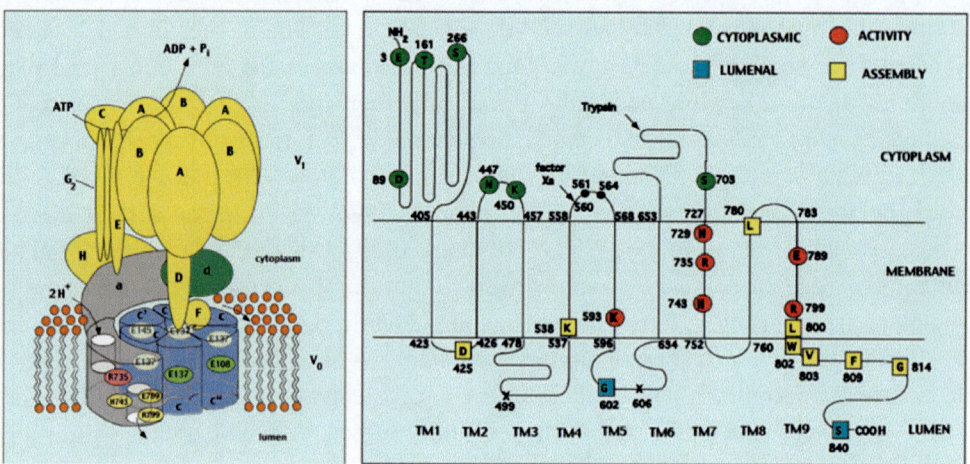

Figure 2. Left: Structural model of V-ATPase from *Saccharomyces cerevisiae*. Right: Topology of subunit *a* from the V_O domain (Kawasaki-Nishi and Forgac, 2003). During proton translocation, the subunits *c*, *c'* and *c*, driven by the ATP hydrolysis in subunits A and B, rotate in the membrane about the central stalk subunit D, *i.e.*, the system resembles a motor. Therefore the *c* subunits are called "rotor" subunits and subunit *a* is called the "stator" subunit. Reprinted with permission from Kawasaki-Nishi and Forgac (2003). Copyright © 2003, Elsevier.

The mutation of histidine residues H729 and H743 of TM7 also affects proton translocation, since it leads to a reduction in 40% of enzyme activity (Kawasaki-Nishi et al., 2003). The transmembrane rotor subunits *c*, *c'* and *c* (see Figure 2) are also involved in proton translocation. Subunits *c* and *c'* are composed of four transmembrane segments and subunit *c* has an additional fifth cytoplasmic segment. The glutamic acid residues of the fourth putative transmembrane segment of subunits *c* and *c'*, and of the second putative transmembrane segment of subunit *c* are of fundamental importance for proton translocation (Wang et al., 2004). Two hemi-channels located in subunit *a* provide the pathway for protons to translocate from the cytoplasm to the lumen (Grabe et al., 2000; Kawasaki-Nishi and Forgac, 2003). It is assumed that rotation of the rotor, due to hydrolysis of ATP in the V_1 domain, forces protonation of the glutamic acid residues located in the centre of the rotor. Protons can access the carboxylic side chain of these residues via the cytoplasmic hemi-channel that is located in the interface between subunit *a* and the rotor. When the *c* subunits rotate the release of another proton into the luminal hemichannel occurs. This release is assisted by arginine R735 of TM7 as it stabilizes the negatively charged side chain of the glutamic acid of the *c* subunit involved.

The cytoplasmic hemi-channel located in subunit *a* is known to act as a binding pocket for bafilomycin, a strong V-ATPase inhibitor (Wang et al., 2005). The potential residues involved in binding are located at the interface between TM4 (of the rotor *c* subunit) and TM7 (of subunit *a*). Inhibition of proton translocation probably occurs when these two segments are constrained to one rigid conformation that prohibits the swiveling of the glutamic acid located in the centre of the rotor.

Table 1. Composition of the cytoplasmic (V_1) and transmembrane (V_O) domains of V-ATPase from *Saccharomyces cerevisiae* (Boekema et al., 1999; Wilkens et al., 1999)

Domain	Subunit	Molecular weight (kDa)	Yeast gene	F-ATPase homologue	Function
V_1	A	70	VMA1	β	Catalytic site, regulation
	B	60	VMA2	α	Non-catalytic site, targeting (?)
	C	40	VMA5	-	Peripheral stalk
	D	34	VMA8	γ	Central Stalk
	E	33	VMA4	δ	Peripheral stalk
	F	14	VMA7	ε	Central stalk
	G	13	VMA10	B	Peripheral stalk
	H	50	VMA13	?	Peripheral stalk

Domain	Subunit	Molecular weight (kDa)	Yeast gene	F-ATPase homologue	Function	Activity related properties
V_O	a	100	VPH1/STV1	a	H⁺ transport, targeting	• R735 (TM7) – essential for proton translocation. • K593 (TM5), H729, H743 (TM7), E789 and R799 (TM9) - required for proton translocation.
	d	38	VMA6	?	Unknown	• Located in the cytoplasmic side of V_O • No transmembrane segments • Bound to the V_O domain upon dissociation of V_1
	c	17	VMA3	c	H⁺ transport, DCCD binding site	• E137 essential for proton translocation
	c′	17	VMA11	c	H⁺ transport	• E145 essential for proton translocation
	c″	21	VMA16	C	H⁺ transport	• E108 essential for proton translocation

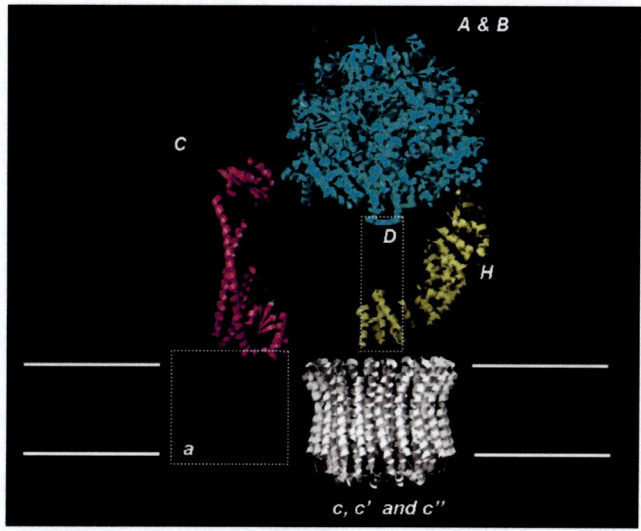

Figure 3. Hypothetical model of the structure of the V-ATPase system build-up according to the proposed topology (Figure 2) taking into account high-resolution structures of subunits available in the PDB databank. Bovine mitochondrial F_1-ATPase (Abrahams et al., 1994), subunit H from *Saccharomyces cerevisiae* V-ATPase (Sagermann et al., 2001), subunit C from *Saccharomyces cerevisiae* V-ATPase (Drory et al., 2004) and rotor subunits *c* from *Enterococcus hirae* V-ATPase (Murata et al., 2005). The structure of subunit *a* is missing, because it is not yet resolved.

These results make subunit *a* a good target to inhibit proton translocation. To design new inhibitors and understand the binding and inhibition process, one needs to know the topology and structure of this subunit. A model of the structure of V-ATPase based on the proposed topology (Figure 2) and on the known high-resolution structures published (Abrahams et al., 1994; Sagermann et al., 2001; Drory et al., 2004; Murata et al., 2005), is depicted in Figure 3.

Structure Determination of Transmembrane Peptides

Despite the advances in both X-ray crystallography and NMR (nuclear magnetic resonance) spectroscopy of transmembrane proteins, the structure of subunit *a* is still unknown (see Figure 3). The presence of approximately 400 residues distributed over nine putative transmembrane regions makes this subunit very challenging to over-express and isolate. An alternative to study entire transmembrane proteins or protein subunits is based on the concept that the primary structure of a protein segment can conserve its conformational information when it is isolated from the entire protein. As a consequence conformational studies of peptides representing transmembrane regions of the protein still report the conformation they adopt in their native environment. This approach was followed in the papers reviewed in this chapter (Duarte et al., 2007a, Duarte et al., 2007b). The efficacy and practicality of this approach is supported by several structural studies of membrane proteins: Ca^{2+}-ATPase (Soulie et al., 1999), F_O-F_1-ATPase (Girvin et al., 1998), potassium ion channel (Ben-Efraim and Shai, 1997), divalent metal transporter protein (Li et al., 2005), bacteriorhodopsin (Orekhov et al., 1994; Katragadda et al., 2001), rhodopsin (Yeagle and Albert, 2002), thrombomodulin (Adler et al., 1995), and G protein coupled receptor (Ding et al., 2001). In this respect, it is interesting to note that in some of these studies the secondary structures obtained for the isolated transmembrane segments were indeed confirmed when the structure of the complete protein was published (Orekhov et al., 1994; Yeagle and Albert, 2002; Nielsen et al., 2003).

One of the major challenges intrinsic to the study of the structure of transmembrane peptides is the selection of the most accurate and relevant environment to solubilize the protein. The solvation chemistry behind a membrane-mimicking solvent has to reproduce in the best way the native environment of the transmembrane peptide under study. In the case of a transmembrane segment peptide three options might occur (not taking into account any residue from connecting loops): i) the segment is fully embedded in the lipid bilayer (see Figure 4, left); ii) the segment is completely surrounded by the transmembrane protein (see Figure 4, right); and iii) the segment, as part of a transmembrane protein, is partially embedded in the bilayer and partially in contact with the surrounding transmembrane segments from the transmembrane proteins. In the case of the first situation, the solvent for the peptide should mimic the solvation shell created by the hydrophobic fatty acid chains of the membrane lipids. In case of the second situation the solvation shell is governed by the interactions with, typically very hydrophobic, amino acid side chains from neighboring protein transmembrane segments. In case of the third situation the solvent/peptide interactions can be depicted as a mixture of interactions i) and ii). Based on the interactions mentioned one can expect for case i) the need of solvents that solvate and stabilize very hydrophobic compounds, *i.e.*, the solvent needs to have a low polarity and a low dielectric constant. In situations ii) and iii), the presence of different amino acid side chains leads to the need of using a solvent that is able to solvate both hydrophobic and hydrophilic solutes (Figure 4).

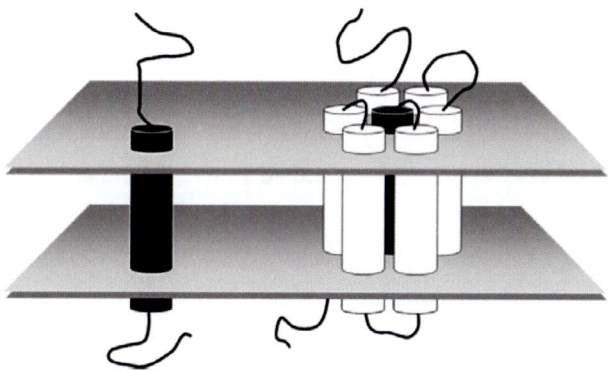

Figure 4. Schematic illustration of the different environments that can surround a transmembrane helical segment peptide (black cylinder). Left: the segment is fully embedded by the lipids in the membrane. Right: the segment is completely surrounded by transmembrane segments (white cylinders) of the corresponding transmembrane protein.

V-ATPase Peptides

Based on the predicted localization of the seventh putative transmembrane segment (TM7) from subunit *a* from yeast (Nishi and Forgac, 2002), two peptides were designed and chemically synthesized: MTM7 (37-residue peptide) and sMTM7 (25-residues peptide) (Figure 5). Both include the putative membrane-spanning section V727 to M753 in which the activity-related amino acid residues (H729, R735 and H743) are located (Nishi and Forgac, 2002). Arginine residue R735 was placed in the centre of the peptide similar to what would be expected for the corresponding membrane segment in its natural environment (Nishi and Forgac, 2002).

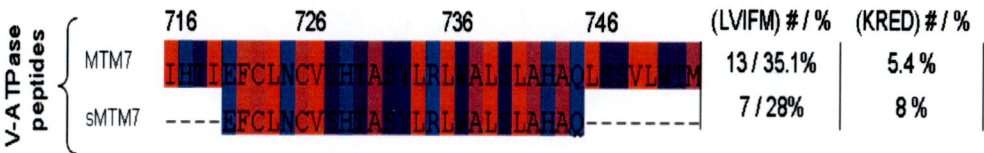

Figure 5. Sequence of the V-ATPase peptides used: peptide MTM7 (peptide mimicking the seventh transmembrane segment of subunit *a* from V-ATPase) and peptide sMTM7 (smaller version of MTM7). The coloring of the residues corresponds with their hydrophobicity: blue – higher hydrophilicity, red – higher hydrophobicity. The hydrophobic (LVIFM) and charged (KRED) amino acid residues are indicated on the right: # – number of residues, % – percentage of total number of residues present in the peptide. The numbering of the residues is according to the numbering of the entire subunit *a* (Nishi and Forgac, 2002).

Peptide MTM7 includes an extension to peptide sMTM7 that represents part of the cytoplasmic and luminal putative turns. Throughout this chapter the numbering of the amino acid residues in peptides MTM7 and sMTM7 will be the same as is used for the native subunit a (Figure 5).

To study the structure of the V-ATPase peptides, nuclear magnetic resonance (NMR) and circular dichroism (CD) spectroscopy were used to identify secondary structure motifs and fold of the peptides under different experimental conditions.

Structural Studies of Peptide MTM7

Circular Dichroism Spectroscopy

Taking into account that TM7 is located in a proteic environment and is surrounded by other transmembrane segments of subunit a and by the transmembrane sections of the rotor subunits of V-ATPase, the peptide is expected to be highly hydrophobic. Indeed, at NMR concentrations (1 to 2 mM) peptide MTM7 is only soluble in SDS micelles and the organic solvents TFE and DMSO. The 2D-NMR spectra of peptide MTM7 in SDS micelles at different ratios show a low signal-to-noise ratio and a severe peak broadening, so no detailed conformational information could be extracted by NMR in these systems. Unfortunately, DMSO has a too high UV cutoff to permit the analysis of the peptide conformation by CD. Therefore the SDS micelle system was used to study the global conformation of the peptide by CD spectroscopy. SDS has been frequently used as a membrane mimetic environment in NMR and CD studies on transmembrane peptides and proteins (Cross and Opella, 1981; Henry et al., 1986; Henry and Sykes, 1987; Pervushin et al., 1991; Killian et al., 1994; Papavoine et al., 1994; Papavoine et al., 1995; Le Maire et al., 2000; Lindberg and Graslund, 2001; Nielsen et al., 2003; Li et al., 2005).

CD spectroscopy was carried out in SDS micelles at peptide:SDS ratios of 1:100 and 1:250. The hydrophobicity index of peptide MTM7 shows that it has a positive hydrophobic index extending from amino acid residue V727 to I757. Consequently, in a micellar environment like SDS, one would expect that the detergent molecules cover the C-terminal part of peptide MTM7 and that the N-terminal region of the peptide is exposed to the aqueous phase. Such a behavior has been found for other transmembrane peptides dissolved in similar micellar systems (Papavoine et al., 1994; Nielsen et al., 2003). However, based on the analysis of the CD data peptide MTM7 has only a relatively low helical content between 21 and 30% for peptide:SDS ratios of 1:100 and 1:250, respectively. This low helical content could be due to the presence of arginine R735 in the middle of the peptide sequence that could interfere with the peptide solubilization in the micelles (Yeagle and Albert, 2002). More likely, peptide MTM7 is expected to be relatively flexible, thereby rapidly undergoing multiple conformational states, which means that longer helices would break into smaller ones (Hesselink et al., 2005) and thus lower CD intensities would be obtained (Manning and Woody, 1991). The low helical content calculated is based on the relatively low CD intensity, the other spectral features of which are typically α-helical. Thus, it is concluded that a relatively large fraction of the MTM7 molecules in the micellar systems dynamically populates the unfolded state (which has an almost zero CD intensity at 222 nm (Park et al., 1992; Hesselink et al., 2005).

In contrast, in the organic solvent TFE peptide MTM7 adopts an α-helical conformation. The spectral minimum at 222 nm is -45,244 deg.cm^2.dmol^{-1}. In addition to this anomalous value, the characteristic α-helical spectral maximum at 190 nm is red shifted to 193 nm. Both observations support that peptide MTM7 contains a longer stretch of helical residues than commonly found in water-soluble globular proteins. Traditional secondary structure analysis packages are based on a comparison of the CD spectrum of interest with a library of CD spectra of water-soluble proteins. However in case of stretched transmembrane α-helical peptides it has been shown that the CD intensity at 222 nm can be more negative than -39,500 deg.cm^2.dmol^{-1} and that the spectral maximum commonly found at 190 nm now exhibits a red shift (Park et al., 1992). From these results we assume that peptide MTM7 in TFE adopts a full α-helical structure possibly due to the natural propensity of the solvent used to induce such a structure. This finding makes TFE a less suitable solvent for NMR studies.

The difference in helical content of peptide MTM7 in SDS systems with peptide-to-SDS ratios of 1:100 and 1:250 can be attributed to the rather low solubility of peptide MTM7 in SDS micelles. At a peptide-to-SDS ratio of 1:100 the peptide is surrounded by a relatively low number of SDS molecules that cover the C-terminal part of MTM7 and provide a local hydrophobic environment in which the C-terminal part of the peptide dynamically populates an α-helical structure according to its α-helix propensity. The other part of the peptide, which is not surrounded by SDS molecules, is not in a favorable stabilizing environment, so it will be unfolded giving rise to no CD signal. Increasing the number of SDS molecules (1:250 sample) permits a new arrangement of the SDS molecules around the peptide and a larger part of peptide MTM7 will be covered by SDS (Le Maire et al., 2000). As a result, a larger part of the peptide dynamically populates the helical state and thus a stronger CD signal at 222 nm is observed. Despite the low helical content detected due to solvent constraints, this result suggests a natural tendency of peptide MTM7 to adopt α-helical structure in the domains stabilized by the SDS molecules. Thermal unfolding CD data obtained for peptide MTM7 in SDS micelles indicate that its unfolding is reversible and has a low cooperativity. Thus, MTM7 folding and unfolding is not a one-step process, but involves an ensemble of different intermediate structural states with similar free energies. The population of these states changes gradually upon increasing the temperature. Thus, the CD results in SDS micelles suggest that the peptide has an inherent propensity to adopt such a secondary structure in its highly hydrophobic natural environment in V-ATPase. However, no conclusive evidence can be obtained about which amino acid residues of MTM7 are involved in helix formation.

NMR Spectroscopy

Although DMSO is known to have denaturing properties (Jackson and Mantsch, 1991), experiments on different transmembrane proteins have shown that structures obtained in DMSO and DMSO-water mixtures accurately describe the structure of the protein or peptide in its native environment (Motta et al., 1991; Yeagle et al., 2000; Bellanda et al., 2001; Yeagle et al., 2001). Based on molecular dynamics simulations, it was recently found that the dual solvation properties of DMSO cause it to be a good membrane-mimicking solvent for transmembrane peptides that do not unfold due to the presence of DMSO (Duarte et al., 2008). As peptide MTM7 is well soluble in DMSO in which it gives rise to reasonable quality NMR spectra, we used DMSO as a solvent to study the conformation of peptide MTM7 by NMR spectroscopy (Figure 6). As NMR tools in our conformational studies, we used the chemical shift index (CSI) and NOE contacts.

The CSI method (Wishart et al., 1992; Wishart and Sykes, 1994) is applied to the $^1H_\alpha$ and $^{13}C_\alpha$ resonances in the NMR spectra and the results are shown in Figure 7. Positive $^{13}C_\alpha$ CSI values indicate a propensity for α-helix, on the other hand negative $^{13}C_\alpha$ CSI values indicate β-sheet conformation. For the $^1H_\alpha$ CSI, negative values point to an α-helix and positive values to a β-sheet conformation. The combination of consecutive $^1H_\alpha$ and $^{13}C_\alpha$ CSI values indicates a propensity for an α-helix configuration for residues T730-A738 and A742-Q745. The helical propensity information for residues T730-A738 is limited due to the lack of assignments of several $^1H_\alpha$ and $^{13}C_\alpha$ nuclei (residues L734, L736 and L739 lack $^1H_\alpha$ and $^{13}C_\alpha$ assignments, and we were not able to assign S732), so no strong evidence of α-helical conformation can be concluded. In Figure 7 also the $d_{\alpha N}(i,i+4)$ and $d_{\alpha N}(i,i+3)$ NOE contacts found for peptide MTM7 in DMSO are presented. The identification of a succession of $d_{\alpha N}(i,i+4)$ and $d_{\alpha N}(i,i+3)$ NOE contacts indicates the presence of an α-helix conformation (Wüthrich, 1976; Wüthrich, 1986).

The combination of the CSI profiles and NOE contacts indicates three α-helical regions in peptide MTM7: C723-A731, Y733-L739 and A742-V749 (Figure 7). For the terminal sections of peptide MTM7 neither structural NOE contacts, nor consistent CSI (T719, L750 and T752) values are found. This is probably due to fraying of the terminal residues. For the two regions between the three helical sections no secondary structure information could be extracted from the NMR data due to cross peak overlap and/or severe cross peak broadening. Two CSI values are exceptional, the amino acid residues V727 and H729 have CSI values that could indicate the presence of a turn, or a helix bend around these residues. However, the CSI values should only be taken as a strong indicator of the helix propensity of the peptide; in fact, NOE contacts are a more reliable indicator of an α-helical conformation and they predict that V727 and H729 reside in a helical segment (Wüthrich, 1976).

The hydrophobicity plot (Figure 8) of the putative TM7 segment and of the adjacent putative loops, shows that the putative cytoplasmic loop has negative hydrophobicity values indicating that these residues are hydrophilic and located in the water phase.

Starting with residue T719 the hydrophobicity values become positive for the first time, indicating that the subsequent section of the putative TM7 segment could be embedded in a hydrophobic environment. There are two small amphipathic oscillations that could indicate the region of TM7 located at the interface between the hydrophobic protein environment and the water phase cytoplasm. Nevertheless, from residue T719 to the luminal section, the average hydrophobicity increases and stays at a high level. Thus, instead of starting at V727 (Kawasaki-Nishi and Forgac, 2003), the putative TM7 segment could already start at T719.

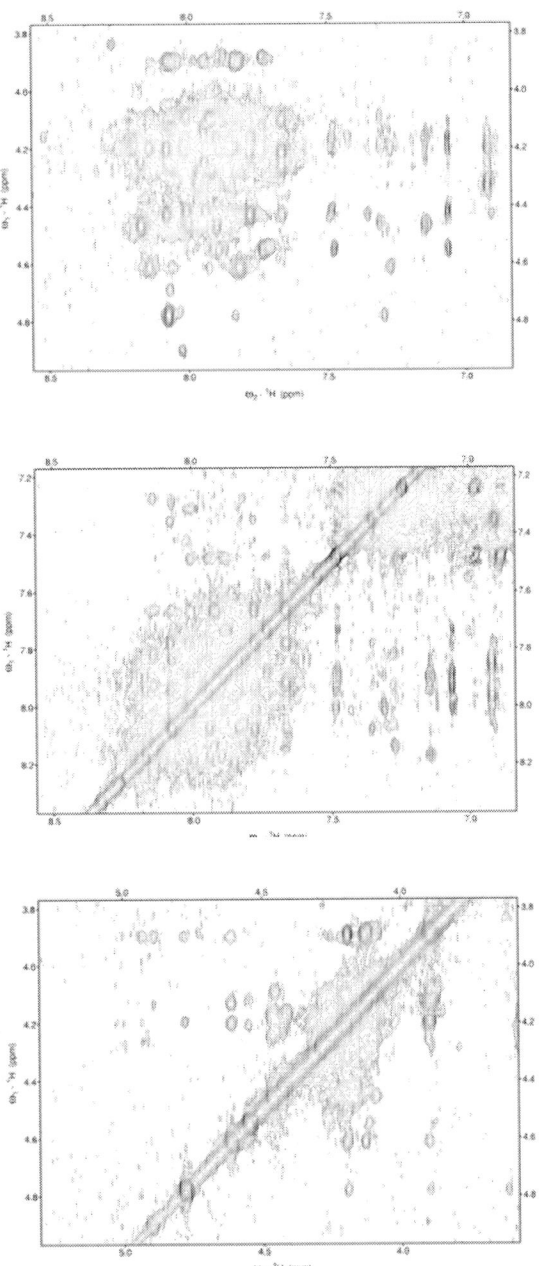

Figure 6. ^1H_N-$^1H_\alpha$ (top), ^1H_N-^1H_N (middle) and $^1H_\alpha$-$^1H_\alpha$ (bottom) regions of the 400 ms 2D NOESY spectrum of peptide MTM7 in d_6-DMSO. NMR spectra were recorded at 750 MHz at 30 °C. Broadening of cross peaks and resonance overlap limit the full assignment of all protons of peptide MTM7. Broadening and overlapping regions are marked with an asterisk. The NMR data were processed using XWINNMR from Bruker. Peak assignment and spectral analysis were carried out using NMRView (Johnson and Blevins, 1994) and Sparky (Goddard, T. D., and Kneller, D. G., University of California, San Francisco). Reprinted with permission from Duarte et al. (2007b). Copyright © 2007, Elsevier.

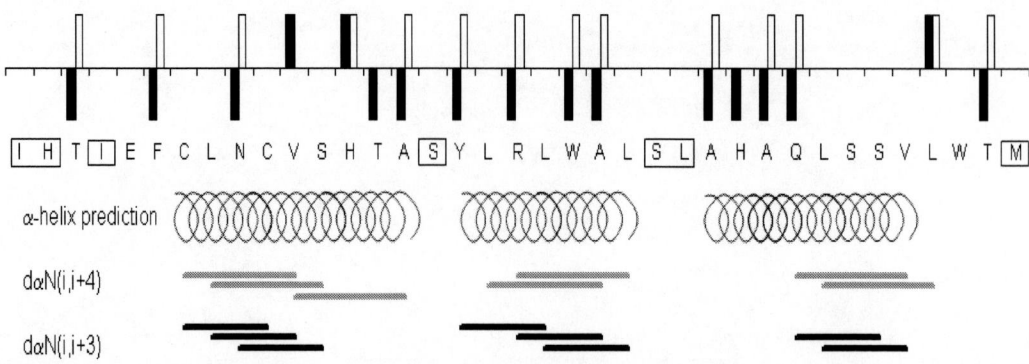

Figure 7. Chemical shift index ($\blacksquare$- $^1H_\alpha$ CSI; $\square$- $^{13}C_\alpha$ CSI) and NOE connectivities ($d_{\alpha N}(i,i+4)$ and $d_\alpha N(i,i+3)$)) of peptide MTM7 in d_6-DMSO. Gray CSI values represent residues with a $^1H_\alpha$ CSI value indicative for a moderate tendency to form helices ($\Delta\delta$(ppm) between -0.05 and -0.10). A consecutive appearance of CSI values of -1 for $^1H_\alpha$ and +1 for $^{13}C_\alpha$ indicate a propensity for an α-helix conformation. Such a sequence is found for residues T730- A738 and A742-Q745. For the residues T730-A738 the information is limited due to some missing assignments. Boxed residues have overlapping resonances and the resonance assignments are ambiguous. The predicted α-helical regions (𝕆𝕆𝕆𝕆𝕆) are based on the combination of CSI data and NOE connectivities. Reprinted with permission from Duarte et al. (2007b). Copyright © 2007, Elsevier.

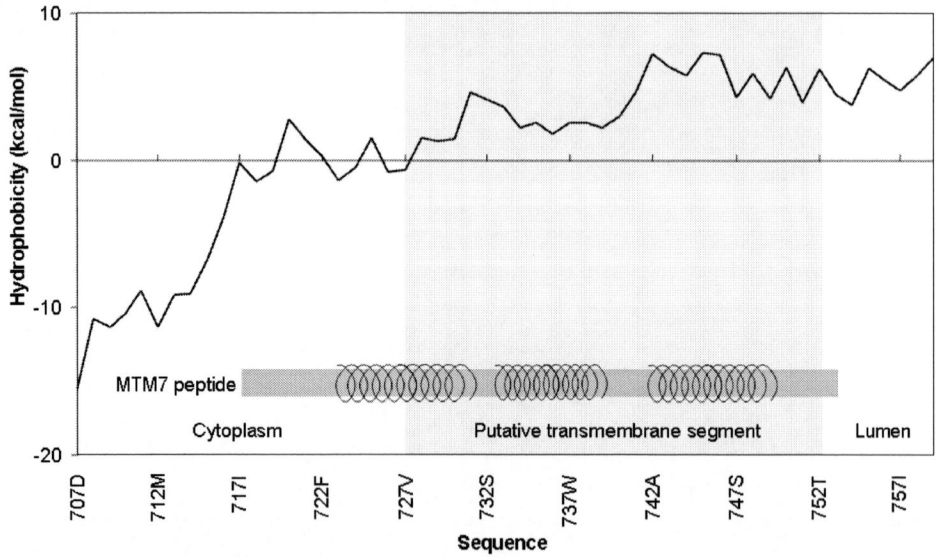

Figure 8. Hydrophobicity plot of the region in which TM7 of V-ATPase from yeast is located. The hydrophobicity is calculated using the Mpex software (Jaysinghe, S., Hristova, K. and White, S. H. (2000) http://blanco.biomol.uci.edu/mpex). The putative TM7 region is marked in yellow and peptide MTM7 is shown by a gray bar. The three helical regions of peptide MTM7 as determined by NMR spectroscopy (Figure 7) are depicted by 𝕆𝕆𝕆𝕆𝕆𝕆. Reprinted with permission from Duarte et al. (2007b). Copyright © 2007, Elsevier.

On the luminal side of TM7 the hydrophobicity is high (Figure 8) and this remains so in the segment beyond the putative TM7. The model for subunit a (Nishi and Forgac, 2002) indicates that TM7 connects to the next transmembrane segment (TM8) via a putative loop composed of 8 residues (from T752 to G760). Due to the high hydrophobicity of this loop, we assume that it will be located in a hydrophobic proteic region. In such a view, the TM7 tryptophan residue at position 751 could act as an anchor (Mall et al., 2002) in the interface between the hydrophobic protein environment and the water phase lumen.

The NMR results of peptide MTM7 in DMSO, combined with the CD data of the peptide in SDS micelles, indicate that the peptide has a high tendency to adopt an α-helical conformation in a hydrophobic environment. Peptide MTM7 in SDS micelles shows a tendency to increase its helical structure with an increase of SDS concentration (1:100 to 1:250). Nevertheless the SDS data show a lower helicity as compared to the NMR results, but they support the observations that peptide MTM7 has a propensity for α-helical conformation. Thus in its natural hydrophobic environment (i.e., subunit a from V-ATPase) the TM7 segment most likely is fully helical, in agreement with recent work from the group of Forgac (Wang et al., 2005). In combination with the hydrophobic data discussed, we propose that the putative TM7 in subunit a is a 32-residue helical segment that spans from T719 (cytoplasmic side) to W751 (luminal side). However, on basis of our data it cannot be excluded that the helical segment contains small non-helical segments. As a result, the new putative TM7 segment is composed of 32 amino acid residues and is within a hydrophobic part of V-ATPase.

Structure Implications

The proposed 32-residue helical seventh transmembrane segment can now be aligned and compared with its neighboring transmembrane subunits, especially with the transmembrane segments from the rotor subunits (c, c' and c) of V-ATPase. The 32-residue helix spans approximately 49 Å and we aligned the putative TM7 along the rotor sub-unit of V-ATPase (Figure 9). TM7 needs to be in contact with the transmembrane segments present in subunits c, c', and c. This structural proximity is required as it forms the basis for the mechanism of proton translocation. This translocation occurs between arginine R735 and the glutamic residues that are present in the subunit c assembly. The height of the rotor in the three-dimensional structure of the rotor subunits from F_1-F_O-ATPase from yeast (Stock et al., 1999) and Na$^+$-V-ATPase from *Enterococcus hirae* (Murata et al., 2005) is 58 and 68 Å, respectively.

Besides the transmembrane helical segments it also comprises the cytoplasmic and luminal-embedded sections of the transmembrane rotor. The height of the rotor is thus larger than that of the proposed TM7. However, if one focuses on the localization and the length of the transmembrane sections of the rotor that interact with TM7, as determined for F_1-F_O-ATPase and Na$^+$-V-ATPase, some similarities are observed. The transmembrane segments found for F_1-F_O-ATPase are composed of 30 or 40 amino acid residues (depending on the segment involved) and are partially embedded in the cytoplasm. The four transmembrane segments present in the rotor of Na$^+$-V-ATPase include 28 to 35 amino acid residues and part of it is proposed to be embedded in the cytoplasm. The proposed TM7 of V-ATPase studied here comprises 32 amino acid residues (T719 – W751), is helical and aligned along the rotor subunits. The length of a fully α-helical transmembrane section this long would be approximately 49 Å. Assuming that arginine R735 is located in the middle of the membrane bilayer as it has to face the functionally important glutamic acid residues of the rotor subunits, and taking into account a bilayer thickness of 39 Å, TM7 extends into the cytoplasm with 9 of its residues and as this region is helical it has a height of approximately to 15 Å (Figure 9). One side of this cytoplasmic part of TM7 interacts with the rotor of V-ATPase and in combination with the other transmembrane segments of subunit *a*. A small section of TM7 is positioned in the lumen and also interacts with the rotor of V-ATPase (Figure 9). From a mechanistic point of view the proposed transmembrane localization of TM7 supports the current model that describes the action of V-ATPase. In this model, two hemi-channels emerge in which proton translocation occurs and the putative TM7 is supposed to be part of the cytoplasmic hemi-channel, where protons are transported into the membrane region. In summary, the results obtained with peptide MTM7 show that the seventh segment of subunit *a* adopts an α-helical structure that is longer than calculated on basis of topology predictions. In the new topology, TM7 spans from the lumen to the cytoplasm were it is stabilized by a hydrophobic proteic environment (Figure 9).

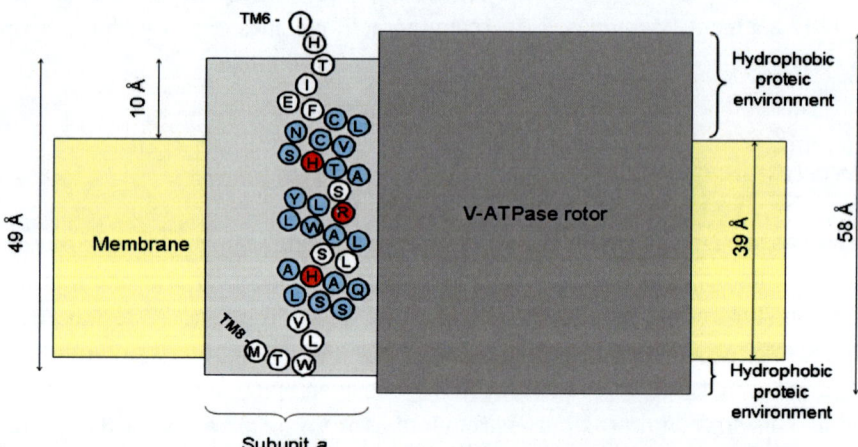

Figure 9. Schematic representation of peptide MTM7 embedded in its natural environment (*i.e.* V-ATPase). The light gray box represents subunit *a*. The TM7 segment of subunit *a* runs from residue T719 up to W751. CD results show that TM7 is helical and this could be confirmed by NMR spectroscopy for the residues colored light blue. For the residues colored white no resonance assignment are available due to cross peak broadening and resonance overlap. The dark gray box represents the V-ATPase rotor and the yellow regions represent the membrane. Arginine residue 735 and histidine residues H729 and H743 that are known to be involved in proton translocation are indicated in red. The height of the light gray box is calculated based on the demonstrated helicity of the comprising residues and assuming a rise of 1.5 Å per residue along the helical axis. The height of the rotor of yeast H^+-V-ATPase is based on the X-ray structure of the rotor subunit of Na^+-V-ATPase (Stock et al., 1999; Murata et al., 2005). Reprinted with permission from Duarte et al. (2007b). Copyright © 2007, Elsevier.

Structural Studies of Peptide sMTM7

NMR Spectroscopy

In performing NMR spectroscopy of peptide sMTM7, the choice of a suitable membrane-mimicking solvent is again a crucial step in the sample preparation. ESR spectroscopy experiments of peptide sMTM7 in SDS micelles were successfully carried out, showing that the peptide adopts mainly an α-helical conformation (Vos et al., 2007). However, 2D NMR experiments require much higher concentrations of peptide sMTM7 as compared to what is needed in ESR studies. Also for this peptide, only DMSO allows the use of the high sMTM7 concentrations (i.e., 2 mM) needed to obtain high-resolution 2D ^{1}H-^{1}H NMR spectra of sufficient quality (Figure 10). Other solvents were tested as well, but the solubility of peptide sMTM7 is either too low, or the obtained signal-to-noise ratio is too poor. The NMR experiments were carried out at 900 MHz to obtain a good sensitivity and dispersion of the resonances involved. In this case, all spin systems (i.e., amino acid residues) were assigned in the TOCSY spectrum and 80% of the NOE contacts observed could be unambiguously assigned in the NOESY spectra (Figure 10).

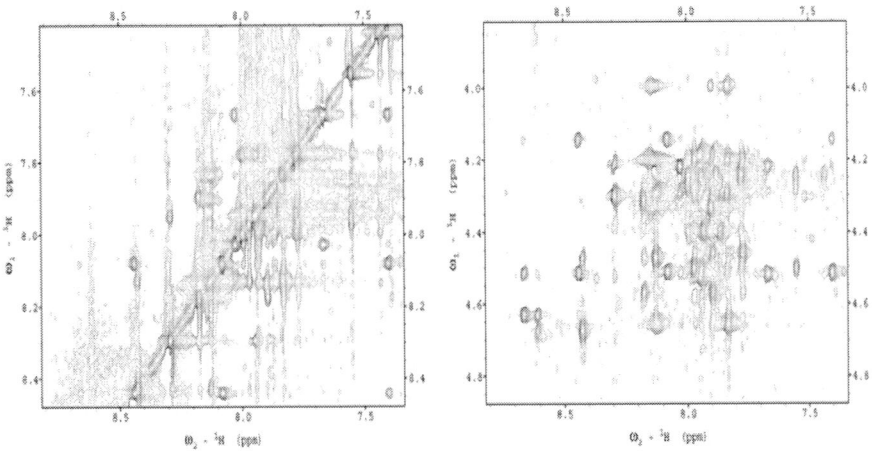

Figure 10. Fingerprint ^{1}H$_N$-^{1}H$_N$ (left) and ^{1}H$_N$-^{1}H$_α$ (right) regions of the 900 MHz 2D-NOESY spectrum of peptide sMTM7 in d_6-DMSO at 30 °C (mixing time of 300 ms). Reprinted with permission from Duarte et al. (2007a). Copyright © 2007, Elsevier.

Secondary Structure

The observation of specific sequential and medium-range NOE contacts can be used to infer the secondary structure of peptides and proteins (Wüthrich, 1976; Wüthrich, 1986). The NOE connectivities relevant to do the latter for peptide sMTM7 (i.e., $d_{αN}(i,i+3)$, $d_{αN}(i,i+4)$ and $d_{αN}(i,i+5)$ connectivities) are shown in Figure 11.

The combination of CSI values and NOE contacts (Figure 11) indicates that peptide sMTM7 predominantly adopts an α-helical structure in the region between C723 and A738. The $d_{αN}(i,i+4)$ and $d_{αN}(i,i+5)$ NOE contacts that characterize α-helicity are not found for residues T730 – A731 and A738 – Q745 of sMTM7 suggesting that in these regions the peptide does not adopt α-helical conformations. The identification of three $d_{\alpha N}(i, i+5)$ contacts (L724 – H729, N725 – T730 and S732 – W737) suggests that in these regions of the peptide a conformational exchange between α-helical and more loosened helical conformation occurs.

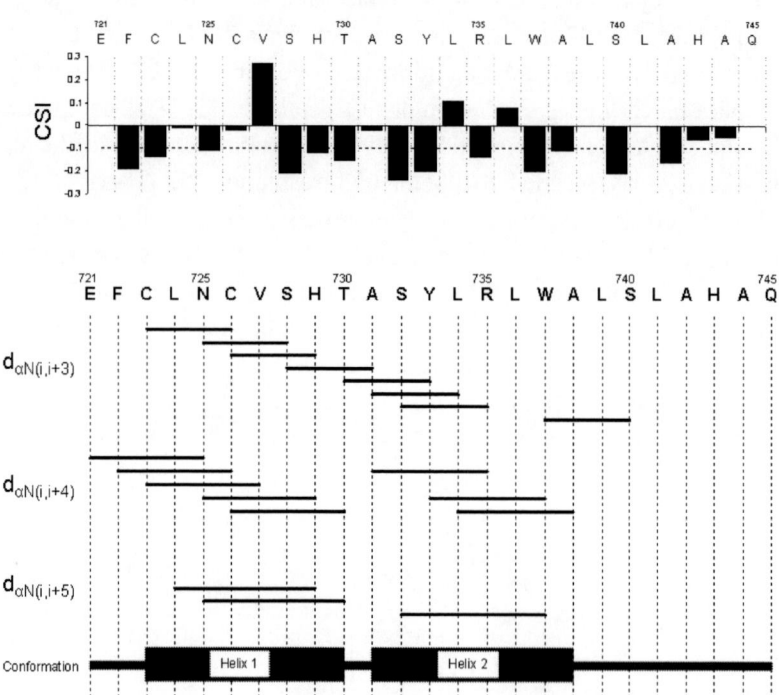

Figure 11. Summary of several secondary structure data obtained for peptide sMTM7 in d_6-DMSO at 30 °C. Top: CSI for $^1H_\alpha$ (■). Residues with CSI values that lie below -0.1 (---) have a high probability to be in an α-helical conformation (Wishart and Sykes, 1994). Many residues have a propensity to be in an α-helix configuration as is inferred from consecutive negative $^1H_\alpha$ CSI values, with residues V727, L734 and L736 being exceptions. Center: NOE connectivities $d_{\alpha N}(i, i+3)$, $d_{\alpha N}(i, i+4)$ and $d_{\alpha N}(i, i+5)$. Bottom: Secondary structure within peptide sMTM7 as deduced from NOE contacts and from the simulated annealing approach that leads to structures at atomic resolution. Reprinted with permission from Duarte et al. (2007a). Copyright © 2007, Elsevier.

A number of 545 distance constraints extracted from the ^1H-^1H-NOESY spectrum of peptide sMTM7 were used as input for a structure calculation procedure (all NOE contacts are deposited in the BioMagResbank under access number BMRB-15025). These constraints include the NOE contacts shown in Figure 11, as well as medium- and long-range NOE contacts identified between side chains of different amino acid residues. The conformational properties of the resulting 20 lowest energy structures of peptide sMTM7 in d_6-DMSO are shown in Figure 12. These structures show that the peptide is composed of two α-helical regions: C726 – H729 and S732 – A738. The two helical segments are separated by a region (T730 – A731) in which coil/bend/turn conformations are predominantly populated.

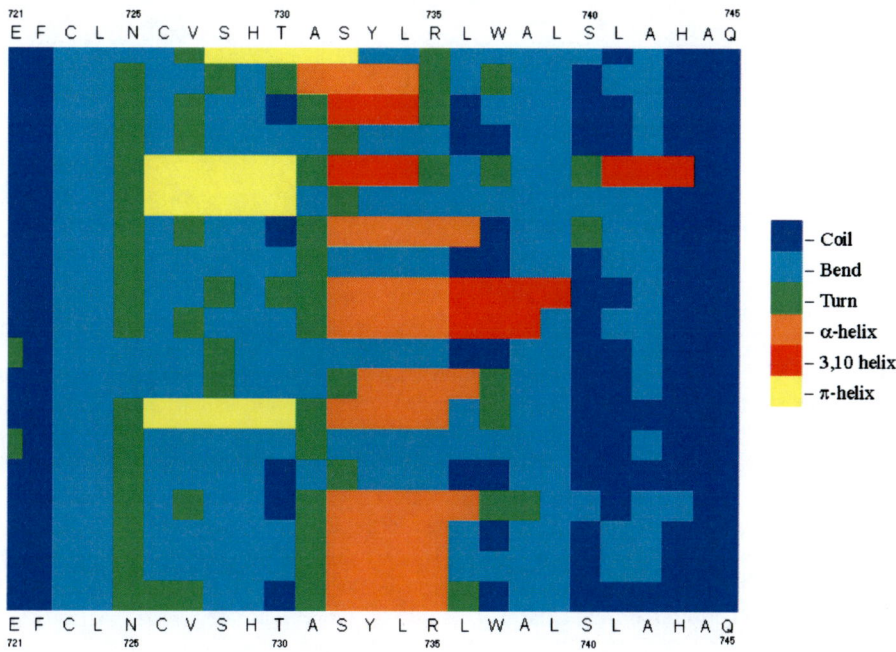

Figure 12. Matrix representation of the conformational properties of the 20 lowest energy structures of peptide sMTM7 as determined by the ARIA software. The horizontal axis represents the sequence of peptide sMTM7 and the vertical axis shows the corresponding secondary structure element in each of the structures calculated. Reprinted with permission from Duarte et al. (2007a). Copyright © 2007, Elsevier.

Structure Calculations

The root-mean-square deviation (RMSD) minimization fits of three different regions of the backbone of the 20 lowest energy structures calculated are shown in Figure 13.

A superimposition of the structures confined to either of the two identified helical regions (C723 – H729 and S732 – A738) leads to relatively low RMSD values thereby confirming the helical character of both sections of sMTM7. These two helical regions act as separate moieties that move independently with respect to one another due to the less rigid section involving T730 – A731 (Figure 13A and B). The existence of such a flexible region is confirmed by the identification of weak long-distance NOE contacts between the side chains of residues located in Helix 1 and Helix 2. These NOE contacts are included in the structure determination procedure. A RMSD minimization of the region T730 – A731 (Figure 13C) shows that both helical regions move independently with respect to one another. The region L739 – Q745 of sMTM7 is considered to be fraying.

In the C-terminal part of peptide sMTM7 no medium nor long-range NOE contacts are detected between residues A738 – Q745 and as a consequence the structure calculations show that this section mainly populates coil/bend/turn conformations, which reflects conformational fraying. C-termini of peptides have stronger fraying properties than N-termini (Miick et al., 1993; Ho et al., 2003). In case of peptide sMTM7 the disulphide bridge that links C723 and C726 contributes to the virtual absence of fraying of the N-terminus (Figure 13A).

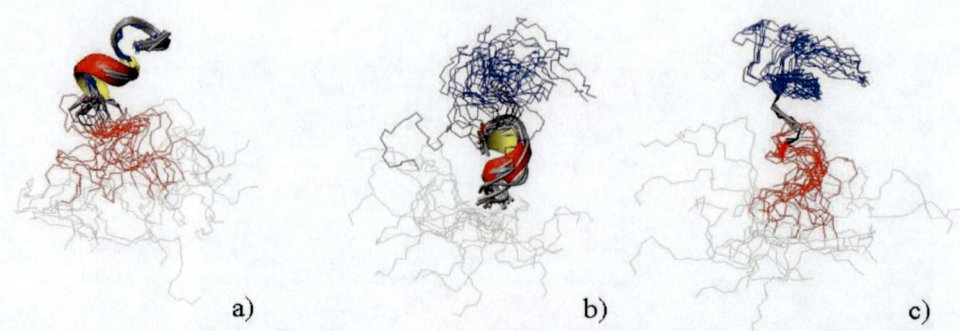

a)   b)   c)

Figure 13. Three RMSD (root-mean-square deviation) minimized superposition of the C_α traces of the 20 lowest energy structures calculated for peptide sMTM7 using the software MOLMOL (Koradi et al., 1996). The RMSD is minimized for the following three regions of the peptide: a) residues C723 – H729 (RMSD: 1.130 Å), b) residues S732 – A738 (RMSD: 3.212 Å), and c) residues T730 – A731 (RMSD: 0.890 Å). The regions with RMSD-minimization are depicted in the ribbon representation, the remaining sections are depicted in their C_α traces. The four regions identified in sMTM7 are differently colored for the purpose of distinction: blue - E721 – H729, black - T730 – A731, red - S732 – A738 and dark grey - A738 – Q745. These structures are deposited in the PDB databank with reference 2NVJ. Reprinted with permission from Duarte et al. (2007a). Copyright © 2007, Elsevier.

The first helical segment of peptide sMTM7 is apparently dynamic as it can adopt turn, bend and α-helical conformations and resembles a loosened α-helix. The second helical segment of peptide sMTM7 adopts α-helical and 3,10-helical conformations. This part of peptide sMTM7 is less dynamic compared to the first helical section as turn and bend structures are hardly populated. Both helical segments are connected by two amino acid residues (T730 and A731) that adopt turn and bend conformations (Figure 12). As a result, both helical segments move independently with respect to one another (Figure 13).

Implications for Proton Channel Function

As discussed in the previous section, NMR studies of peptide MTM7 (Figure 5) show that the C723 – A731 region is helical, but it could not be excluded that this helical segments contains small non-helical segments. The refined study presented for peptide sMTM7 indeed shows that TM7 does not adopt a continuous α-helical structure, but instead it has a flexible non-helical hinge region at T730 – A731. Recently, a flexible region in a peptide from the Na^+,K^+-ATPase was indentified that was correlated with a flexible region in the native protein. In addition, backbone hinges that interrupt transmembrane helical segments have been found for other transmembrane protein (Hunte et al., 2005; Underhaug et al., 2006). The conformational characteristics observed for peptide sMTM7 reflect the intrinsic properties of the peptide. Consequently, it is proposed that the sMTM7 part of TM7 exhibits a similar behavior when it is located in its natural environment, subunit *a* of V-ATPase.

How might the flexible hinge at T730 – A731 affect the proton translocation properties of the sMTM7 region of the V_O domain? The second helical region of peptide sMTM7, which contains arginine R735, needs to be positioned in the centre of the membrane bilayer, thereby facing the central glutamic acids of the rotor (located at TM2 and TM4). As a consequence, the first helical region of peptide sMTM7 is located in the cytoplasmic proton hemi-channel, in agreement with the bafilomycin binding data (see Figure 14).

The flexible region of TM7 (i.e., T730 – A731) that connects two helical segments thus is located near the end of the cytoplasmic hemi-channel (*i.e.*, almost in the centre of the bilayer) (see Figure 14). As region A738 – Q745 does not fray in peptide MTM7 and as it has been shown to be helical in TM7 (Duarte et al., 2007b), this region is depicted as a helix in Figure 14. We speculate that this proposed arrangement of the peptide in the hemi-channel could allow movement of protons to the centre of the rotor via rotation and adjustment of the first helical segment, thereby opening and closing the passage for protons to the centre of the membrane respectively (see blue arrows in Figure 14). This movement could allow the correct orientation of the helical faces expected to be face-to-face during the different steps of proton translocation.

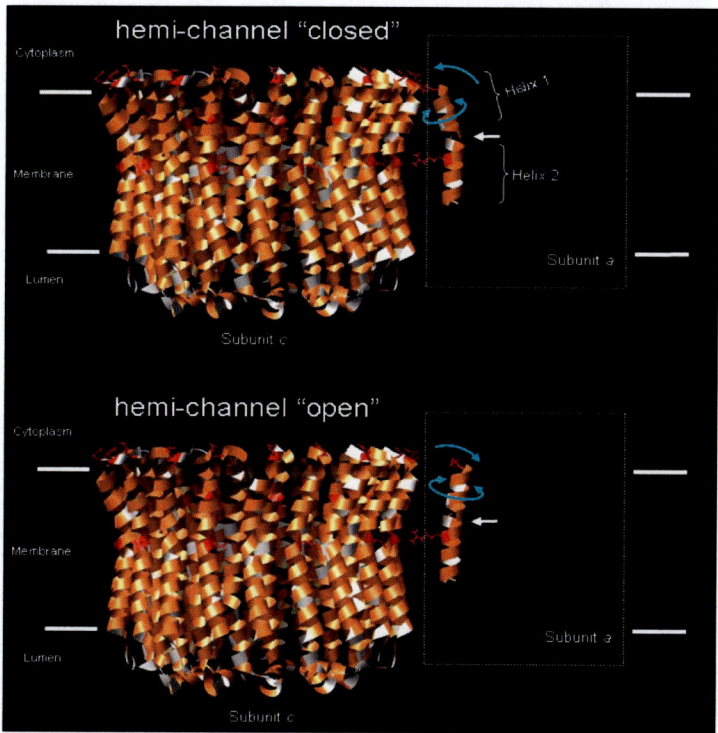

Figure 14. Proposed model for opening and closing of the cytoplasmic hemi-channel of V_O H^+-ATPase. Subunit *c* is represented by the rotor of Na^+-V-ATPase (Murata et al., 2005) (PDB entry: 2BL2). From subunit *a* only the section of TM7 that includes peptide sMTM7 is shown. The membrane boundaries (white horizontal lines) are according to Murata et al., 2005. Peptide sMTM7 is depicted as an α-helix with the exception of residues T730 and A731, which are highlighted by a white arrow and which form a flexible region that can allow Helix 1 and Helix 2 to move independently with respect to one another. The glutamic acids that are located in the rotor and arginine R735 of peptide sMTM7 (depicted as a stick model) are colored red, while the other hydrophilic residues are colored in white. Hydrophobic residues are colored orange. Potential movements of TM7, based on the work presented here, that allow the cytoplasmic hemi-channel to "open" or "close" are indicated by blue arrows. The structures are drawn with the software package Chimera (Pettersen et al., 2004). Reprinted with permission from Duarte et al. (2007a). Copyright © 2007, Elsevier.

Previously, its was proposed that TM7 is a rigid helix and that changes in the orientation of TM4/TM2 relative to TM7 explain the experimental cross-links identified between TM7 and TM4/TM2 (Kawasaki-Nishi et al., 2003). However, the fact that TM7 consists of two helical segments that can rotate independently from one another, as we suggest, also explains the experimental cross-links observed between TM7 and TM4/TM2. Residues T730 and A731 can act as a dynamical ball-and-socket joint, which links two helical segments of sMTM7 in TM7. We propose that the autonomous movement of the N-terminal helical segment, which is positioned in the cytoplasmic hemi-channel, causes the proton translocation channel to open and close thereby enabling proton translocation (see blue arrows in Figure 14). The autonomous movement of the first helical segment of TM7 could also be relevant for the binding of inhibitors to specific amino acid residues of F- and V-ATPases. Since the cytoplasmic loop that connects TM7 to TM6 is quite long (approximately 65 residues) dynamic movement of helix 1 of TM7 could be compensated by a movement further up in this loop. The existence of such a movement opens new opportunities for drug design. Inhibitors that bind to the cytoplasmic loop segment could rigidify it and thereby potentially disable the translocation of protons.

Conclusion

One major task in drug design is the knowledge of the secondary and tertiary structure of the enzyme under study. The topology of the V-ATPase protein complex has been largely established, however, the three-dimensional structure is only known for some individual subunits. For this purpose, two peptides were designed in our work consisting of 25 and 37 amino acid residues (Figure 5), representing the seventh transmembrane segment of subunit *a*, which encompass the proton translocation channel as well as the region of interest for possible inhibitors. Using a combination of NMR and CD spectroscopy the structure of these V-ATPase peptides was studied in different membrane-mimicking environments. Our results indicate that the transmembrane segment of this protein region adopts an α-helical conformation and that this region is longer than proposed by topological studies. Moreover, this segment exhibits a hinge region located near the cytoplasmic end of the channel (Figure 14).

These topologic and structural findings provide a new critical evaluation of the cytoplasmic hemi-channel of subunit *a* as a possible drug target for proton translocation. The longer helical region that spans from the hinge region to the cytoplasmic region and its specific dynamical properties that allow the opening and closing of the proton translocation channel raise two key questions that could be attractive for further research in drug design:

- Can drugs specifically bind to the helical segment changing its rigidity thus affecting proton translocation?
- Can the flexible hinge alone, or together with the helical segment, be specifically targeted by drugs?

The knowhow derived from these questions will allow us to better understand and control the activity on V-ATPase in osteoclast cells, helping in this way the fight against osteoporosis.

Acknowledgments

This work was supported by contract no. QLG-CT-2000-01801 of the European Commission (MIVase – New Therapeutic Approaches to Osteoporosis: targeting the osteoclast V-ATPase).

References

Abrahams, J. P., A. G. W. Leslie, R. Lutter and J. E. Walker (1994). Structure at 2.8 Å resolution of F_1-ATPase from bovine heart mitochondria, *Nature* 370(6491): 621-628.

Adler, M., M. H. Seto, D. E. Nitecki, J. H. Lin, D. R. Light and J. Morser (1995). The structure of a 19-residue fragment from the C-loop of the fourth epidermal growth factor-like domain of thrombomodulin. *J. Biol. Chem.* 270(40): 23366-23372.

Arata, Y., T. Nishi, S. Kawasaki Nishi, E. Shao, S. Wilkens and M. Forgac (2002). Structure, subunit function and regulation of the coated vesicle and yeast vacuolar (H^+)-ATPases. *Biochim. Biophys. Acta* 1555(1-3): 71-74.

Bashford, C. L., R. P. Casey, G. K. Radda and G. A. Ritchie (1975). The effect of uncouplers on catecholamine incorporation by vesicles of chromaffin granules. *Biochem. J.* 148(1): 153-155.

Bellanda, M., E. Peggion, R. Burgi, W. van Gunsteren and S. Mammi (2001). Conformational study of an Aib-rich peptide in DMSO by NMR. *J. Pept. Res.* 57: 97-106.

Ben-Efraim, I. and Y. Shai (1997). The structure and organization of synthetic putative membranous segments of ROMK1 channel in phospholipid membranes. *Biophys. J.* 72(1): 85-96.

Boekema, E. J., J. F. van Breemen, A. Brisson, T. Ubbink Kok, W. N. Konings and J. S. Lolkema (1999). Biological motors: connecting stalks in V-type ATPase. *Nature* 401(6748): 37-38.

Boyer, P. D. (1997). The ATP synthase - a splendid molecular machine. *Ann. Rev. Biochem.* 66: 717-749.

Cross, T. A. and S. J. Opella (1981). Hydrogen-1 and carbon-13 nuclear magnetic resonance of the aromatic residues of fd coat protein. *Biochemistry* 20(2): 290-297.

Ding, F. X., H. Xie, B. Arshava, J. M. Becker and F. Naider (2001). ATR-FTIR study of the structure and orientation of transmembrane domains of the *Saccharomyces cerevisiae* alpha-mating factor receptor in phospholipids. *Biochemistry* 40(30): 8945-8954.

Drory, O., F. Frolow and N. Nelson (2004). Crystal structure of yeast V-ATPase subunit C reveals its stator function. *EMBO reports* 5(12): 1148-1152.

Duarte, A. M. S., W. R. de Jong, R. Wechselberger, C. P. M. van Mierlo and M. A. Hemminga (2007a). Segment TM7 from the cytoplasmic hemi-channel from V_O-H^+- V-ATPase includes a flexible region that has a potential role in proton translocation. *Biochim. Biophys. Acta* 1768(9): 2263-2270.

Duarte, A. M. S., C. J. A. M. Wolfs, N. A. J. van Nuland, M. A. Harrison, J. B. C. Findlay, C. P. M. Van Mierlo and M. A. Hemminga (2007b). Structure and localization of an essential transmembrane segment of the proton translocation channel of yeast H^+-V-ATPase. *Biochim. Biophys. Acta* 1768(2): 218-227.

Duarte, A. M. S., C. P. M. van Mierlo and M. A. Hemminga (2008). Molecular dynamics study of the solvation of an α-helical transmembrane peptide by DMSO, *J. Phys. Chem. B* 112(29), 8664-8671.

Finbow, M. E. and M. A. Harrison (1997). The vacuolar H^+-ATPase: a universal proton pump of eukaryotes. *Biochem. J.* 324(Pt 3): 697-712.

Forgac, M. (1998). Structure, function and regulation of the vacuolar (H^+)-ATPases. *FEBS Lett.* 440(3): 258-263.

Forgac, M. (1999). Structure and properties of the clathrin-coated vesicle and yeast vacuolar V-ATPases. *J. Bioenerg. Biomembr.* 31(1): 57-65.

Girvin, M. E., V. K. Rastogi, F. Abildgaard, J. L. Markley and R. H. Fillingame (1998). Solution structure of the transmembrane H^+-transporting subunit c of the F_1F_O ATP synthase. *Biochemistry* 37(25): 8817-8824.

Grabe, M., H. Y. Wang and G. Oster (2000). The mechanochemistry of V-ATPase proton pumps. *Biophys. J.* 78(6): 2798-2813.

Henry, G. D., J. D. J. O'Neil, J. H. Weiner and B. D. Sykes (1986). Hydrogen exchange in the hydrophilic regions of detergent-solubilized M13 coat protein detected by carbon-13 nuclear magnetic resonance isotope shifts. *Biophys. J.* 49(1): 329-331.

Henry, G. D. and B. D. Sykes (1987). Strategies for the use of NMR spectroscopy in biological macromolecules and assemblies. *Bull. Can. Biochem. Soc.* 24(June): 21-26.

Hesselink, R. W., R. B. M. Koehorst, P. V. Nazarov and M. A. Hemminga (2005). Membrane-bound peptides mimicking transmembrane Vph1p helix 7 of yeast V-ATPase: A spectroscopic and polarity mismatch study. *Biochim. Biophys. Acta* 1716(2): 137-145.

Ho, B. K., A. Thomas and R. Brasseur (2003). Revisiting the Ramachandran plot: Hard-sphere repulsion, electrostatics, and H-bonding in the α-helix. *Protein Sci.* 12: 2508-2522.

Hunte, C., E. Screpanti, M. Venturi, A. Rimon, E. Padan and H. Michel (2005). Structure of a Na^+/H^+ antiporter and insights into mechanism of action and regulation by pH. *Nature* 435(7046): 1197.

Jackson, M. and H. H. Mantsch (1991). Beware of proteins in DMSO. *Biochim. Biophys. Acta* 1078(2): 231-235.

Johnson, B. A. and R. A. Blevins (1994). A computer program for the visualization and analysis of NMR data. *J. Biomol. NMR* 4: 603-614.

Kane, P. M. (2006). The where, when, and how of organelle acidification by the yeast vacuolar H^+-ATPase. *Microbiol. Mol. Biol. Rev.* 70(1): 177-191.

Katragadda, M., J. L. Alderfer and P. L. Yeagle (2001). Assembly of a polytopic membrane protein structure from the solution structures of overlapping peptide fragments of bacteriorhodopsin. *Biophys. J.* 81(2): 1029-1036.

Kawasaki-Nishi, S. and M. Forgac (2003). Proton translocation driven by ATP hydrolysis in V-APTases. *FEBS Lett.* 555: 76-85.

Kawasaki-Nishi, S., T. Nishi and M. Forgac (2003). Interacting helical surfaces of the transmembrane segments of subunits a and c' of the yeast V-ATPase defined by disulfide-mediated cross-linking. *J. Biol. Chem.* 278(43): 41908-41913.

Killian, J. A., T. P. Trouard, D. V. Greathouse, V. Chupin and G. Lindblom (1994). A general method for the preparation of mixed micelles of hydrophobic peptides and sodium dodecyl sulfate. *FEBS Lett.* 348(2): 161-165.

Kirshner, N. (1962). Uptake of catecholamines by a particulate fraction of the adrenal medulla. *J. Biol. Chem.* 237(7): 2311-2317.

Koradi, R., M. Billeter and K. Wüthrich (1996). MOLMOL: a program for display and analysis of macromolecular structures. *J. Mol. Graphics* 14: 51-55.

Lazarova, T., K. A. Brewin, K. Stoeber and C. R. Robinson (2004). Characterization of peptides corresponding to the seven transmembrane domains of human adenosine A2a receptor. *Biochemistry* 43: 12945-12954.

Le Maire, M., P. Champeil and J. V. Moller (2000). Interaction of membrane proteins and lipids with solubilizing detergents. *Biochim. Biophys. Acta* 1508(1-2): 86-111.

Li, F., H. Y. Li, L. H. Hu, M. Kwan, G. H. Chen, Q. Y. He and H. Z. Sun (2005). Structure, assembly, and topology of the G185R mutant of the fourth transmembrane domain of divalent metal transporter. *J. Am. Chem. Soc.* 127(5): 1414-1423.

Lindberg, M. and A. Graslund (2001). The position of the cell penetrating peptide penetratin in SDS micelles determined by NMR. *FEBS Lett.* 497(1): 39-44.

Mall, S., J. M. East and A. G. Lee (2002). Transmembrane alpha helices. *Peptide-lipidinteractions*. D. J. Benos and S. A.Simon. San Diego, Academic Press. 52: 339-370.

Manning, M. C. and R. W. Woody (1991). Theoretical CD studies of polypeptide helices: Examination of important electronic and geometric factors. *Biopolymers* 31(5): 569-586.

Manolson, M., D. Proteau, R. Preston, A. Stenbit, B. Roberts, M. Hoyt, D. Preuss, J. Mulholland, D. Botstein and E. Jones (1992). The VPH1 gene encodes a 95-kDa integral membrane polypeptide required for in vivo assembly and activity of the yeast vacuolar H$^+$-ATPase. *J. Biol. Chem.* 267(20): 14294-14303.

Mellman, I., R. Fuchs and A. Helenius (1986). Acidification of the endocytic and exocytic pathways. *Ann. Rev. Biochem.* 55: 663-700.

Miick, S. M., K. M. Casteel and G. L. Millhauser (1993). Experimental molecular dynamics of an alanine-based helical peptide determined by spin label electron spin resonance. *Biochemistry* 32: 8014-8021.

Motta, A., P. A. Temussi, E. Wunsch and G. Bovermann (1991). A ^{1}H NMR study of human calcitonin in solution. *Biochemistry* 30(9): 2364-2371.

Murata, T., I. Yamato, Y. Kakinuma, A. G. W. Leslie and J. E. Walker (2005). Structure of the rotor of the V-type Na-ATPase from *Enterococcus hirae*. *Science* 308(5722): 654-659.

Nielsen, G., A. Malmendal, A. Meissner, J. V. Moller and N. C. Nielsen (2003). NMR studies of the fifth transmembrane segment of sarcoplasmic reticulum Ca^{2+}-ATPase reveals a hinge close to the Ca^{2+}-ligating residues. *FEBS Lett.* 544(1-3): 50-56.

Nishi, T. and M. Forgac (2002). The vacuolar (H^+)-ATPases-nature's most versatile proton pumps. *Nat. Rev. Mol. Cell. Biol.* 3(2): 94-103.

Njus, D. and G. K. Radda (1979). A potassium ion diffusion potential causes adrenaline uptake in chromaffin-granule 'ghosts'. *Biochem. J.* 180: 579-585.

Orekhov, V. Y., K. V. Pervushin and A. S. Arseniev (1994). Backbone dynamics of (1-71)bacterioopsin studied by two-dimensional ^1H-^{15}N NMR spectroscopy. *Eur. J. Biochem.* 219(3): 887-896.

Papavoine, C. H. M., J. M. A. Aelen, R. N. H. Konings, C.W. Hilbers and F. J. M. van de Ven (1995). NMR studies of the major coat protein of bacteriophage M13. Structural information of gVIIIp in dodecylphosphocholine micelles. *Eur. J. Biochem.* 232(2): 490-500.

Papavoine, C. H. M., R. N. H. Konings, C. W. Hilbers and F. J. M. van de Ven (1994). Location of M13 coat protein in sodium dodecyl sulfate micelles as determined by NMR. *Biochemistry* 33(44): 12990-12997.

Park, K., A. Perczel and G. D. Fasman (1992). Differentiation between transmembrane helixes and peripheral helixes by the deconvolution of circular dichroism spectra of membrane proteins. *Protein Sci.* 1(8): 1032-1049.

Pervushin, K. V., A. S. Arseniev, A. T. Kozhich and V. T. Ivanov (1991). TwodimensionalNMR study of the conformation of (34-65) bacterioopsin polypeptide in SDS micelles. *J. Biomol. NMR* 1(4): 313-322.

Pettersen, E. F., T. D. Goddard, C. C. Huang, G. S. Couch, D. M. Greenblatt, E. C. Meng and T. E. Ferrin (2004). UCSF Chimera - A visualization system for exploratory research and analysis. *J. Comput. Chem.* 25(13): 1605-1612.

Sagermann, M., T. H. Stevens and B. W. Matthews (2001). Crystal structure of the regulatory subunitHof the V-typeATPase of *Saccharomyces cerevisiae*. *Proc. Natl. Acad. Sci. USA.* 98(13): 7134-7139.

Soulie, S., J.-M. Neumann, C. Berthomieu, J. V. Moller, M. le Maire and V. Forge (1999). NMR conformational study of the sixth transmembrane segment of sarcoplasmic reticulum Ca^{2+}-ATPase. *Biochemistry* 38(18): 5813-5821.

Stevens, T. H. and M. Forgac (1997). Structure, function and regulation of the vacuolar (H^+)-ATPase. *Annu. Rev. Cell. Dev. Biol.* 13: 779-808.

Stock, D., A. G. W. Leslie and J. E. Walker (1999). Molecular architecture of the rotary motor in ATP synthase. *Science* 286(5445): 1700-1705.

Underhaug, J., L. O. Jakobsen, M. Esmann, A. Malmendal and N. C. Nielsen (2006). NMR studies of the fifth transmembrane segment of Na^+,K^+-ATPase reveals a nonhelical ion-binding region. *FEBS Lett.* 580(20): 4777.

Vos, W. L., L. S. Vermeer and M. A. Hemminga (2007). Conformation of a peptide encompassing the proton translocation channel of vacuolar H^+-ATPase. *Biophys. J.* 92(1): 138-146.

Wang, Y., T. Inoue and M. Forgac (2004). TM2 but not TM4 of subunit *c* interacts with TM7 of subunit *a* of the yeast V-ATPase as defined by disulfide-mediated crosslinking. *J. Biol. Chem.* 279(43): 44628-44638.

Wang, Y., T. Inoue and M. Forgac (2005). Subunit *a* of the yeast V-ATPase participates in binding of bafilomycin. *J. Biol. Chem.* 280(49): 40481-40488.

WHO,World Health Organization (2007). www.who.gov.

Wieczorek, H., D. Brown, S. Grinstein, J. Ehrenfeld and W. R. Harvey (1999). Animal plasma membrane energization by proton-motive V-ATPases. *BioEssays* 21(8): 637-648.

Wilkens, S., E. Vasilyeva and M. Forgac (1999). Structure of the vacuolar ATPase by electron microscopy. *J. Biol. Chem.* 274(45): 31804-31810.

Wishart, D. S., B. D. Sykes and F. M. Richards (1992). The chemical shift index - A fast and simple method for the assignment of protein secondary structure through NMR spectroscopy. *Biochemistry* 31(6): 1647-1651.

Wishart, D. S. and B. D. Sykes (1994). Chemical shifts as a tools for structure determination. *Methods Enzymol.* 239: 363-392.

Wüthrich, K. (1976). *NMR in biological research: peptides and proteins*. Amsterdam, North-Holland / American Elsevier.

Wüthrich, K. (1986). *NMR of proteins and nucleic acids*. Amsterdam, New York, Wiley.

Yeagle, P. L. and A. D. Albert (2002). Use of NMR to study the three-dimensional structure of rhodopsin. *Methods Enzymol.* 343: 223-231.

Yeagle, P. L., G. Choi and A. D. Albert (2001). Studies on the structure of the Gprotein coupled receptor rhodopsin including the putative G-protein binding site in unactivated and activated forms. *Biochemistry* 40(39): 11932-11937.

Yeagle, P. L., C. Danis, G. Choi, J. L. Alderfer and A. D. Albert (2000). Three dimensional structure of the seventh transmembrane helical domain of the G-protein receptor, rhodopsin. *Mol. Vis.* 27: 6125-6131.

In: Antibiotic Resistance…
Editors: A. R. Bonilla and K. P. Muniz

ISBN 978-1-60741-623-4
© 2009 Nova Science Publishers, Inc.

Chapter XVI

Antibiotic Resistance in Food-Associated Lactic Acid Bacteria

Giorgio Giraffa
Agriculture Research Council
Research Centre for Forage and Dairy Productions
Research Unit "Dairy Products", Via Lombardo 11, 26900 Lodi, Italy

Abstract

The emergence of antimicrobial-resistant microorganisms in both humans and livestock is a growing concern. In recent years, increased focus has been given to food as a carrier of antibiotic resistance (AR) genes. However, there have been few systematic studies to investigate acquired AR in lactic acid bacteria (LAB), which constitute common components of the microbial community of food and play a relevant role in food fermentation. In Europe, the Food Safety Agency (EFSA) received a request to assess the safety of microorganisms throughout the food chain and proposed the Qualified Presumption of Safety (QPS) approach. In the QPS approach, safety assessment will depend upon the body of knowledge available for a given microorganism. Apparently, there are no specific concerns regarding most of the food-associated LAB species, which have a long history of safe use in the food chain, provided that the lack of acquired AR is systematically demonstrated. Consequently, increased efforts have been devoted in recent years to gain more insight into the diffusion of AR phenotypes within food-associated LAB, with particular emphasis on those applied as starter cultures or probiotics. Presently available literature data support the view that, in antibiotic-challenged habitats, LAB (especially enterococci) like other bacteria are involved in the transfer of resistance traits over species and genus borders, with important safety implications. The prevalence of such bacteria with acquired genetically-exchangeable resistances is high in animals and humans that are regularly treated with antibiotics. This led to the European ban of the antibiotics used as growth promoters in animal feed. Such measures should, however, be complemented by a more prudent use of antibiotics in both human and animal clinical therapy.

Introduction

A large variety of antibiotics are currently being used in medicine and veterinary medicine and this has led to the emergence of antibiotic resistance (AR). However, for many years studies on the selection and dissemination of AR have focused mainly on clinically-relevant bacterial species, whereas there have been few systematic studies to investigate the antibiotic susceptibility or the presence of AR genes in commensal bacteria such as lactic acid bacteria (LAB) isolated from food [Mathur and Singh, 2005]. In recent years, debate has centered on links between antimicrobial use in the production of livestock and the emergence of resistant organisms in the human population. Consequently, microbial risk assessment has been used to facilitate scientific investigations into the risks related to the food chain and the possibility that commensal bacteria may play an active role in the spread of AR [Snary et al., 2004]. The main threat associated with AR in commensal bacteria, such as LAB, is the risk of horizontal transfer of its genetic determinants to pathogenic bacteria, thus impairing successful antibiotic treatment of common microbial infections. In this mechanism, antibiotic-resistant LAB (AR-LAB), such as enterococci and several *Lactobacillus* species, act as "reservoirs" of resistance genes, whereas food represents the "physical" carrier for transmission of living AR-LAB from animal and plant sources into the human body [Mathur and Singh, 2005; Ammor et al., 2007].

This chapter reviews the distribution and origin of AR in LAB, the potential mechanisms of transfer, and their role in the dissemination of AR in the animal and human populations.

Emergence and Spread of Antibiotic Resistance

In the last 50 years, the large-scale antibiotic application to treat infectious diseases in humans and animals has led a concomitant occurrence of resistance to antibiotics. Moreover, sub-therapeutic doses of antibiotics have also been massively used in the last two decades as growth promoters in animal husbandry. This latter phenomenon has led to the rapid evolution of AR as a response from bacteria to the dramatic change in their environment introduced by the extensive use of antimicrobials [Mathur and Singh, 2005; Perreten, 2005].

The emergence and spread of AR in bacteria depends on a variety of factors, the most important of which are the presence of resistance genes and the selective pressure caused by the use of antibiotics [Perreten, 2005]. Two public health concerns are associated with this phenomenon: (i) the possibility that AR determinants might be located on genetic mobile elements of either pathogen or commensal bacteria, which would act as reservoirs; (ii) the probability of genetic exchange to other bacteria, especially pathogens.

Intrinsic versus Acquired Resistance

When resistance to an antimicrobial is inherent to a bacterial species, it is generally referred to as "intrinsic resistance" and is typically a species-specific trait. In contrast, when a strain of a typically susceptible species is resistant to a given antimicrobial agent, it is considered to be "acquired resistance". Intrinsic resistance is not horizontally transferable and poses no risks in no-pathogenic bacteria. Acquired resistance can be due to either a mutation of indigenous genes or the acquisition of additional genes (genes acquired by other bacteria via gain of exogenous DNA). In this latter event, resistance has a potential for lateral spread among bacteria [FEEDAP, 2008].

Ecophysiological Aspects of LAB and Their Importance in AR Selection

Lactic acid bacteria (LAB) are a group of Gram-positive bacteria widely found in numerous districts of the human and animal body and in environmental sources (mainly plants). They are the major microflora involved in fermented dairy products, vegetables, and sourdough fermentation and (mainly lactobacilli and pediococci) are part of the starter cultures used in meat fermentation to produce desirable acids and flavor compounds. Moreover, some LAB strains from animal and human intestinal microflora have been adopted as probiotic food supplements [Giraffa, 2004].

The existence of LAB in large numbers in habitats that are regularly challenged with antibiotics (diseased animals, diseased humans, and plants) potentially disposes these bacteria to a selective pressure leading to the development of resistance. There are several known mechanisms for the in vitro horizontal transfer of AR genes in LAB, which involve the presence of mobile elements (such as conjugative or mobilizable plasmids and transposons). Conjugative transposons encoding genes for resistance to tetracycline, erythromycin, chloramphenicol, and kanamycin have been described in *Enterococcus* spp. and streptococci [Mathur and Singh, 2005]. Conjugative plasmids encoding AR genes are common in enterococci but normally have not been observed in starter cultures, most of which stem from the pre-antibiotic era [Teuber et al., 2003].

Antibiotic Resistance Profiles of LAB Isolated from Food

The reported mechanisms of genetic exchange of AR determinants in LAB raised the need to determine the levels of resistance among desired foodborne LAB such as starter, non-starter, and probiotic LAB cultures. This is generally achieved through the determination of the Minimum Inhibitory Concentration (MIC) of the antibiotics for a given microorganism. The distribution of MICs for wild-type strains of a single species appears to be log-normal, and coexistence of wild-type strains and strains with atypically high MICs provides a bimodal distribution of the population. Therefore, profiling MIC distribution within a species is the first step in recognizing strains suspected of carrying acquired resistance traits [Turnidge and Paterson, 2007]. The detection of MIC above a log-normal distribution for a given strain for one or more antimicrobials requires, however, further investigation to make the distinction between acquired and intrinsic resistance. This step is generally carried out by molecular, generally PCR-based, methods to search for genes which can be involved in the horizontal transfer of AR.

The most important LAB for the food industry include the thermophilic *Lactobacillus delbrueckii* subsp. *bulgaricus* and subsp. *lactis*, *Lactobacillus helveticus*, the probiotic *Lactobacillus acidophilus* and bifidobacteria, *Lactobacillus casei*, *Lactobacillus plantarum*, *Streptococcus thermophilus*, *Oenococcus oeni*, and the *Lactococcus* group. Data on acquired AR for these bacteria are, however, still scarce. Antibiotic resistant strains have been reported in most of food-associated LAB, as recently reviewed by Mathur and Singh [2005], although only few studies clearly demonstrate that such resistances are acquired. As a general rule, lactobacilli (especially *L. plantarum*, *L. casei*, and *L. acidophilus*) have a high natural resistance to several antibiotics, such as kanamycin, gentamicin, and vancomycin. However, data from various studies demonstrate the existence of intergenus and interspecies differences and the species-dependency of LAB resistance to the antimicrobial agents [Teuber et al., 2003; Danielsen and Wind, 2003].

Several examples of AR-LAB isolated from food or from the gut of animals exist. Acquired aminoglycoside, erythromycin, and tetracycline resistances have been recently demonstrated in *Lactobacillus* spp. and *O. oeni* strains isolated from wine [Rojo-Bezares et al., 2006]. *Lactobacillus* species from fermented meat products were shown to harbor acquired tetracycline resistance encoded by a plasmid-located *tet*M gene [Gevers et al., 2003]. A bimodal MIC distribution with atypically higher phenotypic resistance to erythromycin, tetracycline, and streptomycin was recently found within seven out of 74 *S. thermophilus* strains [Tosi et al., 2007]. Since the mechanisms of horizontal gene transfer in *S. thermophilus* are poorly studied, the genetic basis of the above reported AR should be carefully evaluated. Conversely, MICs of a number of antibiotics, such as ampicillin, erythromycin, tetracycline, streptomycin, and vancomycin, showed a log-normal distribution (absence of acquired resistance) for *L. delbrueckii* and *L. helveticus* strains isolated from dairy products [Flòrez et al., 2008]. In a recent study, MICs of 16 antimicrobials representing all major antibiotic classes were determined for 473 taxonomically well-characterized isolates of LAB encompassing the genera *Lactobacillus*, *Pediococcus* and *Lactococcus*. Although *in vitro* intra- and interspecies filter-mating experiments failed to show transfer of resistance determinants [Klare et al., 2007], the finding of acquired resistance genes in isolates intended for probiotic or nutritional use highlights once more the importance of testing the antimicrobial susceptibility in documenting the safety of commercial LAB.

Lactic Acid Bacteria with Transferable AR in Food

The presence of LAB with transferable antibiotic resistance in food is of great importance since LAB are used as starter cultures for the production of fermented food. Moreover, a number of meat and dairy products are still produced in Europe with unpasteurized meat and milk, which include the endogenous microflora of the raw material. The finding that conjugative elements of LAB isolated from animals and foods are very similar to elements studied previously in pathogenic streptococci and enterococci [Teuber et al., 1999] supports the view that, in antibiotic challenged habitats, LAB may participate in the communication systems which transfer resistance traits over species and genus border.

Despite molecular biology of LAB started when Gasson and Davies [1980] demonstrated conjugal transfer of the drug resistant plasmid pAMß1 into lactococci, there have been few systematic studies to investigate that acquired antibiotic resistance of LAB in food is transferable. Most data exist for enterococci, whereas the number of reports on lactococci and lactobacilli is limited. In any case, the finding of mobile genetic elements carrying AR in LAB does not explain alone the possible horizontal transfer of such elements to other bacteria. Indeed, not all LAB seem efficient donors and, therefore, may not always act as reservoirs for AR genes. A recent European Project, named Assessment and Critical Evaluation of Antibiotic Resistance Transferability in Food Chain (ACE-ART), provided a critical evaluation of the role of antibiotic use in agriculture and in the prophylaxis and treatment of disease in humans. More specifically, an extensive list of donor bacteria, covering strains belonging to *Bifidobacterium*, *Lactobacillus*, *Lactococcus lactis*, and *S. thermophilus* were tested in model systems for their ability to transfer AR determinants to selected recipients; preliminary results identified strains belonging to all four above mentioned LAB groups that were able to transfer resistance genes [ACE-ART, 2006].

A separate treatment is needed for enterococci. Undoubtedly, species of the genus *Enterococcus* represent the most promiscuous bacterial species discovered within the Gram positive bacteria.

Enterococci: A Case-Study

Enterococci can be readily isolated from foods, including a number of traditional fermented foods. They constitute a large proportion of the autochthonous bacteria associated with the mammalian gastrointestinal tract. Once rejected in the environment by means of human feces, they are able to colonize diverse niches because of their exceptional aptitude to resist or grow in hostile environments. Enterococci are not only associated with warm-blooded animals, but they also occur in soil, surface waters, and on plant and vegetables. By intestinal or environmental contamination, they can then colonize raw foods (e.g. milk and meat) and multiply in these materials during fermentation. Enterococci can also contaminate finished products during food processing. Therefore, many fermented foods made from meat and milk (especially fermented meats and cheeses) contain enterococci [Giraffa, 2007].

Over the last two decades, however, enterococci, formerly viewed as organisms of minimal clinical impact, have emerged as important hospital-acquired pathogens in immune-suppressed patients and intensive care units. The newly accentuated ambiguity concerning the relationships of these bacteria with human beings is related to their enteric habitat, their entering the food chain, their possible involvement in food-borne illnesses due to the presence of virulence factors, such as production of adhesins and aggregation substances, and their antibiotic resistance [for a review, see Giraffa, 2002].

Antibiotic resistance makes enterococci effective opportunists in nosocomial infections. The extremely high level of intrinsic antibiotic resistance within enterococci, coupled with the selective pressure imposed by the use of antibiotics both in clinical therapy and animal husbandry, led to increased selection of strains with acquired resistances. The widespread finding of these microorganisms in raw foods could be the key factor contributing to the spreading of (acquired) antibiotic resistant enterococci (ARE) in both unfermented and fermented foods. ARE have been found in meat products, dairy products, ready-to-eat foods, and even within enterococcal strains proposed as probiotics [Giraffa, 2002]. Once ingested, ARE can survive gastric passage and multiply, thus leading to sustained intestinal carriage.

The resistance to the glycopeptides vancomycin and teicoplanin is the widest known example of acquired AR within enterococci. The use of this class of antimicrobials is of utmost importance in clinical therapy against multiple antibiotic-resistant strains or in the case of allergy to other antibiotics, e.g. ampicillin and penicillin [Morrison et al., 1997]. The chronic use of antibiotics as growth promoters in livestock is a recognized factor acting as selective agent in promoting glycopeptides resistant enterococci. With the emergence of glycopeptide resistance in enterococci (especially *E. faecium*) outside hospitals, a large reservoir of transferable resistance (*van*A gene cluster) was identified in animal husbandry due to the use of avoparcin as feed additive. Similar mechanisms have been suggested for streptogamin, avilamycin, and tylosin resistances. This led to a European ban for use of avoparcin (by 1997) and other growth promoters in animal feeds [Giraffa, 2002].

The evolutionary development of AR in enterococci has been attributed to the presence of effective gene transfer mechanisms through the mobilization of broad range genetic elements, such as conjugative transposons of the Tn*916-1545* family. Enterococci are successful donor organisms for the transfer of AR genes to *Escherichia coli*, *Bacillus subtilis*, *Staphylococcus* spp., and *Listeria monocytogenes* [Mathur and Singh, 2005]. Food-associated enterococci are therefore a reservoir for broad range, efficiently transferable AR.

Antibiotic Resistance: The EFSA Approach

In Europe, the Food Safety Agency (EFSA) received the request to assess the safety of microorganisms throughout the food chain and proposed the Qualified Presumption of Safety (QPS) concept, presumption being defined as "...*an assumption based on reasonable evidence and qualified to allow certain restrictions to apply*" [European Commission, 2003]. In the QPS approach, safety assessment will depend upon the body of knowledge available for a given microorganism. The most recent EFSA opinion on the introduction of a QPS approach to microorganisms used in food/feed states that, on the basis of body of knowledge (also defined as "familiarity"), there are no specific safety concerns regarding most of the food-associated LAB species, which have a long history of apparent safe use in the food chain, provided that the lack of acquired AR is systematically demonstrated. This principle of caution is justified from the finding of mobile genetic elements carrying AR in LAB and the lack of systematic studies on gene transfer mechanisms in these bacteria.

To categorize bacteria as susceptible or resistant, the panel on Additives and Products or Substances used in Animal Feed (FFEDAP) of the EFSA defined also microbiological breakpoints (BP), stating that determination of MICs above the BP levels for a given antimicrobial requires further investigations to distinguish between acquired and intrinsic resistance [European Food Safety Authority, 2007; FEEDAP, 2008]. When resistance has been acquired by a strain belonging to a taxonomic group naturally susceptible to an antimicrobial, the degree of risk of transfer is generally considered to be greater than that associated with intrinsic resistance. The FEEDAP panel definitely considers that bacteria carrying an acquired AR should not be used as feed additives, unless it can be shown that such resistance results from chromosomal mutation.

Conclusion

Lactic acid bacteria have a long history of safe use in food. However, like all other bacteria, LAB are prone to gene exchange to enhance survival in antibiotic-containing environments. Although presently available data indicate that, with the notable exception of enterococci, food-associated species of LAB are rarely involved in genetic transfer of AR determinants, it is expected that a considerable increase of available scientific data (e.g., the aforementioned ACE-ART project) will probably indicate that such bacteria may act as reservoirs and carriers of AR. In the meantime, a series of measures inspired from a principle of precaution should be taken, the most important of which is to systematically test strains for the presence of transferable resistance genes before being used as commercial starters or probiotic cultures in food products. This measure should be complemented by a more prudent use of antibiotics in all fields in which they are used, including agriculture, veterinary and human medicine, and by the use of proper substrates (e.g., pasteurized milk) for food fermentation. Finally, the implementation of HACCP procedures throughout the husbandry and food industries will help to reduce the spread of AR-LAB from animals to humans via the food chain.

References

ACE-ART (2006). Assessment and critical evaluation of antibiotic resistance transferability in food chain. 3rd Open Meeting, Parma, November 16-17.

Ammor, MS, Florez, AB and Mayo, B (2007). Antibiotic resistance in non-enterococcal lactic acid bacteria and bifidobacteria. *Food Microbiology*, *24*, 559-570.

Danielsen, M and Wind, A (2003). Susceptibility of *Lactobacillus* spp. to antimicrobial agents. *International Journal of Food Microbiology 82*, 1-11.

European Commission (2003). On a generic approach to the safety assessment of micro-organisms used in feed/food and feed/food production—A working paper open for comment. http://ec.europa.eu/food/fs/sc/scf/out178_en.pdf.

European Food Safety Authority (2007). Introduction of a Qualified Presumption of Safety (QPS) approach for assessment of selected microorganisms referred to EFSA. *The EFSA Journal*, *587*, 1-16.

FEEDAP (2008). Technical guidance—Update of the criteria used in the assessment of bacterial resistance to antibiotics of human or veterinary importance. *The EFSA Journal*, *732*, 1-15.

Flòrez, AB, Mayo, B, Amtmann, E, Mayer, HK, Korhonen, J, Domig, KJ, Tosi, L, Danielsen, M and Mayrhofer, S (2008). Assessment of the antimicrobial wild-type minimum inhibitory concentration distributions of species of the *Lactobacillus delbrueckii* group. *Dairy Science and Technology*, *88*, 183-191.

Gasson, MJ and Davies, FL (1980). Conjugal transfer of the drug resistance plasmid pAMß1 in the lactic streptococci. *FEMS Microbiology Letters*, *7*, 51-53.

Gevers, D, Danielsen, M, Huys, G and Swings, J (2003). Molecular characterization of *tet*(M) genes in *Lactobacillus* isolates from different types of fermented dry sausage. *Applied and Environmental Microbiology*, *69*, 1270-1275.

Giraffa, G (2002). Enterococci from foods. *FEMS Microbiology Reviews*, *26*, 163-171.

Giraffa, G (2004). Studying the dynamics of microbial populations during food fermentation *FEMS Microbiology Reviews*, *28*, 251-260.

Giraffa, G (2007). Enterococci and dairy products. In: Huy, H editor. *Handbook of Food Production Manufacturing*. New York: John Wiley and Sons Inc.; 85-97.

Klare, I, Konstabel C, Werner, G, Huys, G, Vankerckhoven, V, Kahlmeter, G, Hildebrandt, B, Müller-Bertling, S, Witte, W and Goossens, H. (2007). Antimicrobial susceptibilities of *Lactobacillus*, *Pediococcus* and *Lactococcus* human isolates and cultures intended for probiotic or nutritional use. *Journal of Antimicrobial Chemotherapy*, *59*, 900-912.

Mathur, S and Singh, R (2005). Antibiotic resistance in food lactic acid bacteria—a review. *International Journal of Food Microbiology*, *105*, 281-295.

Morrison, D, Woodford, N and Cookson, B (1997) Enterococci as emerging pathogens of humans. *Journal of Applied Microbiology*, *Suppl. 83*, 89-99.

Perreten, V. (2005). Resistance in the food chain and in bacteria from animals: relevance to human infections. In: White MN, Alekshun MN and McDermott PF editors. *Frontiers in Antimicrobial Resistance: a Tribute to Stuart B. Levy*. Washington DC: ASM Press; ; 446-464.

Rojo-Bezares, B, Sáenz, Y, Poeta, P, Zarazaga, M, Ruiz-Larrea, F, Torres, C (2003). Assessment of antibiotic susceptibility within lactic acid bacteria strains isolated from wine. *International Journal of Food Microbiology, 111,* 234-240.

Snary, EL, Kelly, LA, Davison, HC, Teale, CJ and Wooldridge, M (2004). Antimicrobial resistance: a microbial risk assessment perspective. *Journal of Antimicrobial Chemotherapy*, *53*, 906-917.

Teuber, M, Meile, L and Schwarz, F. (1999). Acquired antibiotic resistance in lactic acid bacteria from food. *Antonie van Leeuwenhoek*, *76*, 115-137.

Teuber, M, Schwartz, F and Meile, L (2003). Antibiotic resistance and transfer in lactic acid bacteria. In: Wood, BJB and Warner, PJ editors. *Genetics of Lactic Acid Bacteria*. New York: Kluwer Academic/Plenum Publishers; 317-354.

Tosi, L, Berruti, G, Danielsen, M, Wind, A, Huys, G and Morelli, L (2007). Susceptibility of *Streptococcus thermophilus* to antibiotics. *Antonie van Leeuwenhoek*, *92*, 21-28.

Turnidge, J and Paterson, DL (2007). Setting and revising antibacterial susceptibility breakpoints. *Clinical Microbiology Reviews*, *20*, 391-408.

In: Antibiotic Resistance…
Editors: A. R. Bonilla and K. P. Muniz

ISBN 978-1-60741-623-4
© 2009 Nova Science Publishers, Inc.

Chapter XVII

Current Status of Antibiotic Resistance in Lactic Acid Bacteria

Leon M. T. Dicks[1], Svetoslav D. Todorov[2]
and Bernadette D. G. M. Franco[2]
[1]Department of Microbiology, University of Stellenbosch,
Stellenbosch, South Africa
[2]Universidade de São Paulo, Faculdade de Ciências Farmacêuticas,
Departamento de Alimentos e Nutrição Experimental,
Laboratório de Microbiologia de Alimentos,
São Paulo, SP, Brazil

Abstract

Lactic acid bacteria (LAB) consist of the genera *Lactobacillus, Carnobacterium, Lactococcus, Enterococcus, Streptococcus, Leuconostoc, Pediococcus, Desemzia, Isobacilum, Paralactobacillus, Tetragenococcus, Trichococcus, Weissella, Oenococcus* and *Melissococcus* and are present in many different habitats, including food and the human and animal intestinal tract. The long history of LAB with fermented foods have bestowed on them GRAS (generally regarded as safe) status. Intestinal strains play an important role in ensuring a healthy microbial balance. Their presence may lead to increased cytokine production and they may even play a role in preventing the growth of carcinogenic cells. A few rare cases of excessive immune stimulation, systemic infections, arthritis and the formation of hepatobiliary lesions have been reported for some strains of LAB. Such symptoms are usually associated with strains penetrating the mucus layer and epithelial cells. Lactic acid bacteria in food and the gastro-intestinal (GI) tract could act as a potential reservoir of antibiotic resistance genes and may participate in the exchange of genes with strains present in same environment to produce multidrug resistant strains. *Lactobacillus, Pediococcus* and *Leuconostoc* spp. have a high natural resistance to vancomycin. Some *Lactobacillus* spp. are by nature resistant to bacitracin, cefoxitin, ciprofloxacin, fusidic acid, kanamycin, gentamycin, metronidazole, nitrofurantoin, norfloxacin, streptomycin, sulphadiazine, teicoplanin, trimethoprim/sulphamethoxazole, and vancomycin. A few cases of *Enterococcus* infection have been associated with abnormal physiological conditions, underlying disease and immunosuppression. *Enterococcus faecalis* is the most dominant species in general GI infections, whereas *Enterococcus faecium* may cause enterococcal bacteremia. Enterococci have intrinsic resistance to cephalosporins, beta-lactams, sulphonamides and low levels of clindamycin and aminoglycosides. Resistance to chloramphenicol, erythromycin, high levels of clindamycin, aminoglycosides, tetracycline, β-lactams (β-lactamase or penicillinase), fluoroquinolones and glycopeptides is usually acquired. Vancomycin-resistant enterococci (VRE) with *van*A, *van*B, *van*C1, *van*C2, *van*C3, *van*D and *van*E genes have led to a number of nosocomial infections. VanA-type strains confer high level inducible resistance to vancomycin and teicoplanin, whereas VanB-type strains display variable levels of inducible resistance. VRE are highly resistant to most antibiotics and successful treatment is a major problem.

The aim of this review is to discuss antibiotic resistance amongst LAB and highlight the genetic determinants involved in horizontal and vertical transfer of resistance genes.

Introduction

Lactic acid bacteria (LAB) are Gram-positive, non-spore forming rods, cocci or cocco-bacilli, i.e. oval shaped (Leroy and de Vuyst, 2004). Apart for the genus *Vagococcus* (Collins et al., 1989), *Lactobacillus ghanensis* (Nielsen et al., 2007), *Lactobacillus nagelii* (Edwards et al., 2000), *Lactobacillus satsumensis* (Endo and Okada, 2005), *Lactobacillus vini* (Rodas et al., 2006), *Lactobacillus agilis* (Weiss et al., 1981), *Lactobacillus mali* (Kaneuchi et al., 1988), *Lactobacillus capillatus* (Chao et al., 2008) and *Lactobacillus ruminis* (Sharpe et al., 1973), all LAB are non-motile. They all produce lactic acid under microaerophilic conditions, and are catalase and oxidase negative (Carr et al., 2002). Some strains exhibit pseudocatalase activity when grown on media rich in heme, such as blood agar (Singh et al., 2007). Carbohydrates are fermented via the Embden Meyerhof Parnas (EMP) pathway to lactic acid and the pentose phosphate pathway to lactic acid, CO_2 and ethanol, depending on the presence of aldolase or phospho ketolase. Several LAB produce bacteriocins (natural antimicrobial peptides) and a vast number of such strains have been isolated in the last two decades (Reviewed by Castellano et al., 2008; Gálvez et al., 2007; Gobbetti et al., 2007).) Some of these strains have probiotic properties, i.e. when ingested in certain numbers, they "exert a positive influence on host physiology and health beyond inherent general nutrition" (Ouwehand et al., 2002). This led to an intense interest in the physiology and genetics of LAB, but also their ability to transfer antibiotic resistance to other strains.

Most enterococci harbor a series of virulence factors and have been associated with a number of human infections (Foulquié-Moreno et al., 2006). Recent reviews have dealt with antibiotic resistance in enterococci of food and human origin (Foulquié-Moreno et al., 2006; Mathur and Singh, 2005). A few cases of bacteremia caused by LAB have been reported (Cannon et al., 2005; Donohue and Salminen, 1996; Gasser, 1994; Husni et al., 1997; Vesterlund et al., 2007). LAB should thus be assessed for safety by conducting studies on their intrinsic properties, pharmacokinetics and interactions with the host (Salminen et al., 1998; Saxelin et al., 2005).

Antibiotics are defined as chemotherapeutic agents with activity against microorganisms (bacteria and fungi) and protozoa (Davey, 2000). The name stems from the Greek phrases αντί (anti or against) and βιοτικός ("biotikos" or "fit for life") and was first used by Selman Waksman in 1942. At that stage the term was used to describe any substance produced by a microorganism that is antagonistic to the growth of other microorganisms in high dilution. The definition of Waksman did not refer to synthetic compounds such as sulfonamides. In general antibiotics are small molecules with molecular weights below 2 kDa.   For centuries humans have been plagued with bacterial diseases such as leprosy, tuberculosis, bubonic plague, sexual transmitted diseases, etc. Most studies were based on empiric knowledge. It is only in the twentieth century that the origin of diseases and the pathogens have been identified and described. The first civilization to use antibiotics was ancient China. The antic Egyptian, Greek, and Arab civilizations used molds and plant extracts to treat bacterial infections. Treatment of malaria (caused by *Plasmodium falciparum*) was only possible in the 17th century when quinine was discovered.

Louis Pasteur and Robert Koch were the first to describe the inhibition of *Bacillus anthracis* by an airborne bacillus (Landsberg, 1949). In 1928 Fleming discovered the antibiotic properties of *Penicillium notatum*. Ten years later Ernst Chain and Howard Florey successfully purified penicillin and shared the Nobel Prize in Physiology with Alexander Fleming (Davey, 2000). In 1939 gramicidin, described by Rene Duboa, was commercialized and used in the Second World War to treat wound infections and ulcers (Van Epps, 2006). Prontosil, discovered by Gerhard Domagk, was successfully used against Gram-positive cocci, but had no effect against enterobacteria. During the twentieth century a number of new antibiotics have been developed, many based on chemical modifications of existing drugs. New generations of β-lactams are typical examples. Some antibiotics (aminoglycosides) are still produced based on isolation from microorganisms.

Mode of Action of Antibiotics

All antibiotics that have been successfully employed for decades as monotherapeutics in the treatment of bacterial infections rely on mechanisms of bacterial growth inhibition which are far more complex than the inhibition of a single enzyme. The targets are often encoded by multiple genes, which mean that the emergence of spontaneous target-related resistance is a comparatively slow process. β-lactam antibiotics, of which penicillin is the best known, targets the family of penicillin-binding proteins (PBPs) present in most bacteria and essential for transpeptidation in peptidoglycan biosynthesis (Scheffers and Pinho, 2005). No β-lactam inhibits all PBPs, but almost all compounds interfere with the activity of more than one essential PBP. Similarly, the quinolones inhibits topo-isomerase II (gyrase), inducing negative supercoils in DNA and topoisomerase IV, decatenating daughter chromosomes after replication (Drlica et al., 2008). Targeting one of these two topo-isomerases is sufficient to prevent growth. However, quinolone levels higher than the inhibitory concentrations for both enzymes are highly effective in preventing the development of antibiotic resistant strains. For glycopeptides the multiple gene aspect is realized by targeting an enzyme substrate, the peptidoglycan precursor lipid II, which has to be assembled and processed by a whole array of enzymes (Kahne et al., 2005). Spontaneous target-related low-level resistance has evolved only rarely in a slow and stepwise process and involves an increase of lipid II concentration rather than direct target mutations. A fourth example is antibiotics that act by binding to the 30S or 50S ribosomal subunits, thereby preventing the translation process. They bind exclusively to ribosomal RNA and not to ribosomal proteins (Connell et al., 2003; Kaul et al., 2006; Schlunzen et al., 2001; Xiong et al., 2000). Since ribosomal RNA is present in multiple copy numbers, the success rate of these antibiotics binding to their target is much higher compared to antibiotics that target single genes. Examples of the latter are rifampin, targeting RNA polymerase (Chopra, 2007); sulfonamides, targeting dihydropteroate synthase (Skold, 2000); trimethoprim, targeting dihydrofolate reductase (Hawser et al., 2006); fusidic acid, targeting elongation factor EF-G (Hansson et al., 2005); and novobiocin, targeting topoisomerase II (Maxwell et al., 2003). These antibiotics are known for rapid resistance mutations in their target genes and are predominantly used in combination and as topical agents. Targets on the surface of bacterial cells are easier to reach. Inhibiting an enzyme by covalent binding rather than competitive inhibition may be more beneficial, especially if (a) competing substrate concentrations are high, (b) the inhibitor acts extracellularly and may diffuse away from its target, and (c) the target needs to be inhibited almost completely to affect cell viability (Brötz-Oesterhelt and Brunner, in press). Quinolones act by initiating a complex cascade of events that lead to chromosome fragmentation (Drlica et al., 2008). A summary of the mode of action ofantibiotics is presented in Figure 1.

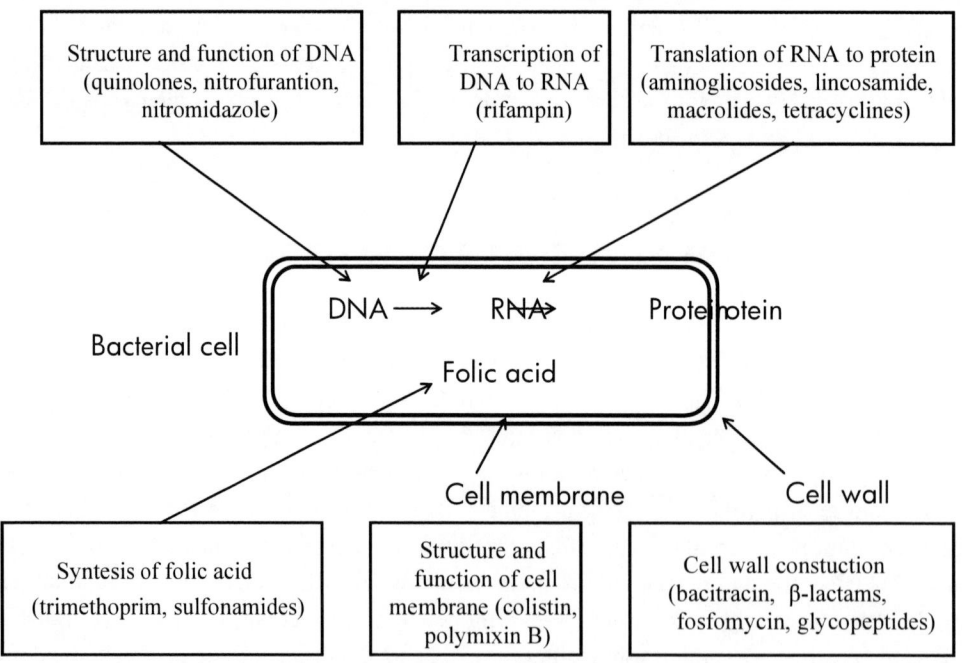

Figure 1. Mode of action of antibiotics.

Aminoglycosides inhibits protein synthesis by attaching to ribosomes. The majority of aminoglycosides are bactericidal. Bacitracin inhibits cell development by interfering with recycling of the membrane carrier, which is needed to add on new cell wall subunits. β-lactam antibiotics such as penicillin, cephalosporin, carbapenems and monobactams disturb cell-wall integrity. Cephalosporins affect target cells in a manner similar to that of penicillin, but have a broader range of applications. Chloramphenicol inhibits protein synthesis by interacting with the 50S bacterial ribosome subunit. Glycopeptides such as vancomycin inhibits cell wall synthesis by interfering with the attachment of new cell wall subunits (muramyl pentapeptides). Macrolides (e.g. erythromycin) and lincosamides (e.g. clindamycin) also bind to 50S bacterial ribosome subunits. Penicillins are involved in the inhibition of the cell wall structure. Quinolones prevents DNA synthesis by interfering with DNA gyrase, an enzyme essential in DNA replication. Rifampin is involved in the inhibition of RNA by suppressing DNA-dependent RNA polymerase. Tetracyclines inhibit protein synthesis by binding to the 30S bacterial ribosome subunit. Trimethoprim and Sulfonamides inhibits metabolism by preventing the synthesis of folic acid.

Antibiotic Resistance - Introduction

The most effective way to avoid development of antibiotic resistant variants is to kill all target cells. If not, the few surviving cells may multiple and recolonise the host, leading to severe infections that are difficult to treat. One of the best examples of antibiotic resistance is found in tuberculoses. Studies conducted in 1984 in the USA have shown that every strain of *Mycobacterium tuberculosis* isolated from patients have become resistant to at least one antibiotic that has been used in treatment of the disease. Over the past decade, a number of multi-drug resistant strains of *M. tuberculosis* have been isolated from patients (Sharma and Mohan, 2004). This clearly acquires the need to develop new-generation antibiotics. Another good example of antibiotic resistance is found in *Staphylococcus aureus*. Glycopeptides such as vancomycin are frequently used to treat methicillin resistant *S. aureus* (MRSA). Over the past decade the number of *S. aureus* strains with intermediate sensitivity to vancomycin (VISA) and strains resistant to vancomycin (VRSA) increased dramatically (Tiwari and Sen, 2006). Genes encoding antibiotic resistance are usually located on plasmids and are thus easily transferred from one cell to the other. Antibiotic resistance may be achieved by a number of different mechanisms, such as (a) a decrease in the uptake of an antibiotic, (b) an increase in the export of an antibiotic, (c) inactivation or modification of the target site, (d) hydrolysis of the antibiotic, (e) modification of the antibiotic, and (f) preventing the activation of an antibiotic (Normark and Normark, 2002).

According to the European Commission (2005), more than 10 million tons of antibiotics have been released into the biosphere since the start of commercial production. This has exerted a very strong selection on the development of resistant strains. Resistance may be inherent to a bacterial genus or species, but may also be acquired through exchange of genetic material, mutations and the incorporation of new genes (Ammor et al., 2007). Teuber (1999) and Salyers et al. (2004) suggested that starter cultures and probiotics may serve as vectors in the transfer of antibiotic resistant genes. Such transfer was documented in other bacterial groups by Levy and Marshall (2004) and Salyers et al. (2004).

Antibiotic Resistance in LAB – The Facts

A great number of different species of LAB are used in industrial fermentation processes and several probiotics are on the market. A number of papers have described LAB that acquired resistance from pathogenic bacteria (Ammor et al., 2007; Mathur and Singh, 2005). Once a strain becomes resistant, the determinant is amplified and may be transmitted to other LAB or even pathogenic bacteria. It is thus important to screen strains for transferable antibiotic resistance, and clear definitions of breakpoint values to discriminate between resistant and susceptible strains have to be in place. Distinguishing between intrinsic (non-specific, nontransferable) and acquired resistance is important and requires comparison of antimicrobial resistance patterns of LAB from different niches (Teuber, 1999).

Antibiotic resistance profiles of LAB are very different. Most species are resistant to metronidazole (MIC $\geq$ 32 mg/ml; Delgado et al., 2005; Flórez et al., 2005), sulphonamides (MIC $\geq$ 256 mg/ml) and trimethoprim (MICs $\geq$ 30 mg/ml; Katla et al., 2001). LAB has limited biosynthetic capabilities. They lack the folic acid synthesis pathway and are thus regarded intrinsically resistant to these agents (Katla et al., 2001). On the other hand, LAB is susceptible to piperacillin and piperacillin plus tazobactam (MICs $\leq$ 16 mg/ml) (Delgado et al., 2005; Flórez et al., 2005; Moubareck et al., 2005). *Lactobacillus, Lactococcus* and *Leuconostoc* species are resistant to high levels of cefoxitin (MICs $\geq$ 30 mg/ml) (Charteris et al., 1998; Delgado et al., 2005; Flórez et al., 2005). Most *Lactobacillus, Pediococcus* and *Leuconostoc* spp. are resistant to high concentrations of vancomycin (MICs $\geq$ 256 mg/ml), whereas most *Lactococcus* isolates are very susceptible (MICs $\leq$ 2 mg/ml) to vancomycin (Danielsen and Wind, 2003; Delgado et al., 2005; Flórez et al., 2005). Resistance of *Lactobacillus, Pediococcus* and *Leuconostoc* spp. to vancomycin is due to the presence of D-Ala-D-Lactate in their peptidoglycan rather than the D-Ala–D-Ala dipeptide (Klein et al., 2000). Such resistance is thus intrinsic in most LAB because the antibiotic's target is absent and not comparable to the transmissible, plasmid encoded vancomycin resistance found in enterococcal species (DeLisle and Perl, 2003). Lactobacilli have a high natural resistance to bacitracin, cefoxitin, ciprofloxacin, fusidic acid, kanamycin, gentamicin, metronidazole, nitrofurantoin, norfloxacin, streptomycin, sulphadiazine, teicoplanin, trimethoprim/sulphamethoxazole, and vancomycin (Danielsen and Wind, 2003). Although homofermentative lactobacilli are sensitive to vancomycin, many strains of *Lactobacillus plantarum, Lactobacillus casei, Lactobacillus salivarius, Lactobacillus leishmannii* and *Lactobacillus acidophilus* are intrinsic resistant to the antibiotic, due to the presence of D-alanine-D-alanine ligase related enzymes (Elisha and Courvalin, 1995). In a recent study (Salminen et al., 2006) strains of *Lactobacillus* isolated from blood samples had low minimum inhibition concentration (MIC) values to imipenem, piperacillin–tazobactam, erythromycin and clindamycin, but revealed variable susceptibility to penicillins and cephalosporins. Lactobacilli are usually sensitive to penicillins (piperacillin and ampicillin) and β-lactamase inhibitors, but more resistant to oxacillin and cephalosporins (cefoxitin and ceftriaxone) due to cell wall synthesis inhibitors (Coppola et al., 2005). Changes in the cell wall impermeability are the main mechanism of resistance since species of this genus lack cytochrome-mediated electron transport (Condon, 1983). However, the cooperation of non-specific mechanisms, such as multidrug transporters (Putman et al., 2001) and defective cell wall autolytic systems (Kim et al., 1982) may also account for differences between strains. Most *Lactobacillus* spp. show a high level of resistance to glycopeptides (vancomycin and teicoplanin). Susceptibility to bacitracin may vary (Coppola et al., 2005; Katla et al., 2001). Lactobacilli are generally susceptible to antibiotics interfering with protein synthesis, such as chloramphenicol, erythromycin, clindamycin and tetracycline, and are more resistant to aminoglycosides (neomycin, kanamycin, streptomycin and gentamicin) (Charteris et al., 1998; Coppola et al., 2005; Zhou et al., 2005). Lactobacilli are in general resistant to most inhibitors of nucleic acid synthesis, including enoxacin, pefloxacin, norfloxacin, nalidixic acid, sulphamethoxazole, trimethoprim, co-trimoxazole and metronidazole (Charteris et al., 1998; Coppola et al., 2005). The antibiotic resistance of *L. plantarum* strains isolated from different niches is listed in Table 1.

Table 1. Resistance to antibiotics reported in some LAB

	Strains	Resistant to	References
Lactobacillus spp.	*L. plantarum*	nalidixic acid, sulpfamethoxazole, tobramycin, ciprofloxacin, compound sulphonamides, oxacillin, amikacin, streptomycin, metronidazole, vancomycin	Todorov and Dicks, 2008
	L. plantarum	ampicillin, augmentin, cefoxitin, cephalotoxin, oxacillin, vancomycin, teicoplanin, clindamycin, rifampicin, tetracycline, kanamycin, ciprofloxacin, nitrofurantoin, trimethoprim	Herreros et al., 2005
	L. plantarum	cloxacillin, vancomycin, gentamicin, kanamycin, neomycin, streptomycin, fusidic acid, nalidixic acid, polymyxin B	Zhou et al., 2005
	L. rhamnosus	cefixime, vancomycin, neomycin, enoxacin, pefloxacin, sulphamethoxazole/trimethoprim	Coppola et al., 2005
	L. rhamnosus	vancomycin, gentamicin, kanamycin, neomycin, streptomycin, fusidic acid, nalidixic acid, polymyxin B	Zhou et al., 2005
	L. rhamnosus GG	cloxacillin, vancomycin, gentamicin, kanamycin, neomycin, streptomycin, fusidic acid, nalidixic acid, polymyxin B	Zhou et al., 2005
	L. rhamnosus LA1	gentamicin, kanamycin, neomycin, streptomycin, fusidic acid, nalidixic acid, polymyxin B	Zhou et al., 2005
	L. reuteri	tetracycline, lincosamide, vancomycin	Kastner et al., 2006, Korhonen et al., 2007
	L. salivarius	vancomycin, tetracycline, kanamycin, streptomycin, clindamycin, tetracycline, erythromycin, trimethoprim, chloramphenicol	Korhonen et al., 2007
	L. agilis	vancomycin, tetracycline	Korhonen et al., 2007

Table 1. (Continued)

	Strains	Resistant to	References
	L. johnsonii	Trimethoprim, tetracycline	Korhonen et al., 2007
	L. gallinarum	Tetracycline	Korhonen et al., 2007
	L. acidophilus	penicillin G, cloxacillin, streptomycin, gentamycin, tetracycline, erythromycin, chloramphenicol	Herrero et al., 1996
	L. acidophilus	kanamycin, streptomycin, fusidic acid, nalidixic acid, polymyxin B	Zhou et al., 2005
	L. delbrueckii	vancomycin, chloramphenicol, tetracycline	Tomé et al., 2008
	L. curvatus	erythromycin, chloramphenicol, gentamicin	Tomé et al., 2008
	L. brevis	penicillin G, cloxacillin, streptomycin, gentamycin, tetracycline, erythromycin, chloramphenicol	Herrero et al., 1996
	L. brevis	ampicillin, cefoxitin, cephalotoxin, oxacillin, vancomycin, teicoplanin, cloramphenicol, clindamycin, rifampicin, tetracycline, kanamycin, ciprofloxacin, nitrofurantoin, trimethoprim	Herreros et al., 2005
	L. casei	penicillin G, cloxacillin, streptomycin, gentamycin, tetracycline, erythromycin, chloramphenicol	Herrero et al., 1996
	L. casei	ampicillin, augmentin, cefoxitin, cephalotoxin, oxacillin, vancomycin, teicoplanin, cloramphenicol, clindamycin, rifampicin, tetracycline, kanamycin, ciprofloxacin, nitrofurantoin, trimethoprim	Herreros et al., 2005
	L. coryniformis	sulfamethoxazole–trimethoprim, penicillin, ampicillin, nalidixic acid, vancomycin	Lara-Villoslada et al., 2007
	L. gasseri	vancomycin, penicillin, ampicillin, nalidixic acid	Lara-Villoslada et al., 2007
Leuconostoc spp.	*L. mesenteroides* subsp. *mesenteroides*	nalidixic acid, sulphamethoxazole, neomycin, tobramycin, ciprofloxacin, amikacin, streptomycin, metronidazole, vancomycin, sulphafurazole	Todorov & Dicks, 2008
	L. mesenteroides	ampicillin, augmentin, cefoxitin, cephalotoxin, oxacillin, vancomycin, teicoplanin, cloramphenicol, clindamycin, rifampicin, tetracycline, kanamycin, ciprofloxacin, nitrofurantoin, trimethoprim	Herreros et al., 2005

	Strains	Resistant to	References
	L. lactis	carbapenem antibiotics	Deye et al., 2003
Oenococcus spp.	*O. oeni*	glycopeptides, cefoxitin, metronidazole, nalidixic acid, gentamicin, kanamycin, streptomycin, nitrofurantoin, sulphadiazine, trimethoprim	Katla et al., 2001; Flórez et al., 2005, Ammor et al., 2007
	O. oeni	glycopeptide (vancomycin), aminoglycosides (streptomycin, gentamicin, and kanamycin), sulfamethoxazole, trimethoprim-sulfamethoxazole, ciprofloxacin, aminoglycosides, glycopeptides and sulfamethoxazole	Rojo-Bezares et al., 2006
Pediococcus spp.	*P. acidilactici*	vancomycin, teicoplanin, streptomycin, kanamycin, tetracycline, doxycycline, ciprofloxacin, sulphamethoxazole, trimethoprim-sulphamethoxazole	Swenson et al., 1990; Danielsen et al., 2007
	P. acidilactici	clindamycin, erythromycin, and streptomycin	O'Connor et al., 2007
	P. acidilactici	chloramphenicol, tetracycline	Tomé et al., 2008
Lactococcus spp.	*L. lactis* subsp. *lactis*	amikacin, ceftazidime, metronidazole, nalidixic acid, neomycin, oxacillin, streptomycin, sulphafurazole, sulphamethoxazole, sulphonamides, tetracycline, tobramycin	Todorov et al., 2007
	L. lactis	tetracycline, clindamycin, erythromycin, macrolide, lincosamide, chloramphenicol, streptogramin B	Walther et al., 2008
	L. lactis	ampicillin, augmentin, cefoxitin, cephalotoxin, oxacillin, vancomycin, teicoplanin, cloramphenicol, clindamycin, rifampicin, tetracycline, kanamycin, ciprofloxacin, nitrofurantoin, trimethoprim.	Herreros et al., 2005
	L. garvieae	Clindamycin, tetracycline, streptomycin, quinupristin–dalfopristin, gentamicin, amikacin	Walther et al., 2008
	L. lactis subsp. *lactis*	rifampicin, streptomycin, spectinomycin	Kojic et al., 2008
Streptococcus spp.	*S. thermophilus*	gentamicin, kanamycin, and streptomycin), trimethoprim and sulphadiazine	Aslim and Beyatli, 2004; Katla et al., 2001; Temmerman et al., 2003.
	S. galloliticum subsp. *macedonicum*	streptomycin, penicillin G, vancomycin	Personal data

Table 1. (Continued)

	Strains	Resistant to	References
Enterococcus spp.	*E. faecium*	nalidixic acid, sulpfamethoxazole, tobramycin, cefuroxime, cefotaxime, compound sulphonamides, oxacillin, cefepime, ceftazidime, ceftriaxone, streptomycin, metronidazole, sulphafurazole	Todorov and Dicks, 2008
	E. faecium	tetracycline, erythromycin, gentamicin, vancomicin	Gomes et al., 2008
	E. faecium	chloramphenicol	Tomé et al., 2008
	E. faecalis	tetracycline, erythromycin, gentamicin, vancomicin	Gomes et al., 2008
	E. italicus	trimethoprim, rifampicin, tetracycline	Fortina et al., 2008

Herreros et al. (2005) observed amongst *L. plantarum* isolates 100% resistance to ampicillin, augmentin, cefoxitin, oxacillin, vancomycin, tetracycline, kanamycin, ciprofloxacin, nitrofurantoin, trimethoprim and teicoplanin, and 50% resistance to cephalotoxin, clindamycin and rifampicin. All strains tested were sensitive to cloranphenicol. In the same study, *Lactobacillus brevis* isolates were 100% resistant to cefoxitin, cephalotoxin, oxacillin, vancomycin, teicoplanin, rifampicin, kanamycin, ciprofloxacin, nitrofurantoin and trimethoprim, 50% were resistant to ampicillin, chloramphenicol and clindamycin, and all were sensitive to augmentin and tetracycline. For *Lactobacillus casei*, all of the tested isolates were resistant to ampicillin, cefoxitin, cephalotoxin, oxacillin, vancomycin, teicoplanin, nitrofurantoin, trimethoprim and cloramphenicol, 66% to augmentin, tetracycline, ciprofloxacin, and 33% to clindamycin, rifampicin and kanamycin (Herreros et al., 2005). Tetracycline resistance was recorded for several strains of *L. plantarum* isolated from raw milk soft cheeses (Teuber, 1999). *Lactobacillus rhamnosus* isolates from Parmigiano Reggiano cheese were resistant to six antibiotics, i.e. cefixime, vancomycin, neomycin, enoxacin, pefloxacin and sulphamethoxazole plus trimethoprim (Coppola et al., 2005). Kastener et al. (2006) reported a tetracyline resistance gene *tet*(W), located on a plasmid in a probiotic strain of *Lactobacillus reuteri* (SD2112). The resistant gene *lnu*(A) (formerly *lin*A) in *L. reuteri* SD2112, related with lincosamide, were recently described (Kastner et al., 2006). A survey on Norwegian yoghurt, sour cream, fermented milk and cheese yielded only one out of 189 isolates resistant to antibiotics. The isolate, identified as a *Lactobacillus* sp. revealed high-level resistance to streptomycin (Katla et al., 2001).

L. plantarum, L. acidophilus, Lactobacillus brevis and *L. casei* isolated from 'home-made' Spanish cheese (Serena, Gamonedo and Cabrales) revealed resistance to penicillin G, cloxacillin, streptomycin, gentamycin, tetracycline, erythromycin and chloramphenicol (Herrero et al., 1996). Tomé et al. (2008) reported two *Lactobacillus delbrueckii* strains, isolated from smoked salmon, with resistance to vancomycin and chloramphenicol. The same authors also described a strain of *Lactobacillus curvatus* resistant to erythromycin, tetracycline, gentamicin and chloramphenicol and a strain of *Pediococcus acidilactici* resistant to chloramphenicol and tetracycline.

All *L. reuteri, L. salivarius* and *L. agilis* isolates from fecal samples of weaning piglets were resistant to vancomycin, while strains of *Lactobacillus johnsonii* and *Lactobacillus gallinarum* were sensitive (Korhonen et al., 2007). Altogether 25 of the 67 isolates in the study of Korhonen et al. (2007) were resistant to trimethoprim, including two strains of *L. johnsonii*. Ciprofloxacin MIC values ≥ 16 μg/ml were recorded for *L. reuteri, Lactobacillus mucosae, L. johnsonii* and *L. gallinarum*. A great majority of the isolates were resistant to tetracycline. When ampicillin or gentamycin resistance was tested by Korhonen et al. (2007), all 67 isolates were sensitive. Only sporadic resistances were observed with erythromycin, clindamycin and streptomycin. Very high MICs were typical to isolates resistant to erythromycin and streptomycin. Only two isolates of *L. salivarius* were sensitive to kanamycin and were multi-resistant, showing simultaneous resistance to vancomycin, streptomycin, clindamycin and tetracycline (Korhonen et al., 2007).

L. coryniformis (Lara-Villoslada et al., 2007) showed intermediate resistance against sulfamethoxazole–trimethoprim, while the results obtained with the other strains of this species suggested full resistance. In the case of *Lactobacillus gasseri*, the assay showed only intermediate sensitivity to vancomycin, while the remaining *L. gasseri* strains seemed to be sensitive. Both strains were susceptible to β-lactam antibiotics such as penicillin or ampicillin, to Gram-positive spectrum antibiotics such as erythromycin and to broad-spectrum antibiotics such as chloramphenicol or tetracycline. In contrast, same strains were resistant to nalidixic acid, a well known antibiotic used in the treatment of Gram-negative bacteria. The most significant difference between *Lactobacillus coryniformis* and *L. gasseri* was the susceptibility to vancomycin, as all strains of *L. coryniformis* were resistant, while those belonging to *L. gasseri* were sensitive. Rojo-Bezares et al. (2006) tested susceptibility to 12 antibiotics in 75 unrelated LAB strains of wine origin (38 *L. plantarum*, three *Lactobacillus hilgardii*, two *Lactobacillus paracasei*, one *Lactobacillus* sp., 21 *Oenococcus oeni*, four *Pediococcus pentosaceus*, two *Pediococcus parvulus*, one *P. acidilactici*, and three *Leuconostoc mesenteroides*). The MIC of the different antibiotics that inhibited 50% of the strains of the *Lactobacillus, Leuconostoc* and *Pediococcus* genera were, respectively, as follows: Penicillin (2.0, ≤0.5, and ≤0.5 μg/ml), erythromycin (≤0.5 μg/ml), chloramphenicol (4.0 μg/ml), ciprofloxacin (64.0, 8.0, and 128.0 μg/ml), vancomycin (≥128.0 μg/ml), tetracycline (8.0, 2.0, and 8.0 μg/ml), streptomycin (256.0, 32.0, and 512.0 μg/ml), gentamycin (64.0, 4.0, and 128.0 μg/ml), kanamycin (256.0, 64.0, and 512.0 μg/ml), sulfamethoxazole (≥1024.0 μg/ml), and trimethoprim (16.0 μg/ml). All 21 strains of *O. oeni* showed susceptibility to erythromycin, tetracycline, rifampicin and chloramphenicol, and exhibited resistance to aminoglycosides, vancomycin, sulfamethoxazole and trimethoprim, that could represent intrinsic resistance. Differences were observed amongst the *O. oeni* strains with respect to penicillin or ciprofloxacin susceptibility. *L. plantarum, L. hilgardii* and *Pediococcus* strains showed high MIC values for ciprofloxacin (MIC ≥ 64.0 μg/ml). The other tested species (*L. paracasei, Lactobacillus* sp. and *L. mesenteroides*) presented a lower MIC range (≤ 2.0 – 8.0 μg/ml). As expected, all the analyzed *Lactobacillus, Leuconostoc* and *Pediococcus* strains showed high vancomycin MIC (≥ 128.0 μg/ml), due to the known intrinsic resistance to glycopeptides of these bacteria (Elisha and Courvalin, 1995; Perichon and Courvalin, 2000), although some lactobacilli do not present this type of intrinsic resistance. The MIC range of tetracycline ranged from 1.0 to $\geq$ 128.0 μg/ml in *L. plantarum* (MIC$_{50}$ of 8.0 μg/ml) and from $\leq$ 0.5 to 32.0 μg/ml in the other LAB species (MIC$_{50}$ of 8.0 μg/ml).

Regarding aminoglycosides (streptomycin, gentamicin and kanamycin), MIC values detected in wine isolates of *L. plantarum*, *L. hilgardii*, *L. paracasei*, *Lactobacillus* sp., *O. oeni*, *P. pentosaceus*, *P parvulus*, *P. acidilactici*, and *L. mesenteroides* were in general very high. A similar observation was reported by Elkins and Mullis (2004) in which lactobacilli show aminoglycoside intrinsic resistance due to membrane impermeability, probably complemented by potential efflux mechanisms. In general, *L. plantarum* and pediococci showed higher MICs for aminoglycosides than the other genera and species (Rojo-Bezares et al., 2006). All LAB strains (Rojo-Bezares et al., 2006) showed high resistance to sulfamethoxazole (MIC $\geq$ 1024.0 μg/ml), similar to the results obtained by others (Charteris et al., 1998; Sidhu et al., 2001a,b) and this fact could reflect intrinsic resistance for this antibiotic. The MIC$_{50}$ of trimethoprim in a study by Rojo-Bezares et al. (2006) was 16.0 μg/ml. The most resistant species to the tested antibiotics in same study were *L. plantarum* and *P. pentosaceus*. With few exceptions, *Lactobacillus* strains showed high MIC values for aminoglycosides (MIC$_{50}$ of streptomycin and gentamicin was 256.0 μg/ml and 64.0 μg/ml, respectively0 and for ciprofloxacin (MIC$_{50}$ of 64 μg/ml], as previously reported (Elkins and Mullis, 2004). Glycopeptide, aminoglycoside and sulfamethoxazole resistance has been formerly described in LAB species (Elisha and Courvalin, 1995; Elkins and Mullis, 2004; Mathur and Singh, 2005), and in all cases it has been associated with their natural and intrinsic resistance, probably due to cell wall structure and membrane impermeability, complemented in some cases by potential efflux mechanisms (Elkins and Mullis, 2004). Results of Zhou et al. (2005) showed that *Lactobacillus* spp. were susceptible to β-lactam antibiotics (penicillin, ampicillin, and cephalothin), Gram-positive spectrum antibiotics (erythromycin and novobiocin) and broad-spectrum antibiotics (chloramphenicol, rifampin, spectinomycin and tetracycline). Olukoya et al. (1993) reported that 80% of *Lactobacillus* strains they tested were resistant to cloxacillin. Similarly, Zhou et al. (2005) found that cloxacillin was much less effective than the other β-lactams, with only one (*L. rhamnosus*) out of 10 strains tested being sensitive. Conversely, almost all of the 10 strains tested by Zhou et al. (2005) were resistant to Gram-negative spectrum antibiotics (fusidic acid, nalidixic acid and polymyxin B) and aminoglycosides (gentamycin, kanamycin, neomycin, and streptomycin). Among antibiotic resistances, vancomycin resistance is of major concern, as it is one of the last antibiotics broadly efficacious against clinical infections caused by multidrug-resistant pathogens (Johnson et al., 1990; Nicas et al., 1989; Woodford et al., 1995). Some LAB however, including strains of *L. casei*, *L. rhamnosus*, *L. plantarum*, *Pediococcous* spp. and *Leuconostoc* spp., are resistant to vancomycin. Such resistance is usually intrinsic, that is, chromosomally encoded and not transmissible (Handwerger et al., 1994; Klein et al., 1998; Ruoff et al., 1988; Swenson et al., 1990). Zhou et al. (2005) reported that all three *L. rhamnosus* strains (including the well known *L. rhamnosus* GG), as well as *L. plantarum* HN045, were resistant to vancomycin.

Transfer of vancomycin resistance from *Lactobacillus* spp. to other bacteria has not been reported in studies of Leclercq et al. (1988) and Quintiliani et al. (1993). However, in enterococci, vancomycin resistance is usually plasmid-encoded and transmissible (Leclercq et al., 1988; Quintiliani et al., 1993). Testing of *L. rhamnosus* HN001 for the presence of the enterococcal *van*A and *van*B genes by PCR using the primers VANA-36F, VANA-992R, VANB-23F and VANB-1016R (Klein et al., 2000) yielded negative results (Zhou et al., 2005). A similar study on *L. rhamnosus* GG yielded the same results (Tynkkynen et al., 1998; Klein et al., 2000). In lactobacilli, not all antibiotic resistances are intrinsic. Some may be plasmid-encoded (Ahn et al., 1992; Fons et al., 1997; Ishiwa and Iwata, 1980; Tannock et al., 1994; Wang and Lee, 1997).

From a total of seven different species included in the genus *Lactococcus*, only two subspecies (*Lactococcus lactis* subsp. *lactis* and *Lactococcus lactis* subsp. *cremoris*) are of industrial importance (Carr et al., 2002). *L. lactis* subsp. *lactis* is usually susceptible to macrolides, bacitracin, erythromycin, lincomycin, novobiocin, teicoplanin and vancomycin, broad-spectrum antibiotics such as rifampicin, spectinomycin and chloramphenicol, and β-lactams such as penicillin, ampicillin, amoxicillin, piperacillin, ticarcillin and imipenem. Susceptibility to tetracycline, cephalothin, nitrofurantoin and cefotetan is variable (Ammor et al., 2007). Most lactococcal species are resistant to metronidazole, cefoxitin, trimethoprim, Gram-negative spectrum antibiotics including polymyxin B, nalidixic acid and fusidic acid, and the aminoglycosides gentamicin and kanamycin (Flórez et al., 2005; Herrero et al., 1996; Temmerman et al., 2003). *L. lactis* subsp. *lactis* HV219, isolated from human vagina and a potential probiotic, was resistant to amikacin, ceftazidime, metronidazole, nalidixic acid, neomycin, oxacillin, streptomycin, sulphafurazole, sulphamethoxazole, sulphonamides, tetracycline and tobramycin (Todorov et al., 2007). A strain of *L. lactis* subsp. *lactis* described as a bacteriocin producer was found to be resistant to rifampicin, streptomycin and spectinomycin (Kojic et al., 2008). While *L. lactis* subsp. *lactis* is non-pathogenic and used as starter culture for the production of dairy products, *Lactococcus garvieae* has emerged as an animal pathogen (Teuber, 1995). The species causes mastitis in cows and is a fish pathogen (Devriese et al., 1999; Eyngor et al., 2004; Pitkälä et al., 2004). *L. garvieae* has also been associated with human infections such as septicemia, osteomyelitis and endocarditis in immunocompromised patients (James et al., 2000; Mofredj et al., 2000). In *L. lactis* subsp. *lactis*, resistances to tetracycline, clindamycin, macrolide, lincosamide, streptogramin B, chloramphenicol and erythromycin were reported (Walther et al., 2008). All *L. garvieae* isolates studied by Walther et al. (2008) displayed resistance to clindamycin (> 8.0 mg/ml) which has been described to be intrinsic to this species and proposed to be a selective criterion to distinguish between *L. garvieae* and *L. lactis* subsp. *lactis* (Elliott and Facklam, 1996). In the same study (Walther et al., 2008), 14 isolates of *L. garvieae* displayed resistance to tetracycline and contained the *tet*(M) or *tet*(S) gene. Resistances to streptomycin and decreased susceptibility to quinupristin–dalfopristin were also found. The two *L. garvieae* strains (CWM1003 and CWM1004) which displayed resistance to streptomycin showed simultaneously decreased susceptibility to gentamicin (4.0 mg/ml) and amikacin (32.0 mg/ ml) (Walther et al., 2008).

Herreros et al. (2005) tested 18 LAB isolated from Armada cheese for antibiotic susceptibility. No strain was totally susceptible to all antibiotics and multiple resistance to most antibiotics was observed (Herreros et al., 2005). This is in accordance with various reports indicating that LAB are normally resistant to the principal types of antibiotics, such as β-lactam, cephalosporins, aminoglycosides, quinolone, imidazole, nitrofurantoin and fluoroquinolines (Halami et al., 2000). Herreros et al. (2005) observed that from nine tested *L. lactis* subsp. *lactis* isolates, three were resistant to ampicillin and tetracycline, four to augmentin and cephaotoxin, five to cefoxitin, vancomycin and clindamycin, six to teicoplanin, cloranphenicol, kanamycin and ciprofloxacin, seven to rifampicin, eight to nitrofurantoin and oxacillin, and nine to trimethoprim.

Not much is known about the antibiotic susceptibility of *S. thermophilus*, apart from a few studies that have shown that some strains are sensitive to chloramphenicol, tetracycline, erythromycin, cephalothin, quinupristin/dalfopristin and ciprofloxacin. The species shows moderate to high resistance to aminoglycosides (gentamicin, kanamycin, and streptomycin), trimethoprim and sulphadiazine (Aslim and Beyatli, 2004; Katla et al., 2001; Temmerman et al., 2003). Variable susceptibility to penicillin G, ampicillin and vancomycin has been reported (Aslim and Beyatli, 2004; Katla et al., 2001; Temmerman et al., 2003). Resistance to penicillin G, ampicillin and vancomycin is a problem, as consumption of live *S. termophilus* via yoghurt is increasing and there is a potential for transfer of this resistance to pathogenic bacteria in the human gastrointestinal tract. *Streptococcus galloliticum* subsp. *macedonicum* exhibits resistance to streptomycin, penicillin G and vancomycin (personal data), similarly to the resistance reported for *Streptococcus termophilus* (Aslim and Beyatli, 2004; Katla et al., 2001; Temmerman et al., 2003). The strain of *S. macedonicus* studied by Lombardi et al. (2004) was not resistant to cefalotine, cefuroxime, clindamycin, co-trimoxazol (trimethoprim+sulfametoxazol), erythromycin, gentamicin, penicillin G, tetracycline or vancomycin.

The absence of antibiotic resistance can be considered a positive trait for bacteria used in food production. A total of 64 strains of *S. thermophilus* were studied by Tosi et al. (2007) for susceptibility to erythromycin, clindamycin, streptomycin, gentamicin, tetracycline and ampicillin. Most strains displayed low MICs to erythromycin (0.25 to 1.0 μg/ml) and tetracycline (0.125 to 1.0 μg/ml). However, four strains were able to grow at 256.0 μg/ml erythromycin. These strains also exhibited atypical resistance to tetracycline with MICs ranging from 16.0 to 32.0 μg/ml. An additional four strains were resistant to the same level of tetracycline, but were susceptible to erythromycin. The MIC values for streptomycin ranged from 4.0 to 32.0 μg/ml, except for one strain being resistant to 128.0 μg/ml. One of the erythromycin resistant strains was also resistant to clindamycin (MIC > 256.0 μg/ml). All other examined strains showed clindamycin MICs between 0.03 and 0.125 μg/ml. No gentamicin or ampicillin resistant strains were observed as MICs ranged from 2.0 to 16.0 μg/ml and from 0.03 to 0.5 μg/ml for gentamicin and ampicillin, respectively.

Limited information has been published on the antibiotic susceptibility of *Pediococcus* spp. Penicillin G, imipenem, gentamicin, netilmicin, erythromycin, clindamycin, rifampin, chloramphenicol, daptomycin and ramoplanin are usually active against *Pediococcus* spp. (Danielsen et al., 2007; Swenson et al., 1990; Tankovic et al., 1993; Temmerman et al., 2003; Zarazaga et al., 1999), although susceptibility levels are species dependent. On the contrary, pediococci are intrinsically resistant to glycopeptides (vancomycin and teicoplanin) and to streptomycin, kanamycin, tetracycline (especially *P. acidilactici*), doxycycline, ciprofloxacin, sulphamethoxazole and trimethoprim-sulphamethoxazole (Table 1) (Swenson et al., 1990; Danielsen et al., 2007).

Some *Pediococcus* strains are resistant to all β-lactams, aminoglycosides, macrolides, tetracyclines and quinolones (Tankovic et al., 1993; Temmerman et al., 2003). *P. acidilactici* NCIMB 6990 (producer of pediocin AcH) is resistant to clindamycin, erythromycin and streptomycin. Genes encoding resistance are located on the plasmid harbouring the bacteriocin operon (O'Conner et al., 2007). Zarazaga et al. (1999) tested ten strains of *P. pentosaceus* and two strains of *P. acidilactici* for susceptibility to 13 antimicrobial agents. One strain was resistant to macrolides, but the mechanism of resistance could not be elucidated. Tankovic et al. (1993) determined the MIC of 25 strains of *P. acidilactici* and nine strains of *P. pentosaceus* and observed that only one strain was resistant to erythromycin while all strains were resistant to tetracycline. Erythromycin resistance was related to the plasmid associated with an erythromycin resistance methylase B [*erm*(B)] gene, while no tetracycline resistance gene could be detected (Tankovic et al., 1993).

Swenson et al. (1990) studied 20 strains of *P. acidilactici* and three strains of *P. pentosaceus*. They found one *P. acidilactici* strain with resistance to erythromycin and clindamycin, which indicates that an *erm* gene was present. Another *P. acidilactici* strain had an erythromycin MIC of 4.0 μg/ml, which was higher than the other strains tested. The strain was susceptible to clindamycin. The tetracycline MICs ranged from 4.0 to 64.0 μg/ml, which suggests intrinsic resistance (Swenson et al., 1990).

Danielsen et al. (2007) observed variable results for antibiotic susceptibility to erythromycin, tetracycline and trovafloxacin in pediococci, depending on the time of incubation (from 1 do 6 days). It is possible that the antibiotics are not stable for that long or a building of resistence is involved. *P. damnosus* NCIMB 701835 and *P. parvulus* NCIMB 701834 did not grow on ISO-sensitest supplemented with horse blood, but when tested on MRS, the MICs were similar to the MICs obtained on ISO-sensitest supplemented with horse blood. The MIC for aminoglycosides was approximately tenfold higher when cells were grown on MRS. An inhibitory effect of MRS on aminoglycosides and increased MIC for certain antibiotics have been reported previously (Huys et al., 2002). *P. damnosus, P. parvulus* and *P. dextrinicus* were the most susceptible to aminoglycosides, while *P. acidilactici* and *P. pentosaceus* were the most resistant. *P. acidilactici* and *P. pentosaceus* appear to differ in susceptibility to erythromycin. (*P. acidilactici* has higher MICs than *P. pentosaceus*) and to trovafloxacin (*P. pentosaceus* has higher MICs than *P. acidilactici*). *P. acidilactici* NCIMB 6990 had an erythromycin MIC of ≥ 256.0 μg/ml and a synercid MIC of 24.0 μg/ml, due to the presence of an *erm*(B) gene (Danielsen et al., 2007).

Leuconostoc species (including *O. oeni*) are usually resistant to glycopeptides, cefoxitin, metronidazole, nalidixic acid, gentamicin, kanamycin, streptomycin, nitrofurantoin, sulphadiazine and trimethoprim and susceptible to rifampicin, chloramphenicol, erythromycin, clindamycin and tetracycline (Flórez et al., 2005; Swenson et al., 1990) (Table 1). Resistance to carbapenem has been reported for a strain of *Leuconostoc lactis* associated with human ventriculitis infection (Deye et al., 2003). A study on antibiotic resistance of LAB isolated from Armada cheese has shown a multiple resistance to most antibiotics (Herreros et al., 2005). Herreros et al. (2005) observed that 50% from tested *L. mesenteroides* was resistant to ampicillin, augmentin, cephalotoxin, clindamicin and rifampicin, and all were resistant to cefoxitin, oxacillin, vancomycin, teicoplanin, cloranphenicol, tetracycline, kanamycin, ciprofloxacin, nitrofurantoin and trimethoprim.

Antibiotic susceptibility of 21 strains of *O. oeni* (Rojo-Bezares et al., 2006) was studied by disk diffusion method, and also by agar dilution method in the case of the aminoglycosides. No growth inhibition was observed for any of the *O. oeni* strains when disks of glycopeptide (vancomycin), aminoglycosides (streptomycin, gentamycin, and kanamycin), sulfamethoxazole and trimethoprim-sulfamethoxazole were used, pointing absence of the related antibiotic resistance genes. On the other hand, growth inhibition was observed for all *O. oeni* strains when the disks of erythromycin, chloramphenicol, tetracycline, and rifampicin were used. For the nitrocefin test, no strain expressed β-lactamase activity. Results regarding ciprofloxacin were variable, as fifteen strains showed resistance and six were sensitive to the antibiotic. According to these results, *O. oeni* seems to have intrinsic resistance to aminoglycosides, glycopeptides and sulfamethoxazole, as is the case of lactobacilli, pediococci and *Leuconostoc* spp. (Mathur and Singh, 2005). *O. oeni* strains were uniformly susceptible to erythromycin, tetracycline, cloramphenicol and rifampicin (Rojo-Bezares et al., 2006).

Antibiotic resistance in genus *Enterococcus* is controversial. Enterococci have a long history of application in food production (Schillinger et al., 1996) due to their favorable metabolic activities (lipolysis, esterolysis, citrate utilization, etc.) contributing to the typical taste and flavor of fermented foods (Centeno et al., 1996; Giraffa and Carminati 1997; Manolopoulou et al., 2003). However some *Enterococcus* strains are human and animal pathogens. The control of enterococci in food processing has assumed a different importance in the recent years, as the conviction of the harmlessness of these bacteria has been partly changed by the increase of their incidence in nosocomial infections. Some of them were associated with important medical cases related with endocarditis, bacteremia, intra-abdominal and pelvic infections and infections in the urinary tract and central nervous system (Foulquié-Moreno et al., 2006). The presence of vancomycin-resistant enterococci (VRE), partly due to the use of avoparcin as feed additive in animal husbandry, represents a significant threat to public health, as glycopeptides are considered to be the last resource - drugs in the treatment of enterococcal infections. Moreover, VRE are frequently resistant to many standard antibiotics commonly used to treat these illnesses (Landman and Quale, 1997). Antibiotic resistance trends among *E. faecalis* and *E. faecium* have been extensively reviewed (Bonten et al., 2001; Cetinkaya et al., 2000;; Franz et al., 2003; Huycke et al., 1998; Klare et al., 2003). Specific cause for concern and a contributing factor to pathogenesis of enterococci is their antibiotic resistance to a large variety of antibiotics (Landman and Quale, 1997; Leclercq, 1997; Murray, 1990). It was shown that enterococci are normally intrinsically resistant to a large number of antibiotics. The resistance is mediated by genes located on the chromosome, in contrast to acquired resistance that is mediated by genes residing on plasmids or transposons (Clewell, 1990; Murray, 1990). Examples of intrinsic antibiotic resistance include resistance to cephalosporins, β-lactams, sulphonamides and low levels of clindamycin and aminoglycosides, while examples of acquired resistance include resistance to chloramphenicol, erythromycin, high levels of clindamycin and aminoglycosides, tetracycline, high levels of β-lactams, fluoroquinolones and glycopeptides, such as vancomycin (Leclercq, 1997; Murray, 1990). Vancomycin resistance is of special concern because this antibiotic is considered a last option for treatment of infections caused by multiple resistant enterococci Vancomycin resistant *Enterococcus* spp. in hospitals led to infections that could not be treated with conventional antibiotic therapy. Antibiotic resistance alone cannot explain the virulence of enterococci. The pathogenesis of most infections follows a common sequence of events involving colonization and adhesion to host tissues, invasion of the tissue and resistance to both nonspecific and specific defense mechanisms of the host. The pathogen must produce pathological changes either directly by toxin production or indirectly by inflammation (Johnson, 1994). In the past, enterococci were considered to possess subtle virulence traits that were not easily identified (Jett et al., 1994).

For applications of enterococci in foods, antibiotic resistance is of special concern because genetic determinants of resistance in these bacteria are generally located on conjugative plasmids or transposons, prone to genetic exchange (Hasman et al., 2005; Zanella et al., 2006). Multi-resistance has been more commonly reported for *E. faecalis* due to its notorious ability to acquire and transfer antibiotic-resistance genes (Çitak et al., 2004; McBride et al., 2007). Gomes et al. (2008) reported that the prevalence of antibiotic resistance was higher for *E. faecalis* compared to *E. faecium* isolates. In the same study (Gomes et al., 2008) *E. faecalis* showed resistance to tetracycline (31%), erythromycin (10%) and gentamicin (22.5%). Multi-resistance (gentamicin, erythromycin and tetracycline) was observed for three *E. faecalis* isolates. There were *E. faecium* isolates resistant to tetracycline (6.5%) and erythromycin (9%). Moreover, three *E. faecium* isolates were vancomycin-resistant (MIC 256.0 mg/ml) but sensitive to the other antibiotics tested. The MIC for all gentamicin-resistant isolates was 4500.0 mg/ml (high-level resistance), whereas it ranged from 32.0 to 256.0 mg/ml for tetracycline and from 16.0 to 4256.0 mg/ml for erythromycin. The three vancomycin-resistant *E. faecium* isolates did not harbor the *van*A or *van*B genes and it was hypothesized that other resistance genes (*van*D, E or G) could be involved. The frequency found in the study of Gomes et al. (2008) for antibiotic resistance are lower than those previously reported by Çitak et al. (2004) who found 86.1% of the enterococci isolated from Turkish white cheese were vancomycin resistant, and by Harada et al. (2004) who reported an overall prevalence of enterococci resistant to tetracycline in broiler chickens superior to 85%. However, Abriouel et al. (2008) reported an overall prevalence of antibiotic-resistant *E. faecium* in vegetables lower than reported in miscellaneous foods. The results presented here indicate that foods could not be ruled out as a potential source for spreading antibiotic-resistant strains. Sparo et al. (2008) studied the sensitivity of *E. faecium* strains, isolated from dry-fermented sausages, to ampicillin, tetracycline, chloramphenicol, vancomycin and teicoplamin. Resistance to high levels of the aminoglucosides gentamicin and streptomycin could be ruled out. No β-lactamase activity was detected for *E. faecalis* CECT7121 (Sparo et al., 2008). Tomé et al. (2008) reported resistance to chloramphenicol by a strain of *E. faecium* isolated from cold-smoked salmon, evaluated for its potential application as biopreservative.

The biotechnological and safety properties of the novel enterococcal species of dairy origin, *Enterococcus italicus*, were investigated by Fortina et al. (2008). The strains of the species showed technological characteristics related to their use as adjunct cultures in the production of artisanal cheeses. They were susceptible or poorly resistant to several clinical relevant antibiotics. All strains were susceptible to kanamycin and ampicillin. They were inhibited at the break-point level of chloramphenicol (MIC 8.0 µg/ml), gentamicin (MIC 512.0 µg/ml) and streptomycin (MIC 1024.0 µg/ml). A low resistance to vancomycin was observed (break-point 8.0 µg/ml). All strains were resistant to a high level of trimethoprim (ranging from 150.0 to 500.0 µg/ml) and rifampicin (ranging from 50.0 to 200.0 µg/ml). Regarding tetracycline resistance (Tcr), the response was variable within the species. Three strains showed a low level of resistance (20.0 µg/ml), whereas the remaining four isolates showed MIC values > 150.0 µg/ml. In general the low resistance rates detected in the new enterococcal species are remarkable. All strains were susceptible or poorly resistant to 6 antibiotics, comprising the clinical relevant antibiotics ampicillin, vancomycin and gentamicin and a low incidence of resistance towards tetracycline was observed. The strains showed a common resistance to rifampicin and trimethoprim; this fact suggests that these resistances could be intrinsic to the species. If further studies will provide that the genetic determinant caring resisatnce are not related with mobile genetic elements, the risk of horizontal genetic transfer of rifampicin and trimethoprin resistance to other organisms can be considered as minimal. β-Haemolysis, as well as gelatinase activity, was not observed in any of the tested strains (Fortina et al., 2008). Transfer of resisatnce to antimicrobial substances is an essential mechanism in LAB if they need to adapt and survive in specific environments. Among the resistance mechanisms, enzymatic inactivation of the antibiotics, restricted import of antibiotics, active export of antibiotics or target modifications may be better target point in the future research.

An overuse of antibiotics in the treatment and prophylaxis of bacterial infections might be the principal factor with regard to bacterial resistance to such medicines and explain the high resistance levels shown by the strains. In addition, other practices aiming increased production on farms may also favor the development of resistance among bacteria that infect animals (Lukášová and Šustáčková, 2003).

From raw milk, bacteria may be transferred into raw milk cheeses. Indeed, resistance to various antibiotics has been detected in strains of different species of LAB isolated from craft-made Spanish cheeses (Herrero et al., 1996). Thus, cheeses produced from raw milk or with starters resistant to antimicrobials may act as vectors of antibiotic resistant human pathogens.

Genetic Basis of Antibiotic Resistance in LAB

Application of antibiotics in human and veterinary medicine and farmers' practice has increased drastically over the last few decades. Uncontrolled application of antibiotics lead to the selection of drug resistant bacterial strains, which now requires research and development of new antibiotics. This could be based on modifications of already existing drugs, or the discovery of completely new generation antimicrobial agents, such as bacteriocins.

Scientific studies suggest that viable LAB, included as part of our diet, or used in combination with other antimicrobial agents, may be an answer to the control of several diseases. However, these living organisms may contain antibiotic resistance genes and act as vectors of these genes to pathogenic bacterial species. They can also be a bridge for interspecies transfer of such genes. The effect of uncontrolled application of probiotics may be similar to that achieved by the uncontrolled application of antibiotics in the last decades, leading to the development of multidrug resistant strains. It is important that scientists act responsibly and ethically, applying strict scientific criteria when developing new products.

Several genes encoding antibiotic resistance have been detected from genome studies. Some of these genes are located in the bacterial chromosome, but they may also be present on plasmid DNA. If present on plasmids, the genes are easily transfered to other cells by horizontal gene transfer. On the other hand, some researchers pointed out that antibiotic resistance genes located on the genome also need to be taken in consideration when the safety of a strain is evaluated. The dissemination of antibiotic resistance genes can reduce the therapeutic possibilities in infectious diseases. Given the presence of such genes in LAB and indirect evidence that these genes could be transferred along the food chain (Ahn et al., 1992; Gevers et al., 2003; Jacobsen et al., 2007; Morelli et al., 1988; Tannock, 1987; Teuber et al., 1999), it is important to look for the presence of transferable antibiotic resistance genes in LAB strains that are, or shall be used as, probiotics for human or animal consumption or as starter cultures for fermented food or animal feed.

The issue of antibiotic resistance was taken very seriously in the construction of an antibiotic sensitive derivative of a (probiotic) *L. reuteri* ATCC 55730 by selective removal or curing of the resistance plasmids (Vankerckhoven et al., 2008). The presence of potential transferable resistance genes in many LAB species is well established (Table 2). The nucleotide sequence identity of most determinants encountered in LAB to genes previously described in distinct bacterial groups suggests that resistance emerged in microorganisms other than LAB, to which they were somehow transferred via mobile genetic elements.

The antibiotic resistance genes give a better chance to species, including LAB to survive, and from an evolutionary point of view, they have a very positive role in their life cycle. From a human point of view these genes are undesirable. Lactobacilli are generally susceptible to antibiotics inhibiting the synthesis of proteins, such as chloramphenicol, erythromycin, clindamycin and tetracycline, and more resistant to aminoglycosides (neomycin, kanamycin, streptomycin and gentamicin) (Charteris et al., 1998; Coppola et al., 2005; Zhou et al., 2005). However, strains resistant to these antibiotic agents have been also identified (Charteris et al., 1998; Danielsen and Wind, 2003; Delgado et al., 2005; Flórez et al., 2005), and several genes providing such resistance have been studied; e.g., a chloramphenicol resistance gene (*cat*) has been detected in *L. reuteri* (Lin et al., 1996) and *L. plantarum* (Ahn et al., 1992); different erythromycin-resistance genes (*erm*) have been found in many species (Cataloluk and Gogebakan, 2004; Fons et al., 1997; Tannock et al., 1994) (Table 2) as well as a number of tetracycline resistance genes – *tet*(K, M, O, Q, S, W, 36) (Chopra and Roberts, 2001; Villedieu et al., 2003; Roberts, 2005; Torres et al., 2005; Huys et al., 2006) (Table 2). The *tet*(S) gene in *L. plantarum* probiotic strain CCUG 43738 is located on a plasmid of 14-kbp (Huys et al., 2006). Noteworthy is the genetic organization of *erm*(B) in *L. johnsonii* G41, which seems to have become inserted into the chromosome from a plasmid-encoded *erm*(B) locus of *E. faecalis* (Flórez et al., 2006). The presence of *tet*(W) (tetracycline) and lincosamide *lnu*(A) (lincosamide) resistance genes in the *L. reuteri* probiotic strain SD 2112 (Kastner et al., 2006) has also to be highlited.

Table 2. Detection of antibiotic resistance genes in species of LAB

Species	Antibiotic resistance genes	References
E. casseliflavus	*van*(A), *van*(C2), *van*(B)	Shaghaghi et al., 2007
E. faecalis	*tet*(M), *tet*(O), *tet*(S), *tet*(K), *tet*(L), *erm(*A), *erm*(B), *erm*(C), *mef*(A), *mef*(E); *msr*(A/B), *ere(*A). *ere*(B), *cat, van*(C), *van*(A), *van*(B), *van*(D), *van*(E), *van*(G)	Fines et al., 1999 Flórez et al., 2006 Gevers et al., 2003a Hummel et al., 2007 Huys et al., 2004 Jacobsen et al., 2007 Leclercq et al., 1989, 1992 Perichon et al., 1997
E. faecium	*van*(C), *van*(A), *van*(B), *van*(D), *van*(E), *van*(G), *tet*(M), *tet*(O), *tet*(S), *tet*(K), *tet*(L), *erm*(A), *erm*(B), *erm*(C), *mef*(A), *mef*(E); *msr*(A/B), *ere(*A). *ere*(B), *cat*	Fines et al., 1999 Gomes et al., 2008 Hummel et al., 2007 Leclercq et al., 1989, 1992 Perichon et al., 1997 Shaghaghi et al., 2007
E. gallinarum	*van*(C1), *van*(A), *van*(B)	Shaghaghi et al., 2007
E. italicus	*tet*(S), *tet*(L), *tet*(M) , *tet*(K)	Fortina et al., 2008 Hummel et al., 2007 Huys et al., 2004 Maietti et al., 2007
L. acidophilus	*aaa*(6')*Ie-aph*(2")*Ia, tet*(M), *erm*(B), *gyr*(A)	Catalouk and Gogebakan, 2004 Ouoba et al., 2008 Tenorino et al., 2001
L. alimentarius	*tet*(M)	Gevers et al., 2003
L. animalis	*erm*(B)	Martel et al., 2003
L. casei	*aph*(3')-III, *aad*(A), *aad*(E), *aad*(A), *tet*(M), *erm*(B)	Catalouk and Gogebakan, 2004 Ouoba et al., 2008
L. coryniformis	*van*A, *van*B	Lara-Villoslada et al., 2007
L. crispatus	*erm*(B), *tet*(M)	Strøman et al., 2003
L. curvatus	*tet*(M)	Gevers et al., 2003
L. fermentum	*erm*(B), *erm*(LF), *vat*(E-1), *tet*(M)	Cataloluk and Gogebakan, 2004 Fons et al., 1997 Gfeller et al., 2003
Lac. garvieae	*tet*(M), *tet*(S), *erm*(B), *mdt*(A)	Flórez et al., 2008a,b Teuber et al., 1999 Walther et al., 2008
L. gasseri	*tet*(M), *erm*(B), *van*(A), *van*(B)	Catalouk and Gogebakan, 2004 Lara-Villoslada et al., 2007
L. johnsonii	*erm*(B), *tet*(M), *erm*(B)	Catalouk and Gogebakan, 2004 Flórez et al., 2006 Martel et al., 2003
Species	Antibiotic resistance genes	References
L. lactis	*tet*(M), *tet*(S), *erm*(B), *mdt*(A), *catp*C223, *str,*	Flórez et al., 2008ab Perreten et al., 2001 Putman et al., 2001 Teuber et al., 1999 Walther et al., 2008

Species	Antibiotic resistance genes	References
L. lactis subsp. *lactis*	*tet*(S), *tet*(M), *mdt*(A), *cat*, *str*, *erm*(T)	Ammor et al., 2007 Chopra and Roberts, 2001 Perreten et al., 1997 Perreten et al., 2001 Raha et al., 2002
L. paracasei	*aph*(3')-III, *aad*A	Ouoba et al., 2008
L. paraplantarum	*gyr*(A), *tet*(S)	Ouoba et al., 2008
L. plantarum	*cat*, *tet*(S), *tet*(M), *aac*(6')-*aph*(2''), *ant*(6), *aph*(3')-IIIa, *erm*(B), *cat*-TC, *gyr*(A), *aad*(E)	Ahn et al., 1992 Catalouk and Gogebakan, 2004 Danielsen, 2002 Gevers et al., 2003 Huys et al., 2006 Ouoba et al., 2008 Rojo-Bezares et al., 2006
L. reuteri	*tet*(W), *tet*(S), *lnu*(A) (formerly *lin*A), *cat*, *aph*(3')-III, *aad*A, *aad*E, *erm*(B), *erm(T)*, *cat*-TC, *gyr*(A)	Axelsson et al., 1988 Kastner et al., 2006 Lin and Chung, 1999 Lin et al., 1996 Martel et al., 2003 Ouoba et al., 2008 Tannock et al., 1994
L. rhamnosus	*tet*(M), *erm*(B)	Catalouk and Gogebakan, 2004
L. sakei	*tet*(M)	Gevers et al., 2003
L. salivarius	*aaa*(6')-*aph*(2''), *erm*(B)	Martel et al., 2003 Tenorio et al., 2001
L. delbrueckii subsp. *bulgaricus*	*bac*(R), *van*(R), *nov*(R), *kan*(R), *spi*(R), *str*(R)	Rivals et al., 2007
Lactobacillus spp.	*tet*(M), *tet*(O), *erm*(T), *tet*(K), *tet*(M), *tet*(S), *tet*(W), *tet*(36)	Chopra and Roberts, 2001 Danielsen, 2002 Roberts, 2005 Villedieu et al., 2003 Whitehead and Cotta, 2001
Leuc. citreum	*tet*(S)	Gevers, 2002
O. oeni	*aph*(3')-IIIa, *aac*(6')-*aph*(2'')	Rojo-Bezares et al., 2006
P. acidilactici	*erm*(B), *aaa*(6')-*aph*(2''), *erm*(AM), *aad*(E)	Danielsen et al., 2007 O'Connor et al., 2007 Rojo-Bezares et al., 2006 Tankovic et al., 1993 Tenorio et al., 2001 Zarazaga et al., 1999
P. parvulus	*tet*(L), *aac*(6')-*aph*(2''), *ant*(6), *aac*(60)Ie-*aph*(200)Ia	Rojo-Bezares et al., 2006 Tenorio et al., 2001
S. thermophilus	*erm*(B)	Aslim and Beyatli, 2004

aac=aminoglycoside acetyltransferase; *ant* = aminoglicoside adenyllyltransferase; *aph* = aminoglycoside phosphotransferase; *aph*(3')-III, *aad*, *aad* = aminoglycoside; *bac* = bacitracin resistance gene; *cat* = chloramphenicol acetyltransferase; *erm* = erythromycin resistance gene; *kan* = kanamycin resistance gene; *lmr*P = secondary multidrug transporter; *lnu* = lincosamide resisatnce gene; *mdt* = multiple drug transporter; *nov* = novobiocin resistance gene; *spi* = spiramycin resistance gene; *str* = streptomycin resistance gene; *str* = streptomycin resistant gene; *tet* = tetracycline resistence gene; *van* = vancomycin resistance gene; *vat* = streptogramin A acetyltransferase

Lactobacilli are usually resistant to most inhibitors of nucleic acid synthesis, including enoxacin, pefloxacin, norfloxacin nalidixic acid, sulphamethoxazole, trimethoprim, co-trimoxazole and metronidazole (Charteris et al., 1998; Coppola et al., 2005). Most resistances to these antibiotics seem to be intrinsic. As observed with the lactobacilli, single strains of *L. lactis* have been shown to be resistant to chloramphenicol, clindamycin, streptomycin, erythromycin and tetracycline (Flórez et al., 2005; Raha et al., 2002; Temmerman et al., 2003).

Resistance determinants to all these antimicrobial agents have been found in lactococci (Perreten et al., 1997ab; Raha et al., 2002). *L. lactis* subsp. *lactis* K214, isolated from raw-milk soft cheese, was found to contain at least three different plasmid-encoded antibiotic resistance determinants (for tetracycline [*tet*(S)], chloramphenicol and streptomycin) (Perreten et al., 1997ab). And other tetracycline resistant strains have been shown to harbor the *tet*(M) (Chopra and Roberts, 2001). In addition to the dedicated resistance mechanisms mentioned, general detoxification systems in *L. lactis* subsp. *lactis* may contribute to enhancing the MICs of otherwise susceptible lactococcal strains.

A secondary multidrug transporter *Lmr*P has been implicated in the resistance of *L. lactis* to a broad range of clinically important antibiotics (Putman et al., 2001). Cells expressing *Lmr*P showed increased resistance to lincosamide, streptogramin, tetracycline and the 14- and 15-C member lactone ring macrolides. Further, Perreten et al. (2001) discovered an efflux gene, *mdt*(A), in *L. lactis* subsp. *lactis* K214, which confers increased resistance to macrolides, lincosamides, streptogramins and tetracyclines in *L. lactis* and *E. coli*.

A relationship has been reported between antibiotic resistance and the possession of plasmids in *S. thermophilus* species (Aslim and Beyatli, 2004). Recently, four out of 70 *S. thermophilus* strains were found to be resistant to erythromycin due to the presence of a rRNA methylase [*erm*(B)] gene (Aslim and Beyatli, 2004).

Rivals et al. (2007) studied the acquisition of different antibiotic resistances and the corresponding physiological responses to cold stress of *L. delbrueckii* subsp. *bulgaricus* strain CFL1. In this study, six resistant mutants were spontaneously obtained and studied depending on the target of the antibiotic: (i) bacitracin and vancomycin (*bac*R, *van*R, wall synthesis), (ii) novobiocin (*nov*R, DNA replication), and (iii) kanamycin, spiramycin, streptomycin (*kan*R, *spi*R, *str*R, RNA translation). The mutations modified growth and cold stress response at three different physiological levels: (i) *van*R and *spi*R mutants showed significant lower growth rates compared to the wild type strain; (ii) *van*R and *bac*R mutants displayed a slightly higher resistance to freezing-thawing challenge whereas *str*R and *spi*R mutants were more sensitive compared to the wild type; (iii) the recovery of acidification activity after freezing and during frozen storage was improved by considering the *nov*R strain, but not with the *van*R and *spi*R mutants. Thus, acquisition of some antibiotic resistance by spontaneous mutation led to modification on the cold stress response. The hypothesis formulated by authors of a unique cellular thermostat is discussed regarding the diversity of the tested antibiotics (Rivals et al., 2007).

The 10 877 bp plasmid pMD5057 caring the tetracycline resistance from *L. plantarum* 5057 was sequenced. The replication region found on this plasmid was homologus to other plasmids isolated from LAB while the tetracycline resistance region [containing (*tet*(M) gene] had high homology to sequences obtained from *Clostridium perfringens* and *S. aureus*

(Danielsen, 2002). A *Lactobacillus* IS-element was found within the tetracycline resistant region. The same plasmid was found to contain three open reading frames with unknown functions (Danielsen, 2002). According to Danielsen (2002) this was the first report on the sequence of the antibiotic resistance plasmid from *L. plantarum*. The question regarding this plasmid and its tetracycline resistance gene is if this gene was transferred to *L. plantarum* from *C. perfringens* or *S. aureus* and how it can not be in similar risk for transfer or other antibiotic resistance genes in the similar way.

Lactobacillus spp. isolated from fermented dry sausages have been reported to harbor *tet*(M), a tetracycline resistance gene (Gevers et al., 2003b).

Antibiotic resistance genes were studied in several strains isolated from wine (*L. plantarum*, *L. hilgardii*, *L. paracasei*, *Lactobacillus* sp, *O. oeni*, *P. pentosaceus*, *P. parvulus*, *P. acidilactici*, and *L. mesenteroides*) by PCR and sequencing, and the following genes were detected: *erm*(B) (in one *P. acidilactici*), *tet*(M) (in one *L. plantarum*), *tet*(L) (in one *P. parvulus*), *aac*(6')-*aph*(2") (in four *L. plantarum*, one *P. parvulus*, one *P. pentosaceus* and two *O. oeni*), *ant*(6) (in one *L. plantarum*, and two *P. parvulus*), and *aph*(3')-IIIa (in one *L. plantarum* and one *O. oeni*). This was the first report, according to Rojo-Bezares et al. (2006), that *ant*(6), *aph* (3')-IIIa and *tet*(L) genes were found in *Lactobacillus* and *Pediococcus* strains and that antimicrobial resistance genes were reported in *O. oeni* strains (Rojo-Bezares et al., 2006).

Probiotic bacteria and starter cultures of *Lactobacillus* and *Weissella* of African and European origins were studied by Ouoba et al. (2008) and compared for their susceptibility to antimicrobials. The study included determination of MICs for 24 antimicrobials, detection of resistance genes by PCR reactions using specific primers and sequencing of positive amplicons. Variations were observed and high levels of intrinsic resistance were found among the tested species (Ouoba et al., 2008). Positive amplicons were obtained for resistance genes encoding aminoglycoside [*aph*(3')-III, *aad*A, *aad*E] and tetracycline [*tet*(S)] from isolates from Europe and macrolide [*erm*(B)] from an isolate from Africa. However, only the *erm*(B) gene found in *L. reuteri* L4:12002 from Africa contained a homologous sequence to previously published sequences. This gene could be transferred in vitro to enterococci. Higher prevalence of phenotypic resistance for aminoglycoside was found in isolates from Europe (Ouoba et al., 2008). The concern raised by this study is the fact that *L. reuteri* is well recommended probiotic species applied in several probiotic preparations all over the World.

For LAB data defining breakpoints for antimicrobials and data on prevalence of antimicrobial resistance are rare and (in some point) a bit controversial. These results of the difference in the methods applied and of the culture media used that can have an influence in the determination of the MICs. This fact points to the usefulness of the detection of antibiotic resistance genes as a gold standard in determination of the resistance profile of LAB.

Production of LAB fermented foods is a traditional process and these products have potential to be used as probiotic products, because of high levels of LAB with possible health beneficial effects (Lei et al., 2006). One important factor in the selection of probiotic bacteria is the investigation of the possibility of the bacteria to host and transfer resistance genes. According Ouoba et al. (2008) their study is are the first published on prevalence of antimicrobial resistant determinants in LAB isolated from African traditional foods. The susceptibility of the studied LAB by Ouoba et al. (2008) to antimicrobials as well as their ability to host and transfer resistance genes was variable according to the isolate and the antimicrobial. The reduced susceptibility towards trimethoprim, sulphamethoxazole and apramycin indicates intrinsic resistance to these antimicrobials. For quinolones, amino acids variations similar to those reported by Hummel et al. (2007) were observed in the QRDR amino acids sequences of the *gyr*A. However, none of the variation observed has been reported to be associated with increase in quinolones resistance (Hummel et al., 2007). High level resistance to quinolones in Gram-positive bacteria are linked to a substitution in the *gyr*A QRDR sequence of 83-ser to Arg or Glu-87 to either Gly or Lys (Petersen and Jensen, 2004). Such substitutions did not occur among the ciprofloxacin-resistant bacteria studied. However other variations in the QRDR of *par*C i.e. substitution of Ser-80 with Leu/Ileu could be responsible for high level resistance to quinolone (Petersen and Jensen, 2004). Variations observed at species level for the susceptibility to glycopeptides have been previously identified among LAB (Danielsen and Wind, 2003) and do not indicate an acquisition of antimicrobial resistance towards glycopeptides. The reduced susceptibility to the cephalosporin and cefpodoxime can be attributed to intrinsic resistance of the different species since none of these bacteria were resistant to penicillin (first generation β-lactam) (Ouoba et al., 2008).

The major financial and societal costs caused by the increas in the antibiotic resistance in pathogenic microorganisms are a well-known problem. The attenuation of this problem is complicated by commercial bacteria that may act as reservoirs for antibiotic resistance determinants found in pathogens (Levy and Marshall, 2004; Salyers and Shoemaker, 1996). This statement is supported by the fact that the same type of genes encoding resistance to, for example, tetracycline, erythromycin, chloramphenicol, streptomycin and streptogramin have been found in commercial lactococci and lactobacilli as well as in potentially pathogenic enterococci and pathogenic streptococci (Teuber, 1999). A very important similarity in resistance genes has also been observed for tetracycline-resistant in *L. plantarum*, *L. sakei* subsp. *sakei*, *L. sakei* subsp. *carnosum*, *L. alimentarium* and *L. curvatus*. It is important to point the closely genetic relation of these strains. All these strains have been isolated from Belgian fermented dry sausages (Gevers et al., 2000, 2003a). Partial sequencing of the tetracycline resistance genes detected in all the species revealed two sequence homology groups (SHGs) with 99.6% identity to *tet*(M) genes of *E. faecalis* and *Neisseria meningitidis* (SHG I) and of *S. aureus* (SHG II) (Gevers et al., 2003a; Huys et al., 2004).

A survey (Kastner et al., 2006) was carried out in Switzerland to determine the current antibiotic resistance situation of microbial food additives. Two hundred isolates of different species (*Lactobacillus* spp., *Staphylococcus* spp., *Bifidobacterium* spp., *Pediococcus* spp.) from 90 different sources were typed by molecular and other methods. They were screened for phenotypic resistances by disk diffusion method to 20 antibiotics. Twenty-seven isolates was showed resistance that are not related with intrinsing features of the respective genera were further analyzed by microarray hybridization as a tool to trace back phenotypic resistances to specific genetic determinants. Their presence was finally verified by PCR amplification or Southern hybridization. This study resulted in the detection of the tetracycline resistance gene *tet*(K) in five different *Staphylococcus* isolates used as starter cultures in meat preparations and the *tet*(W) in the probiotic cultures *Bifidobacterium lactis*

DSM 10140 and *L. reuteri* SD 2112 as detected on the plasmid. The lincosamide resistance *lnu*(A) was found in *L. reuteri* SD 2112 (Kastner et al., 2006).

The aminoglycoside resistance gene *aac*(60)Ie-*aph*(200)Ia has been reported in some *Pediococcus* species from animal and wine origin, including *P. pentosaceus* and *P. parvulus* (Tenorio et al., 2001). Genetic determinants for macrolides resistance [*erm*(AM) genes] have been analyzed in *P. acidilactici* strains (Tankovic et al., 1993; Zarazaga et al., 1999), and one of these genes was found to be encoded on a 46-kbp non-transferable plasmid (Tankovic et al., 1993). An *erm*(B) gene has been associated to a 11.6-kbp plasmid in a *P. acidilactici* strain (Danielsen et al., 2007). The complete nucleotide sequence of pEOC01, a plasmid (11 661 bp) from *P. acidilactici* NCIMB 6990 encoding resistance to clindamycin, erythromycin, and streptomycin was determined. The plasmid, which also replicates in *Lactococcus* and *Lactobacillus* species contains 16 putative open reading frames (ORFs), including regions annotated to encode replication, plasmid maintenance and multidrug resistance functions. Based on the analysis the plasmid replicates via a theta replicating mechanism closely related to those of many larger *Streptococcus* and *Enterococcus* plasmids. Interestingly, genes homologous to a toxin/antitoxin plasmid maintenance system are present and are highly similar to the omega–epsilon–zeta operon of *Streptococcus* plasmids. The plasmid contains two putative antibiotic resistance homologs, an *erm*(B) gene encoding erythromycin and clindamycin resistance, and a streptomycin resistance gene, *aad*(E). Of particular note is the *aad*(E) gene which holds 100% identity to an *aad*E gene found in *Campylobacter jejuni* plasmid but which probably originated from a Gram-positive source (O'Connor et al., 2007). This observation is significant since it provides evidence of recent horizontal transfer of streptomycin resistance from a lactic acid bacterium to a Gram-negative intestinal pathogen. This allow to infer a role for such plasmids for dissemination of antibiotic resistance genes possibly in the human gut (O'Connor et al., 2007).

Forty-one strains of *L. lactis* and 31 strains of *L. garvieae*, isolated from bovine milk, were tested for susceptibility to 17 antibiotics and screened for the presence of antibiotic resistance genes using microarray. Resistance to tetracycline, clindamycin, erythromycin, streptomycin, nitrofurantoin was found. The tetracycline-resistant *L. garvieae* and *L. lactis* harbored *tet*(M) and *tet*(S). It was observed that *L. lactis* resistant to clindamycin was simultaneously resistant to erythromycin and was harboring a *erm*(B) gene. The multidrug transporter *mdt*(A), originally described in *L. lactis*, was detected for the first time in *L. garvieae* and does not confer decreased susceptibility to erythromycin nor tetracycline in this species. *mdt*(A) of *L. garvieae* contains one mutation in each antiporter motif C, which is known to play an essential role in drug efflux antiporters. This suggests that the mutations found in the C-motifs of *mdt*(A) from *L. garvieae* may be responsible for susceptibility. The study revealed the presence of antibiotic resistance genes in non-pathogenic and pathogenic lactococci from bovine milk products, including a mutated transporter in *L. garvieae*. While the antibiotic resistance situation of *Lactococcus* isolated from milk is not well documented, resistant strains have been reported to be present in raw milk cheese (Teuber et al., 1999; Flórez et al., 2008ab). One of these strains, *L. lactis* K214, harbored a multidrug resistance plasmid pK214 which contains the tetracycline resistance gene *tet*(S), the chloramphenicol resistance acetyltransferase gene *catp*C223, the streptomycin adenylyl transferase gene *str* and the multidrug transporter gene *mdt*(A) (Perreten et al., 1997). *mdt*(A) was shown to confer resistance to macrolides, lincosamides, streptogramins and tetracycline in *L. lactis* (Perreten et al., 2001) and has not been detected in other species to date. Specific PCR and sequencing showed that a *tet*(M) gene was present in two tetracycline-resistant *L. lactis* strains isolated from raw milk, starter-free cheese. Hybridisation experiments using as a probe an internal segment of the gene obtained by PCR associated *tet*(M) with plasmids of around the same size (30 kbp) in both strains. Molecular analysis of the tetracycline resistance loci, including the upstream and downstream regions of the genes, showed them to be identical to one other and to the *tet*(M) encoded by the conjugative transposon Tn916. Amplification of Tn916-derived segments suggested that the transposon was complete in the two *L. lactis* strains. Further, curing of the tetracycline resistance was accompanied by a reduction in size of the plasmids comparable to that expected for Tn916. Tetracycline resistance could be transferred by conjugation to plasmid-free *Lactococcus* and *Enterococcus* strains. However, no plasmid DNA was detected among the transconjugants while both *tet*(M) and transposon-related sequences were amplified by PCR. This suggested that only the transposon was mobilized to the bacterial chromosome (Flórez et al., 2008).

Walther et al. (2008) studied *Lactococcus* species isolated from bovine milk and their antibiotic resistance with focus on the presence of *mdt*(A) gene – a mutated multidrug transporter in *L. garvieae* strains. All *L. garvieae* isolates displayed resistance to clindamycin (> 8 mg/ml) which has been described to be intrinsic to this species, and they proposed the detection of this characteristic to be used as a selective criterion to distinguish between *L. garvieae* and *L. lactis* (Elliott and Facklam, 1996). However, the presence of the MLSB resistance gene *erm*(B) in *L. lactis* shows that the use of clindamycin is no longer appropriate to differentiate between both species. Fourteen *L. garvieae* isolates displayed also resistance to tetracycline ($\geq$ 32 mg/ml) (45.2%) and contained the *tet*(M) or *tet*(S) genes. Resistances to streptomycin (> 64 mg/ml) (6.5%) and decreased susceptibility to quinupristin–dalfopristin (> 8 mg/ml) (9.7%) were also found. The two *L. garvieae* strains CWM1003 and CWM1004 which displayed resistance to streptomycin showed simultaneously decreased susceptibility to gentamicin (4 mg/ml) and amikacin (32 mg/ ml). The resistance mechanism for these drugs remained unknown (Walther et al., 2008).

Vancomycin resistance can be intrinsic (*van*C) or acquired (*van*A, *van*B, *van*D, *van*E, *van*G) (Leclercq et al., 1989; Leclecq et al., 1992; Perichon et al., 1997; Fines et al., 1999). The most frequent transferable vancomycin-resistant phenotypes are *van*A which are associated with an increased level of inducible vancomycin resistance and cross-resistance to teicoplanin, and *van*B which usually display variable levels of inducible resistance to vancomycin only (Cetinkaya et al., 2000).

There is special concern about the application of *E. faecium* as part of starter cultures used for preparation of several traditional fermented foods products in Mediterranean countries. In the study of Shaghaghi et al. (2007) weres evaluated Enterococcal isolates from Iran. All *E. gallinarum* isolates carried *van*C1 gene with 64 (65%) and 14 (14%) isolates concomitantly harboring either *van*A or *van*B gene, respectively. Some *E. casseliflavus* concomitantly harbored *van*A and *van*C2 or *van*B and *van*C2. Typing the total enterococci isolates with a high resolution biochemical fingerprinting method showed a high diversity (Di=0.91). Shaghaghi et al. (2007) have shown, by biochemical fingerprinting, the presence of highly diverse glycopeptide resistant *E. gallinarum* and *E. casseliflavus* that have captured *van*A and *van*B under natural conditions. According to Shaghaghi et al. (2007) this is the first report in that geographical region showing high frequency of antibiotic resistant enterococcal population in particular *E. gallinarum,* carrying assorted vancomycin resistance genes.

In the study of Maiettia et al. (2007) the antibiotic susceptibility and the incidence of virulence factors among 30 *E. italicus* isolates originating mainly from different Italian cheeses were tested. Although not all 30 isolates showed unique genotypes, PCR fingerprinting evidenced a notable genotypic diversity among the *E. italicus* collection under study. All isolates were susceptible to vancomycin, gentamicin, erythromycin, ampicillin, chloramphenicol and bacitracin. Five isolates corresponding to three unique genotypes exhibited phenotypic resistance to tetracycline with MICs ranging from 64 – 256 mg/ml. By PCR-based detection, the genetic basis of the TetR phenotype in these strains was linked to the *tet*(S) gene whereas detection of *tet*(L), *tet*(M) and the integrase element into of the Tn916/Tn1545 family of transposons were negative. Likewise, none of the strains appeared to contain any of the tested virulence genes [(*gel*(E), *asa*(I), *cpd*, *agg*, *cyl*(A), *cyl*(B), *cyl*(M), *ace* and *hyl*(Efm)]. The results of this study warrant further research on the environmental dissemination of TetR *E. italicus* and on the potential transferability of its *tet*(S) genes (Maiettia et al., 2007). *E. italicus* strains were associated with low virulence profiles, as verified by screening for the presence of 33 different genes encoding antibiotic resistance and known virulence factors in the genus *Enterococcus* (Fortuna et al., 2007). From the data obtained the presence of *E. italicus* strains in cheeses (Fortuna et al., 2007) and data reported by Maiettia et al. (2007) results in a low health risk and that within the species new safe adjunct cultures for the dairy industry could be found (Fortina et al., 2008).

Fortina et al. (2008) did a survey on biotechnological potential and safety of the novel *Enterococcus* spp. of dairy origin, *E. italicus*. The strains tested harbored an RP (ribosomal protection protein) *tet* gene, according to the resistance phenotype. However, while the majority of the enterococcal strains showed the presence of *tet*M gene (Huys et al., 2004; Hummel et al., 2007), in *E. italicus*, *tet*(S) seems the dominant *Tcr* determinant. In all cases *tet*(S) was associated with the *tet*(K) gene, encoding an efflux pump protein (EP); both RP and EP genes have been referred as important mechanisms of tetracycline resistance and have been described frequently associated in the same strain (Aarestrup et al., 2000; Del Campo et al., 2003). The 4 isolates (Fortina et al., 2008) for which a highest MIC was detected (150 μg/ml) also harbored the *tet*(M). The combined presence of these genes could explain the higher level of Tcr exhibited by the strains. In Several enterococci and streptococci from clinical and food origin the *tet*(M) gene detected was more frequently related to conjugative transposomes, particularly to members of the broad host range Tn916-Tn1545 conjugative transposom family (Clewell et al., 1995; Huys et al., 2004). Interestingly, the *tet*M positive *E. italicus* strains did not contain the int-Tn gene, indicating that these strains could use a different mechanism, other than conjugative transposition, for the dissemination of *tet*M genes. Although a high incidence of gentamicin-resistance has been shown among food enterococci and a chloramphenicol resistance is often associated with Tcr (Teuber et al., 1999; Franz et al., 2001; Hummel et al., 2007), *E. italicus* strains seem to be free of the respective determinants, according to the phenotypic data. The *E. italicus* isolates did not possess any of the *van* genes tested (Fortina et al., 2008).

The genetic determinants responsible for the resistance against tetracycline [*tet*(K), *tet*(L), *tet*(M), *tet*(O) and *tet*(S)], erythromycin (*erm*A,B,C; *mef*A,E; *msr*A/B; and *ere*A,B) and chloramphenicol (*cat*) of 38 antibiotic resistant *E. faecium* and *E. faecalis* strains from food were characterized (Hummel et al., 2007). In addition, the transferability of resistance genes was also assessed using filter mating assays. The *tet*(L) determinant was the most commonly detected among tetracycline-resistant enterococci (94% of the strains), followed by the *tet*(M), which occurred in 63.0% of the strains. *tet*(K) occurred in 56.0% of the resistant strains, while for *tet*(O) and *tet*(S) could not be detected. The integrase gene of the Tn916-1545 family of transposons was present in 81.3% of the tetracycline resistant strains, indicating that resistance genes might be transferable by transposons. All chloramphenicol-resistant strains carried a *cat* gene, and 81.8% of the erythromycin-resistant strains carried the *erm*B gene. Two (9.5%) of the 21 erythromycin-resistant strains, which did not contain *erm*A,B,C, *ere*A,B and *mph*A genes harbored the *msr*C gene encoding an erythromycin efflux pump, which was confirmed by sequencing the PCR amplicon. In addition, all *E. faecium* strains contained the *msr*C gene, but none of the *E. faecalis* strains. Transfer of the genetic determinants for antibiotic resistance could only be demonstrated in one filter mating experiment, where both *tet*(M) and *tet*(L) were transferred from *E. faecalis* FAIR-E 315 to the *E. faecalis* OG1X recipient strain. Results of Hummel et al. (2007) show the presence of various types of resistance genes as well as transposon integrase genes associated with transferable resistances in enterococci, indicating a potential for gene transfer in the food environment (Hummel et al., 2007).

The analysis of the probiotic strains *L. coryniformis* CECT5711 and *L. gasseri* CECT5714 for the presence of the *van*A and *van*B genes by PCR using specific primers gave negative results in both cases (Lara-Villoslada et al., 2007).

Mobile Genetic Elements – The Fundament of the Transfer of Antibiotic Resistance

Bacterial cells use a complex array of mechanisms to share and spread resistance determinants. The main mechanisms of horizontal transfer in bacteria in natural environments are believed to be conjugation and transduction via bacteriophages (Kleinschmidt et al., 1993). In conjugation, plasmids may be important in spreading of antibiotic resistance (Kleinschmidt et al., 1993; Grillot-Courvalin et al., 2002). Lactococci posses an indigenous conjugation system (Gasson and Fitzgard, 1994). Information regarding the lactobacilli and native conjugation system is limited. The transfer of resistance (plasmid and transposon mediated) between LAB and from LAB to other Gram-positive or Gram-negative bacteria has been reported. *Enterococcus* spp. are well known for conjugation (Clewell and Weaver, 1989). Enterococci may also be very good donors for antibiotic resistance gene transfer to lactiobacilli (Shrago and Dobrogosz, 1988) and other enterococci (Rice et al., 1998). Gevers et al. (2003b) reported the possibility for *in vitro* transfer of resistance to tetracycline between donor of *Lactobacillus* spp. and *E. faecalis* as receptor. Some of the isolates studied by Gevers et al. (2003b) transferred their resistance genes to *Lactococcus lactis* subsp. *lactis*.

When reporting data on antimicrobial resistance, one has to clearly distinguish between natural (intrinsic or inherent) and acquired resistance. Natural antibiotic resistance is in the majority of cases non-transferable and present in (nearly) all members of the WT (wild type) population of a given taxonomic group. In contrast, bacterial strains with acquired antibiotic resistances are characterized by MICs that are clearly higher than the normal MIC range of the WT population of a given taxonomic group. Acquired resistances result (A) from mutations or accumulation of mutations in the organism's own DNA that finally leads to resistance against the corresponding antibiotic or (B) from acquisition of transferable resistance genes from donors. Foreign DNA can be acquired by conjugation, transduction or transformation. Acquired antibiotic resistances due to the acquisition of exogenous DNA can potentially be transferred by plasmids or (conjugative) transposons to other bacterial species or genera. Acquired antibiotic resistance due to mutations of housekeeping chromosomal genes most probably represents a low risk of horizontal dissemination. Only few probiotics for human consumption or starter cultures of fermented food or feed products will be classified as resistant (''acquired or mutational''). The participants discussed methods to demonstrate horizontal gene transfer. It was concluded that transfer of acquired resistance genes may occur under proper experimental conditions, and that failure to demonstrate *in vitro* horizontal gene transfer does not exclude the risk of dissemination of genes. In other words, while negative transfer experiments do not provide evidence for the absence of transfer, standardized transfer methods would be helpful to estimate whether the probability for resistance transfer is low or high. In fact, there are no standardized methods to demonstrate transfer of resistance genes, and there are substantial inter- and intra-laboratory variations. On the other hand, several authors have recently shown that transfer of resistance genes occurs more frequently *in vivo* than *in vitro* (Jacobsen et al., 2007; Tannock, 1987). One possible approach for eliminating antibiotic resistance is selective removal or curing of plasmids coding for antibiotic resistance (Huys et al., 2006). It was concluded that this is an interesting approach for currently used probiotics with acquired transferable resistance genes. However, several participants did remark that the cured strain would phenotypically and genotypically be different from the parent strain, and that the impact of the genetic changes on the probiotic properties should be assessed. Consensus was reached among the participants that micro-organisms not belonging to the WT distributions of relevant antimicrobials should not be developed as future products for consumption by humans or animals without proper risk assessment. However, further research is needed on characterization of acquired resistance mechanisms and transferability of resistance genes and on methods for determining transferability. Ultimately, this research should generate data that can be used to establish risk assessment criteria. Besides being widespread commercial bacteria, lactococci have an important application as fermentation starter cultures for cheese manufacture. Several gene transfer mechanisms have been found in lactococci (Gasson, 1990), including an aggregation mediated high frequency conjugation system.

In the work of Lampkowska et al. (2008), the pAMβ1 plasmid (26.5 kb) served as a model for transfer of a mobile conjugative element between two lactococcal strains. The plasmid, which was originally isolated from *E. faecalis*, was chosen for the study due to its self-transmissibility and constitutive MLS resistance (Clewell et al., 1974). Moreover, pAMβ1 has already been shown to be transfered via conjugation to *Bacillus*, *Clostridium*,

Staphylococcus, *Enterococcus*, *Lactobacillus* and *Lactococcus* (Cocconcelli et al., 1985; Gasson and Davies, 1980; Hespell and Whitehead, 1991; Morelli et al., 1988; Sasaki et al., 1988; Shrago et al., 1986; Tannock, 1987; Vescovo et al., 1983). An important factor in risk assessment of antibiotic resistance genes is to test their ability to transfer. In the same study (Lampkowska et al., 2008) it was initiated the optimization and validation (in the inter-laboratory experiment) of a conjugation protocol for studing plasmid transfer between lactococcal species, and assessing the comparability of obtained results (Lampkowska et al., 2008). The ability of *L. reuteri* from Africa to transfer the erythromycin resistance gene *erm*(B) to closely related bacteria was investigated by conjugation by Ouoba et al. (2008).

Lactobacillus spp. isolated from fermented dry sausages have been reported able to harbor *tet*(M), a tetracycline resistance gene (Gevers et al., 2003b). The possibility for *in vivo* transfer of resistance to macrolide from *Lactobacillus* to enterococci has been documented by Jacobsen et al. (2007) indicating that *Lactobacillus* spp. can be a vector in the spread of antimicrobial resistance.

What is the chance to transferring antibiotic resistance genes to some pathogenic bacteria? In the developing world diarrhea is a major cause of morbidity and mortality of children (Bryce et al., 2005). Among the most well documented beneficial health effects of LAB are the shortening of periods of diarrhea (Rosenfeldt et al., 2002a,b). Progress is needed in the development of treatments that shorten, alleviate or even prevent diarrhea in the developing world. In addition to this, in an African setting there is a need for effective, acceptable, cheap and easily accessible products for prevention or treatment of diarrhea (Lei and Jakobsen, 2004).

Two wild-type strains of *L. plantarum* previously isolated from dry fermented sausages were analyzed for their ability to transfer antibiotic resistance plasmids in the gastrointestinal tract (Jacobsen et al., 2007). For this purpose, authors used gnotobiotic rats as an *in vivo* model. Rats were initially inoculated with the recipient *E. faecalis* JH2-2 at a concentration of 10^{10} CFU/ml. After a week, either of the two donors *L. plantarum* DG 522 (harbouring a *tet*(M)-containing plasmid of c. 40 kb) or *L. plantarum* DG 507 [harbouring a *tet*(M)-containing plasmid of c. 10 kb and an *erm*(B)-containing plasmid of c. 8.5 kb] was introduced at concentrations in the range of 10^8–10^{10} CFU/ml. Two days after donor introduction, the first transconjugants (TCs) were detected in fecal samples. The detected numbers of *tet*(M)-TCs were comparable for the two donors. In both cases, this number increased to c. 5.10^2 CFU/g faeces towards the end of the experiment. For *erm*(B)-TCs, the number was significantly higher and increased to c. 10^3 CFU/g faeces. According to Jacobsen et al. (2007) they were the first showing *in vivo* transfer of wild type antibiotic resistance plasmids from *L. plantarum* to *E. faecalis* (Jacobsen et al., 2007).

VRE (Vancomycin resistant Enterococci) are widespread in hospitals in the United States. The incidence of VRE bloodstream infections in the United States rose from 0.4% in 1989 to 25.2% in 1999 (National Nosocomial Infections Surveillance, 1999), with a concomitant rapid increase of VRE among *E. faecium* isolates (60% *E. faecium* versus 2% *E. faecalis*) (Wisplinghoff et al., 2004). It is generally admitted that VRE in the United States have emerged as a result of antibiotic use in hospitals (Menichetti, 2005). In Europe, the prevalence of VRE varies widely among countries and seems to be high in Italy and the United Kingdom (Menichetti, 2005). Isolates of VRE have been recovered from various animal sources in different European countries (Klare et al., 1995). This reservoir has been linked to the use of avoparcin in livestock (Aarestrup, 1999; Bager et al., 1997; Wegener et al., 1999), and suggests gene transfers between animals and humans via contamination over the food chain). This link is further supported by the presence of genotypically indistinguishable *van*A gene clusters in isolates of VRE from human and nonhuman sources (Simonsen et al., 1998; Jensen et al., 1999; Stobberingh et al., 1999) and by a decrease in VRE colonization rates in the European Union after avoparcin have been banned (Quednau et al., 1998; Klare et al., 1999; Kuhn et al., 2005; van den Bogaard and Stobberingh, 1999). Resistance of enterococci of clinical origins to other antimicrobial compounds of clinical interest is also a major concern, particularly with the increasing detection rates of antibiotic resistant *E. faecium* isolates (Treitman et al., 2005).

Acknowledgments

Dr. Svetoslav D. Todorov was supported by CAPES, Ministry of Education, Brazilian Government, Brasilia, Brazil.

References

Aarestrup, F. M. (1999). Association between the consumption of antimicrobial agents in animal husbandry and the occurrence of resistant bacteria among food animals. *International Journal of Antimicrobial Agents, 12*, 279–285.

Aarestrup, F. M., Agerso, Y., Gerner-Smidt, P., Madsen, M. and Jensen, L.B. (2000). Comparison of antimicrobial resistance phenotypes and resistance genes in *Enterococcus faecalis* and *Enterococcus faecium* from humans in the community, broilers, and pigs in Denmark. *Diagnostic Microbiology and Infection Diseases, 37*, 127–137.

Abriouel, H., Ben Omar, N., Molinos, A. C., López, R. L., Grande, M. J., Martínez-Viedma, P., Ortega, E., Cañamero, M. M. and Gálvez, A. (2008). Comparative analysis of genetic diversity and incidence of virulence factors and antibiotic resistance among enterococcal populations from raw fruit and vegetable foods, water and soil, and clinical samples. *International Journal of Food Microbiology, 123*, 38–49.

Ahn, C., Collins-Thompson, D., Duncan, C. and Stiles, M. E. (1992). Mobilization and location of the genetic determinant of chloramphenicol resistance from *Lactobacillus plantarum* caTC2R. *Plasmid, 27*, 169–176.

Ammor, M.S., Flóres, A.B. and Mayo, B. (2007). Antibiotic resistance in not-enterococcal lactic acid bacteria and bifidobacteria. *Food Microbiology, 24*, 559-570.

Aslim, B. and Beyatli, Y. (2004). Antibiotic resistance and plasmid DNA contents of *Streptococcus thermophilus* strains isolated from Turkish yoghurts. *Turkish Journal of Veterinary and Animal Science, 28*, 257–263.

Axelsson, L. T., Ahrne, S. E. I., Andersson, M. C. and Stahl, S. R. (1988). Identification and cloning of a plasmid-encoded erythromycin resistance determinant from *Lactobacillus reuteri*. *Plasmid, 20,* 171-174.

Bager, F., Madsen, M., Christensen, J. and Aarestrup, F. M. (1997). Avoparcin used as a growth promoter is associated with the occurrence of vancomycin-resistant *Enterococcus faecium* on Danish poultry and pig farms. *Preventative Veterinary Medicine, 31*, 95-112.

Bonten, M. J. M., Austin, D. J. and Lipsitch, M. (2001). Understanding the spread of antibiotic resistant pathogens in hospitals: Mathematical models as tools for control. *Clinical infectious diseases, 33*, 1739-1746.

Brötz-Oesterhelt, H. and Brunner, N.A. How many modes of action should an antibiotic have? *Current Opinion in Pharmacology* (in press).

Bryce, J., Boschi-Pinto, C., Shibuya, K., Black, R. E., the WHO Child Health Epidemiology Reference Group (2005). WHO estimates of the causes of death in children. *The Lancet, 365*, 1147–1157.

Cannon, J. P., Lee, T. A., Bolanos, J. T. and Danziger, L. H. (2005). Pathogenic relevance of Lactobacillus: a retrospective review of over 200 cases. *European Journal of Microbiological Infectious Disease, 24*, 31–40.

Carr, F. J., Chill, D. and Maida, N. (2002). The lactic acid bacteria: a literature survey. *Critical Review in Microbiology, 28*, 281–370.

Castellano, P., Belfiore, C., Fadda, S. and Vignolo, G. (2008). A review of bacteriocinogenic lactic acid bacteria used as bioprotective cultures in fresh meat produced in Argentina. *Meat Science, 79*, 483-499.

Cataloluk, O. and Gogebaken, B. (2004). Presebce of drug resistance in intestinal lactobacilli of dairy and human origin. *FEMS Microbiology Letters, 236*, 7–12.

Centeno, J. A., Menéndez, S. and Rodriguez-Otero, J. L. (1996). Main microbial flora present as natural starters in Cebreiro raw cow's-milk cheese (Northwest Spain). *International Journal of Food Microbiology, 33*, 307–313.

Cetinkaya, Y., Falk, P. and Mayhall, C.G. (2000). Vancomycin-resistant enterococci. *Clinical Microbiology Reviews, 13*, 686-698.

Chao, S. H., Tomii, Y., Sasamoto, M., Fujimoto, J., Tsai, Y.C. and Watanabe, K. (2008). *Lactobacillus capillatus* sp. nov., a motile bacterium isolated from stinky tofu brine. *International Journal of Systematic and Evolutionary Microbiology, 58*, 2555–2559.

Charteris, W. P., Kelly, P. M., Morelli, L. and Collins, J. K. (1998). Antibiotic susceptibility of potentially probiotic *Lactobacillus* species. *Journal of Food Protection, 61*, 1636–1643.

Chopra, I. and Roberts, M. (2001). Tetracycline antibiotics: mode of action, applications, molecular biology, and epidemiology of bacterial resistance. *Microbiology and Molecular Biology Reviews, 65*, 232–260.

Chopra, I. (2007). Bacterial RNA polymerase: a promising target for the discovery of new antimicrobial agents. *Current Opinion in Investigation of Drugs, 8*, 600-607.

Çitak, S., Yucel, N. and Orhan, S. (2004). Antibiotic resistance and incidence of *Enterococcus* species in Turkish white cheese. *International Journal of Dairy Technology, 57*, 27-35.

Clewell, D. B. and Weaver, K. E. (1989). Sex pheromones and plasmid transfer in *Enterococcus faecalis*. *Plasmid, 21*, 175–184.

Clewell, D. B. (1990). Movable genetic elements and antibiotic resistance in enterococci. *European Journal of Clinical Microbiology and Infectious Diseases, 9*, 90–102.

Clewell, D. B., Flannagan, S. E. and Jaworski, D. D. (1995). Unconstrained bacterial promiscuity: the Tn916–Tn1545 family of conjugative transposons. *Trends in Microbiology, 3,* 229–236.

Clewell, D. B., Yagi, Y., Dunny, G. M. and Schultz, S. K. (1974). Characterization of three plasmid deoxyribonucleic acid molecules in a strain of *Streptococcus faecalis*: identification of a plasmid determining erythromycin resistance. *Journal of Bacteriology, 117,* 283–289.

Cocconcelli, P. S., Morelli, L. and Vescovo, M. (1985). Conjugal transfer of antibiotic resistances from *Lactobacillus* to *Streptococcus lactis*. *Microbiol. Aliment. Nutr. 3,* 163–165.

Collins, M. D., Ash, C., Farrow, J. A. E., Wallbanks, S. and Williams, A. M. (1989). 16S Ribosomal ribonucleic acid sequence analysis of lactococci and related taxa. Description of *Vagococcus fluvialis* gen. nov., sp. nov. *Journal of Applied Bacteriology, 67,* 453–460

Condon, S. (1983). Aerobic metabolism of lactic acid bacteria. *Irish Journal of Food Science and Technology, 7,* 15–25.

Connell, S. R., Tracz, D. M., Nierhaus, K.H. and Taylor, D.E. (2003). Ribosomal protection proteins and their mechanism of tetracycline resistance. *Antimicrobial Agents and Chemotherapy, 47,* 3675-3681.

Coppola, R., Succi, M., Tremonte, P., Reale, A., Salzano, G. and Sorrentino, Z. (2005). Antibiotic susceptibility of *Lactobacillus rhamnosus* strains isolated from Parmegiano Reggiona cheese. *Le Lait, 85,* 193–204.

Danielsen, M. and Wind, A. (2003). Susceptibility of *Lactobacillus* spp. to antimicrobial agents. *International Journal of Food Microbiology, 82,* 1–11.

Danielsen, M. (2002). Characterization of the tetracycline resistance plasmid pMD5057 from *Lactobacillus plantarum* 5057 reveals a composite structure. *Plasmid, 48,* 98–103.

Danielsen, M., Simpson, P. J., O'Connor, E. B., Ross, R. P. and Stanton, C. (2007). Susceptibility of *Pediococcus* spp. to antimicrobial angents. *Journal of Appllied Microbiology, 102,* 384-389.

Davey, P.G. (2000). "Antimicrobial chemotherapy". In Ledingham, J.G.G. and Warrell, D.A. (Eds.), Concise Oxford Textbook of Medicine. Oxford: Oxford University Press, 1475. ISBN 0192628704.

Del Campo, R., Ruiz-Garbajosa, P., Sanchez-Moreno, M. P., Baquero, F., Torres, C., Canton, R. and Coque, T. M. (2003). Antimicrobial resistance in recent faecal enterococci from healthy volunteers and food handlers in Spain: genes and phenotypes. *Microbial Drug Resistance, 9,* 47–60.

Delgado, S., Flórez, A. B. and Mayo, B. (2005). Antibiotic susceptibility of *Lactobacillus* and *Bifidobacterium* species from the human gastrointestinal tract. *Current Microbiology, 50,* 202–207.

DeLisle, S. and Perl, T. M. (2003). Vancomycin-resistant enterococci: a road map on how to prevent the emergence and transmission of antimicrobial resistance. *Chest 123,* 504S–518S.

Devriese, L. A., Hommez, J., Laevens, H., Pot, B., Vandamme, P. and Haesebrouck, F. (1999). Identification of aesculin-hydrolyzing streptococci, lactococci, aerococci and enterococci from subclinical intramammary infections in dairy cows. *Veterinary Microbiology, 70*, 87–94.

Deye, G., Lewis, J., Patterson, J. and Jorgensen, J. (2003). A case of *Leuconostoc ventriculitis* with resistance to carbapenem antibiotics. *Clinical Infectious Diseases, 37*, 869–870.

Donohue, D. and Salminen, S. (1996). Safety of probiotic bacteria. Asia Pacific *Journal of Clinical Nutrition, 5*, 25–28.

Drlica, K., Malik, M., Kerns, R. J. and Zhao, X. (2008). Quinolone-mediated bacterial death. *Antimicrobial Agents and Chemotherapy, 52*, 385-392.

Edwards, C. G., Collins, M. D., Lawson, P. A. and Rodriguez, A. V. (2000). *Lactobacillus nagelii* sp. nov., an organism isolated from a partially fermented wine. *International Journal of Systematic and Evolutionary Microbiology, 50*, 699–702.

Elisha, B. G. and Courvalin, P. (1995). Analysis of genes encoding dalanine: d-alanine ligase-related enzymes in *Leuconostoc mesenteroides* and *Lactobacillus* spp. *Gene, 152*, 79–83.

Elkins, C. A. and Mullis, L. B. (2004). Bile-mediated aminoglycoside sensibility in *Lactobacillus* species likely results from increased membrane permeability attributable to cholic acid. *Applied and Environmental Microbiology, 70*, 7200–7209.

Elliott, J. A. and Facklam, R. R. (1996). Antimicrobial susceptibilities of *Lactococcus lactis* and *Lactococcus garvieae* and a proposed method to discriminate between them. *Journal of Clinical Microbiology, 34*, 1296–1298.

Endo, A. and Okada, S. (2005). *Lactobacillus satsumensis* sp. nov., isolated from mashes of shochu, a traditional Japanese distilled spirit made from fermented rice and other starchy materials. *International Journal of Systematic and Evolutionary Microbiology, 55*, 83–85

European Commission, 2005. Opinion of the Scientific Panel on Additives and Products of Substances used in Animal Feed on the updating of the criteria used in the assessment of bacteria for resistance to antibiotics of human or veterinary importance. EFSA J. 223, 1–12.

Eyngor, M., Zlotkin, A., Ghittino, C., Prearo, M., Douet, D. G., Chilmonczyk, S. and Eldar, A. (2004). Clonality and diversity of the fish pathogen *Lactococcus garvieae* in Mediterranean countries. *Applied and Environmental Microbiology, 70*, 5132–5137.

Fines, M., Perichon, B., Reynolds, P., Sahm, D.F. and Courvalin, P. (1999). *Van*E, a new type of acquired glycopeptide resistance in *Enterococcus faecalis* BM4405. *Antimicrobial agents and Chemotherapy, 43*, 2161-2164.

Flórez, A. B. and Mayo, B. (2006). Microbial diversity and succession during the manufacture and ripening of traditional, Spanish, blue-veined Cabrales cheese, as determined by PCR-DGGE. *International Journal of Food Microbiology, 110*, 165–171.

Flórez, A. B., Ammor, M. S. and Mayo, B. (2008a). Identification of *tet*(M) in two *Lactococcus lactis* strains isolated from a Spanish traditional starter-free cheese made of raw milk and conjugative transfer of tetracycline resistance to lactococci and enterococci. *International Journal of Food Microbiology, 121*, 189–194.

Flórez, A. B., Ammor, M. S., Mayo, B., van Hoek, A. H., Aarts, H. J. and Huys, G. (2008b). Antimicrobial susceptibility profiles of 32 type strains of *Lactobacillus, Bifidobacterium,*

Lactococcus and *Streptococcus* spp. *International Journal of Antimicrobial Agents, 31,* 484–486.

Flórez, A. B., Delgado, S. and Mayo, B. (2005). Antimicrobial susceptibility of lactic acid bacteria isolated from a cheese environment. *Canadian Journal of Microbiology, 51,* 51–58.

Fons, M., Hege, T., Ladire, M., Raibaud, P., Ducluzeau, R. and Maguin, E. (1997). Isolation and characterization of a plasmid from *Lactobacillus fermentum* conferring erythromycin resistance. *Plasmid, 37,* 199–203.

Fortina, M. G., Ricci, G., Borgo, F., Manachini, P. L., Arends, K., Schiwon, K., Abajy, M.Y. and Grohmann, E. (2008). A survey on biotechnological potential and safety of the novel *Enterococcus* species of dairy origin, *E. italicus. International Journal of Food Microbiology, 123,* 204–211.

Fortina, M. G., Ricci, G., Borgo,F. Manachini, P. L. (2007). Rapid identification of *Enterococcus italicus* by PCR with primers targeted to 16S rRNA gene. *Letters in Applied Microbiology, 44,* 443–446.

Foulquié-Moreno, M. R., Sarantinopoulos, P., Tsakalidou, E. and De Vuyst, L. (2006). The role and application of enterococci in food and health. *International Journal of Food Microbiology, 106,* 1–24.

Franz, C. M. A. P., Stiles, M. E., Schleifer, K. H. and Holzapfel, W. H. (2003). Enterococci in foods—a conundrum for food safety. *International Journal of Food Microbiology, 88,* 105–122.

Franz, C. M., Muscholl-Silberhorn, A. B., Yousif, N. M. K., Vancanneyt, M., Swings, J. and Holzapfel, W. H. (2001). Incidence of virulence factors and antibiotic resistance among Enterococci isolated from food. *Applied and Environmental Microbiology, 67,* 4385–4389.

Gálvez A., Abriouel, H., López, R. L. and Bem Omar, N. (2007). Bacteriocin-based strategies for food biopreservation. *International Journal of Food Microbiology, 120,* 51-70.

Gasser, F. (1994). Safety of lactic-acid bacteria and their occurrence in human clinical infections. *Bulletin de L'Institut Pasteur, 92,* 45–67.

Gasson, M. (1990). In vivo genetic systems in lactic acid bacteria. *FEMS Microbiology Reviews, 87,* 43–60.

Gasson, M. J. and Davies, F. L. (1980). Conjugal transfer of the drug resistance plasmid pAMß1 in the lactic streptococci. *FEMS Microbiology Letters, 7,* 51–53.

Gasson, M. J. and Fitzgard, G. F. (1994). Gene transfer systems and transposition. In: Gasson, M. J. and de Vos, W. M. (Eds.), Genetics and Biotechnology of Lactic Acid Bacteria. Blackie Academics and Professional, London, pp. 1–51.

Gevers, D. (2002). Tetracycline resistance in lactic acid bacteria isolated from fermented dry sausages. Ph.D Thesis. Gent University, Gent, Belgium.

Gevers, D., Danielsen, M., Huys, G. and Swings, J. (2003a). Molecular characterization of *tet*(M) genes in *Lactobacillus* isolates from different types of fermented dry sausage. *Applied and Environmental Microbiology, 69,* 1270–1275.

Gevers, D., Huys, G. and Swings, J. (2003b). In vitro conjugal transfer of tetracycline resistance from *Lactobacillus* isolates to other Gram-positive bacteria. *FEMS Microbiology Letters, 225,* 125–130.

Gevers, D., Huys, G., Devlieghere, F., Uyttendaele, M., Debevere, J. and Swings, J. (2000). Isolation and identification of tetracycline resistant lactic acid bacteria from prepacked sliced meat products. *Systematic and Applied Microbiology, 23*, 279–284.

Giraffa, G. and Carminati, D. (1997). Control of *Listeria monocytogenes* in the rind of Taleggio, a surface-smear cheese, by a bacteriocin from *Enterococcus faecium* 7C5. *Science Alimentaier, 17*, 383–391.

Gobbetti, M., De Angelis, M., Di Cagno, R., Minervini, F. and Limitone, A. (2007). Cell–cell communication in food related bacteria. *International Journal of Food Microbiology, 120,* 34-45.

Gomes, B. C., Esteves, C.T., Palazzo, I. C. V., Darini, A. L. C., Felis, G.E., Sechi, L.A., Franco, B.D.G.M. and De Martinis, E.C.P. (2008). Prevalence and characterization of *Enterococcus* spp. isolated from Brazilian foods. *Food Microbiology, 25*, 668–675.

Grillot-Courvalin, C., Goussard, S. and Courvalin, P. (2002). Wild-type intracellular bacteria deliver DNA intomammalian cells. *Cellular Microbiology, 4,* 177–186.

Halami, P. M., Chandrashekar, A. and Nand, K. (2000). *Lactobacillus farciminis* MD, a newer strain with potential for bacteriocin and antibiotic assay. *Letters in Applied Microbiology, 30*, 197–202.

Handwerger, S., Pucci, M. J., Volk, K. J., Liu, J. P. and Lee, M.S. (1994). Vancomycin-resistant *Leuconostoc mesenteroides* and *Lactoacillus casei* synthesize cytoplasmic peptidoglycan precursors that terminate in lactate. *Journal of Bacteriology*, 176, 260-264.

Hansson, S., Singh, R., Gudkov, A. T., Liljas, A., Logan, D.T. (2005). Structural insights into fusidic acid resistance and sensitivity in EF-G. *Journal of Molecular Biology, 348,* 939-949.

Harada, T., Mito, Y., Otsuki, K. and Murase, T. (2004). Resistance to gentamicin and vancomycin in enterococcal strains isolated from retail broiler chickens in Japan. *Journal of Food Protection, 67*, 2292–2295.

Hasman, H., Villadsen, A. G. and Aarestrup, F. M. (2005). Diversity and stability of plasmids from glycopeptide-resistant *Enterococcus faecium* (GRE) isolated from pigs in Denmark. *Microbial Drug Resistance, 11*, 178–184.

Hawser, S., Lociuro, S. and Islam, K. (2006). Dihydrofolate reductase inhibitors as antibacterial agents. *Biochemical Pharmacology, 71*, 941-948.

Herrero, M., Mayo, B., Ganzales, B. and Suarez, J. E. (1996). Evaluation of technologically important traits in lactic acid bacteria isolated from spontaneous fermentations. *Journal of Applied Bacteriology, 81*, 565–570.

Herreros, M. A., Sandoval, H., González, L., Castro, J. M., Fresno, J. M. and Tornadijo. M. E. (2005). Antimicrobial activity and antibiotic resistance of lactic acid bacteria isolated from Armada cheese (a Spanish goats' milk cheese). *Food Microbiology, 22*, 455–459.

Hespell, R. B. and Whitehead, T. R. (1991). Introduction of Tn916 and pAMß1 into *Streptococcus bovis* JB1 by conjugation. *Applied and Environmental Microbiology, 57*, 2710–2713.

Hummel, A., Holzapfel, W. H. and Franz, C. M. A. P. (2007). Characterisation and transfer of antibiotic resistance genes from enterococci isolated from food. *Systematic and Applied Microbiology, 30*, 1–7.

Husni, R. N., Gordon, S. M., Washington, J. A. and Longworth, D. L. (1997). *Lactobacillus* bacteremia and endocarditis: review of 45 cases. *Clinical Infectious Diseases*, *25*, 1048–1055.

Huycke, M.M., Sahm, D.F. and Gilmore, M.S. (1998). Multiple-drug resistant Enterococci: The nature of the problem and an agenda for the future. *Emerging Infectious Diseases, 4,* 239-249.

Huys, G., D'Haene, K., and Swings, J. (2002). Influence of the culture medium on antibiotic susceptibility testing of food-associated lactic acid bacteria with the agar overlay disc diffusion method. *Letters in Applied Microbiology, 34,* 402-406.

Huys, G., D'Haene, K., and Swings, J. (2006). Genetic basis of tetracycline and minocycline resistance in potentially probiotic *Lactobacillus plantarum* strain CCUG 43738. *Antimicrobial Agents and Chemotherapy, 50,* 1550-1551.

Huys, G., D'Haene, K., Collard, J.-M. and Swings, J. (2004). Prevalence and molecular characterization of tetracycline resistance in *Enterococcus* isolates from food. *Applied and Environmental Microbiology, 70,* 1555–1562.

Ishiwa, H. and Iwata, S. (1980). Drug resistance plasmids in *Lactobacillus fermentum. Journal of General and Applied Microbiology, 26,* 71–74.

Jacobsen, L., Wilcks, A., Hammer, K., Huys, G., Gevers, D., and Andersen, S. R. (2007). Horizontal transfer of *tet*(M) and *erm*(B) resistance plasmids from food strains of Lactobacillus plantarum to *Enterococcus faecalis* JH2-2 in the gastrointestinal tract of gnotobiotic rats. *FEMS Microbiology Ecology, 59,* 158-166.

James, P. R., Hardman, S. M. and Patterson, D. L. (2000). Osteomyelitis and possible endocarditis secondary to *Lactococcus garvieae*: a first case report. *Postgraduation Medical Journal, 76,* 301–303.

Jensen, L. B., Hammerum, A. M., Poulsen, R. L. and Westh, H. (1999). Vancomycin-resistant *Enterococcus faecium* strains with highly similar pulsed-field gel electrophoresis patterns containing similar Tn1546-like elements isolated from a hospitalized patient and pigs in Denmark. *Antimicrobial Agents and Chemotherapy, 43,* 724–725.

Jett, B. D., Huycke, M. M. and Gilmore, M. S. (1994). Virulence of enterococci. *Clinical Microbiology Reviews, 7,* 462–478.

Johnson, A. P. (1994). The pathogenicity of enterococci. *Journal of Antimicrobials and Chemotherapy, 33,* 1083–1089.

Johnson, A. P., Uttley, A. H. C., Woodford, N. and George, R. C. (1990) Resistance to vancomycin and teicoplanin – an emerging clinical problem. *Clinical Microbiology Reviews, 3,* 280-291.

Kahne, D., Leimkuhler, C., Lu, W. and Walsh, C. (2005). Glycopeptide and lipoglycopeptide antibiotics. *Chemistry Reviews, 105,* 425-448.

Kaneuchi, C., Seki, M. and Komagata, K. (1988). Taxonomic Study of *Lactobacillus mali* Carr and Davis 1970 and Related Strains: Validation of *Lactobacillus mali* Carr and Davis 1970 over *Lactobacillus yamanashiensis* Nonomura 1983. *International Journal of Systematic Bcteriology,* 269-272.

Kastner, S., Perreten, V., Bleuler, H., Hugenschmidt, G., Lacroix, C. and Meile, L. (2006). Antibiotic susceptibility patterns and resistance genes of starter cultures and probiotic bacteria used in food. *Systematic and Applied Microbiology, 29,* 145–155.

Kastnera, S., Perretenb, V., Bleulera, H., Hugenschmidta, G., Lacroixa, C. and Meile, L. (2006). Antibiotic susceptibility patterns and resistance genes of starter cultures and probiotic bacteria used in food. *Systematic and Applied Microbiology, 29,* 145–155

Katla, A. K., Kruse, H., Johnsen, G. and Herikstad, H. (2001). Antimicrobial susceptibility of starter culture bacteria used in Norwegian dairy products. *International Journal of Food Microbiology, 67,* 147–152.

Kaul, M., Barbieri, C. M., Pilch, D. S. (2006). Aminoglycoside-induced reduction in nucleotide mobility at the ribosomal RNA A-site as a potentially key determinant of antibacterial activity. *Journal of American Chemistry Society, 128,* 1261-1271.

Kim, K. S., Morrison, J. O. and Bayer, A. S. (1982). Deficient autolytic enzyme activity in antibiotic-tolerant lactobacilli. *Infections and Immunology, 36,* 582–585.

Klare, I., Badstubner, D., Konstabel, C., Bohme, G., Claus, H. and Witte, W. (1999). Decreasing incidence of *Van*A-type vancomycin-resistant enterococci isolated from poulty meat and from fecal samples of human in the community after discontinuation of avoparcin usage in animal husbandry. *Microbial Drug Resistance-Mechanisms Epidemiology and Disease, 5,* 45-52.

Klare, I., Heier, H., Claus, H., Bohme, G., Marin, S., Seltmann, G., Hakenbeck, R., Antanassova, V. and Witte, W. (1995). *Enterococcus faecium* strains with *van*A-mediated high-level glycopeptide resistance isolated from animal foodstuffs and fecal samples of humans in the community. *Microbial Drug Resistance-Mechanisms Epidemiology and Disease, 1,* 265-272.

Klare, I., Konstabel, C., Badstubner, D., Werner, G. and Witte, W. (2003). Occurrence and spread of antibiotic resistances in *Enterococcus faecium*. *International Journal of Food Microbiology, 88,* 269-290.

Klein, G., Hallman, C., Casas, I. A., Abad, J., Louwers, J. and Reuter, G. (2000). Exclusion of *van*A, *van*B and *van*C type glycopeptide resistance in strains of *Lactobacillus reuteri* and *Lactobacillus rhamnosus* used as probiotics by polymerase chain reaction and hybridization methods. *Journal of Applied Microbiology, 89,* 814–815.

Klein, G., Pack, A. and Reuter, G. (1998). Antibiotic resistance patterns of enterococci and occurrence of vancomycin-resistant enterococci in raw minced beef and pork in Germany. *Applied and Environmental Microbiology, 64,* 1825–1830.

Kleinschmidt, J., Soeding, B., Teuber, M. and Neve, H. (1993). Evaluation of horizontal and vertical gene transfer and stability of heterologus DNA in *Streptococcus thermophylus* isolated from yoghurt and yoghurt starter cultures. *Systematic and Applied Microbiology, 16,* 287-295.

Kojic, M., Jovcic, B., Begovic, J., Fira, D. and Topisirovic, L. (2008). Large chromosomal inversion correlated with spectomycin in *Lactococcus lactis* subsp. *lactis* bv. *diacetylactis* S50. *Canadian Journal of Microbiology, 54,* 143-149.

Korhonen, J. M., Sclivagnotis, Y. and von Wright, A. (2007). Characterization of dominant cultivable lactobacilli and their antibiotic resistance profiles from faecal samples of weaning piglets. *Journal of Applied Microbiology, 103,* 2496-2503.

Kuhn, I., Iversen, A., Finn, M., Greko, C., Burman, L. G., Blanch, A. R., Vilanova, X., Manero, A., Taylor, H., Caplin, J., Dominguez, L., Herrero, I. A., Moreno, M. A. and Mollby, R. (2005). Occurrence and relatedness of vancomycin-resistant enterococci in animals, humans, and the environment in different European regions. *Applied and Environmental Microbiology, 71*, 5383-5390.

Lampkowska, J., Louise, F. L., Monaghan, A., Toomey, N., Schjørring, S., Jacobsen, B., van der Voet, H., Andersen, S. R., Bolton, D., Aarts, H., Krogfelt, K. A., Wilcks, A. and Bardowski, J. (2008). A standardized conjugation protocol to asses antibiotic resistance transfer between lactococcal species. *International Journal of Food Microbiology, 127,* 172–175.

Landman, D. and Quale, J. M. (1997). Management of infections due to resistant enterococci: a review of therapeutic options. *Journal of Antimicrobials and Chemotherapy, 40,* 161–170.

Landsberg, H. (1949). Prelude to the discovery of penicillin. Isis, 40, 225–227.

Lara-Villoslada, F., Sierra, S., Martín, R., Delgado, S., Rodríguez, J. M., Olivares, M. and Xaus, J. (2007). Safety assessment of two probiotic strains, *Lactobacillus coryniformis* CECT5711 and *Lactobacillus gasseri* CECT5714. *Journal of Applied Microbiology, 103,* 175–184.

Leclercq, R. (1997). Enterococci acquire new kinds of resistance. *Clinical Infectious Diseases, 24 (Suppl. 1),* S80– S84.

Leclercq, R., Derlot, E., Duval, J. and Courvalin, P. (1988). Plasmid-mediated resistance to vancomycin and teicoplanin in *Enterococcus faecium. New England Journal of Medicine, 319,* 157–161.

Leclercq, R., Derlot, E., Weber, M., Duval, J. and Courvalin, P. (1989). Transferable vancomycin and teicoplanin resistance in *Enterococcus faecium. Antimicrobial Agents and Chemotherapy, 33,* 10–15.

Leclercq, R., Dutkamalen, S., Duval, J. and Courvalin, P. (1992). Vancomycin resistance gene Vanc is specific to *Enterococcus gallinarium. Antimicrobial Agents and Chemoterapy, 36,* 2005-2008.

Lei, V. and Jakobsen, M. (2004). Microbiological characterization and probiotic potential of koko and koko sour water, African spontaneously fermented millet porridge and drink. *Journal of Applied Microbiology, 96,* 384–397.

Lei, V., Friis, H. and Michaelsen, K.F. (2006). Spontaneously fermented millet product as a natural probiotic treatment for diarrhoea in young children: an intervention study in Northern Ghana. *International Journal of Food Microbiology, 110,* 246–253.

Leroy, F. and de Vuyst, L. (2004). Lactic acid bacteria as functional starter cultures for the food fermentation industry. *Trends in Food Science and Technology, 15,* 67–78.

Levy, S. B. and Marshall, B. (2004). Antibacterial resistance world wide: causes, challenges and responses. *Nature Medicine Reviews, 10,* S122–S129.

Lin, C. F., Fung, Z. F., Wu, C. L. and Chung, T. C. (1996). Molecular characterization of a plasmid borne (pTC82) chloramphenicol resistance determinant (cat-Tc) from *Lactobacillus reuteri* G4. *Plasmid, 36,* 116–124.

Lin, C.F. and Chung, T.C. (1999). Cloning of erythromycin-resistance determinants and replication origins from indigenous plasmids of *Lactobacillus reuteri* for potential use in construction of cloning vectors. *Plasmid 42,* 31–41.

Lombardi, A., Gatti, M., Rizzotti, L., Torriani, S., Andrighetto, C. and Giraffa, G. (2004). Characterization of *Streptococcus macedonicus* strains isolated from artisanal Italian rawmilk cheeses. *International Dairy Journal, 14*, 967–976.

Lukášová, J. and Šustáčková, A. (2003). Enterococci and antibiotic resistance. *Acta Veterinaria Brno, 72*, 315–323.

Maiettia, L., Bonvinia, B., Huysb, G. and Giraffa, G. (2007). Incidence of antibiotic resistance and virulence determinants among *Enterococcus italicus* isolates from dairy products. *Systematic and Applied Microbiology, 30*, 509–517.

Manolopoulou, E., Sarantinopoulos, P., Zoidou, E., Aktypis, A., Moschopoulou, E., Kandarakis, I. G. and Anifantakis, E. M. (2003). Evolution of microbial populations during traditional Feta cheese manufacture and ripening. *International Journal of Food Microbiology, 82,* 153-161.

Martel, A., Meulenaere, V., Devriese, L. A., Decostere, A. and Haesebrouck, F. (2003). Macrolide and lincosamide resistance in the gram-positive nasal and tonsillar flora of pigs. *Microbial Drug Resistance, 9,* 293–297.

Mathur, S. and Singh, R. (2005). Antibiotic resistance in food lactic acid bacteria. *International Journal of Food Microbiology, 105,* 281–295.

Maxwell, A. and Lawson, D. M. (2003). The ATP-binding site of type II topoisomerases as a target for antibacterial drugs. *Current Topics in Medical Chemistry, 3*, 283-303.

McBride, S. M., Fischetti, V. A., LeBlanc, D. J., Moellering Jr., R. C. and Gilmore, M. S. (2007). Genetic Diversity among *Enterococcus faecalis*. PLoS ONE, 2: e582. doi:10.1371/journal.pone.0000582.

Menichetti, F. (2005). Current and emerging serious Gram-positive infections. *Clinical Microbiology and Infection, 11*, 22-28.

Mofredj, A., Baraka, D., Cadranel, J. F., LeMaitre, P., Kloeti, G. and Dumont, J. L. (2000). *Lactococcus garvieae* septicemia with liver abscess in an immunosuppressed patient. *American Journal of Medicine, 109*, 513–514.

Morelli, L., Sarra, P. G. and Bottazzi, V. (1988). In vivo transfer of pAM-beta-1 from *Lactobacillus reuteri* to *Enterococcus faecalis*. *Journal of Applied Bacteriology, 65,* 371–375.

Moubareck, C., Gavini, F., Vaugien, L., Butel, M. J. and Doucet-Populaire, F. (2005). Antimicrobial susceptibility of bifidobacteria. *Journal of Antimicrobials and Chemotherapy, 55*, 38–44.

Murray, B. E. (1990). The life and times of the *Enterococcus*. *Clinical Microbiology Reviews, 3*, 46–65.

Nicas, T. I., Cole, C. T., Preston, D. A., Schabel, A. A. and Nagarajan, R. (1989) Activity of glycopeptides against vancomycin-resistant Gram-positive bacteria. *Antimicrobial agents and Chemoterapy, 33*, 1477-1481.

Nicas, T. I., Wu, C. Y. E., Hobbs, J. N., Preston, D. A., Allen, N. E. (1989). Characterization of vancomycin resistance in *Enterococcus faecium* and *Enterococcus faecalis*. *Antimicrobial Agents and Chemoterapy, 33*, 1121-1124.

Nielsen, D. S., Schillinger, U., Franz, C. M. A. P., Bresciani, J., Amoa-Awua, W., Holzapfel, W. H. and Jakobsen, M. (2007). *Lactobacillus ghanensis* sp. nov., a motile lactic acid bacterium isolated from Ghanaian cocoa fermentations. *International Journal of Systematic and Evolutionary Microbiology, 57,* 1468-1472.

Normark, B. H. and Normark, S. (2002). Evolution and spread of antibiotic resistance. *Journal of Internal Medicine, 252,* 91–106.

O'Connor, E. B., Ross, R. P. and Hill, C. (2007). Application of bacteriocins in the food industry. In: Riley, M. A. and Gillor, O. (Eds.), Research and Applications in Bacteriocins. Horizon Bioscience Scientific Press.

Olukoya, D. K., Ebigwei, S. I., Adebawo, O. O. and Osiyemi, F. O. (1993). Plasmid profiles and antibiotic susceptibility patterns of *Lactobacillus* isolated from fermented foods in Nigeria. *Food Microbiology, 10,* 279–285.

Ouoba, L. I. I., Lei, V. and Jensen, L.B. (2008). Resistance of potential probiotic lactic acid bacteria and bifidobacteria of African and European origin to antimicrobials: Determination and transferability of the resistance genes to other bacteria. *International Journal of Food Microbiology, 121,* 217–224.

Ouwehand, A. C., Salminen, S. and Isolauri, E. (2002). Probiotics: an overview of beneficial effects. *Antonie Van Leeuwenhoek International Journal of General and Molecular Microbiology, 82,* 279–289.

Perichon, B. and Courvalin, P. (2000). Update on vancomycin resistance. *International Journal of Clinical Practice, 115,* 88–93.

Perichon, B., Reynolds, P. and Courvalin, P. (1997). VanD-type glycopeptide-resistant *Enterococcus faecium* BM4339. *Antimicrobial Agents and Chemoterapy, 41,* 2016-2018.

Perreten, V., Kolloffel, B. and Teuber, M., (1997a). Conjugal transfer of the Tn 916-like transposon Tn FO1 from *Enterococcus faecalis* isolated from cheese to other Gram-positive bacteria. *Systematic and Applied Microbiology, 20,* 27– 38.

Perreten, V., Schwarz, F. V., Teuber, M. and Levy, S. B. (2001). *Mdt* (A), a new efflux protein conferring multiple antibiotic resistance in *Lactococcus lactis* and *Escherichia coli. Antimicrobial Agents and Chemotherapy, 45,* 1109– 1114.

Perreten, V., Schwarz, F., Cresta, L., Boeglin, M., Dasen, G. and Teuber, M. (1997b). Antibiotic resistance spread in food. *Nature, 389,* 801–802.

Petersen, A. and Jensen, L.B. (2004). Analysis of *gyr*A and *par*C mutations in enterococci from environmental samples with reduced susceptibility to ciprofloxacin. *FEMS Microbiology Letters, 231,* 73–76.

Pitkälä, A., Haveri, M., Pyorala, S., Myllys, V. and Honkanen-Buzalski, T. (2004). Bovine mastitis in Finland 2001 - Prevalence, distribution of bacteria, and antimicrobial resistance. *Journal of Dairy Science, 87,* 2433-2441.

Putman, M., van Veen, H. W., Degener, J. E. and Konings, W. N. (2001). The lactococcal secondary multidrug transporter *Lmr*P confers resistance to lincosamides, macrolides, streptogramins and tetracyclines. *Microbiology, 147,* 2873–2880.

Quednau, M., Ahrné, S., Petersson, A. C. and Molin, G. (1998). Antibiotic-resistant strains of *Enterococcus* isolated from Swedish and Danish retailed chicken and pork. *Journal of Applied Microbiology, 84,* 1163– 1170.

Quintiliani R., Nightingale, C. H. and Sullivan, M. C. (1993). Use of pharmacodynamic concepts in developing cost effective dosing method for piperacillin. *Clinical Therapeutics, 154 (Supplement A),* 44-49.

Raha, A. R., Ross, E., Yusoff, K., Manap, M. Y. and Ideris, A. (2002). Characterisation and molecular cloning of an erythromycin resistance plasmid of *Lactococcus lactis* isolated from chicken cecum. *Journal of Biochemistry, Molecular Biology and Biophysics, 6,* 7–11.

Rice, L. B., Carias, L. L., Donskey, C. L. and Rudin, S. D. (1998). Transferable, plasmid-mediated *Van*B-type glycopeptide resistance in *Enterococcus faecium. Antimicrobial Agents and Chemotherapy, 42,* 963–964.

Rivals, J. P., Beal, C., Thammavongs, B., Gueguen, M. and Panoff, J.-M. (2007). Cryotolerance of *Lactobacillus delbrueckii* subsp *bulgaricus* CFL1 is modified by acquisition of antibiotic resistance. *Cryobiology, 55,* 19-26.

Roberts, M. C. (2005). Update on acquired tetracycline resistance genes. *FEMS Microbiology Letters, 245,* 195–203.

Rodas, A. M., Chenoll, E., Macián, M.C., Ferrer, S., Pardo, I. and Aznar, R. (2006). *Lactobacillus vini* sp. nov., a wine lactic acid bacterium homofermentative for pentoses *International Journal of Systematic and Evolutionary Microbiology, 56,* 513–517.

Rojo-Bezares, B., Sáenz, Y., Poeta, P., Zarazaga, M., Ruiz-Larrea, F. and Torres, C. (2006). Assessment of antibiotic susceptibility within lactic acid bacteria strains isolated from wine. *International Journal of Food Microbiology, 111,* 234–240.

Rosenfeldt, V., Michaelsen, K. F., Jakobsen, M., Larsen, C. N., Møller, P. L., Pedersen, P., Tvede, M., Weyrehter, N. H., Valerius, N. H. and Paerregaard, A. (2002a). Effect of *Lactobacillus* strains in young children hospitalized with acute diarrhea. *Pediatric Infectious Disease Journal, 21,* 411–416.

Rosenfeldt, V., Michaelsen, K. F., Jakobsen, M., Larsen, C. N., Møller, P. L., Tvede, M., Weyrehter, H., Valerius, N. H., and Paerregaard, A. (2002b). Effect of probiotic *Lactobacillus* strains on acute diarrhea in a cohort of non-hospitalized children attending day-care centers. *Pediatric Infectious Disease Journal, 21,* 417–419.

Ruoff, K. L., Kuritzkes, D. R., Wolfson, J. S., Ferraro, M. J. (1988). Vancomycin-resistant Gram-positive bacteria isolated from human sources. *Journal of Clinical Microbiology, 26,* 2064-2068.

Salminen, M. K., Rautelin, H., Tynkkynen, S., Poussa, T., Saxelin, M., Valtonen, V. and Jarvinen, A., (2006). *Lactobacillus* bacteremia, species identification, and antimicrobial susceptibility of 85 blood isolates. *Clinical Infectious Diseases, 42,* 35–44.

Salminen, S., Von Wright, A., Morelli, L., Marteau, P., Brassard, D., DeVos, W. M., Fonden, R., Saxelin, M., Collins, K., Mogensen, G., Birkeland, S. E. and Mattila- Sandholm, T. (1998). Demonstration of safety of probiotics. *International Journal of Food Microbiology, 44,* 93–106.

Salyers, A. A. and Shoemaker, N. B. (1996). Resistance gene transfer in anaerobes: New insights, new problems. *Clinical Infectious Diseases, 23,* S36-S43.

Salyers, A. A., Gupta, A. and Wang, Y. (2004). Human intestinal bacteria as reservoirs for antibiotic resistance genes. *Trends in Microbiology, 12,* 412–416.

Sasaki, Y., Taketomo, N. and Sasaki, T. (1988). Factors affecting transfer frequency of pAMß1 from *Streptococcus faecalis* to *Lactobacillus plantarum*. *Journal of Bacteriology, 170,* 5939–5942.

Saxelin, M., Tynkkynen, S., Mattila-Sandholm, T. and de Vos, W. (2005). Probiotic and other functional microbes: from markets to mechanisms. *Current Opinion in Biotechnology, 16,* 1–8.

Scheffers, D. J. and Pinho, M.G. (2005). Bacterial cell wall synthesis: new insights from localization studies. *Microbiology and Molecular Biology Reviews, 69,* 585-607.

Schillinger, U., Geisen, R. and Holzapfel, W.H. (1996). Potential of antagonistic microorganisms and bacteriocins for the biological preservation of foods. *Trends in Food Science and Technology, 7,* 158–164.

Schlunzen, F., Zarivach, R., Harms, J., Bashan, A., Tocilj, A., Albrecht, R., Yonath, A. and Franceschi, F. (2001). Structural basis for the interaction of antibiotics with the peptidyl transferase centre in eubacteria. *Nature, 413,* 814-821.

Shaghaghi, B. Talebi, M., Katouli, M., Moellby, R., Kuehn, I. and Pourshafie, M. R. (2007). Phenotypic diversity of multiple antibiotic resistant enterococci with emphasis on *Enterococcus gallinarum* carrying *van*A and *van*B genes. *Water and Soil Pollution, 186,* 255-261.

Sharma, S. K. and Mohan, A. (2004). Multidrug-resistant tuberculosis. *Indian Journal of Medical Research, 120,* 354-376.

Sharpe, M. E., Latham, M. J. and Gravie, E. I. (1973). Two new species of *Lactobacillus* isolated from the rumen, *Lactobacillus ruminis* sp. nov. and *Lactobacillus vitulinus* sp. nov. *Journal of General Microbiology, 77,* 37–49.

Shrago, A. W. and Dobrogosz, W. J. (1988). Conjugal transfer of group-B streptococcal plasmids and comobilization of *Escherichia coli–Streptococcus* shuttle plasmids to *Lactobacillus plantarum*. *Applied and Environmental Microbiology, 54,* 824–826.

Shrago, A. W., Chassy, B. M. and Dobrogosz, W. J. (1986). Conjugal plasmid transfer (pAMß1) in *Lactobacillus plantarum*. *Applied and Environmental Microbiology, 53,* 574–576.

Sidhu, M. S., Heir, E., Sorum, H. and Holck, A. (2001a). Genetic linkage between resistance to quaternary ammonium compounds and beta-lactam antibiotics in food-related *Staphylococcus* spp. *Microbial Drug Resistance-Mechanisms Epidemiology and Diseases, 7,* 363-371.

Sidhu, M. S., Langsrud, S. and Holck, A. (2001b). Disinfectant and antibiotic resistance of lactic acid bacteria isolated from the food industry. *Drug Resistance-Mechanisms Epidemiology and Diseases, 7,* 73-83.

Simonsen, G. S., Haaheim, H., Dahl, K. H., Kruse, H., Lovseth, A., Olsvik, O. and Sundsfjord, A. (1998). Transmission of *Van*A-type vancomycin-resistant enterococci and *van*A resistance elements between chicken and humans at avoparcin-exposed farms. *Drug Resistance-Mechanisms Epidemiology and Diseases, 4,* 313-318.

Singh, U. P., Tyagi, P. and Upreti, S. (2007). Manganese complexes as models for manganese-containing pseudocatalase enzymes: Synthesis, structural and catalytic activity studies. *Polyhedron, 26,* 3625-3632.

Skold, O. (2000). Sulfonamide resistance: mechanisms and trends. *Drug Resist Updat, 3,* 155-160.

Sparo, M., Nuñez, G. G., Castro, M., Calcagno, M. L., Allende, M. A.G., Ceci, M., Najle, R. and Manghi, M. (2008). Characteristics of an environmental strain, *Enterococcus faecalis* CECT7121, and its effects as additive on craft dry-fermented sausages. *Food Microbiology, 25,* 607–615.

Stobberingh, E., van den Bogaard, A., London, N., Driessen, C., Top, J. and Willems, R. (1999). Enterococci with glycopeptide resistance in turkeys, turkey farmers, turkey slaughterers, and (sub)urban residents in the South of the Netherlands: Evidence for transmission of vancomycin resistance from animals to humans? *Antimicrobial Agents and Chemoterapy, 43,* 2215-2221.

Strøman, P., Muller, C. C. and Sorensen, K. I. (2003). Heat shock treatment increases the frequency of loss of an erythromycin resistance-encoding transposable element from the chromosome of *Lactobacillus crispatus* CHCC3692. *Applied and Environmental Microbiology, 69,* 7173–7180.

Swenson, J. M., Facklam, R. R. and Thornsberry, C. (1990). Antimicrobial susceptibility of vancomycin-resistant *Leuconostoc, Pediococcus,* and *Lactobacillus* species. *Antimicrobial Agents and Chemotherapy, 34,* 543–549.

Tankovic, J., Leclercq, R. and Duval, J. (1993). Antimicrobial susceptibility of *Pediococcus* spp. and genetic basis of macrolide resistance in *Pediococcus acidilactici* HM3020. *Antimicrobial Agents and Chemotherapy, 37,* 789–792.

Tannock, G. W., Luchansky, J. B., Miller, L., Connell, H., Thodeandersen, S., Mercer, A. A. and Kalenhammer, T. R. (1994). Molecular characterization of a plasmid borne (pGT633) erythromycin resistance determinant (*erm*GT) from *Lactobacillus reuteri* 100-63. *Plasmid, 31,* 60–71.

Tannock, G.W. (1987). Conjugal transfer of plasmid pAM beta1 in *Lactobacillus reuteri* and between lactobacilli and *Enterococcus faecalis*. *Applied and Environmental Microbiology, 53,* 2693–2695.

Temmerman, R., Pot, B., Huys, G. and Swings, J. (2003). Identification and antibiotic susceptibility of bacterial isolates from probiotic products. *International Journal of Food Microbiology, 81,* 1–10.

Tenorio, C., Zarazaga, M., Martínez, C. and Torres, C. (2001). Bifunctional enzyme 60-N-aminoglycoside acetyltransferase-200-O-aminoglycoside phosphotransferase in *Lactobacillus* and *Pediococcus* isolates of animal origin. *Journal of Clinical Microbiology, 39,* 824–825.

Teuber, M. (1995). The genus *Lactococcus*. In: Wood, B. J. B. and Holzapfel, W. H. (Eds.), The Genera of Lactic Acid Bacteria. Blackie Academic and Professional, London, pp. 173– 234.

Teuber, M. (1999). Spread of antibiotic resistance with food-borne pathogens. *Cellular and Molecular Life Science, 56,* 755–763.

Tiwari, H. K. and Sen, M. R. (2006). Emergence of vancomycin resistant *Staphylococcus aureus* (VRSA) from a tertiary care hospital from northern part of India. *BMC Infectious Diseases, 6,* 156-162 doi:10.1186/1471-2334-6-156.

Todorov, S. D., Botes, M., Danova, S.T. and Dicks, L. M. T. (2007). Probiotic properties of *Lactococcus lactis* subsp. *lactis* HV219, isolated from human vaginal secretions. *Journal of Applied Microbiology, 103,* 629–639.

Tomé, E., Gibbs, P. A. and Teixeira, P. C. (2008). Growth control of *Listeria innocua* 2030c on vacuum-packaged cold-smoked salmon by lactic acid bacteria. *International Journal of Food Microbiology, 121,* 285-294.

Torres, C., Rojo-Bezares, B., Sáenz, Y., Zarazaga, M. and Ruiz-Larrea, F. (2005). Antibiotic resistance phenotypes and mechanisms of resistance in lactic acid bacteria of oenological origin. Eighth Symposium on Lactic Acid Bacteria: Genetics, metabolism, and applications. FEMS, Egmond aan Zee, The Netherlands.

Tosi, L., Berruti, G., Danielsen, M., Wind, A., Huys, G. and Morelli, L. (2007). Susceptibility of *Streptococcus thermophilus* to antibiotics. *Antonie Van Leeuwenhoek International Journal of General and Molecular Microbiology, 92,* 21-28.

Treitman, A. N., Yarnold, P. R., Warren, J. and Noskin, G. A. (2005). Emerging incidence of *Enterococcus faecium* among hospital isolates (1993 to 2002). *Journal of Clinical Microiology, 43,* 462-463

Tynkkynen, S., Singh, K. V. and Varmanen, P. (1998). Vancomycin resistance factor of *Lactobacillus rhamnosus* GG in relation to enterococcal vancomycin resistance (*van*) genes. *International Journal of Food Microbiology, 41,* 195-204.

Van den Bogaard, A. E. and Stobberingh, E. E. (1999). Antibiotics in animal feeds and the emergence and dissemination of bacterial resistance in man. *Antibiotic Therapy and Control of Antimicrobial Resistance in Hospitals,* 6th Maurice Rapin Colloquium, OCT 22-23, 1998 Les Baux Provence, France, 51-60.

Van Epps, H.L. (2006). René Dubos: unearthing antibiotics. Journal of Experimental Medicine, 203, 259. doi:10.1084/jem.2032fta.

Vankerckhoven, V., Huys, G., Vancanneyt, M., Vael, C., Klare, I., Romond, M.-B., Entenza, J. M., Moreillon, P., Wind, R. D., Knol, J., Wiertz, E., Pot, B., Vaughan, E. E., Kahlmeter, G. and Goossens, H. (2008). Biosafety assessment of probiotics used for human consumption: recommendations from the EU-PROSAFE project. *Trends in Food Science and Technology, 19,* 102-114.

Vescovo, M., Morelli, L., Bottazzi, V. and Gasson, M. J. (1983). Conjugal transfer of broad-hostrange plasmid pAMß1 into enteric species of lactic acid bacteria. *Applied and Environmental Microbiology, 46,* 753–755.

Vesterlund, S., Vankerckhoven, V., Saxelin, M., Goossens, H., Salminen, S. and Ouwehand, A. C. (2007). Safety assessment of *Lactobacillus* strains: Presence of putative risk factors in faecal, blood and probiotic isolates. *International Journal of Food Microbiology, 116,* 325-331.

Villedieu, A., Díaz-Torres, M. L., Hunt, N., McNab, R., Spratt, D. A., Wilson, M. and Mullany, P. (2003). Prevalence of tetracycline resistance genes in oral bacteria. *Antimicrobial Agents and Chemotherapy, 47,* 878–882.

Walther, C., Rossano, A., Thomann, A. and Perreten, V. (2008). Antibiotic resistance in *Lactococcus* species from bovine milk: Presence of a mutated multidrug transporter *mdt*(A) gene in susceptible *Lactococcus garvieae* strains. *Veterinary Microbiology, 131,* 348–357.

Wang, T.T. and Lee, B.H. (1997). Plasmids in *Lactobacillus*. *Critical Review in Biotechnology, 17*, 227–272.

Wegener, H. C., Aarestrup, F. M., Jensen, L.B., Hammerum, A. M. and Bager, F. (1999). Use of antimicrobial growth promoters in food animals and *Enterococcus faecium* resistance to therapeutic antimicrobial drugs in Europe. *Emerging Infectious Diseases, 5,* 329-335.

Weiss, N., Schillinger, U., Laternser, M. and Kandler, O. (1981). *Lactobacillus sharpeaea* sp. nov. and *Lactobacillus agilis* sp. nov., two new species of homofermentative, meso-diaminopimelic acid-containing lactobacilli isolated from sewage. Zentralblatt fur Bakteriologie und Hygiene I Abteilung Oiginale C-Allgemeine Angewandte und Okologische Mikrobiologie C2, 242-253.

Whitehead, T. R. and Cotta, M. A. (2001). Sequence analyses of a broad hostrange plasmid containing ermT from a tylosin-resistant *Lactobacillus* sp. isolated from swine feces. *Current Microbiology 43*, 17–20.

Wisplinghoff, H., Bischoff, T., Tallent, S. M., Seifert, H., Wenzel, R. P. and Edmond, M. B. (2004). Nosocomial bloodstream infections in US hospitals: Analysis of 24,179 cases from a prospective nationwide surveillance study. *Clinical Infectious Diseases, 39,* 309-317.

Woodford, N., Jones, B. L., Baccus, Z., Ludlam, H. A. and Brown, D. F. (1995). Linkage of vancomycin and high-level gentamicin resistance genes on the same plasmid in a clinical isolate of *Enterococcus faecalis*. *Journal of Antimicrobials and Chemotherapy, 35*, 179–184.

Xiong, L., Kloss, P., Douthwaite, S., Andersen, N. M., Swaney, S., Shinabarger, D. L. and Mankin, A. S. (2000). Oxazolidinone resistance mutations in 23S rRNA of *Escherichia coli* reveal the central region of domain V as the primary site of drug action. *Journal of Bacteriology, 182,* 5325-5331.

Zanella, R. C., Lima, M. J. C., Tegani, L. S., Hitomi, A., Brandileone, M. C. C., Palazzo, I. C. V. and Darini, A. L. C. (2006). Emergence of VanB phenotype-vanA genotype in vancomycin-resistant enterococci in Brazilian hospital. *Brazilian Journal of Microbiology, 37,* 117–118.

Zarazaga, M., Sáenz, Y., Portillo, A., Tenorio, C., Ruiz-Larrea, F., Del Campo, R., Baquero, F. and Torres, C. (1999). In vitro activities of ketolide HMR3647, macrolides, and other antibiotics against *Lactobacillus, Leuconostoc*, and *Pediococcus* isolates. *Antimicrobial Agents and Chemotherapy, 43*, 3039–3041.

Zhou, J. S., Pillidge, C. J., Gopal, P. K. and Gill, H. S. (2005). Antibiotic susceptibility profiles of new probiotic *Lactobacillus* and *Bifidobacterium* strains. *International Journal of Food Microbiology, 98,* 211–217.

In: Antibiotic Resistance...
Editors: A. R. Bonilla and K. P. Muniz

ISBN 978-1-60741-623-4
© 2009 Nova Science Publishers, Inc.

Chapter XVIII

Nanobiotics to Combat Bacterial Drug Resistance

Sampath C. Abeylath and Edward Turos

Department of Chemistry, University of South Florida,
Tampa, FL,USA

Abstract

One of the major medical advances of the 20th century has been the development of effective antibiotics which have had a profound impact on the quality of human life. The ability to treat and cure deadly infections and bacterial diseases has forever changed our medical profession and way of life, providing unprecedented relief from pain, suffering, and death due to microbial infection. However, consistent overuse and misuse of powerful broad-spectrum antibiotics over several decades has added to and indeed accelerated the spread of microbial drug resistance. Resistance mechanisms have been found for every class of antibiotic agent used clinically. A major global healthcare problem relates to serious infections caused by bacteria having resistance to commonly used antibiotics. Not only are such infections typically more severe than those of antibiotic-responsive ones, they also require more aggressive interventive measures and are thus significantly more difficult and expensive to treat. Consequently, as we enter the 21st century, a pressing need exists for novel approaches to effectively deal with drug-resistant microbes and the health problems they pose. Nature may provide answers to help guide us, in the form of viral warriors known as bacteriophages, as a means to control and subdue pathogenic bacteria in their natural habitat. Like phages, which emerged presumably through a long evolutionary process, researchers now are acquiring the capabilities to target and neutralize deadly bacteria with *nano*particle-based anti*biotics*, or *nanobiotics*. This chapter discusses the different types of nanobiotics being investigated for delivering and improving therapeutic efficacy of a wide assortment of anti-infectives. The emphasis will be on nanoparticle containers or vehicles to overcome bacterial drug resistance that in essence protect and deliver various classes of antibiotic drugs, including β-lactams, fluoroquinolones, gentamycin, and vancomycin. A brief synopsis is provided on the role nanobiotics could play in drug discovery and development.

Introduction

The term *nanobiotics* is explicitly defined herein to refer to *particles measuring 1-350 nanometers in size and having antibacterial capabilities*.[1] The matrix of the particle may possess antibiotic effects itself, or carry an antibiotic drug within its interior or on its surface that can act upon a bacterial target. There are a variety of possible scenarios for how a nanoparticle may exert antibacterial action. Direct interaction with a microbe on the cell membrane could disrupt cellular function, such as the uptake of essential nutrients or intercellular communication, or induce microbes to clump unnaturally into non-viable, morphologically disrupted coagulates. Most commonly, antibacterial effects arise from the presence of an attached (or entrapped) antibiotic compound within (or on the surface) of the nanoparticle, which transfers the drug to the microbe upon contact. Likewise, there are all sorts of materials that can make up the nanoparticle matrix, and as such, the opportunities for developing nanobiotics with specified functions are seemingly endless.

Nanoparticles as Delivery Vehicles

Various types of drug delivery strategies have been explored with many different classifications of pharmacological agents, for the purpose of improving therapeutic efficacy through more favorable drug bioavailability, serum stability and pharmacokinetics. A representative listing can be found in the cited references.[2-50] The basic premise is a very simple one conceptually: to encase the drug within the protective matrix of a suitable delivery scaffold. Options for this are quite diverse, in terms of the materials that can be used for the delivery vehicle and the classes of therapeutic drug that could potentially be delivered, as well as with respect to biodegradation of the vehicle or targeting to a particular site in the body. An early example entailed the use of a natural macromolecule (DNA) in combination with an anticancer drug, doxorubicin, in an attempt to reduce undesirable cytotoxic effects of the chemothereutic agent in healthy human tissue.[51,52] The first systems used as drug delivery containers, developed in the early 1970s, consisted of microspheres and microcapsules that allowed drugs to be placed inside, and then implanted into the human body to release the active drug near the target site.[13] This was then followed by the use of colloidal particulates less than a micron in size having greater mobility in the body and thus better ability to actually carry, or deliver, a drug systemically. It was found, however, that after intravenous administration most colloidal particles are quickly scavenged by phagocytic cells in the liver and spleen, depending on the size and surface characteristics of the particulates, and concentrated there for elimination.[32] These early particulates thus had limited utility as drug carriers due to rapid clearance from the body as a result of plasma proteins depositing onto their surface, and subsequently recruiting phagocytes for disposal by the reticulo-endothelial system (RES). Stealth systems then came about by modifying the surface of the particles with surfactants that provided protection from these proteins, thus greatly enhancing the serum lifetimes (Figure 1).[19,30] This allowed for a longer period of controlled drug release. Couvreur′s early work with nanoparticles to deliver the anticancer compound doxorubicin demonstrated that the adsorption of doxorubicin onto poly(isobutyl cyanoacrylate) nanoparticles significantly reduced mortality and weight loss of mice under a variety of treatment regimens, and also diminished cardiotoxicity of the cancer drug due to poor uptake of the nanoparticle by the myocardium.[53] Target-seeking drug carriers have also been devised, by layering onto the surface of the vehicle a monoclonal antibody or other recognition elements that provide for specific recognition of a cellular target.[5,9,31]

Nanoparticles constitute another major category of delivery vehicles for a wide assortment of drug types and biomedical applicatiions.[8-49] By strict definition, these carriers may have dimensions of 1-1000 nm, but most of those reported in the literature are generally 5-350 nm in diameter, and can be made from essentially any type of biocompatible substance. The morphological and physical properties of nanoparticles can also vary across a broad spectrum, as can their methods of preparation. The different types of nanoparticle systems that have been studied so far for delivery of antibiotics are depicted schematically in Figure 2.

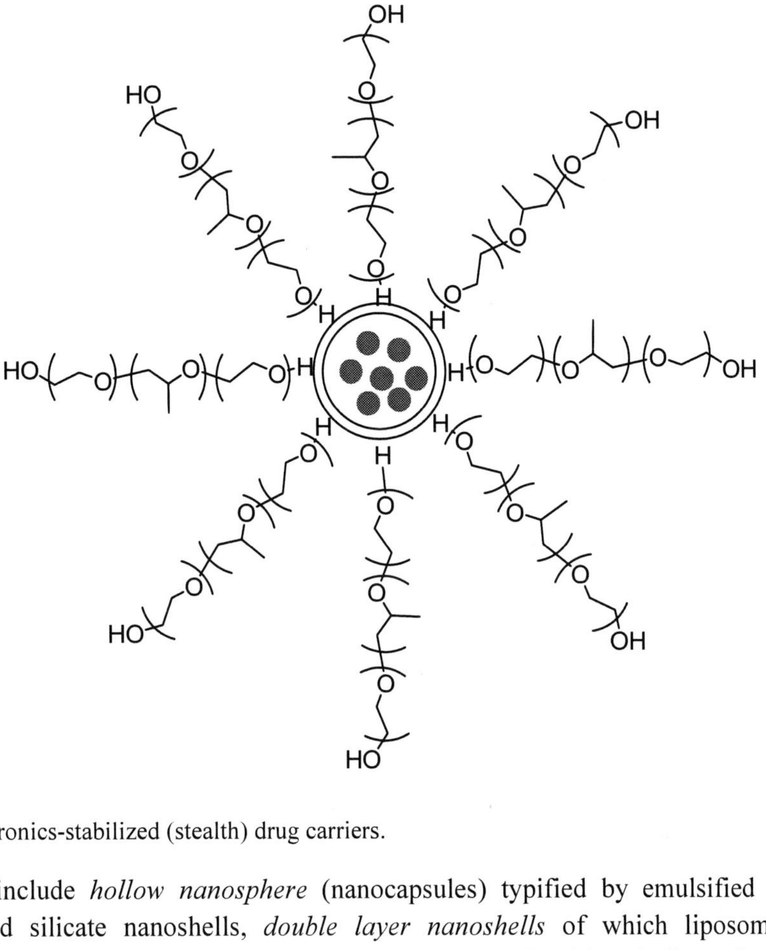

Figure 1. Pluronics-stabilized (stealth) drug carriers.

These include *hollow nanosphere* (nanocapsules) typified by emulsified oil-in-water droplets and silicate nanoshells, *double layer nanoshells* of which liposomes are one example, *solid core nanoparticles* such as those made of gold and silver, *hyperbranched nanoparticles* made of dendritic skeletal networks, and *perforated nanoparticles* that include emulsified organopolymers.

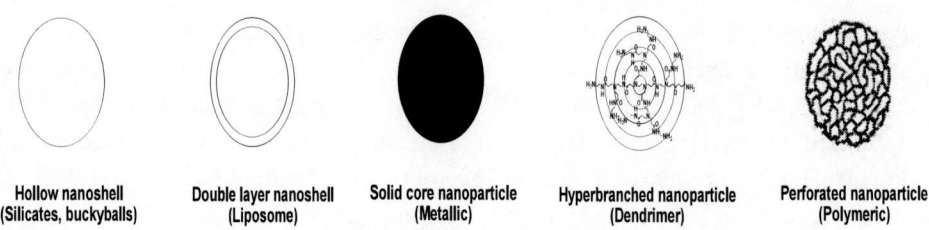

Hollow nanoshell | Double layer nanoshell | Solid core nanoparticle | Hyperbranched nanoparticle | Perforated nanoparticle
(Silicates, buckyballs) | (Liposome) | (Metallic) | (Dendrimer) | (Polymeric)

Figure 2. General types of nanoparticles used for antibiotics delivery (nanobiotics).

Hollow nanoshells and *double layer nanoshells* generally function as capsules by entrapping compounds inside their protected interior environment, but also can adsorb molecules onto their surface through either electrostatic interactions or covalent attachment. *Solid core* (metallic) nanoparticles have no empty regions in their interior, and can only carry molecules on their exterior. These uniformly shaped spherical particles generally measure only about 5 nm in diameter, but their large surface area enables a large number of molecules to be appended to the outside, or to be used as a rigid scaffold for building larger nanoscale structures. *Hyperbranched and perforated nanoparticles* are primarily polymeric matrices onto which drug molecules can either be chemically attached, or entrapped within the crevices of the matrix. It is fair to say that while some of these nanoparticle systems may have never been specifically designed for antibacterial drug delivery, or to overcome antibiotic resistance mechanisms per se, they appear to be very well suited for this purpose. Many of the developments in nanoparticle design and utility for antibiotic applications are relatively recent, yet often can be traced back to the very beginning of the antibiotics era. A short description of each nanoparticle system, as it applies to antibacterials, allows one to see what some of the described applications have been and where further opportunities may lie.

Nanoshells can be made of any polymeric material that can form a netlike structure with an empty interior cavity. To create this, the outer shell is made by polymerizing an appropriate monomeric substance around a solid core, which serves as a template for the polymerization. An excellent example of this was recently described by Stenzel and colleagues in the synthesis of novel polygalactose nanocages.[54] Initially, an amphiphilic block copolymer, poly(lactide)-*block*-poly(6-*O*-acryloyl-R-D-galactopyranose), was created in aqueous solution as micelles having pendent galactose moieties covering the surface. Using hexandiol diacrylate, these glycosylated micelles were then cross-linked using a reversible addition fragmentation chain transfer (RAFT) process to construct stable nanoparticle aggregates. The inner PLA core was then degraded away by aminolysis with hexylamine to afford the desired glycopolymer as hollow nanoballs. The authors hope to use these glycosylated nanoshells for drug delivery applications. *Inorganic nanoshells* can likewise be constructed by crafting a durable polymeric substance such as silicate around a solid core material such as calcium carbonate or a gold nanoparticle, with subsequent chemical erosion of the core to leave behind the intact silica shell.[42,48] These hollow nanoshells can be used to entrap a drug molecule inside for slow release, as will be discussed in more detail later. *Fullerenes*, such as C_{60}, constitute yet another type of nanoshell consisting of an impenetrable outer shell of interconnected carbon atoms onto which drug molecules can be chemically attached to the outer periphery. The van der Waals diameter of a

C_{60} molecule is about 1 nanometer (nm), which borders on the lower limit of a nanoparticle. These are interesting materials with intriguing physical properties, that can be exploited for drug delivery applications, but so far, they have not been employed to any great extent for antibiotics delivery. There is a report that an aqueous mixture of C_{60} and poly(vinylpyrrolidone) shows antibacterial activity upon photoirradiation, suggesting that this combination could serve as a potentially exploitable photoinduced antibacterial agent.[40] Additionally, cationic fullerenes can be light-activated and may be used as novel antimicrobial photosensitizers [41].

Liposomes have been studied as carriers of biologically active compounds since 1971 and evaluated intensively across various disease categories for drug delivery applications.[9] Liposomal nanoparticles consist of phospholipid bilayers with an aqueous phase in the center due to the hydrophilic heads of the liposome organizing towards the bulk aqueous media, and the hydrophobic tails lining up inwards. In water, this creates a relatively stable bilayer wherein a water-soluble drug such as penicillin can be entrapped within the aqueous core, while lipophilic molecules can concentrate in the lipophilic bilayer region. How liposomes function as delivery vehicles depends on the type of cells they interact with, but the premise is that delivery of an antibiotic occurs through endocytosis, which follows the initial interaction of the liposome with the cell membrane, either through a mediated or passive fusion of the lipoproteins, a process which inevitably releases the encapsulated drug. One of the drawbacks of liposomes is their stability, which may be difficult to control in terms of programmed drug release. Pegylated variants now exist that provide stealth properties and much longer serum lifetimes.[30] Hydrogels consist of polymer strands such as polyacrylic acid and poly(vinyl alcohol) that spontaneously form colloids in water.[36] As for liposomes, antibiotics can be entrapped inside the crosslinked matrix of hydrogels and be released in a controlled manner.[55] Indeed, a few antibiotics including gentamycin sulfate and vancomycin hydrochloride have been introduced inside hydrogels based on polyacrylic acid-gelatin constructs. The size ranges of these capsules are 2-2.5 mm in length and about 1 mm in width, well beyond the dimensions of even microparticles.[35] Nevertheless, the premise is that hydrogel-based systems can be developed for in vivo nanobiotic applications.

Metal nanoparticles have also been explored for a variety of drug delivery applications, including antibiotics. Their small (5 nm), spherical size and large, activated metal surface provide a facile means for coordinating drug molecules either through surface charges or covalent thiol linkages. Gold nanoparticles modified with cationically charged surface residues on are somewhat toxic due to their cidal interactions with cell membranes, while anionically charged groups are non-toxic.[56] Silver nanoparticles are also commonly employed for antibiotic applications, partly because they have bactericidal activity on their own, which may be the result of blocking cellular processes that affect bacterial survival.[57] The biocidal concentration of silver nanoparticles is nanomolar while silver ions is μmolar, indicating much stronger antimicrobial activity despite possibly having similar modes of action.[58] The antimicrobial activity of colloidal silver depends on the dimensions of the particles, with smaller ones having a greater effect. Panacek's studies showed that silver nanoparticles of average size of 25 nm have strong antimicrobial and bactericidal activity against both Gram-positive and Gram-negative bacteria, including multi-drug resistant microbes such as methicillin-resistant *S. aureus*. Silver nanoparticles combined with poly(methyl methacrylate) nanofiber composites have been found to kill bacterial three times more effectively than $AgNO_3$, and nine times that of silver sulfadiazine.[59] The silver nanofiber composite showed excellent biocidal potential against both Gram-positive bacteria (*S. aureus*) as well as Gram-negative bacteria (*Escherichia coli*). Thus, the material making up the matrix (including the exterior surfactant and surface residues) may endow the nanoparticle with antimicrobial behavior, and a secondary mode of action, that complements that of the antibiotic it may carry, which is an important attribute when dealing with multi-drug resistant bacteria.

Dendrimeric nanoparticles have unique chemical structures that make them highly suitable for drug delivery.[5,6] These are hyperbranched polymers or polymer-like assemblies comprised of co-centric layers of functionality, such as the polyamidoamino (PAMAM) structure shown in Figure 3 [60].

The interior crevices of dendrimers are well-suited for encapsulation of guest molecules and through chemical synthesis heteroatomic functionality (such as amines, carbonyls) can be suitably tailored for enhanced entrapment and delivery. The multivalent outer regions of more advanced (higher-generation) dendrimers, which have greater branching, can contain likewise reactive functional groups such as amines or carboxylic acids that permit sequestering of molecules through entrapment or covalent attachment. So far, however, this design has not been adequately explored. Tomalia has reported the preparation of PAMAM dendrimer-silver complexes that have strong antimicrobial activity against various Gram positive bacteria through a slow release of silver ions [61].

Polylysine-based dendrimers having mannosyl surface groups can inhibit adhesion of *E. coli* to horse blood cells, possibly making these nanostructures as antibacterial agents [62].

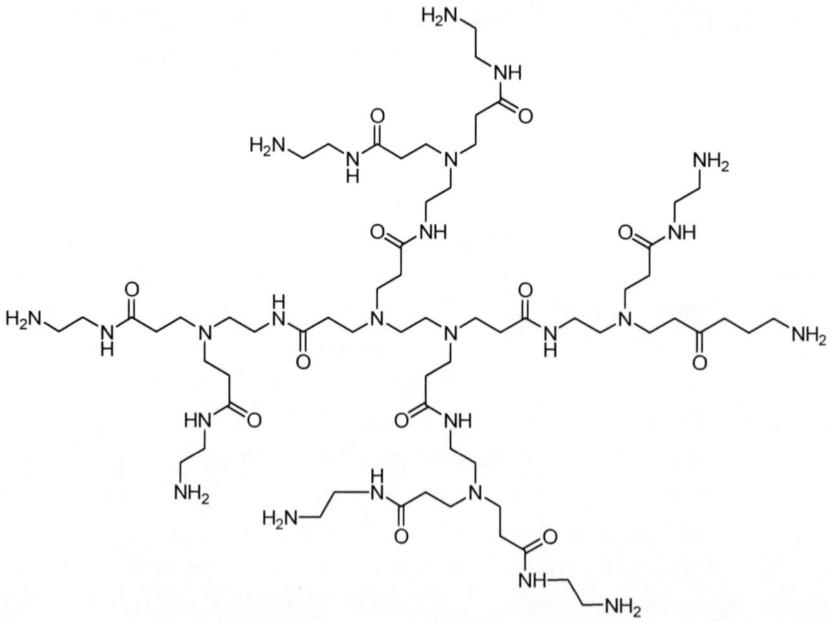

Figure 3. Example of a hyperbranched polyamidoamino (PAMAM) building block used to assemble dendrimeric nanoparticles.

In another study aimed at designing dendrimers that can sequester deadly bacterial carbohydrate-binding entities such as cholera toxin and *Escherichia coli* heat-labile toxin, a glycodendrimer was investigated and found to have pentavalent binding to cell surface glycolipids (GM1 gangliosides) [63]. Thus, carbohydrated dendrimer nanoparticles can be designed for selectively binding to and inhibiting glycosyl receptors on bacterial membranes, a feature that is well-suited for targeting of pathogenic bacteria and antibiotics. Dendrimers can also have potent antimicrobial activity on their own, without the need to carry antibacterial drugs, by virtue of their surface charge.[64-66] Such antibacterial dendrimers generally contain cationic surface functionalities such as amines or tetraalkyl ammonium groups which destabilize the bacterial cell membrane to induce cell lysis. Although only a few studies on the *in vivo* toxicity of dendrimers have been reported, dendrimer solutions injected into mice seem to be non-toxic [60,67].

Polymeric nanoparticles form a separate class of nanobiotic systems comprised of emulsified nanospheres in aqueous media, which can be made in a variety of ways from an assortment of monomeric building blocks such as those shown in Figure 4 [6-37].

Various methods for producing drug-carrying nanoparticles have been developed [3], including spray drying and ultra-fine milling, which give broad distributions of particle sizes [68], nanoprecipitation [69], and emulsion polymerization.[70] Nanoparticles are typically more stable than liposomes in biological fluids and during storage. Nanoparticles can have favorable pharmacological properties for drug delivery due to their biocompatibility, biodegradability, consistent morphology and uniquely small size that allows for targeted delivery.[9] Different tissues and organs respond to nanoparticles of specific size ranges. Nanoparticles under 100 nm in size can avoid being recognized by the RES and get into bone marrow, whereas those > 300 nm are quickly picked up by phagocytes (except for the stealths) and are not able to penetrate into heart and lung tissue.[71,72] Nanoparticles emulsified in water can usually be delivered orally and be readily absorbed in the gastrointestinal tract, in a manner through which the nanoparticle protects the drug from degradation while inside.[73] Once absorbed, the nanoparticles can serve as a drug reservoir in releasing the antibiotic over a prolonged period. This certainly has implications for overcoming drug resistance mechanisms in that the nanoparticles can navigate the sensitive antibiotic molecules through the regions around the resistant bacteria where hydrolyzing enzymes conduct surveillance. Nanoparticles can also be administered through intravenous, subcutaneous and intraperitoneal injection, which may have advantages depending on whether the resistant infection is localized in skin, certain tissues, or is systemic. Nanoparticles may also exhibit controlled release of antibiotics [25].

Polyacrylate-based nanoparticles have been studied as drug carriers since the 1970s, with Kreuter and Speiser showing the use of polyacrylamide nanoparticles forming in the presence of antigens that led to a novel vaccine adjuvant.[15] Three years later, Couvreur's laboratory reported on a series of poly(alkyl cyanoacrylate) (PACA) nanoparticles that are bioresorbable, and are being used as surgical glues.[16] Couvreur developed and investigated in detail PACA nanoparticles over a 30-year period, and has studied their use extensively with a wide variety of drugs (including antibiotics) both *in vitro* and *in vivo*.[29] Poly(alkyl cyanoacrylate) and polyacrylate nanoparticles are readily prepared in water at pH 3 by emulsion polymerization.[70]

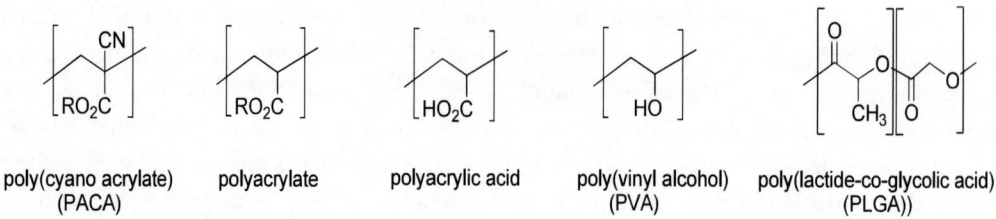

poly(cyano acrylate)   polyacrylate   polyacrylic acid   poly(vinyl alcohol)   poly(lactide-co-glycolic acid)
        (PACA)   (PVA)   (PLGA))

Figure 4. Polymeric platforms used to prepare emulsified nanoparticles for antibiotics delivery.

The procedure requires the use of surfactants to prevent aggregation and to control a uniform particle size distribution. Methods for the characterization and purification of polymeric nanoparticles have been described.[74] The effect of surfactant structure and charge on toxicity and antimicrobial activity of polyacrylate nanoparticle emulsions, as well as methods for purifying and removing unwanted toxic impurities, have likewise been investigated.[75] Most recently, studies on in vivo bioactivity of polyacrylate nanoparticles have been reported.[76] Couvreur has developed biodegradable nanoparticle frameworks that can be used for intracellular targeting of antibiotics.[77] Many types of lipophilic and water-soluble drugs, including various antibacterial classes, can be carried inside or on the surface of the nanoparticle, either through covalent attachment to the nanoparticle matrix, or by encapsulation or surface association. These will be described in more detail later the chapter.

Chitosan nanoparticles represent another popular drug delivery vehicle [39,40], which has recently started to find applications in the antibiotics area.[78-95] Chitosan is a non-toxic biopolymer prepared by saponification of the N-acyl side chain of chitin, a natural substance obtained commercially from crab shells and shrimp (Figure 5).

Although chitosan polymer itself has antimicrobial properties, through the effects of its polycationic nature on bacterial membrane stability and permeability, its low solubility in water and need for low pH (below 6.5) somewhat limits its drug delivery capabilities.[79-84] A number of studies on the effect of structure, degree of N-acylation, size, and derivatization on antibacterial activity has been described in the literature.[85-93] Recently, however, chitosan nanoparticles have been made that offer consider promise for antibacterial applications, particularly with regards to overcoming microbial drug resistance [94-96]. Qi and colleagues have evaluated the antibacterial activity of chitosan nanoparticles and copper-loaded chitosan nanoparticles against a variety of common microorganisms, including *E. coli*, *S. choleraesuis*, *S. typhimurium*, and *S. aureus*.[78] Copper ion was adsorbed onto the chitosan nanoparticle surface by ion-exchange, and characterized structurally by a number of physical methods.

The copper-free chitosan nanoparticles measured from 28 to 49 nm with an average of diameter of around 40 nm, while the copper-complexed nanoparticles were much larger, measuring on average 257 nm with a broad size distrubution from 65 to 664 nm. Both are insoluble in water, dilute acid and dilute base, with a positively-charged surface The bioactivity of both nanoparticle systems was impressive, with minimum inhibitory concentration (MIC) values below 0.25 ug/mL and minimum bactericidal concentration (MBC) values of around 1 ug/mL.

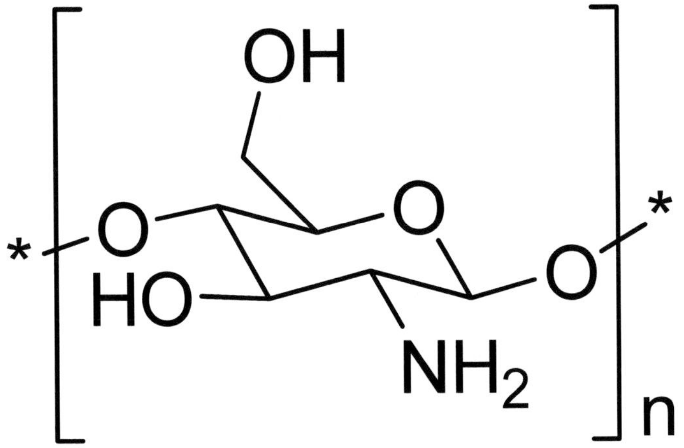

Figure 5. Chitin.

Atomic force microscopy confirmed that the chitosan nanoparticles disrupted the bacterial cell membranes, leading to leakage of cytoplasmic contents. Thus, the chitin nanoparticles were considerably more bioactive than chitin polymer, undoubtedly testimony to the fact that it is much smaller in size and compact in cationic charge and able to interact more aggressively towards the bacterial membrane. The copper-adsorbed chitosan nanoparticles, in turn, were about twice as strong in activity than the chitosan nanoparticles. It was suggested by the authors that this slight enhancement in activity of the copper-entrapped nanoparticles could be due to their enlarged size, greater cationic surface charge, or the possible slow release of copper ion by the matrix into the bacterial membrane, but this has not yet been confirmed. While antimicrobial activity appears to be fairly uniform across gram-positive and gram-negative microbes, multi-drug-resistant microbes were not tested in this initial study. A further caveat is that the microbiological assays were done in 0.25% acetic acid (due to the insoublity of the nanoparticles in neutral pH) and bioactivity was said to be lower in aqueous solution. In follow-up to this work, Chen and coworkers investigated N-oleoyled chitosan particles, which could be prepared by oil-in-water (O/W) emulsification, against *E. coli* and *S. aureus*, as a function of varying the chitosan molecular weight, degree of substitution, concentration of the nanoparticles, and pH.[97] Although described as being self-assembled nanoparticles, information about the actual particle size range was not reported, nor was the surface charge. The antibacterial effects of the N-oleoylated chitosan dispersion were considerably weaker than that of chitosan nanoparticles or the copper-coordianted nanoparticles, with MIC values being from 31 to 125 ug/mL for *E. coli* and 125 ug/mL for *S. aureus*. Antibacterial activity against *E. coli* decreased with increasing molecular weight of the chitosan used, but not for *S. aureus*. Cell membrane disruption and leakage caused by the N-oleoyl chitosan O/W dispersion was observed.

A conceptually different type of nanoparticle construct having cidal effects on bacteria was described by Ghadiri, in which a mixture of different D and L cyclic peptides self-assemble into elongated nanotubes.[98] The investigators found that six- and eight-residue cyclic D,L-α-peptides are cidal to both Gram-positive and/or Gram-negative bacterial membranes but not to mammalian cells, by causing an increase of membrane permeability, loss of transmembrane ion potential, and rapid cell death. The effectiveness of this class of materials as selective antibacterial agents was demonstrated against a lethal MRSA infection in mice. Cyclic peptides are proteolytically stable, easy to synthesize, and can potentially be matched to interact specifically with discrete membrane components.

Bacteriophages- Nature´s Very Own Nanobiotics

With the widespread development of antibiotic resistance in pathogenic bacteria, the use of bacteriophages (phages) has long been recognized as an alternative to small molecule antibiotics in safely controlling bacterial infections. Phages are bacterial viruses, usually measuring between 20 and 200 nm in size, and consisting of a DNA or RNA genome hidden within a tough protein coat called a capsid (Figure 6).[99] The first known therapeutic use of phages in humans dates back to World War I (1919) with a flurry of early interest in antibacterial therapy. However, a lack of understanding of basic phage biology led to a series of clinical failures, and excitement soon waned when the era of antibiotics arrived in the 1930s and 1940s. Like all viruses, phages are metabolically inert in their extracellular form, reproducing only after infecting suitable host bacteria.[100] When a bacteriophage comes upon a target bacterium, its tail fibers search the outer cell surface for the molecular features that distinguish it as a suitable host, and subsequently bind to the surface before injecting its genetic material into the cell. There are two main groups of bacteriophages – *lytic* and *lysogenic* – differing in how they get their host to replicate their genetic information. *Lytic* bacteriophages instruct the machinery in the host cell to synthesize more bacteriophages, until the point that the bacterium bursts to release fully viable progeny viruses to begin the cycle again. Each cycle takes an average of 30 minutes and produces 50–400 phages, and is repeated until all the bacteria are consumed. *Lysogenic* bacteriophages attach their genetic strands directly onto the bacterial DNA where it gets replicated along with the bacteria nucleic acid. Phage DNA can be cut free from the host's DNA at any time, which in turn instructs the host cell to continue replicating phage in this manner until newly formed bacteriophages are released without damaging the infected cell. The killing effect of the lytic phages make them particularly attractive as antibacterials. Bacteriophages have the advantage in that they cannot infect mammalian cells, but selectively target and act upon selected bacteria. This action is, in fact, so highly specific and regulated that it can ensure one bacterial species or, in some cases, even just a single strain of bacteria, is acted upon.[101]

Phages have several characteristics that make them potentially attractive therapeutic agents: they are (i) extremely effective in lysing targeted pathogenic bacteria, (ii) they are generally safe, as underscored by their extensive clinical use in Eastern Europe and the former Soviet Union and the commercial sale of phages in the 1940s in the United States, and (iii) they are able to be quickly modified to combat the emergence of newly emerging bacterial threats.[102] Now, as the problem of antibiotic resistance becomes ever more acute, bacteriophages are being re-evaluated as the basis of new therapeutic strategies.

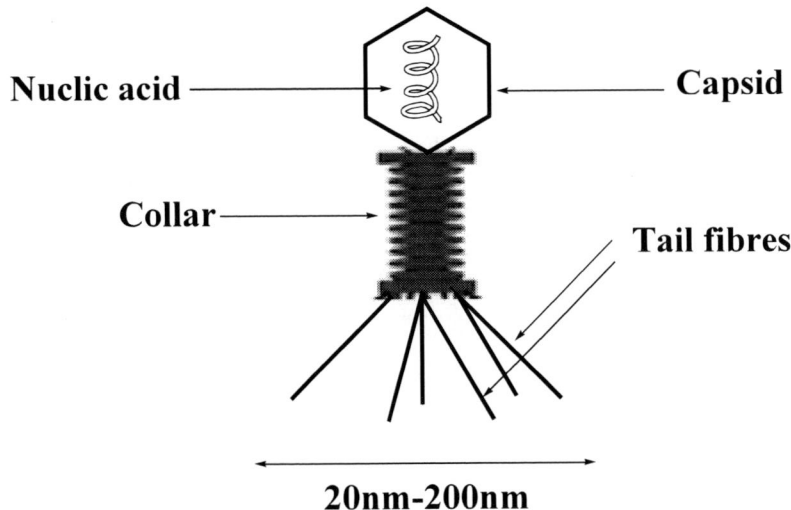

Figure 6. A schematic representation of a bacteriophage.

There is some concern in phages having the ability to also transfer virulence genes and those mediating resistance to antibiotics to other bacteria. Yet, it is this specificity and efficiency in how phages identify their bacterial targets that inspire designers of synthetic nanoparticles for use against selected pathogenic microorganisms.

More recently, synthetically-modified viral nanoparticles such as cowpea mosaic virus have been investigated as a means to construct durable nanoblocks having "addressable" surface functionality.[103,104] Although these chemically-mutated viruses appear to be directed towards materials research applications, their potential for use in nanobiology and drug delivery is likewise apparent.

Nanoparticles as Antibiotic Drug Delivery Vehicles

So far, the vast majority of reported studies and applications using nanoparticle drug carriers have been for targeted delivery of cancer chemotherapeutics to mammalian cells. However, the use of nanoparticles for antibiotics delivery have also been studied, albeit to a much lesser degree.[12] The employment of nanoparticles for delivery of antibiotics is thus a relatively young and under-explored area of investigation. The vast majority of studies on nanoparticles as antibiotic carriers have been restricted to only a few well-known antibiotic drugs, such as ciprofloxacin and penicillin. More recently, efforts have centered on the development of drug delivery approaches to overcome bacterial drug resistance, such as for new lipophilic β-lactam antibiotics [105] and delivery to intracellular pathogens which are dormant.[106] However, the vast majority of research reported so far has not been specifically focused on multi-drug resistance mechanisms, and thus an opportunity exists to do so. The following section provides a short discussion .on the most common classes of antibiotics available for use with nanoparticles, and the problem of multi-drug bacterial resistance.

Classes of Antibiotics and their Modes of Action: The entire history of humankind can be regarded from a medical perspective as a continuing struggle for survival against infectious diseases, which are still the second-leading cause of death worldwide and the third cause of death in developed countries.[107,108] Since the introduction of penicillin into clinical use in the early 1940's, a number of new classes of antibiotic compounds have been developed in pharmaceutical laboratories which have likewise contributed to improvement of human health. Before commercial antibiotics were available, bacterial infections such as meningitis and endocarditis were almost uniformly fatal, and common infections such as *Staphylococcus aureus* bacteraemia had a mortality of 80%.[109] Antibiotics are specifically defined as naturally-occurring compounds produced by actinomycetes, fungi, or bacteria that interfere with some essential bacterial structure or process, preventing their growth, virulence or replication (bacteriostatic effects), or survival (bactericidal effects), with no deleterious effects on the eukaryotic host.[110] Most classes of antibiotics have been chemically modified in the laboratory to confer better drug properties. Thus, in addition to the natural antimicrobial compounds, a large number of semi-synthetic and fully-synthetic compounds have been generated by chemists which kill or inhibit the growth of various bacteria. For the sake of this discussion, we will not distinguish between the natural and synthetically-derived antibacterials, but instead, refer generically to all as antibiotics. Antibiotics are usually classified on the basis of their chemical structure and mode of action, with the main classes being the β-lactams, cyclic peptides, aminoglycosides, tetracyclines, macrolides, lincosamides, oxazolidinones, quinolones, as well as sulfa drugs (Figure 7). These act upon one of four primary cellular processes in bacteria: (i) cell wall biosynthesis, (ii) protein biosynthesis, (iii) nucleic acid biosynthesis, and (iv) folate biosynthesis.[111]

Cell wall biosynthesis inhibitors: Both Gram-positive and Gram-negative bacteria are surrounded by a cell wall, composed mainly of a peptidoglycan: a strong net-like polymer responsible for maintaining the shape and size of the bacterial cell and for resisting the high intracellular osmotic pressure. The cell wall also serves as a physical barrier to separate the contents inside the cell from the extracellular environment. The glycan component of this rigid cell wall structure consists of alternating units of *N*-acetylmuramic acid (NAM) and *N*-acetylglucosamine (NAG), with a short peptide stem being attached to NAM via its nitrogen side chain. In cell wall biosynthesis, these short peptide fragments in adjacent glycan strands are important, in that at the appropriate time of presentation outside the cell membrane, are enzymatically crosslinked together to produce the characteristic web-like structure of the peptidoglycan. These final steps of peptidoglycan biosynthesis occur extracellularly through biochemical processes that are mediated by enzymes associated with the cellular membrane. Most commonly referred to as penicillin-binding proteins (PBPs), their main function is to crosslink peptide chains between adjoining glycan strands. *β-Lactam antibiotics* such as the penicillins (1) are bactericidal agents that inhibit bacterial cell wall crosslinking. Penicillin is morphologically similar to the D-alanyl-D-alanine terminus of the pentapeptide attached to *N*-acetylmuramic acid, and fits neatly inside the active site of the PBP. It is here that penicillin irreversibly binds to the protein by acylating the catalytic serine residue. This event disrupts cell wall synthesis by blocking transpeptidation of the nascent peptidoglycan, thus causing the bacterial cells to become more permeable to water and eventually lyse open.[112-115] Cyclic peptides such as *vancomycin* (2), an antibiotic used as a last resort against drug-resistant bacterial infections, also target the pentapeptide terminus undergoing enzymatic crosslinking. Vancomycin, however, binds tightly to the terminal D-alanyl-D-alanine residue and thereby keeps it from entering the active site of the PBPs. This substrate sequestration leads to the failure of peptidoglycan crosslinks, making the cell wall susceptible to osmolysis.[116]

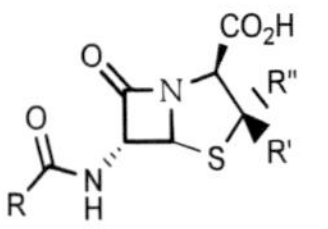

Penicillin (1)

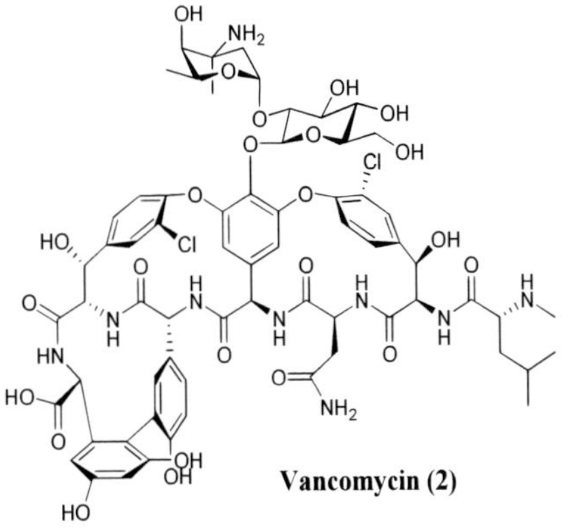

Vancomycin (2)

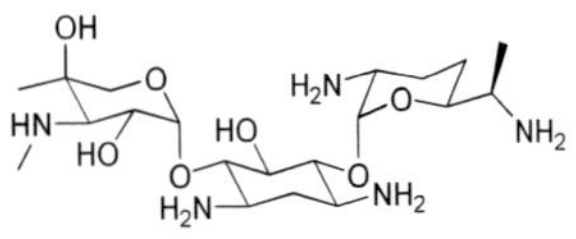

Gentamicin (3)

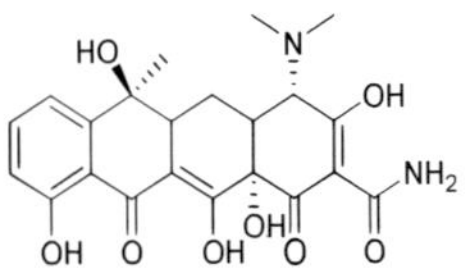

Tetracycline (4)

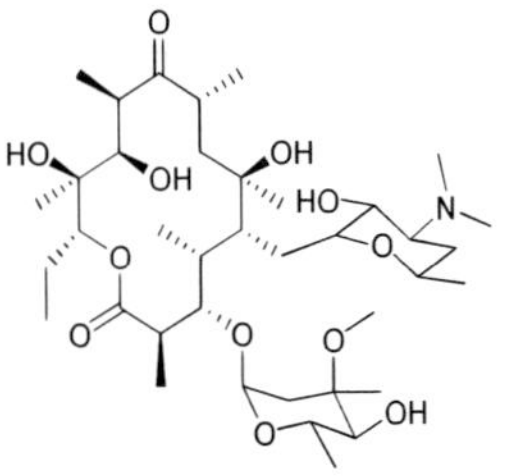

Erythromycin A (5)

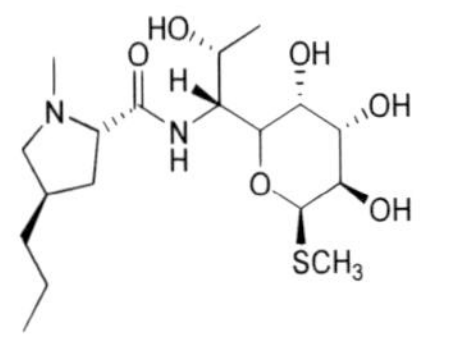

Lincomycin (6)

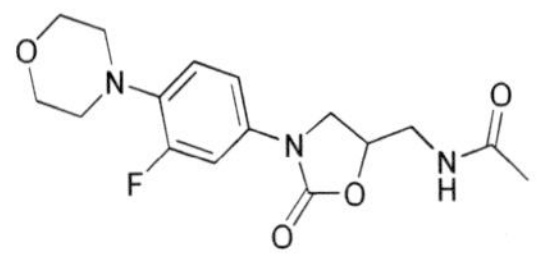

Linezolid (7)

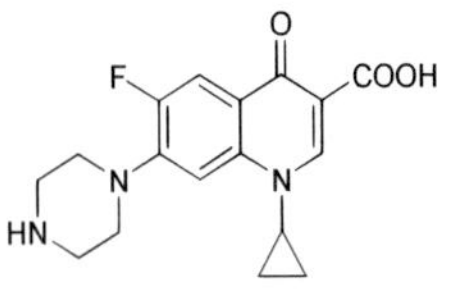

Ciprofloxacin (8)

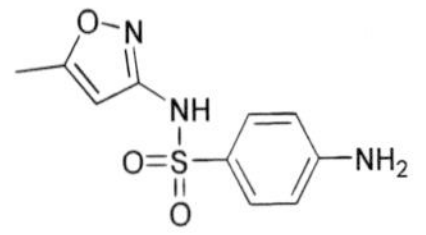

Sulfamethoxazole (9)

Figure 7. Common classes of antibiotics: β-lactams (1), cyclic peptides (2), aminoglycosides (3), tetracyclines (4), macrolides (5), lincosamides (6), oxazolidinones (7), quinolones (8), and sulfa antibiotics (9).

Protein biosynthesis inhibitors: The polynucleic acids direct the formation of proteins needed by the cell through catalysis by the 30S and 50S ribosomal subunits.[117] These two units come together to initiate the protein synthesis and separate when synthesis is complete. There are many highly regulated steps involved in protein biosynthesis, which includes initiation, elongation, and termination. The cellular machinery of prokaryotes differs substantially from their eukaryotic counterpart, enabling certain antibiotics to be effective and selective for bacteria. *Aminoglycosides* such as gentamycin (3) and *tetracylines* (4) interact with the conserved sequences of the 30S subunit while *macrolides* such as erythromycin A (5) and *lincosamides* like lincomycin (6) associate with the 50S subunit.[118-120] Although the mode of action of *oxazolidinones* such as linezolid (7) is not completely clear, it has been shown that they also bind to the 50S ribosomal subunit and have no affinity for the 30S subunit.[121]

Nucleic acid biosynthesis inhibitors: DNA replication is an essential process for all organisms. Bacterial chromosomal DNA is packed in a highly twisted (supercoiled) state in the cell, and dramatically changes its structure during the replication process.[122] The enzymes involved in the interconversion of topologically different forms of DNA are called topoisomerases. The DNA topoisomerases are classified into type I and type II. Type I topoisomerase transiently breaks one of the twin DNA strands while type II topoisomerase cleaves both strands at the same time. The *quinolones* such as ciprofloxacin (8) target type II topoisomerase, DNA gyrase, and affects the double-strand cleavage/double-strand religation equilibrium in the gyrase catalytic reaction, in such a way that the cleaved complex accumulates by stabilization in the presence of the quinolone.[123]

Folate inhibitors: Sulfa antibiotics (9), or para-aminophenylsulfonamides, kill bacteria by interfering with folic acid metabolism by virtue of their structural similarity to the natural cellular substrate, para-aminobenzoic acid.[124] Sulfamethoxazole selectively inhibits folate biosynthesis by forming a product that cannot be a substrate for the dihydropteroate synthase enzyme, an enzyme possessed by bacteria but not humans.

Antibiotic resistance: Antibacterial drugs have been in clinical use for more than 60 years and their extensive availability in hospitals and throughout the global community has created major pressures for bacteria to become more drug-resistant. Antibiotic resistance is an evolutionary response for bacteria to avoid being killed off by the therapeutic agent.[125] It seems that whatever antibacterial drug is used, bacteria quickly adapt by developing resistance, thus highlighting the need for more innovative approaches that can provide longer-term solutions to this ever-growing problem. One of the more recent areas of investigation towards this goal lies in the development of delivery platforms that improve the effectiveness of antibiotics while trying to minimize the onset of further resistance.

Clinically significant resistance appears after months to years after a new antibiotic is introduced into medical use.[126,127] For example, penicillin resistance was detected a few years after its clinical debut in 1942 [128], and streptomycin, a year after its discovery in 1944.[129,130] In the exceptional case of vancomycin, its resistance appeared almost 30 years (in 1987) after its clinical introduction.[131] The long delay was likely due in part to limited use of vancomycin in the first 25 years, since the other effective antibiotics were available during the "antibiotics era" of the 1950s through the 1960s. But then indiscriminate use of antibiotics resulted in the emergence of methicillin-resistant *Staphylococcus aureus* (MRSA), which exhibits multi-antibiotic resistance against many structurally unrelated antibiotics.[132] In turn, vancomycin-resistant *Enterococci* (VRE) appeared in 1986 due to widespread use of vancomycin, which was regarded as the antibiotic of last resort.[133,134] Then the discovery of partially vancomycin-resistant strains of *S. aureus* in 1997 led to the first case of fully vancomycin-resistant *S. aureus*.[135].

Antibiotic resistance can be either intrinsic (natural) or acquired. An example of intrinsic resistance is *Pseudomonas aeruginosa*, an opportunistic pathogen whose low membrane permeability is likely a main reason for its innate protection from many antibiotics.[136,137]

Acquired resistance is caused by acquisition of a plasmid and/or transposon that harbors determinants for resistance, or by chromosome mutation.[129,134] The major mechanisms of antibiotic resistance are (i) prevention of accumulation of antibiotics in the cytoplasm by decreasing cellular uptake or increasing efflux out of the cell, (ii) inactivation of antibiotics by hydrolysis or structural modification, (iii) alteration of the cellular target in order to reduce affinity for antibiotics, and (iv) over-produce the enzyme to compensate for antibiotic activity.[126,129,136,138].

Preventing access of antibiotics to their cellular targets results from decreasing the influx or increasing the efflux of antibiotics across biological membranes.[136,139] *P. aeruginosa*, once again, exemplifies this mechanism of antibiotic resistance. Mutants lacking an outer membrane porin channel, OprD2, decrease the uptake of carbapenem, a β-lactam antibiotic, and increase resistance to this antibiotic by ensuring low accessibility of the drug to its target, penicillin-binding protein.[136,140] A mutation resulting in over-expression of a multi-drug efflux pump, MexAB-OprM, renders this organism resistant to a wide variety of structurally unrelated antibiotics.[141,142] Since a loss-of-function mutation in the MexAB-OprM efflux pump causes hypersensitivity toward various antibiotics, the intrinsic resistance of this organism appears to be due mainly to an active efflux of antibiotics.[141,143] From the first indication that plasmid-coded tetracycline resistance in *E. coli* is due to energy-dependent efflux of the drug [139], this mechanism of antibiotic resistance, namely transmembrane efflux of antibiotics, led to the recognition of the widespread presence of multi-drug efflux pumps in bacteria evoking resistance to clinically important drugs.[136,137] Overcoming this obstacle has been very difficult.

Enzymatic inactivation of antibiotics either by hydrolysis or by modification provides another major mechanism of resistance in pathogenic bacteria to natural antibiotics such as β-lactams and aminoglycosides.[126,129] There are four known classes of β-lactamases, the primary cause of acquired resistance to β-lactam antibiotics. In their active site, these hydrolytic enzymes contain either a serine residue (classes A, C, D) or a coordinated metal ion (Zn^{2+}) (class B) that mediates the hydrolytic cleavage of the β-lactam ring.[144] The serine β-lactamases cleave penicillins by first forming covalent penicilloyl-*O*-serine intermediates that are then hydrolyzed to inactive by-products.[145] In contrast to β-lactams, the aminoglycoside antibiotics do not possess hydrolytically fragile groups. Thus, the enzymatic inactivation strategy for aminoglycoside-resistant bacteria is to modify the OH and NH_2 groups of the aminoglycosides.[146,147] Aminoglycosides bind specifically to regions on the 30S ribosome subunit near the site for aminoacyl-tRNA binding by forming strong hydrogen bonds through the hydroxyl and amino groups.[148,149] This high affinity of aminoglycosides for rRNA inhibits protein biosynthesis. Enzymatic modification of aminoglycosides disrupts the hydrogen bonding sufficiently to lower the affinity of the drugs for rRNA, and enhance resistance.

Although definitive evidence for the origin of the antibiotic-resistant determinants remains to be found, such resistance determinants most probably are acquired by pathogenic bacteria from a pool of resistance genes in other microbial genera, including antibiotic-producing organisms. β-Lactamase was identified in 1940, several years before the introduction of penicillin into clinical use, indicating that there may have already been a pool of antibiotic resistant genes existing in Nature [150].

In contrast to enzymatic inactivation of natural antibiotics, no enzymes that hydrolyze or modify man-made antibiotics such as sulfonamides, trimethoprim, and quinolones have been found. The mechanism of antibiotic resistance for these synthetic antibiotics and those natural products such as rifampicin, where inactivating enzymes have not been identified, is commonly achieved by target alterations. The most common mechanism of target alteration is the acquisition of new genes, carried on plasmids or transposons, which result in enzymatic modification of the normal target so that it does not bind the antibiotics. The erythromycin family of macrolides and the streptogramin B family exemplify this mechanism of antibiotic resistance.[126,151] In erythromycin-resistant bacteria, the exocyclic amino group of a specific adenine residue, A2058, in 23S rRNA is mono- or dimethylated by an Erm (erythromycin-ribosome methylation) methyltransferase, resulting in cross-resistance to macrolides, lincosamides, and streptogramin B (MLS$_B$ phenotype). [152,153] This modification reduces the affinity of the rRNA for the antibiotics but does not interfere with protein biosynthesis. The recent crystal structure of the 50S subunit of the ribosome complexed with erythromycin revealed the importance of hydrogen bonds between erythromycin and A2058 of 23S rRNA. [120] Erm is the major resistance mechanism in erythromycin-resistant *Staphylococcus aureus* and is present in erythromycin-producing organisms as a mechanism of self-protection.[151,152] Another example of target alteration can be seen in VRE. Five clinical phenotypes of vancomycin resistance have been identified so far, VanA, VanB, VanC, VanD and VanE.[155] The enzymes in VanA, VanB, and VanD resistance are involved in reprogramming of the peptidoglycan termini from D-Ala-D-Ala to D-Ala-D-lactate, which decreases the binding affinity of vancomycin to its native target (D-Ala-D-Ala) by 1000-fold, leading to a high vancomycin resistance.[156] On the other hand, VanC and VanE replaces the terminal D-Ala with D-Ser, leading to low-level resistance.[157].

Bacterial resistance to β-lactam antibiotics can be caused not only by β-lactamase, but also by alteration (or mutation) of penicillin binding proteins to lower the binding affinity of β-lactam drugs.[126,138] Unlike many other pathogens, *Streptococcus pneumoniae* does not employ β-lactamases as the major mechanism of resistance to β-lactams, but rather depends on the structural variation of PBPs. The most highly β-lactam-resistant clinical isolates produce altered forms of high-molecular weight PBPs that have reduced affinity for β-lactams.[158-161] Evidence shows that MRSA has acquired the *mecA* gene, which encodes a new PBP, termed PBP2' (also PBP2A), having relatively low affinity for all β-lactams.[126,138]

There is now a pressing need for ways to combat (or capitalize on) antibiotic resistance mechanisms, and to develop novel drug delivery approaches for targeting microbial pathogens, such as MRSA. The employment of nanoparticle carriers for antibiotic delivery has included a variety of different systems. Nanoparticles hold significant promise for both drug delivery and modification of the mechanism of action needed to overcome antibiotic resistance. We discuss in the following sections the use of nanoparticles as a means to enhance the performance of antibiotics against drug-resistant bacteria.

β-Lactam-Based Nanobiotics

Given the widespread use of β-lactam antibiotics and their profound success over the years in treating bacterial infections, it is not surprising to also find longstanding interest in combining them with nanoparticles. Couvreur's laboratory has done extensive work in this field, having more than three decades of investigation into poly(cyano acrylate) nanoparticles and their use as antibiotic carriers. These can conveniently be made by anionic polymerization in water in the presence of suitable surfactants.[9,11,23,25,29,53,77] One such example includes the use of poly(isohexyl cyanoacrylate) (PICA) nanoparticles for the non-covalent entrapment of ampicillin. Conveniently, these nanoparticle emulsions can be freeze-dried to remove the water, providing nanoparticle powders that are stable in storage and can then be readily reconstituted by addition of water. The size of the nanoparticles prepared in this manner depend on the amount of drug loading- ranging from around 130 nm for no drug, to about 200 nm for 2 mg/ml of loaded ampicillin. Freeze-drying does not affect nanoparticle size or its properties. Efficiency of drug loading into the nanoparticle matrix, and subsequent drug release, both depend on the type of cyanoacrylate ester used to build the nanoparticle matrix. Interestingly, encapsulation of ampicillin into polyisohexyl cyanoacrylate nanoparticles significantly enhances efficacy of the drug by 120-fold in treating intracellular infections in mice.[23] Mice infected with *Salmonella typhimurium* responded to merely 0.8 mg of ampicillin bound to the nanoparticles in the same way as three 32 mg doses of ampicillin itself. Similarly, these nanoparticles increased bioactivity of the β-lactam by 20 times in treating *L. monocytogenes* infection. Ultrasonic autoradiography indicated that the nanoparticles diffuse through the human cell to target the cell wall of the bacteria living inside.[106] This impressive activity enhancement is thought to be due to not only improved cellular uptake of the water-soluble antibiotic when carried by the nanoparticle, but also to an increase in concentration of drug by capture of the nanoparticles in the liver and spleen where the infection microbe resides. Thus, these nanoparticles help in the delivery of β-lactams to intracellular bacteria, especially those taking up residence in the RES organs.

Poly(ethyl cyanoacrylate) (PECA) nanoparticles have likewise been investigated as a means to entrap β-lactam antibiotics for use as colloidal suspensions in aqueous media [17,18]. More recently, Fontana employed pluronics (non-ionic polyoxyethylenepolyoxypropylene block co-polymers) of different molecular weight ranges to produce amoxicillin-loaded poly(cyano acrylate) nanoparticles of around 350 nm.[19] Different drug concentrations do not alter the size of these particles, which are stable at physiological pH for at least 5 hours but rapidly degrade in acidic media. Release of ampicillin is thus dependent on the pH and the surfactant structure, with quicker release occurring for less hydrophilic and larger molecular weight pluronics as surfactant. The hydrolysis of the ester side chain of the poly(alkyl cyanoacrylate) is the main degradation mechanism, which can be catalyzed by esterase hydrolysis at pH 7.4. Antimicrobial activity of PECA nanoparticles was found to be equal to or greater than that of free ampicillin, but studies against resistant microbes have not been reported. Fontana later introduced amoxicillin-loaded PECA nanoparticles which are surface coated with pluronic F68. For these, particle size is dependent on the molecular weight of the PEG additive, but is generally

200-320 nm. Uptake by phagocytes is greatly reduced for the PEG-coated (stealth) nanoparticles compared with non-pegylated systems, thus increasing dramatically the serum half-life and drug carrier capabilities. These PECA nanoparticles may be particularly useful for site-specific delivery of β-lactams to the stomach.

More recently, the Turos laboratory developed a facile chemical procedure for preparing antibacterially-active polyacrylate nanoparticles, which enhances the water-solubility and antibacterial properties of highly lipophilic N-thiolated β-lactam antibacterials.[120,162,163] In this method, the water-insoluble antibiotic was first converted to an acrylated form, then dissolved in a mixture of liquid monomers (butyl acrylate and styrene) before being emulsified with a surfactant and polymerized in the presence of a water-soluble radical initiator (Figure 8). This procedure affords much smaller polyacrylate-styrene nanoparticles (45 nm) as emulsions, which enhance the performance of water-insoluble antibiotics which passively target sites within the bacterial cell. These nanoparticle antibiotics were found to have promising in vitro antibacterial properties against MRSA and *B. anthracis*.

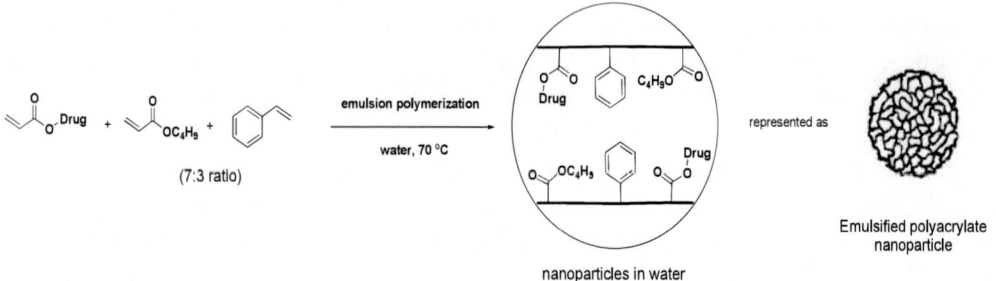

Figure 8. Emulsion polymerization of acrylated β-lactam drug monomers to make antibiotic-conjugated poly(butyl acrylate-styrene) nanoparticle emulsions in water.

As a consequence of the emulsion polymerization, all of the antibiotic is covalently attached to the polymeric matrix of the nanoparticle, and can only be released as an active drug by hydrolysis of the linkage. The nature of this linkage seems to be critical for activity, since the order of in vitro antimicrobial activity follows that of hydrolytic sensitivity.

This polymer-based nanotechnology has also been demonstrated to rejuvenate antibacterial activity of water-soluble penicillins against β-lactamase-producing forms of *S. aureus*.[164] Penicillin-containing polyacrylate nanoparticles, prepared by free radical emulsion polymerization in water using either acrylated penicillin monomers (for covalent attachment to the nanoparticle matrix) or penicillin esters (for encapsulation into the nanoparticle), retain their full antimicrobial properties in the presence of ultrahigh concentrations of β-lactamase. This "protective" effect is illustrated in the microbiological experiment shown in Figure 9. Microbiological assays performed against a penicillin-susceptible strain of *S. aureus* in the absence of added penicillinase protein (left image) versus in the presence of 100 μg of penicillinase added to the agar (right image) compare the effects of the nanoparticle on antimicrobial activity. In this experiment, penicillin G loses all of its antimicrobial activity (bottom right disk on each plate) when penicillinase protein is mixed into the agar, while the penicillin nanoparticles (labeled NP) retain their full activity at all concentrations tested. Moreover, the in vitro bioactivity of these nanopenicillins depends on the structure of the penicillin derivative used, as well as on the type of functionality linking the penicillin to the polymeric framework. The order of in vitro bioactivity observed in the assays follows the ease of cleavability of the penicillin molecule from the polyacrylate chain, with imide > ester > amide (Figure 10).

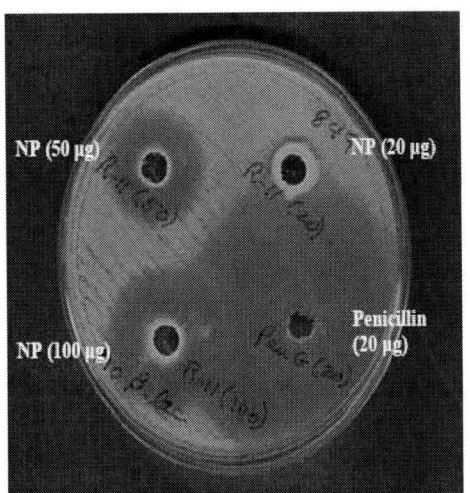 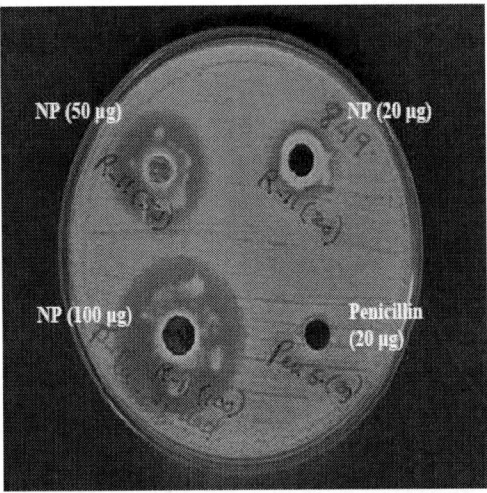

Figure 9. Kirby–Bauer assays of penicillin-conjugated polyacrylate nanoparticles (NP) against S. aureus in the absence (left) versus presence (right) of β-lactamase protein, demonstrating the protective properties of polyacrylate nanoparticles on penicillin.

The Turos group also has recently described *glyco*sylated polyacrylate *nano*particles as anti*biotics* (termed *glyconanobiotics*) and evaluated their *in vitro* antibacterial capabilities against two dangerous pathogenic microbes, MRSA and *B. anthracis* [165]. Examples include the use of water-insoluble N-thiolated β-lactam antibacterials as well as the more highly water-soluble penicillin, attached to the nanoparticle framework through a series of cleavable ester linkages (Figure 11). This illustrates the possibility of employing relatively large, chemically-sensitive acrylated monomers and carbohydrate motifs for the formation of emulsified polyacrylate nanoparticles.

imide-linked > ester-linked > amide-linked

Figure 10. Relative bioactivities of penicillin-bound polyacrylate nanoparticles reflect the propensity for hydrolytic cleavage of the linker.

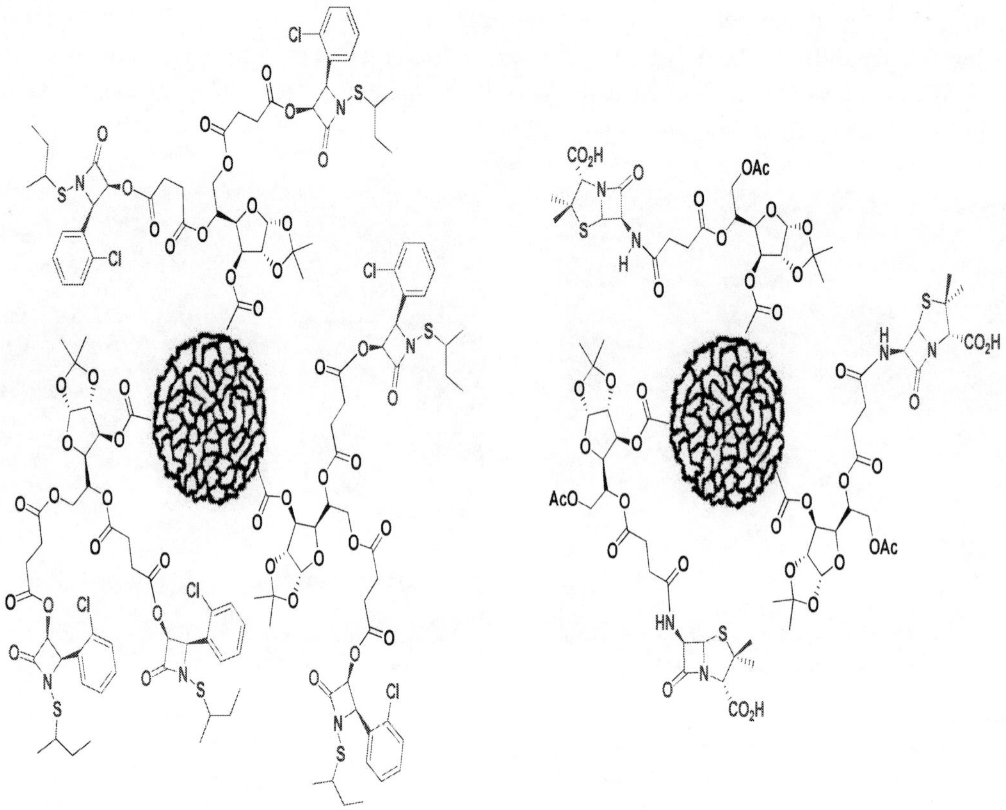

Figure 11. Synthesis of β-lactam-conjugated glycosylated nanoparticles.

Emulsions made of benzathine penicillin G-containing poly(lactide-co-glycolic acid) (PLGA) nanoparticles can be formed by spontaneous emulsification, providing biodegradable nanostructures which measure < 200 nm in size that entrap the β-lactam drug present in the media.[166] This process gives very high (85%) encapsulation efficiency of the drug, which can be released systemically within about two hours.

Silver nanoparticles are interesting on their own right because of their intrinsic antimicrobial properties and non-toxicity to human tisssue.[61,167,168] Therefore, coupling an antibiotic onto the surface provides the opportunity to perhaps enhance the bioactivity of both the silver as well as the antibiotic through synergistic enhancement. The β-lactam drug, amoxicillin, is a good representative since its structure contains a number of heteroatomic groups which can chelate onto the surface of the silver nanoparticles, as depicted in Figure 12. These silver nanoparticles can act upon bacteria via a combination of mechanisms, and thus provide an effective strategy to overcome antimicrobial resistance. The synergistic effects of amoxicillin-silver nanoparticles are illustrated in Figure 13.[169] The bars corresponding to the silver nanoparticles (nanosilver) and amoxicillin alone (a, b) show some reduction in the number of bacterial colonies, but the combination of the two (c,d) provides for nearly total destruction. A similar effect was seen for silver nanoparticles coated with Cefoperazone, a third-generation semisynthetic cephalosporin antibiotic, against MRSA [170].

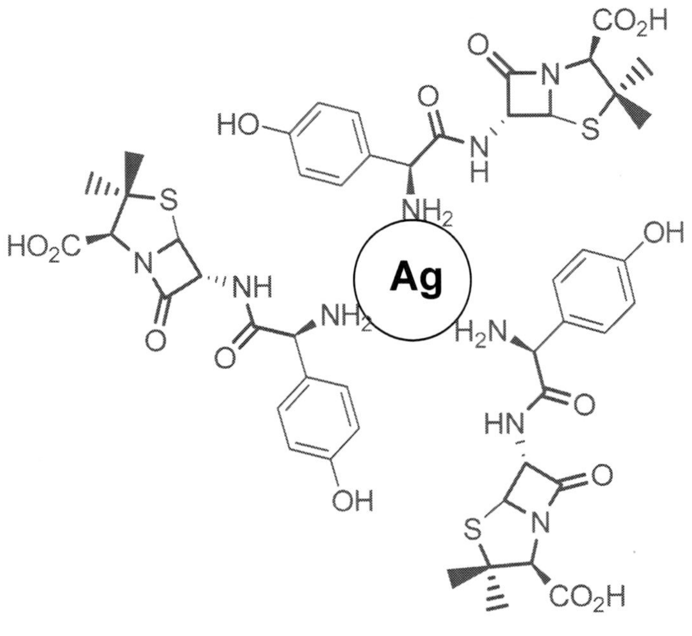

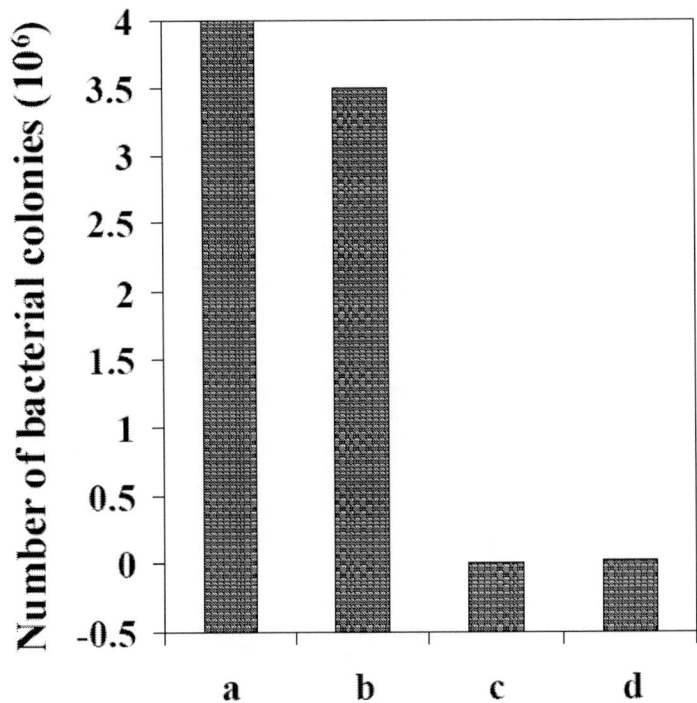

Figure 12. Amoxicillin-coated silver nanoparticles.

Figure 13. Effect of combining the β-lactam antibiotic amoxicillin with nanosilver on *E. coli*. a) 5 μg/ml nanosilver; b) 150 μg/ml amoxicillin; c) 150 μg/ml amoxicillin plus 5 μg/ml nanosilver; d) 150 μg/ml amoxicillin plus 10 μg/ml nanosilver.

Chen and coworkers investigated porous hollow silica nanoparticles as drug carriers due to their extremely high chemical and thermal stability, and huge surface area for drug adsorption.[42] These unusual nanoparticles are made by using calcium carbonate as a template for the silica lattice to form as an aqueous suspension, which when evaporated produce spherical nanoparticles with a diameter of 60-70 nm. The outer wall of the silica particle itself is about 10 nm thick. The cephalosporin, cefradine, has been used to coat the inside surface crevices of the porous silica particles.

The pores burst-release ~ 74% of the entrapped drug within 20 minutes. The employment of these fascinating nanoparticle constructs specifically for drug-resistant bacteria has not been reported.

Aminoglycoside-Based Nanoparticles

The use of gold nanoparticles as drug delivery carriers has been demonstrated to improve efficacy of aminoglycosides against Gram-positive and Gram-negative bacteria like *S. aureus*, *M. luteus*, *E. coli* and *P. aeruginosa*.[43] Since the gold nanoparticles themselves do not possess antimicrobial activity, this activity enhancement is probably due to the high antibiotic concentration localized on the surface of the nanoparticle.(Figure 14). Transmission electron microscopy indicates that while the bare gold nanoparticles are 12 15 nm in diameter, in the presence of streptomycin, gentamycin, or neomycin the nanoparticles have a tendancy to form larger aggregates of varying size.

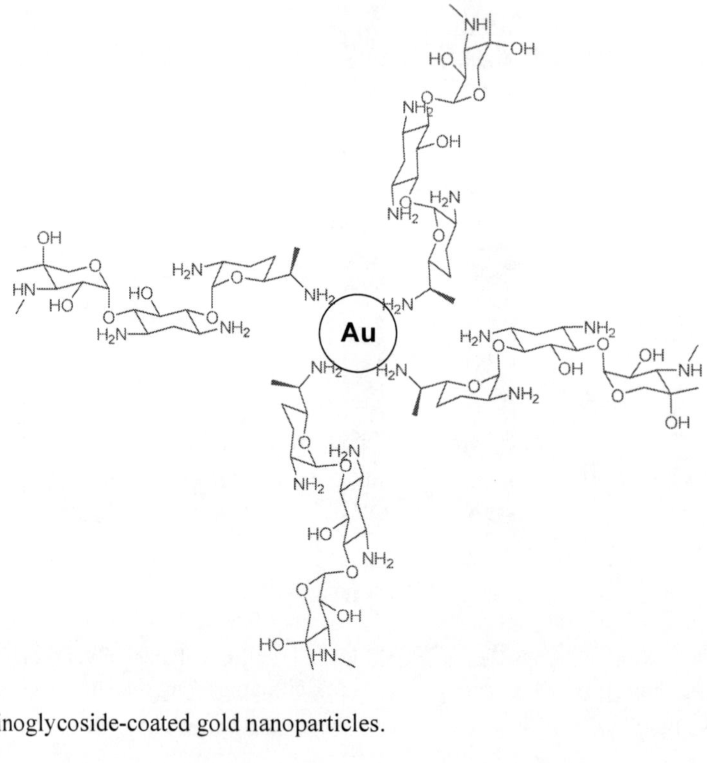

Figure 14. Aminoglycoside-coated gold nanoparticles.

Gentamycin sulfate can likewise be loaded into biodegradable PLGA nanoparticles, which in turn have been found to possess good activity against *S. aureus*. This may be useful for treating intracellular *Brucella* infections due to the likely uptake by phagocytes.[27] The potential for oral administration of streptomycin employing streptomycin-encapsulated PLG nanoparticles has been examined.[21] More than a twenty-fold increase in the relative bioavailability of PLG by oral delivery of PLG-encapsulated streptomycin compared to intramuscular injection of the free drug was found. In *Mycobacterium tuberculosis* H 37 Rv infected mice, eight doses of the oral streptomycin-encapsulated LPG nanoparticle formulation administered weekly were comparable to 24 intramuscular injections of free streptomycin.

Ciprofloxacin-Based Nanoparticles

In his investigations of emulsified poly(cyano acrylate) nanoparticles, Couvreur prepared ciprofloxacin variants in which most of the antibiotic drug content is entrapped within the nanoparticle matrix.[22] It was determined, however, that 30% of the drug content was bound covalently to the polymer chain, as a result of the anionically-induced polymerization. The authors noted that poly(isobutyl cyanoacrylate) nanoparticles containing ciprofloxacin are more active than the free drug itself in reducing colony forming units in human macrophages infected with *M. avium* complex. It has been hypothesized that entrapment of ciprofloxacin inside the nanoparticles could improve intracellular retention and distribution within infected compartments [9].

Nah and colleagues have recently found that ciprofloxacin-encapsulated PLGA nanoparticles possess inherently lower in vitro bioactivity than ciprofloxacin itself, but greater in vivo effects due to slow, sustained release of the antibiotic from the nanoparticle.[28] Ludwig and his coworkers synthesized ciprofloxacin-loaded PLGA nanoparticles measuring about 210 nm in size by high-pressure homogenization.[171] A study on the effects of added viscosifying agent to the nanopaticle solution on ciprofloxacin release was conducted, and the rate of drug leakage was dependent on differences in viscoelastic behaviour of the polymer employed. It was thus concluded that the selection of the polymer used to control viscosity of the nanoparticle eye drop solution is important in obtaining the optimal drug concentration for ocular applications.

Abeylath and Turos reported the synthesis and antimicrobial properties of poly(butyl acrylate-styrene) nanoparticles having ciprofloxacin (colored red) attached to the matrix through a cleavable linker (colored blue), as shown in Figure 15.[165] The size of these nanoparticles average around 45 nm when sodium dodecyl sulfate (3 mole percent) is used as surfactant. Strong anti-MRSA and anti-Bacillus bioactivity is observed during the preliminary testing of these *glyco*sylated *nanobiotics* (*glyconanobiotics*).

The laboratories of Cheng and Xu studied polyamidoamine-based dendrimers as a means for solubilizing water-insoluble quinolone antibiotics, nadifloxacin and prulifloxacin.[44] Their results demonstrated that encapsulation of the quinolones inside the dendrimer matrix afforded excellent solubility of these drugs, and similar antibacterial activity to that of the free drugs themselves, suggesting that PAMAM dendrimers might be suitable antibiotic carriers.

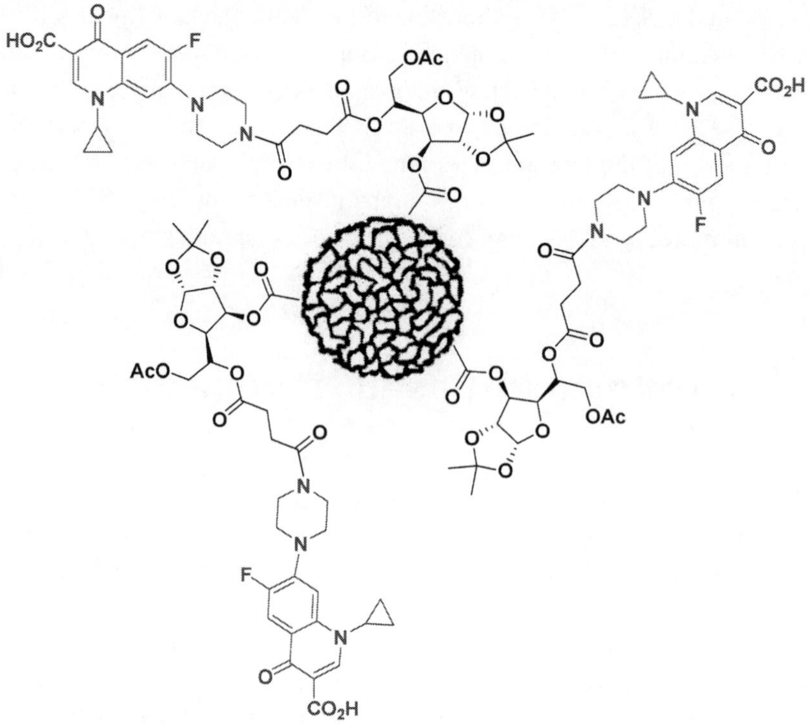

Figure 15. Ciprofloxacin-conjugated poly(butyl acrylate-styrene) nanoparticles for MRSA and *Bacillus anthracis.*

It is suggested that that the dendrimers might enhance penetration of the drug through the bacterial membrane. Since only one microbe was tested, it is not known if the dendrimers could enhance bioactivity against other microbes or drug-resistant strains. The authors do provide caution, however, about questions of toxicity in the use of dendrimers for antibiotics delivery, but are hopeful that structural modification of the dendrimer may overcome this issue.

Liposomes have likewise been investigated as a means to encapsulate ciprofloxacin.[45] For this study, large unilamellar liposomes measuring 200 nm in diameter were used to investigate the physicochemical properties affecting the retention and location of the antibiotic within the liposomal structure. Nuclear magnetic resonance (NMR) studies show that approximately 90% of the drug molecules is actually inside the aqueous interior of the liposomes, where the molecules self-associate through π-stacking. The ciprofloxacin concentrations in this aqueous environment can exceed 250 mM, which is about 100 times higher than that reached in bulk aqueous media before precipitation occurs. Curiously, only a very small proportion of the entrapped drug partitions into the inner monolayer wall of the liposome. The rapid leakage of encapsulated ciprofloxacin from liposomes may account for why these nanoparticles have not been as widely investigated for antibiotics delivery as one might anticipate, compared to cancer drug delivery. Moreover, the consequence of liposomal entrapment on antimicrobial activity or bacterial drug resistance do not appear to have been investigated. Analogous molecular uptake and release experiments have been reported for model fluoroquinolones in hydrogels [46].

Ciprofloxacin-coated gold nanoparticles have also been reported.[47] The nature of binding of the drug molecule to the gold was investigated by voltammetric and spectroscopic methods, which indicate that the nitrogen atom of the piperazine ring binds strongly to the surface of the gold nanoparticles (Figure 16).

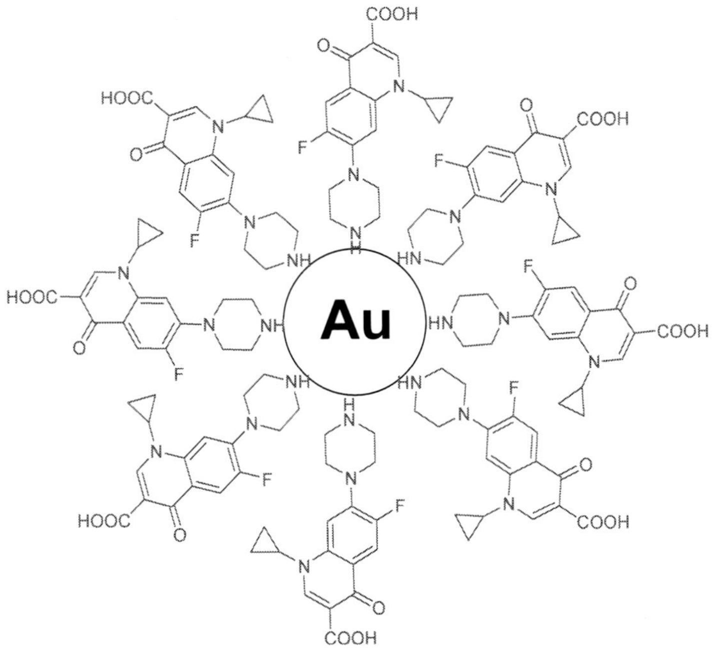

Figure 16. Ciprofloxacin-gold nanoassembly.

Pradeep´s laboratory have described the preparation of ciprofloxacin-encapsulated silica nanoshells by using gold nanoparticles as a structural template. First, ciprofloxacin molecules can be surface-coated onto the gold nanoparticles, and a shell of silicon dioxide is then constructed around this before the gold is excravated through cyanide-leaching.[48] The result is a silica shell or "nanobubble" effectively encasing a reservoir of ciprofloxacin molecules. TEM images of the cip@SiO$_2$ nanoshells show particles of averaging ~15 nm in diameter. These interesting constructs have subsequently been found to improve the antibacterial activity of the loaded antibiotic, mainly due to the enhanced penetration into the bacterial cells.[49] Against *Escherichia coli* DH5R, the nanobiotics showed better antibacterial activity compared to free ciprofloxacin, while identical activities of the free and nanoparticle-bound drug were found for *Lactococcus lactis* MG 1363.

Biologically active polymer core/shell nanoparticles, formed by self-associating the hydrophilic and hydrophobic segments of the amphiphilic polymer have been synthesized by Lu and Yang´s teams for ciprofloxacin delivery across the blood-brain barrier [50].

These nanobiotics may provide a promising treatment for brain infections. Single-dose nanoparticle delivery systems for prolonged release of ciprofloxacin have recently been studied by Jain and Banerjee, using albumin, gelatin, chitosan, and solid lipid nanoparticles as carriers.[39] Results suggest that chitosan nanoparticles and solid nanoparticles may act as particularly promising carriers for sustained ciprofloxacin release in ocular and skin infections.

Vancomycin-Based Nanoparticles

The development of strategies capable of rapidly identifying infectious microbes in clinical samples would facilitate proper treatment of deadly infections and help avoid the spread of antimicrobial drug-resistance. Towards this end, there are many opportunities where research in nanotechnology and nanomaterials can aid in the detection and identification of infectious agents, as well as the ability to selectively target therapeutics to the infection site. One approach that has been investigated is to modify the surface of nanoparticles with ligands that can bind strongly to specific sites, such as membrane-bound proteins and carbohydrated receptors, thereby bringing the nanoparticle into close contact with the bacterial cell (Figure 17).

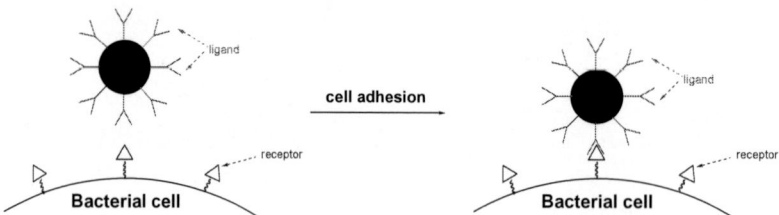

Figure 17. Schematic depiction of a surface-modified nanoparticle interacting with bacterial receptors on the cell surface.

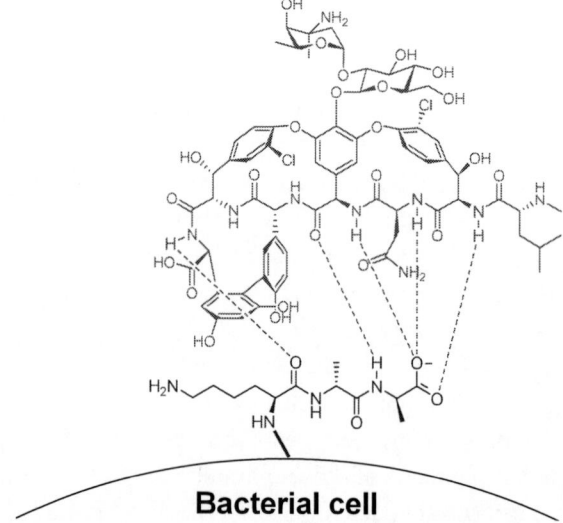

Figure 18. Cartoon representation of the vancomycin-D-alanyl-D-alanine interaction on the surface of a bacterial cell.

Vancomycin-conjugated nanoparticles have been found ideally-suited to serve as affinity probes to selectively trap pathogens. Vancomycin is capable of strongly interacting with a broad range of Gram-positive bacteria through hydrogen bonding between its heptapeptide backbone and the D-alanyl-D-alanine end of the pre-cross-linked peptidoglycan of bacterial cells (Figure 18). Hence, through this type of specific interaction with the bacterial cell wall, vancomycin has emerged as an attractive bacterial targeting agent.

Gold nanoparticles having vancomycin bound via distinct orientations, as shown in Figure 19, have been employed in magnetic confinement assays to isolate a variety of Gram-positive and Gram-negative bacteria from aqueous solution [172,173].

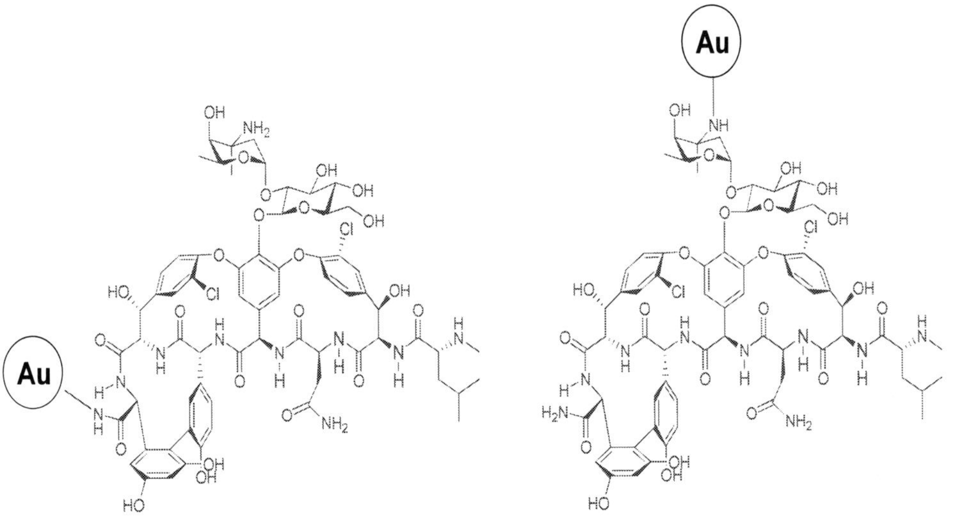

Figure 19. Vancomycin-bound gold nanoparticles.

Most recently, Bing Xu and colleagues demonstrated that such vancomycin-coated gold nanoparticles significantly enhance *in vitro* antibacterial activity of the antibiotic against vancomycin-resistant enterococci (VRE) strains and *E. coli* (a Gram-negative microbe).[174] The investigators suggest that these vancomycin-bound nanoparticles may act as a rigid polyvalent inhibitor in which the high concentration of vancomycin (estimated to be around 31 vancomycin molecules per nanoparticle) on the gold surface may interact with multiple vancomycin binding sites on the surface of the bacterial cell. Curiously, cysteine-coated gold nanoparticles (used as a control) also show similar activity against *E. faecium*, albeit two-fold lower (4-8 ug-mL), yet still considerably more active than vancomycin itself (MIC >128 ug/mL). The activity of the cysteine-loaded nanoparticles and the mode of interaction with the bacterial membrane is thought to differ from that of the vancomycin-bound system.

Collectively, these studies with vancomycin-coated gold nanoparticles illustrate an additional way that antibiotic-coated nanoparticles might be used to target bacterial cells and to counter antimicrobial drug resistance, through polyvalent inhibition of membrane receptor sites. The small size (4-5 nm) and constant shape of gold nanoparticles make them an ideal model system to investigate multivalency in drug delivery applications and in materials research development.

Sulfa-Based Nanoparticles

Cheng and Wuen recently reported the employment of polyamidoamine dendrimers to solubilize the sulphonamide antibiotic, sulfamethoxazole.[175] Their preliminary studies have shown that like for the quinolone dendrimers (described above) these increase the in vitro antibacterial activity of sulfamethoxazole against *E. coli* and provide for sustained release. Other microbes were not investigated in this study, so it is not known whether the dendrimers carrying the sulphonamide antibiotic could also improve the spectrum of bioactivity to other pathogenic bacteria or to drug-resistant strains.

Conclusion

Science fiction writers and those in the entertainment industry have for many years depicted the future of medicine to be based on sub-microscopic robots patrolling the blood stream and immune system looking for the causes of human disease. These nanorobots were portrayed to be outfitted with all the requisite "intelligence" and tools needed to fix whatever problems they came upon to treat disease, or destroy invaders such as deadly viruses and bacteria. While medicine has not yet achieved such a level of sophistication, those visionary depictions do not lie all that far beyond today's horizon. Indeed, researchers are rapidly learning how to design nanoscopic materials with functionality to perform a number of complicated operations, including targeted drug or gene delivery and cellular repair. Rapid advances in nanomaterials and nanomedicines are bringing these once-imaginary creations into reality, and nanobiotics certainly fit well within this fascinating paradigm.

The sheer diversity of materials and chemical frameworks that can be used to create nanoparticle matrices, and their countless biomedical applications that could potentially be developed, should give nanobiotics a prominent niche in the drug development arena. But clearly, we are only at the very beginning of what could surely become an exciting era of research and development into nanoparticle biology and design. Nanotechnologies applied to antibiotics delivery still trail far behind those investigated already for anticancer agents, but could certainly capitalize on many of the findings and ongoing investigations in that field, such as toxicity, biodistribution and pharmacokinetics parameters, cellular targeting and biostability. For use against bacteria, we need to know more about how to target cells better, what drives those interactions, what the effects of these interactions might be on cellular viability and communication, so we can deliver the nanobiotic to the specific microbial cell (or even human cell) of interest. At the present time, there is still a dearth of clinical data on the use of nanoparticles as antibiotics, and much more investigation must still be carried out to assess human toxicity and side effects, as well as therapeutic efficacy across a broader range of infection types. Nevertheless, the evidence gathered so far certainly indicates great promise in the use of nanoparticles for systemic applications and infection control.[17,23,53,76] Indeed, at this point, the development of nanoparticle-based technologies for medicine (referred to as *nanomedicine*) is still largely investigational, and a plethora of safety issues associated with nanomaterials in general exist that will require caution and continuing study.[176] The interaction of nanoparticles with human tissue as well as with microbial cells is an expanding field of research, but has remained largely underexplored with regards to antibiotics delivery or the treatment of infectious diseases. Until the risks of nanoparticles on human health have been adequately assessed, their roles in human therapy will likely remain rather limited. Nonetheless, even in the short-term, novel applications of certain nanoparticles may be found in topical treatments for optical infections, minor skin infections, abrasions and burns, as antibacterial coatings on surgical stents and implant devices, and as antimicrobial actives in cosmetics.[4,8] The most substantitive value, though, of nanobiotics will most certainly be borne out in various systemic applications involving drug-resistant pathogenic diseases. Therapeutic utility will ultimately be dictated by the types of nanoparticles being used and the drugs they carry (if any), as well as on their size, shape, stability, concentration, drug loading and drug release properties, cell recognition capabilities, biotoxicity, pharmacodynamics and biodistribution properties. Each nanoparticle system may be unique with respect to each of these parameters (and others), and thus need to be investigated independently, but answers to these questions will eventually reveal what biomedical applications may lie just down the road. Through creative design, it may be possible to minimize or even overcome certain risks, such as those due to cellular or systemic toxicity, or coagulation throughout the vasculature or RES organs, thereby enabling a wide assortment of biomedical applications. This allows drug designers and nanoparticle architects to tailor their antibiotics to the nanoparticle vehicle, and vice versa. The ingenuity will drive these developments, as will the data obtained through further experimentation.

Precisely how nanobiotics may fit into drug discovery and development is well worth pondering, particularly with respect to overcoming or even avoiding the continuing onset of drug resistance. In its most simplistic form as a drug carrier, the nanoparticle may alter the way the drug enters the cell or its exposure to enzymes and other destructive components that might degrade the drug before it can act. A most notable example already noted is for penicillin-bound nanoparticles, which shield the β-lactamase-sensitive drug molecule from degradation by penicillin-resistant bacteria.[105] Acting as a chaperone, the nanoparticle can deliver the antibiotic directly into the bacterial membrane or even the cytoplasm, with drug release occurring there (perhaps mediated by esterases), which ensures delivery of high concentrations of drug inside the bacterial cell and also the possibility that the drug could act on the PBP's as it effuses outward from the cell. This changes the very manner in which the antibiotic may normally function, and overcome the mechanism of resistance that had been developed by the microbe towards that class of antibiotic. Thus, an obsolete family of drugs may be made useful again, or to become effective against microbes otherwise resistant to the free drug. All of this, once validated and recognized, feeds directly into the de novo design of new antibiotics and prodrugs. The small, uniform size of nanoparticles may enable delivery of antibiotics to localities within the human body where infections are typically difficult to treat, such as the brain, gastrointestinal tract, heart tissue, and intracellular sites. Getting the proper antibiotic to the specific site of infection, rather than to unaffected tissue where the drug does no good and is deplenished and diluted, helps to not only increase effective concentration where the drug is actually needed, but also reduces its exposure to communal bacteria and to the onset of drug resistance. Targeted drug delivery, a more advanced realm of nanoparticles research, in effect exploits the attachment of recognizable ligands onto the surface of the nanoparticle, similar to that used by vancomycin-coated nanoparticles and viruses, to recognize specific cell types and microbes of interest.

Intracellular bacterial infections represent another challenging, yet largely unexplored, area of investigation for nanoparticle-based antibiotics and drug delivery. [177] Nanoparticles may be effective in reaching dormant, "persistent" bacteria hiding within human cells, as demonstrated by Couvreur in the case of penicillin-loaded nanoparticles.[106] Nanobiotics have likewise been shown to enable antibacterials to be carried into macrophages as a means to eradicate intracellular pathogens in the liver and spleen. Thus, opportunities seem ripe for development of "smarter" nanobiotics that can both recognize specific human tissue or organs, and deliver a suitable antibiotic or packet of antibiotics to the targeted microbe with high precision and effectiveness. Much more is sure to come through further innovation and creative investigation into nanoparticles as microbiocides (e.g., silver nanoparticles, chitosan nanoparticles, dendrimers, peptidyl nanotubes, etc.) and antibiotic delivery vehicles.

Another yet unexplored aspect of nanobiotics that could surely hold significant promise for controlling drug resistance, and overcoming deadly infections, is the employment of multi-drug containing nanoparticles. Incorporation of two to several different classes of antibacterial drugs into a nanoparticle ensures controlled delivery of the antibiotics so they reach the same microbe together, hitting multiple bacterial targets or cellular processes simultaneously as a means to overcome resistance pathways. In essence, these multi-modal nanobiotics would deliver to the same target cell a complete cocktail of complementary antibiotics or their prodrugs, releasing them into the microbe all at once in a burst, or through a controlled manner that could be pre-engineered into the design of the nanoparticle. Thus, it is important to know what drugs to be able to release first, at what concentration and cellular site, and how to time the release of second or third antibiotics. The types of nanoparticles to use for this kind of chemotherapy, and the materials employed to contain the drug (or even layering different materials on the same nanoparticle matrix as a way to control delivery), are all critical elements in the design process.

It is hopeful and reasonable to think that human ingenuity and careful experimentation will allow us to create sophisticated, effective nanobiotics capable of detecting and treating bacterial disease while overcoming or delaying drug resistance pathways. Many of these discoveries will likely become apparent over the next few years, as nanobiotics as a discipline further expands and develops, adding yet another new weapon to the arsenal in Man's ongoing battle with infectious diseases.

References and Notes

[1]   This definition contrasts from that found in various published forums and ubiquitously on the internet, where the term *nanobiotic* refers to almost any material having some effect on a biological or pharmacological process. These ambiguous usages are confusing, and include nanometer-sized robots in the blood to treat human disease, and antibiotics that kill nanobacteria associated with deleterious calcium deposits, among a host of many other unrelated topics.

[2]   Allen, T.M.; Cullis, P.R. Drug delivery systems: entering the mainstream. *Science* 2004, *303*, 1818-1822.

[3]   Langer, R. New methods of drug delivery. *Science* 1990, *249*, 1527-1533.

[4]   Le Bourlais, C.; Acar, L.; Zia, H.; Sado, P. A.; Needham, T.; Leverge, R. Ophthalmic drug delivery systems- recent advances. *Prog. Retin. Eye Res.* 1998, *17*, 33-58.

[5]   Boas, U.; Heegaard, P. M. H. Dendrimers in drug research. *Chem. Soc. Rev.* 2004, *33*, 43-63.

[6]   Elizabeth, R.; Gillies, J.; Frechet, M. J. Dendrimers and dendritic polymers in drug delivery. *Drug Discov. Today* 2005, *10*, 35-43.

[7]   Kreuter, J. In *Micro-encapsulation in Medicine and Pharmacy*. M. Donbrow, Ed., CRC Press, Boca Raton, FL, 1992.

[8]   Zimmer, A.; Kreuter, J. Microspheres and nanoparticles used in ocular delivery systems. *Adv. Drug Deliv. Rev.* 1995, *16*, 61-73.

[9]   Huguette, P. A.; Andremont, A.; Couvreur, P. Targeted delivery of antibiotics using liposomes and nanoparticles: research and applications. *Int. J. Antimicrob. Agents* 2000, *13*, 155-168.

[10]   Kreuter, J. Nanoparticle-based drug delivery systems. *J. Control. Release* 1991, *16*, 169 -176.

[11]   Couvreur, P.; Dubernet, C.; Puisieux, F. Controlled drug delivery with nanoparticles: current possibilities and future trends. *Eur. J. Pharm. Biopharm.* 1995, *41*, 2–13.

[12]   Allémann, E.; Gurny, R.; Doelker, E. Drug-loaded nanoparticles - preparation methods and drug targeting issues. *Eur. J. Biopharm.* 1993, *39*, 173-191.

[13]   Ravi Kumar, M.N.V. Nano and microparticles as controlled drug delivery devices. *J. Pharm. Pharm. Sci.* 2000, *3*, 234-258.

[14]   Abeylath, S.; Turos, E. Drug delivery approaches to overcome bacterial resistance to β-lactam antibiotics. *Exp. Opin. Drug Deliv.* 2008, *5*, 931-949.

[15]   Kreuter, J.; Speiser, P. P. New adjuvants on a poly(methyl methacrylate) base. *Infect Immun.* 1976, *13*, 204-210.

[16]   Couvreur, P.; Kante, B.; Roland M.; Guiot, P.; Bauduin, P.; Speiser, P. Polycyanoacrylate nanocapsules as potential lysosomotropic carriers: preparation, morphological and sorptive properties. *J. Pharm. Pharm.* 1979, *31*, 331-332.

[17]   Cavallaro, G. M.; Fresta, G.; Giammona, G.; Villari, P. A. Entrapment of β-lactams antibiotics in polyethyl cyanoacrylate nanoparticles: studies on the possible in vivo application of this colloidal delivery system. *Int. J. Pharm.* 1994, *111*, 31-41.

[18]   Fontana, G.; Pitarresi, G.; Tomarchio, V. Carlisi, B.; Biagio, P. L. S. Preparation, characterization and in vitro antimicrobial activity of ampicillin-loaded poly(ethyl cyanoacrylate) nanoparticles. *Biomaterials* 1998, *19*, 1009-1117.

[19]   Fontana, G.; Licciardi, M.; Mansueto, S. Schillaci, D.; Giammona, G. Amoxicillin-loaded poly(ethyl cyanoacrylate) nanoparticles: influence of PEG coating on the particle size, drug release rate and phagocytic uptake. *Biomaterials* 2001, *22*, 2857-2865.

[20]   Turos, E.; Shim, J.Y.; Wang, Y.; Greenhalgh, K.; Reddy, G. S. K.; Dickey, S.; Lim, D. V. Antibiotic-conjugated polyacrylate nanoparticles: New opportunities for development of anti-MRSA agents. *Bioorg. Med. Chem. Lett.* 2007, *17*, 53-56.

[21] Pandey, R.; Khuller, G. K. Nanoparticle-based oral drug delivery system for an injectable antibiotic- streptomycin. *Chemotherapy* 2007, *53*, 437–441.

[22] Page-Clisson, M. E.; Pinto-Alphandary, H.; Ourevitch, M.; Andremont, A.; Couvreur, P. Development of ciprofloxacin-loaded nanoparticles: physicochemical study of the drug carrier. *J. Control. Release* 1998, *56*, 23-32.

[23] Fattal, E.; Youssef, M.; Couvreur, P.; Andremont, A. Treatment of experimental salmonellosis in mice with ampicillin-bound nanoparticles. *Antimicrob. Agents Chemother.* 1989, *33*, 1540 -1543.

[24] Williams, J.; Lansdown, R.; Sweitzer, R.; Romanowski, M.; LaBell, R.; Ramaswami, R.; Unger, E. Nanoparticle drug delivery system for intravenous delivery of topoisomerase inhibitors. *J. Control. Release* 2003, *91*, 167-172.

[25] Fourage, M.: Dewulf, M.; Couvreur, P.; Roland, M.; Vranckx, H. Development of dehydroemetine nanoparticles for the treatment of visceral leishmaniasis. *J. Microencapsulation* 1989, *6*, 29-34.

[26] Soppimath, K.S.; Aminabhavi, T.M.; Kulkami, A.R.; Rudzinski, W.E. Biodegradable polymeric nanoparticles as drug delivery devices. *J. Control. Release* 2001, *70*, 1-20.

[27] Prior, S.; Gamazo, C.; Irache, J. M.; Merkle, H. P.; Gander, B. Gentamicin encapsulation in PLA/PLGA microspheres in view of treating *Brucella* infections. *Int. J. Pharm.* 2000, *196*, 115-125.

[28] Jeong, Y.; Nab, H.; Seo, D.; Kim, D.; Lee, H.; Jang, M.; Na, S.; Roh, S.; Kim, S.; Nah, J. Ciprofloxacin-encapsulated poly(dl-lactide-*co*-glycolide) nanoparticles and its antibacterial activity. *Int. J. Pharm.* 2008, *352*, 317–323.

[29] Vauthier, C.; Dubernet, C.; Fattal, E.; Pinto-Alphandary, H.; Couvreur, P. Poly(alkyl cyanoacrylates) as biodegradable materials for biomedical applications. *Adv. Drug Deliv. Rev.* 2003, *55*, 519-548.

[30] Gabizon, A.; Catane, R.; Uziely, B.; Kaufman, B.; Safra, T.; Cohen, R.; Martin, F.; Huang, A.; Barenholz, Y. Prolonged circulation time and enhanced accumulation in malignant exudates of doxorubicin encapsulated in polyethylene-glycol coated liposomes. *Cancer Res.* 1994, *54*, 987-992.

[31] Huwyler, J.; Wu, D.; Paradridge, W. M. Brain drug delivery of small molecules using immunoliposomes. *Proc. Natl. Acad. Sci. USA* 1996, *93*, 14164-14169.

[32] Fernandez-Urrusuno, R.; Fattal, E.; Rodrigues, J. M.; Feger, J.; Bedossa, P.; Couvreur, P. Effect of polymeric nanoparticle administration on the clearance activity of the mononuclear phagocyte system in mice. *J. Biomed. Mat. Res.* 1996, *31*, 401-408.

[33] Lobenberg, R.; Kreuter, J. Macrophage targeting of azidothymidine: a promising strategy for AIDS therapy. *AIDS Res. Hum. Retroviruses* 1996, *12*, 1709-1715.

[34] Chun, L. Poly(L-glutamic acid)-anticancer drug conjugates. *Adv. Drug Deliv. Rev.* 2002, *54*, 695-713.

[35] Changez, M.; Koul, V.; Dinda, A. K. Efficacy of antibiotics-loaded interpenetrating network (IPNs) hydrogel based on poly(acrylic acid) and gelatin for treatment of experimental osteomyelitis: in vivo study. *Biomaterials* 2005, *26*, 2095-2104.

[36] Risbud, M. V.; Hardikar, A. A.; Bhat, S.V.; Bhode R. R. pH-sensitive freeze-dried chitosan-polyvinyl pyrrolidone hydrogels as controlled release system for antibiotic delivery. *J. Control. Release* 2000, *68*, 23 -30.

[37] Patel, V. R.; Amiji, M. M. Preparation and characterization of freeze-dried chitosan-poly(ethylene oxide) hydrogels for site-specific antibiotic delivery in the stomach. *Pharm. Res.* 1996, *13*, 588-593.

[38] Janes, K. A.; Fresneau, M. P.; Marazuela, A.; Fabra, A.; Alonso, M. J. Chitosan nanoparticles as delivery systems for doxorubicin. *J. Control. Rel.* 2001, *73*, 255-267.

[39] Jain, D.; Banerjee, R. Comparison of ciprofloxacin hydrochloride-loaded protein, lipid, and chitosan nanoparticles for drug delivery. *J. Biomed. Mat. Res. Part B: Applied Biomaterials* 2007, *86B*, 105-112.

[40] Kai, Y.; Komazawa, Y.; Miyajima, A.; Miyata, N.; Yamakoshi, Y. Fullerene as a novel photoinduced antibiotic. *Fullerenes, Nanotubes and Carbon Nanostructures* 2003, *11*, 79-87.

[41] Tegos, G.; Demidova, T.; Arcila-Lopez, D.; Lee, H.; Wharton, T.; Gali, H.; Hamblin, M. Fullerenes as light-activated antimicrobial agents. Cationic fullerenes are effective and selective antimicrobial photosensitizers. *Chem. Biol.* 2005, *12*, 1127-1135.

[42] Chen, J. F.; Ding, H. M.; Wang, J. X.; Shao, L. Preparation and characterization of porous hollow silica nanoparticles for drug delivery application. *Biomaterials* 2004, *25*, 723-727.

[43] Grace, A. N; Pandian, K. Antibacterial efficacy of aminoglycosidic antibiotics protected gold nanoparticles-A brief study. *Colloids and Surfaces A: Physicochem. Eng. Aspects* 2007, *297*, 63–70.

[44] Cheng, M.; Qu, H.; Ma, M.; Xu, Z.; Xu, P.; Fang, Y.; Xu, T. Polyamidoamine (PAMAM) dendrimers as biocompatible carriers of quinolone antimicrobials: an in vitro study. *Eur. J. Med. Chem.* 2007, *42*, 1032-1038.

[45] Maurer, N.; Wong, K. F.; Hope, M. J.; Cullis, P.R. Anomalous solubility behavior of the antibiotic ciprofloxacin encapsulated in liposomes: a ^{1}H NMR study. *Biochim. Biophysica Acta* 1998, *1374*, 9-20.

[46] Vilches, A.P.; Kairuz, A. J.; Alovero, F.; Olivera, M. E.; Allemandi, D. A.; Manzo, R.H. Release kinetics and up-take studies of model fluoroquinolones from carbomer hydrogels. *Int. J. Pharm.* 2002, *246*, 17-24.

[47] Tom, R. T.; Suryanarayanan, V.; Reddy, P. G., Baskaran, S.; Pradeep, T. Ciprofloxacin-protected gold nanoparticles. *Langmuir* 2004, *20*, 1909 -1914.

[48] Rosemary, M. J.; Suryanarayanan, V.; Reddy, P. G.; MacLaren, I.; Baskaran, S.; Pradeep, T. Ciprofloxacin@SiO2: fluorescent nanobubbles. *Proc. Indian Acad. Sci., Chem. Sci.* 2003, *115*, 703-709.

[49] Rosemary, M. J.; MacLaren, I.; Pradeep T. Investigations of the antibacterial properties of ciprofloxacin@SiO2. *Langmuir* 2006, *22*, 10125-10129.

[50] Liu, L.; Guo, K.; Lu, J.; Venkatraman, S. S.; Luo, D.; Ng, K. C.; Ling, E.; Moochhala, S.; Yang, Y. Biologically active core/shell nanoparticles self-assembled from cholesterol-terminated PEG-TAT for drug delivery across the blood-brain barrier. *Biomaterials* 2008, *29*, 1509-1517.

[51] Trouet, A.; Deprez-De Campeneere, D.; De Duve, C. Chemotherapy through lysosomes with a DNA-daunorubicin complex. *Nature New Biol.* 1972, *239*, 110-112.

[52] Trouet, A.; Deprez-De Campeneere, D.; De Smedt-Malengreaux, M.; Atassi, G. Experimental leukemia chemotherapy with a "lysosomotropic" adriamycin-DNA complex. *Eur. J. Cancer.* 1974, *10*, 405-411.

[53] Kante, B.; Couvreur, P.; Guiot, P.; Dubois-Crack, G.; Roland, M.; Mercier, M.; Speiser, P. Toxicity of polyalkylcyanoacrylate nanoparticles I: free nanoparticles. *J. Pharm. Sci.* 1982, *71*, 786-790.

[54] Ting, S. R. S.; Gregory, A. M.; Stenzel, M. H. Polygalactose containing nanocages: the RAFT process for the synthesis of hollow sugar balls. *Biomacromolecules* 2009, *10*, 342-352.

[55] Martens, P. J.; Bryant, S. J.; Anseth, K. S. Tailoring the degradation of hydrogels formed from multivinyl poly(ethylene glycol) and poly(vinyl alcohol) macromers for cartilage tissue engineering. *Biomacromolecules* 2003, *4*, 283-292.

[56] Goodman, C. M.; Mccusker, C. D.; Yilmaz, T.; Rotello, V. M. Toxicity of gold nanoparticles functionalized with cationic and anionic side chains. *Bioconjug. Chem.* 2004, *15*, 897-900.

[57] Panacek, A.; Kvitek, L.; Prucek, R.; Kolar, M.; Vecerova, R.; Pizurova, N.; Sharma, V. K.; Nevecna, T.; Zboril, R. Silver colloid nanoparticles: synthesis, characterization, and their antibacterial activity. *J. Phys. Chem. B* 2006; *110*, 16248-16253.

[58] Dibrov, P.; Dzioba, J.; Gosink, K. K.; Hase, C. C. Chemiosmotic mechanism of antimicrobial activity of Ag + in *Vibrio cholerae. Antimicrob. Agents Chemother.* 2002, *46*, 2668-2670.

[59] Kong, H.; Jang, J. Antibacterial properties of novel poly(methyl methacrylate) nanofiber containing silver nanoparticles. *Langmuir* 2007, *24*, 2051-2056.

[60] Roberts, J. C.; Bhalgat, M. K.; Zera, R. T. Preliminary biological evaluation of polyamidoamine (PAMAM) starburst dendrimers. *J Biomed. Mater. Res.*, 1996, *30*, 53–65.

[61] Balogh, L.; Swanson, D. R.; Tomalia, D. A.; Hangauer, G. L.; McManus, A. T. Dendrimer−silver complexes and nanocomposites as antimicrobial agents. *Nano Lett.* 2001, *1*, 18-21.

[62] Nagahori, N.; Lee, R. T.; Nishimura, S.; Page, D.; Roy, R.; Lee, Y. C. Inhibition of adhesion of type 1 fibriated *Escherichia coli* to highly mannosylated ligands. *Chembiochem*, 2002, *3*, 836–844.

[63] Schengrund, C. "Multivalent" saccharides: development of new approaches for inhibiting the effects of glycosphingolipid-binding pathogens. *Biochem. Pharm.* 2003, *65*, 699-707.

[64] Chen, C. Z.; Cooper, S. L.. Interactions between dendrimer biocides and bacterial membranes. *Biomaterials* 2002, *23*, 3359–3368.

[65] Chen, C. C.; Beck-Tan, N. C.; Dhurjati, P.; van Dyk, T. K.; LaRossa, R. A.; Cooper, S. L. Quaternary ammonium functionalized poly(propylene imine) dendrimers as effective antimicrobials: structure-activity studies. *Biomacromolecules* 2000, *1*, 473–480.

[66] Chen, C. Z.; Cooper, S. L. Recent advances in antimicrobial dendrimers. *Adv. Mater.*, 2000, *12*, 843–846.

[67] Bourne, N.; Stanberry, L. R.; Kern, E. R.; Holan, G.; Matthews, B.; Bernstein, D. I. Dendrimers, a new class of candidate topical microbicides with activity against herpes simplex virus infection. *Antimicrob. Agents Chemother.* 2000, *44*, 2471–2474.

[68] Reverchon, E.; Della Porta, G. Production of antibiotic micro- and nano-particles by supercritical antisolvent precipitation. *Powder Technol.* 1999, *106*, 23-29.

[69] Reis, C. P.; Neufeld, R. J.; Ribeiro, A. J.; Veiga, F. Nanoencapsulation I. Methods for preparation of drug-loaded polymeric nanoparticles. *Nanomed. Nanotechnol. Biol. Med.* 2006, *2*, 8-21.

[70] Gilbert, R.G. *Emulsion Polymerization: A Mechanistic Approach*, Academic Press: London, 1995.

[71] Jani, P.; Halbert, W.; Langridge, J.; Florence, A. T. The uptake and translocation of latex nanospheres and microspheres after oral administration to rats. *J. Pharm. Pharm.* 1989, *41*, 809-812.

[72] Jani, P.; Halbert, G. W.; Langridge, J.; Florence, A. T. Nanoparticle uptake by the rat gastrointestinal mucosa: quantitation and particle size dependency. *J. Pharm. Pharm.* 1990, *42*, 821-826.

[73] Cui, Z.; Mumper, R. J. The effect of co-administration of adjuvants with a nanoparticle-based genetic vaccine delivery system on the resulting immune responses. *Eur. J. Pharm. Biopharm.* 2003, *55*, 11-18.

[74] Venier-Julienne, M. C.; Benoi, J. P. Preparation, purification and morphology of polymeric nanoparticles as drug carriers. *Pharm. Acta Helv.* 1996; *71*, 121-128.

[75] Garay-Jimenez, J.; Young, A.; Gergeres, D.; Greenhalgh, K.; Turos, E. Methods for purifying and detoxifying sodium dodecyl sulfate stabilized nanoparticles. *Nanomedicine* 2008, *4*, 98-105.

[76] Greenhalgh, K.; Turos, E. In vivo studies of polyacrylate nanoparticle emulsions for topical and systemic applications. *Nanomedicine.* 2009, *5*, 49-54.

[77] Couvreur, P.,Fattal, E.; Alphandary, H.; Puisieux, F.;Andremont, A. Intracellular targeting of antibiotics by means of biodegradable nanoparticles. *J. Control. Release* 1992, *19*, 259 -267.

[78] Qi, L.; Xu, Z.; Jiang, X.; Hu, C.; Zou, X. Preparation and antibacterial activity of chitosan nanoparticles. *Carbohyd. Res.* 2004, *339*, 2693-2700.

[79] Rabea, E. I.; Badawy, M. E.-T.; Stevens, C. V.; Smagghe, G.; Steurbaut, W. Chitosan as antimicrobial agent: applications and mode of action. *Biomacromolecules* 2003, *4*, 1457-1465.

[80] Liu, H.; Du, Y. M.; Wang, X. H.; Sun, L. P. Chitosan kills bacteria through cell membrane damage. *Int. J. Food Microbiol.* 2004, *95*, 147-155.

[81] Ueno, K.; Yamaguchi, T.; Sakairi, N.; Nishi, N.; Tokura, S. Antimicrobial activity of fractionated chitosan oligomers. *Adv. Chitin Sci.* 1997, *2*, 156-161.

[82] Jeon, Y. J.; Park, P.J.; Kim, S.K. Antimicrobial effect of chitooligosaccharides produced by bioreactor. *Carbohyd. Polym.* 2001, *44*, 71-76´

[83] Koide, S. S. Chitin-chitosan: Properties, benefits and risks. *Nut, Res.* 1998, *18*, 1091-1101;

[84] Sudarshan, N. R.; Hoover, D. G.; Knorr, D. Antibacterial action of chitosan. *Food Biotech.* 1992, *6*, 257-272.

[85]   Liu, N.; Chen, X.G.; Park, H.J.; Liu, C G.; Liu, C. S.; Meng, X. H., Yu, L. J. Effect of
       MW and concentration of chitosan on antibacterial activity of *Escherichia coli*.
       Carbohyd. Polym. 2006, *64*, 60-65.

[86]   Liu, X. F.; Guan, Y. L.; Yang, D. Z.; Li, Z.; Yao, K. D. Antibacterial action of chitosan
       and carboxymethlyated chitosan. *J. Appl. Polym. Sci.* 2001, *79*, 1324-1335.

[87]   Park, P. J; Je, J. Y.; Byun, , H. G.; Moon, S. H.; Kim, S. K. Antimicrobial activity of
       hetero-chitosan and their oligosaccharides with different molecular weights. *J.
       Microbio. Biotech.* 2004, *14*, 317-323.

[88]   Li, Y.; Chen, X. G.; Liu, N.; Liu, C. S.; Liu, C. G.; Meng, X. H.; Yu, L. J.; Kennedy, J.
       F. Physicochemical characterization and antibacterial property of chitosan acetates.
       Carbohyd. Polym. 2007, *67*, 227-232.

[89]   Choi, B. K.; Kim, K. Y.; Yoo, Y. J.; Oh, S. J.; Choi, J. H.; Kim, C. Y. In vitro
       antimicrobial activity of chitooligosaccharide mixture against *Actinobacillus
       actinomycetimcomitans* and *Streptococcus mutans*. *Int. J. Antimic. Agents* 2001, *18*,
       553-557.

[90]   Fujimoto, T.; Tsuchiya, Y.; Terao, M.; Nakamura, N.; Yamamoto, M. Antibacterial
       effects of chitosan solution against *Legionella pheumophila*, *Escherichia coli*, and
       Staphylococcus aureus. *Int. J. Food Microbiol.* 2006, *112*, 96-101.

[91]   No, H. K.; Park, N. Y.; Lee, S. H.; Meyers, S. P. Antibacterial activity of chitosan and
       chitosan oligomers with different molecular weights. *Int. J. Food Microbio.* 2002, *74*,
       65-72.

[92]   Zheng, L. Y.; Zhu, J. F. Study on antimicrobial activity of chitosan with different
       molecular weights. *Carbohyd. Polym.* 2003, *54*, 527-530.

[93]   Yoshihiko, O.; Mayumi, S.; Takahiro, A.; Hiroyuki, S.; Yoshihiro, S.; Ichiro, N.;
       Tetsuaki, T. Antimicrobial activity of chitosan with different degrees of acetylation and
       molecular weights. *Biocontrol Sci.* 2003, *8*, 25-30.

[94]   Liu, C. G.; Desai, K. G.; Chen, X. G.; Park, H. J. Linoleic acid-modified chitosan for
       formation of self-assembled nanoparticles. *J. Agricult. Food Chem.* 2005, *53*, 437-441.

[95]   Li, Y. Y.; Chen, X. G.; Liu, C. S.; Cha, D. S.; Park, H. J.; Lee, C. M. Effect of the
       molecular mass and degree of substitution of oleoylchitosan on the structure,
       rheological properties, and formation of nanoparticles. *J. Agricult. Food Chem.* 2007,
       55, 4842-4847.

[96]   Chen, X. G.; Lee, C. M.; Park, H. J. O/W emulsification for the self-aggregation and
       nanoparticle formation of linoleic acid-modified chitosan in the aqueous system. *J.
       Agricult. Food Chem.* 2003, *51*, 3135-3139.

[97]   Xing, K.; Chen, X. G.; Li, Y. Y.; Liu, C. S.; Liu, C. G.; Cha, D. S.; Park, H. J.
       Antibacterial activity of oleoyl-chitosan nanoparticles: a novel antibacterial dispersion
       system. *Carbohyd. Polym.* 2008, *74*, 114-120.

[98]   Fernandez-Lopez, S.; Kim, H.-S.; Choi, E. C.; Delgado, M.; Granja, J. R.; Khasanov,
       A.; Kraehenbuehl, K.; Long, G.; Weinberger, D. A.; Wilcoxen, K. M.; Ghadiri, M. R.
       Antibacterial agents based on the cyclic D,L-α-peptide architecture. *Nature*, 2001, *412*,
       452-455.

[99]   Clark, J. R.; March, J. B. Bacteriophages and biotechnology: vaccines, gene therapy
       and antibacterials. *Trends Biotechnol.* 2006, *24*, 112-118.

[100] Marks, T.; Sharp, R. Bacteriophages and biotechnology: a review. *J. Chem. Technol. Biotechnol.* 2000, *75*, 6-17.

[101] Sandeep, K. Bacteriophage precision drug against bacterial infections. *Curr. Sci.* 2006, *90*, 631-633.

[102] Sulakvelidze, A.; Alavidze, Z.; Morris, J. G. Bacteriophage therapy. *Antimicrob. Agents Chemother.* 2001, *45*, 649-659.

[103] Wang, Q.; Lin, T.; Tang, L.; Johnson, J. E.; Finn, M. G. Icosahedral virus particles as addressable nanoscale building blocks. *Angew. Chem.* 2002, *114*, 477-480; *Angew. Chem. Int. Ed.* 2002, *41*, 459-462.

[104] Kaltgrad, E.; Gupta, S. S.; Punna, S.; Huang, C.-Y.; Chang, A.; Wong, C.-H.; Finn, M. G.; Blixt, O. Anti-carbohydrate antibodies elicited by polyvalent display on a viral scaffold. *ChemBioChem* 2007, *8*, 1455-1462.

[105] Turos, E.; Reddy, G. S. K.; Greenhalgh, K.; Ramaraju, P.; Abeylath, S. C.; Jang, S.; Dickey, S.; Lim, D. V. Penicillin-bound polyacrylate nanoparticles: restoring the activity of β-lactam antibiotics against MRSA. *Bioorg. Med. Chem. Lett.* 2007, *17*, 3468-3472.

[106] Balland, O.; Pinto-Alphandary, H.; Viron, A.; Puvion, E.; Andremont, A.; Couvreur, P. Intracellular distribution of ampicillin in murine macrophages infected with *Salmonella typhimurium* and treated with (3H) ampicillin-loaded nanoparticles. *J. Antimicrob. Chemother.* 1996, *37*, 105-115.

[107] Cohen, M. Changing pattern of infectious disease. *Nature* 2000, *406*, 762-767.

[108] Fauch, A. S. Infectious diseases: considerations for the 21st century. *Clin. Infect. Dis.* 2001, *32*, 675-685.

[109] Mandell, G.; Bennett, J.; Dolin, R. Principles and practice of infectious diseases. 5th ed., Churchill Livingstone, Philadelphia, 2000, pp. 2065-2092.

[110] Walsh, C. Antibiotics, action, origins, resistance. ASM Press, Washington, DC, 2000: pp. 3-49.

[111] Walsh, C. Where will new antibiotics come from? *Nat. Rev. Microbiol.* 2003, *1*, 65-70.

[112] Waxman D.J.; Strominger J.L. Sequence of active site peptides from the penicillin-sensitive D-alanine carboxypeptidase of *Bacillus subtilis*. *J. Biol. Chem.* 1980, *255*, 3964-3976.

[113] Frere J.M.; Nguyen-Disteche M.; Coyette J.; Joris B. Interaction with the penicillin binding proteins. The chemistry of β-lactams. Blackie Academic and Professional, NewYork. 1992. pp. 148-197.

[114] Ghuysen J.M.; Charlier P.; Coyette J.; Duez, C.; Fonze, E.; Fraipont, C.; Goffin, C.; Joris, B.; Nguyen-Disteche, M. Penicillin and beyond: evolution, protein fold, multimodular polypeptides, and multiprotein complexes. *Microb. Drug. Resist.* 1996, *2*, 163-175.

[115] Goffin C.; Ghuysen J. M. Multimodular penicillin-binding proteins: an enigmatic family of orthologs and paralogs. *Microbiol. Mol. Biol. Rev.* 1998, *62*, 1079-1093.

[116] Williams, D.H. The glycopeptide story: how to kill the deadly 'superbugs'. *Nat. Prod. Rep.* 1996, *13*, 469-477.

[117] Mueller F.; Doring T.; Erdemir T.; Greuer B.; Junke N.; Osswald, M.; Rinke-Appel, J.; Stade, K.; Thamm, S.; Brimacombe, R. Getting closer to an understanding of the three-dimensional structure of ribosomal RNA. *Biochem. Cell. Biol.* 1995, *73*, 767-773.

[118] Carter, A. P.; Clemons, W. M.; Brodersen, D. E.; Morgan-Warren, R. J.; Wimberly, B. T.; Ramakrishnan, V. Functional insights from the structure of the 30S ribosomal subunit and its interactions with antibiotics. *Nature* 2000, *407*, 340-348.

[119] Brodersen, D. E.; Clemons, W. M.; Carter, A. P.; Morgan-Warren, R. J.; Wimberly, B. T.; Ramakrishnan, V. The structural basis for the action of the antibiotics tetracycline, pactamycin, and hygromycin B on the 30S ribosomal subunit. *Cell* 2000, *103*, 1143-1154.

[120] Schlunzen, F.; Zarivach, R.; Harms, J.; Bashan, A.; Tocilj, A.; Albrecht, R.; Yonath, A.; Franceschi, F. Structural basis for the interaction of antibiotics with peptidyl transferase centre in eubacteria. *Nature* 2001, *413*, 814-821.

[121] Zhou C. C.; Swaney S. M.; Shinabarger D. L.; Stockman B. J. ^{1}H nuclear magnetic resonance study of oxazolidinone binding to bacterial ribosomes. *Antimicrob. Agents Chemother.* 2002, *46*, 625–629.

[122] Sherratt, D. J. Bacterial chromosome dynamics. *Science* 2003, *301*, 780-785.

[123] Maxwell, A. DNA gyrase as a drug target. *Trends Microbiol.* 1997, *5*, 102-109.

[124] Mascaretti, O. A. Bacteria versus antibacterial agents, an integrated approach. ASM Press, Washington, DC, 2003, pp. 289-328.

[125] Kotra L. P.; Mobashery S. β-lactam antibiotics, β-lactamases and bacterial resistance. *Bull. Inst. Pasteur* 1998, *96*, 139-150.

[126] Walsh, C. Molecular mechanisms that confer anti-bacterial drug resistance. *Nature* 2000, *406*, 775-781.

[127] Livermore, D. Can better prescribing turn the tide of resistance ? *Nat. Rev. Microbiol.* 2004, *2*, 73-78.

[128] Travis, J. Reviving the antibiotic miracle? *Science* 1994, *264*, 360-362.

[129] Davies, J. Inactivation of antibiotics and the dissemination of resistance genes. *Science* 1994, *264*, 375-382.

[130] Waksman, S. A.; Reily, H. C.; Schatz, A. Strain specificity and production of antibiotic substances. V. Strain resistance of bacteria to antibiotic substances, especially to streptomycin. *Proc. Natl. Acad. Sci. USA.* 1945, *31*, 157-164.

[131] Murray, E. Vancomycin resistant *enterococci. Am. J. Med.* 1997, *102*, 284-293.

[132] Neu, H. C. The crisis in antibiotic resistance. *Science* 1992, *257*, 1064-1073.

[133] Williams, D. H. The glycopeptide story: how to kill the deadly 'superbugs'. *Nat. Prod. Rep.* 1996, *13*, 469-477.

[134] Coates, A.; Hu, Y.; Bax, R.; Page, C. The future challenges facing the development of new antimicrobial drugs. *Nat. Rev. Drug Discovery* 2002, *1*, 895-910.

[135] Sievert, D. M.; Boulton, M. L; Stoltman, G.; Johnson, D.; Stobierske, M. G.; Downes, F. P.; Somsel, P. A.; Rudrik, J. T.; Brown, W.; Hafeez, W.; Lundstorm, T.; Flanagan, E.; Johnson, R.; Mitchell, J. *Staphylococcus aureus* resistant to vancomycin: United States, 2002. *Morbid. Mortal. Wkly. Rep..* 2002, *51*, 565-567.

[136] Nikaido, H. Prevention of drug access to bacterial targets: permeability barriers and active efflux. *Science* 1994, *264*, 382-388.

[137] Nakae, T. Role of membrane permeability in determining antibiotic resistance in *Pseudomonas aeruginosa*. *Microbiol. Immunol.* 1995, *39*, 221-229.

[138] Spratt, B. G. Resistance to antibiotics mediated by target alterations. *Science* 1994, *264*, 388-393.

[139] McMurry, L.; Petrucci, R. E. Jr.; Levy, S. B. Active efflux of tetracycline encoded by four genetically different tetracycline resistance determinants in *Escherichia coli*. *Proc. Natl. Acad. Sci.* USA 1980, *77*, 3974-3977.

[140] Yoneyama, H.; Nakae, T. Cloning of the protein D2 gene of *Pseudomonas aeruginosa* and its functional expression in the imipenem-resistant host. *FEBS Lett.* 1991, *283*, 177-179.

[141] Poole, K.; Krebes, K.; McNally, C.; Neshat, S. Multiple antibiotic resistance in *Pseudomonas aeruginosa*: evidence for involvement of an efflux operon. *J. Bacteriol.* 1993, *175*, 7363-7372.

[142] Morshed, S. R. M.; Lei, Y.; Yoneyama, H.; Nakae, T. Expression of genes associated with antibiotic extrusion in *Pseudomonas aeruginosa*. *Biochem. Biophys. Res. Commun.*, 1995, *210*, 356-362.

[143] Yoneyama, H.; Ocaktan, A.; Tsuda, M.; Nakae, T. The role of *mex*-gene products in antibiotic extrusion in *Pseudomonas aeruginosa*. *Biochem. Biophys. Res. Commun.*, 1997, *233*, 611-618.

[144] Babic, M.; Hujer, A. M.; Bonomo, R. A. What's new in antibiotic resistance? Focus on β-lactamases. *Drug Res. Updates* 2006, *9*, 142-156.

[145] Fisher, J.; Belasco, J. G.; Khosla, S.; Knowles, J. R. β-Lactamase proceeds *via* an acyl-enzyme intermediate: interaction of the *Escherichia coli* RTEM enzyme with cefoxitin. *Biochemistry* 1980, *19*, 2895-2901.

[146] Kotra, L. P.; Haddad, J.; Mobashery, S. Aminoglycosides: perspectives on mechanisms of action and resistance and strategies to counter resistance. *Antimicrob. Agents Chemother.* 2000, *44*, 3249-3256

[147] Wright, G. E. Aminoglycoside-modifying enzymes. *Curr. Opin. Microbiol.* 1999, *2*, 499-503.

[148] Carter, A. P.; Clemons, W. M.; Brodersen, D. E.; Morgan-Warren, R. J.; Wimberly, B. T.; Ramakrishnan, V. Functional insights from the structure of the 30S ribosomal subunit and its interactions with antibiotics. *Nature* 2000, *407*, 340-348.

[149] Brodersen, D. E.; Clemons, W. M.; Carter, A. P.; Morgan-Warren, R. J.; Wimberly, B. T.; Ramakrishnan, V. The structural basis for the action of the antibiotics tetracycline, pactamycin, and hygromycin B on the 30S ribosomal subunit. *Cell* 2000, *103*, 1143-1154.

[150] Abraham, E. P.; Chain, E. An enzyme from bacteria able to destroy penicillin. *Nature* 1940, *146*, 837-837.

[151] Bussiere, D.; Muchmore, S. W.; Dealwis, C. G.; Schluckebier, G.; Nienaber, V. L.; Edalji, R. P.; Walter, K. A.; Ladror, U. S.; Holzman, T. F.; Abad-Zapatero, C. Crystal structure of ErmC', and rRNA methyltransferase which mediates antibiotic resistance in bacteria. *Biochemistry* 1998, *37*, 7103-7112.

[152] Weisblum, B. Erythromycin resistance by ribosome modification. *Antimicrob. Agents Chemother.* 1995, *39*, 577-585.

[153] Skinner, R.; Cundliffe, E.; Schmidt, F. J. Site of action of a ribosomal RNA methylase responsible for resistance to erythromycin and other antibiotics. *J. Biol. Chem.* 1983, *258*, 12702-12705.

[154] Schlunzen, F.; Zarivach, R.; Harms, J.; Bashan, A.; Tocilj, A.; Albrecht, R.; Yonath, A.; Franceschi, F. Structural basis for the interaction of antibiotics with the peptidyl transferase center in eubacteria. *Nature* 2001, *413*, 814-821.

[155] Cetinkaya, Y.; Falk, P.; Mayhall, C. G. Vancomycin-resistant *enterococci*. *Clin. Microbiol. Rev.* 2000, *13*, 686-707.

[156] Bugg, T. D.; Wright, G. D.; Dutka-Malen, S.; Arthur, M.; Couvalin, P.; Walsh, C. T. Molecular basis for vancomycin resistance in *Enterococcus faecium* BM4147: biosynthesis of a depsipeptide peptidoglycan precursor by vancomycin resistance proteins VanH and VanA. *Biochemistry* 1991, *30*, 10408-10415.

[157] Park, I. S.; Lin, C. H.; Walsh, C. T. Bacterial resistance to vancomycin: overproduction, purification, and characterization of VanC2 from *Enterococcus casseliflavus* as a D-Ala-D-Ser ligase. *Proc. Natl. Acad. Sci. USA* 1997, *94*, 10040-10044.

[158] Nagai, K.; Davies, T. A.; Jacobs, M. R.; Appelbaum, P. C. Effects of amino acid alterations in penicillin-binding proteins (PBPs) 1a, 2b, and 2x on PBP affinities of penicillin, ampicillin, amoxicillin, cefditoren, cefuroxime, cefprozil, and cefaclor in 18 clinical isolates of penicillin-susceptible, -intermediate, and –resistant pneumococci. *Antimicrob. Agents Chemother.* 2002, *46*, 1273-1280.

[159] Zighelboim, S.; Tomasz, A. Penicillin-binding proteins of multiply antibiotic-resistant South African strains of *Streptococcus pneumoniae. Antimicrob. Agents Chemother.* 1980, *17*, 434-442.

[160] Hakenbeck, R.; Grebe, T.; Zahner, D.; Stock, J. B. β-Lactam resistance in *Streptococcus pneumoniae*: penicillin-binding proteins and non-penicillin-binding proteins. *Mol. Microbiol.* 1999, *33*, 673-678.

[161] Hakenbeck, R.; Ellerbrock, H.; Briese, T.; Handwerger, S.; Tomasz, A. Penicillin-binding proteins of penicillin-susceptible and –resistant pneumococci: immunological relatedness of altered proteins and changes in peptides carrying the beta-lactam binding site. *Antimicrob. Agents Chemother.* 1986, *30*, 553-558.

[162] Turos, E.; Long, T. E.; Konaklieva, M. I.; Coates, C.; Shim, J.Y.; Dickey, S.; Lim, D. V.; Cannons, A. N-Thiolated β-lactams: novel antibacterial agents for methicillin-resistant *Staphylococcus aureus. Bioorg. Med. Chem. Lett.* 2002, *12*, 2229-2231.

[163] Revell, K. D.; Heldreth, B.; Long, T.E.; Jang, S.; Turos, E. *N*-Thiolated β-lactams: studies on the mode of action and identification of a primary cellular target in *S. aureus. Bioorg. Med. Chem.* 2007, *15*, 2453-2467.

[164] Turos, E.; Reddy, G. S. K.; Greenhalgh, K.; Ramaraju, P.; Abeylath, S. C.; Jang, S.; Dickey, S.; Lim, D. V. Penicillin-bound polyacrylate nanoparticles: restoring the activity of β-lactam antibiotics against MRSA. *Bioorg. Med. Chem. Lett.* 2007, *17*, 3468-3472.

[165] Abeylath, S. C.; Turos, E.; Dickey, S.; Lim, D. L. Glyconanobiotics: novel carbohydrated nanoparticle antibiotics for MRSA and *Bacillus anthracis. Bioorg. Med. Chem.* 2008, *16*, 2412-2418.

[166] Santos-Magalhaes, N. S.; Pontes, A.; Pereira, V. M. W.; Caetano, M. N. P. Colloidal carriers for benzathine penicillin G: nanoemulsions and nanocapsules. *Int. J. Pharm.* 2000, *208*, 71-80.

[167] Diaz, H. V. R.; Batdorf, K. H.; Fianchinin, M. Diyabalanage, H. V. K.; Carnahan, S.; Mulcahy, R.; Rabiee, A.; Nelson, K.; Waasbergen, L. Antimicrobial properties of highly fluorinated silver(I) tris(pyrazolyl)borates. *J. Inorg. Biochem.* 2006, *100*, 158-160.

[168] Ramstedt, M.; Cheng, N.; Azzaroni, O. Mossialos, D.; Mathieu, H. J.; Huck, W. T. S. Synthesis and characterization of poly(3 sulfopropylmethacrylate) brushes for potential antibacterial applications. *Langmuir* 2007, *23*, 3314-3321.

[169] Li, P.; Li, J.; Wu, C.; Wu, Q.; Li, J. Synergic antibacterial effects of β-lactam antibiotic combined with silver nanoparticles. *Nanotechnology* 2005, *16*, 1912-1917.

[170] De Souza, A.; Mehta, D.; Leavitt, R. W. Bactericidal activity of combinations of silver-water dispersion with 19 antibiotics against seven microbial strains. *Curr. Sci.* 2006, *91*, 926-929.

[171] Diilen, K.; Weyenberg Vandervoort, J.; Ludwig, A. The influence of the use of viscosifying agents as dispersion media on the drug release properties from PLGA nanoparticles. *Eur. J. Pharm. Biopharm.* 2004, *58*, 539-549.

[172] Kell, J. A.; Stewart, G.; Ryan, S.; Peytavi, R.; Boissinot, M.; Huletsky, A.; Bergeron, M. G.; Simard, B. Vancomycin-modified nanoparticles for efficient targeting and preconcentration of gram-positive and gram-negative bacteria. *ACS Nano* 2008, *2*, 1777-1788.

[173] Gu, H.; Ho, P.; Tsang, K. W. T.; Wang, L.; Xu, B. Using biofunctional magnetic nanoparticles to capture vancomycin-resistant *Enterococci* and other gram-positive bacteria at ultra low concentration. *J. Am. Chem. Soc.* 2003, *125*, 15702-15703.

[174] Gu, H.; Ho, P. L.; Tong, E.; Wang, L.; Xu, B. Presenting vancomycin on nanoparticles to enhance antimicrobial activities. *Nano Letters* 2003, *3*, 1261-1263.

[175] Ma, M.; Cheng, Y.; Xu, Z.; Xu, P.; Qu, H.; Fang, Y.; Xu, T.; Wen, L. Evaluation of polyamidoamine (PAMAM) dendrimers as drug carriers of anti-bacterial drugs using sulfamethoxazole (SMZ) as a model drug. *Eur. J. Med. Chem.* 2007, *42*, 93-98.

[176] Buzea, C.; Pacheco, I. I.; Robbie, K. Nanomaterials and nanoparticles: Sources and toxicity *Biointerphases* 2007, *2*, MR17-MR71.

[177] Lewis, K., Persister cells, dormancy, and infectious disease. *Nat. Rev. Microbiol.* 2007, *5*, 48-56.

In: Antibiotic Resistance…
Editors: A. R. Bonilla and K. P. Muniz

ISBN 978-1-60741-623-4
© 2009 Nova Science Publishers, Inc.

Chapter XIX

Veterinary Antibiotics and Their Possible Impact on Resistant Bacteria in the Environment

Nicole Kemper[*]
Certified Veterinary Specialist in Microbiology
Certified Veterinary Specialist in Animal Hygiene
Institute of Animal Breeding and Husbandry,
Christian-Albrechts-University Kiel
Hermann-Rodewald-Str. 6, D-24118 Kiel,
Germany

Abstract

In this chapter, recent studies on the fate of antibiotics, and especially antibiotics used in animal husbandry, are evaluated under the aspect of potential risks for human health. Because the assumed quantity of antibiotics excreted by animal husbandry adds up to thousands of tons per year, major concerns about their degradation in the environment have risen during the last decades. One main problem with regard to the excessive use of antibiotics in livestock production is the potential promotion of resistance and the resulting disadvantages in the therapeutic use of antimicrobials. Since the beginning of antibiotic therapy, more and more resistant bacterial strains have been isolated from environmental sources showing one or multiple resistance. After administration, the medicines, their metabolites or degradation products reach the terrestrial and aquatic environment indirectly by the application of manure or slurry to areas used agriculturally or directly by pasture-reared animals excreting directly on the land.

After surface run-off, driftage or leaching in deeper layers of the earth, their fate and the impact on environmental bacteria remains rather unknown. Especially against the background of increasing antibiotic resistance, the scientific interest in antimicrobially

[*] Tel: ++49-431-880-4533; Fax: ++49-431-880-5265; nkemper@tierzucht.uni-kiel.de

active compounds in the environment and the possible occurrence of resistant bacteria has increased permanently. On the one side, scientific interest has focused on the behaviour of antibiotics and their fate in the environment, on the other hand, their impact on environmental and other bacteria has become an issue of research. With the advances of modern analytical methods, studies using these new techniques provide accurate data on concentrations of antimicrobial compounds and their residues in different organic matters. Some antibiotics seem to persist a long time in the environment, especially in soil, while others degrade very fast. Not only are the fate of these pharmaceuticals, but also their origin and their possible association with resistant bacteria objects of scientific interest.

This chapter presents an overview of the present studies on the use of veterinary antibiotics in agriculture, on the occurrence of antibiotic compounds and resistant bacteria in soil and water and clearly demonstrates the need for further studies.

Introduction

The use of veterinary pharmaceuticals in livestock production has aroused major public health concerns during recent years. Besides other human, animal and environmental impairments, the emergence and spread of resistant bacteria is particularly considered as a daunting risk. In human as well as in veterinary medicine, antibiotics are used to treat and prevent disease. Antibiotics are defined as naturally-occurring, semi-synthetic and synthetic compounds with antimicrobial activity that can be applied parentally, orally or topically. From the immoderate appliance of antibiotics, resulting in environmental contamination with original substances or derivatives, three main risks are discussed: besides the indirect impact on human and animal health via resistant micro-organisms, direct organic damage is feared. Additionally, the influences on the biotic environment are a matter of concern. An overview on the presence and behaviour of antibiotics in the aquatic and terrestrial environment was provided by Kemper (2008); major parts of this chapter are based on this review article.

Both in human and veterinary medicine, the call for rational antibiotic therapy is based on considerations regarding the increased occurrence of resistance. A continuous debate about resistance promotion has taken place since the late 1960s, when the Swann Committee concluded that antibiotics used in human medicine or those promoting cross resistance should not be used as growth promoters in animals (Swann Committee, 1969). The main groups of important antibiotics used as therapeutics and administered today in human and veterinary medicine are listed in Figure 1.

In Europe, the banning of antibiotic growth promoters was administered as a precaution because the agricultural use of antibiotics might act as an important source of resistance in bacteria affecting humans (European Parliament and Council, 2003). Opinions on this ban are still extremely diverse. On the one hand, the theoretical hazard to human health which has arisen from the use of growth-promoting antibiotics can not be denied; but on the other hand, the facts, examined independently without political or commercial influence, seem to show actual risk as extremely small or even zero in many cases (Phillips et al., 2004). Nevertheless, as long as these facts remain unknown, all circumstances leading to a close interaction between antibiotics, bacteria, animals and humans have to be considered with regard to increasing resistance.

class	compounds	primary usage	potential side effects
aminoglycosides	apramycin	pigs only	
	gentamycin	all animals, humans	neurotoxic
	kanamycin	dogs, pigs, cattle, horses	nephrotoxic
	neomycin	all animals	ototoxic, nephrotoxic
	sisomycin	humans only	ototoxic, nephrotoxic
	spectinomycin	pigs, cattle, poultry, sheep	
	streptomycin	obsolete	
ß-lactams: penicillins	amoxicillin	all animals	
	ampicillin	all animals	
	azlocillin	humans	
	benzylpenicillin	all animals	
	cloxacilin	cattle	
	dicloxacilin	cattle	
	flucloxacillin	humans	
	methicillin	humans	
	mezlocillin	humans	allergic reactions
	nafcillin	humans	
	oxacillin	cattle	
	piperacillin	humans	
	phenoxymethylcillin	humans	
	penicillin G	humans	
cephalosporines	cefalexin	dogs	
	cefalotin	humans	
	cefazolin	humans	
	ceftiofur	cattle, pigs	cross allergic reactions to
	cefotaxim	humans	ß-lactams
	cefotiam	humans	
	cefquinom	cattle, pigs	
fluorochinolones	ciprofloxacin	humans	
	enrofloxacin	all animals	arthropathies in young
	marbofloxacin	all animals	animals
	flumequin	humans	
	ofloxacin	humans	
lincosamides	clindamycin	dogs, humans	gastro-intestinal problems
	lincomycin	pigs, cats, dogs, cattle	
macrolides	azithromycin	humans	
	clarithromycin	humans	
	erythromycin	humans, cattle, chicken	
	roxithromycin	humans	
	spiramycin	all animals	
	tylosin	animals only	
	vancomycin	humans	
sulphonamides	sulphanilamide	humans	
	sulphadimethoxine	cattle, pigs, chicken	nephrotoxic
	sulphadimidine	cattle, sheep, chicken	
	sulphamethoxazole	humans	
	sulphapyridine	pigs	
trimethoprim		in combination with sulphonamides	
tetracyclines	chlortetracycline	cattle, pigs	hepatotoxic
	doxycycline	humans, cats, dogs	
	oxytetracycline	humans, cattle, sheep, pigs	
	tetracycline	humans, horse, sheep, pigs	

Figure 1. Important antibiotics in human and animal medicine (Kemper, 2008).

Antibiotic Resistance in Zoonotic Bacteria

The main interest regarding the use of antimicrobials in human and animal treatment is the development of resistant bacteria strains representing a health risk to humans and animals. New resistance mechanisms, multi-drug resistance or combinations of resistance and the possible horizontal spread of resistance between different species of bacteria have attracted scientific attention recently. As antibiotic resistance protects antibiotic-producing organisms from their own products, and other originally susceptible organisms from competitive attack, it is as ancient as antibiotics. It can be a natural property of the bacteria or acquired as a secondary mechanism. Briefly, antimicrobial resistance is defined as the capacity of bacteria to survive exposure to a defined concentration of an antimicrobial substance (Acar and Rostel, 2001). In applied microbiological laboratory diagnostics, this definition is extended by bacterial mechanisms governing higher minimum inhibitory concentration (MIC) than the original wild bacteria (Acar and Rostel, 2001).

In general, any application of antibiotics, no matter for which purpose, has the potential to lead to bacterial resistance. As an answer to selection pressure, resistance develops when the selecting substance is in prolonged contact with the bacterial population at sub-inhibitory concentrations, allowing the bacteria to survive. The chance to meet this correct sub-inhibitory concentration is the greater, the larger antibiotics are distributed in an ecosystem, regardless of whether animals, humans or the environment are affected. Not only direct therapeutic use of antibiotics, but also indirect contact with them might enhance the resistance of bacteria, not taking into account the bacteria's origins: resistance genes have been isolated from human pathogens, bacteria of animal origin, and environmental bacteria (Angulo et al., 2004; Levy, 1997; van den Bogaard and Stobberingh, 1999). Although there is a growing concern over the potential development of resistance when antimicrobial substances are released in the environment, the effects that environmental changes may have on the populations dynamics of bacteria an their antibiotic resistance have attracted far less attention (Martinez, 2008). Moreover, international travel and trade in animals and food are supposed to increase the risk of antimicrobial resistance world-wide (Acar and Rostel, 2001).

High level resistance can be generated by the co-operation of several resistance mechanisms. Genes governing resistance are newly combined via mutation, mainly in chromosomes, or acquired by horizontal transmission on transposons or plasmids. Plasmids or transposons, ofter carrying more than one marker of resistance, are considered as main systems transferring resistance from one donor-bacterium to another recipient-bacterium (Acar and Rostel, 2001). It has to be stressed that resistance is mainly located on mobile genetic elements such as plasmids, transposons, integrons, gene cassettes and bacteriophages, indirectly transporting the ability for resistance from non-pathogens to pathogenic micro-organisms. Only less than 5% of antibiotic resistance is located on chromosomal-based determinants (Nwosu, 2001). Thus, even if the main risk of provoking resistance has to be seen in connection with the clinical application of antibiotics and the abundance of certain pathogens in a restricted area such as a hospital or stables, the influence of bacteria located elsewhere cannot be denied. Resistance can be transferred to environmental bacteria. This is supported by several studies showing resistance patterns in bacteria isolated from soils (Onan and LaPara, 2003; Sengeløv et al., 2003). The impact of this potential transfer from non-pathogenic to pathogenic bacteria is a complex and difficult task for future research.

Recently, gram-negative bacteria with extended-spectrum ß-lactamase and multiresistant pneumococcal bacteria have been isolated from hospitals all over the world, representing a serious therapeutic problem in human medicine (Lee et al., 2001; Morris and Masterton, 2002). The most studied location of emergence of resistance is indeed the digestive tract of humans and animals with its huge amounts of bacteria and the obligatory presence of antibiotics after administration (Acar and Rostel, 2001). However, also the application of veterinary antibiotics in livestock production is suspected to significantly contribute to the selection for strains resistant to antibiotics used in human medicine. As mentioned above, not only the transfer of resistant pathogenic bacteria, but also the transfer of non-pathogenic resistant bacteria and their genes encoding resistance represent major problems. Transmission of these strains might be performed via direct contact with animals or via the food-chain to the consumers. There is accumulating evidence that antibiotic-resistant bacteria from cattle, pigs and poultry enter the food chain and can therefore transfer resistance genes to human commensals present in the human digestive tract (Dzidic et al., 2008; Perreten et al., 1997; Teuber et al., 1999; Wegener, 2003; World Health Organisation, 1997). The transfer of resistance genes among bacteria belonging to the physiological flora of the human colon is described by several studies (Davison, 1999; Ochmann et al., 2000). This transfer grows to a problem when accomplished with potentially pathogenic bacteria (Dzidic et al., 2008),

Increasing resistance has been noticed in the food-borne pathogens *Campylobacter* species (spp.) and *Salmonella* spp, particularly to fluorochinolones and third generation cephalosporins. In *Salmonella* spp. and *Escherichia coli*, multi-drug resistance is a worrying possibility, as well. Examples for zoonotic bacteria, presenting a health risk to humans, and known resistance in these pathogens are listed in Figure 2.

The current state of knowledge of bacterial resistance development and transfer has been documented in recent reviews (McDermott et al., 2003; White et al., 2002; Witte, 2000). Besides this, antibiotics may also represent a human health risk as allergic substances (Mellon et al., 2001). Allergic reactions can be evoked by some antibiotics such as penicillin, transferred into the organisms by oral or parenteral routes. Additionally, cases of serious photoallergic reactions and chronic photosensitive dermatitis have been reported after the administration of olaquindox (Schauder, 1989).

Regarding environmental issues, antibiotic resistance can be used as indicator for faecal source determination, for example in the analysis of effluents from sewage treatment plants (Hagedorn et al., 1999; Pillai et al., 1997; Wiggins, 1996). For instance, there have been attempts to use antibiotic resistance as indicator in faecal streptococci: in a study by Wiggins et al. (1999), antibiotic resistance analysis was conducted to identify the origin of the samples, classified in cattle, human, poultry and wild. Although some isolates were misclassified, the authors conclude that resistance patterns are strong indicators for different sources of pollution. Actually, the information contained in the resistance patterns seems strong enough to use for classification of unknown isolates from polluted waters, which may contain mixtures of different sources.

species	clinical disease in humans	possible resistance against	literature
Escherichia coli	diarrhoea, urinary tract infections, septicaemia	ß-lactams tetracyclines streptomycin/spectinomycin sulphonamides cimethoprim chinolones chloramphenicoles gentamycin/kanamycin/neo-mycin	(Angulo et al., 2004; Bundesinstitut für Risikobewertung, 2004)
Salmonella spp.	diarrhoea	ß-lactams tetracyclines streptomycin/spectinomycin sulphonamides cimethoprim chinolones chloramphenicole gentamycin/kanamycin/neo	(Angulo et al., 2004; Davis et al., 2007; Hensel & Helmuth, 2005)
Campylobacter spp.	diarrhoea, neuronal damages as sequels	ciprofloxacin tetracyclines doxycycline erythromycin trimethoprim sulphamethoxazole	(Angulo et al., 2004; Bae et al., 2005; Luber et al., 2003; Senok et al., 2007)

Figure 2. Resistance in zoonotic bacteria (Kemper, 2008).

Antibiotics in Livestock Farming

In livestock farming, antimicrobial agents have been used since the early 1950s to treat infections and improve growth and feed efficiency. Before the ban of growth promoters, in Europe especially pigs and poultry were treated with the majority of antibiotics administered in agricultural livestock production, while other species received only one percent of prescriptions (Ungemach, 2000). The amounts of antibiotics used in one year can only be calculated roughly: in 1999, 13,288 tons of antibiotics were used in the EU and Switzerland, of which 29% were used in veterinary medicine, 6% as growth promoters and 65% were used in human medicine [European Federation of Animal Health (FEDESA), 2001]. However, an actual decline in antibiotics used in agricultural has been recorded since the prohibition of growth promoters in 2006. In the U.S.A, the percentage of antibiotics used in livestock farming was 70% out of a total of approximately 16,200 tons (Union of concerned scientists, 2001).

Animal performance in livestock production, and therefore economic output, is significantly decreased by diseases. The intention of the use of antibiotics is to limit progression of disease in the population. Following the National Committee for Clinical Laboratory Standards (2002), herd or flock antibiotic use can be described by the terms of therapy, control, prevention and growth promotion. Therapy includes all antibiotic treatment of animals showing frank clinical disease. If antimicrobial treatment is administered to a herd or flock in which morbidity and/or mortality has exceeded baseline norms, it is defined as a control, whereas prevention is the use of antibiotics in animals considered to be at risk, but before showing the onset of disease or identification of causal agents. The administration of an antimicrobial over a period of time, usually as a feed additive, to growing animals is defined as growth promotion, resulting in improved physiological performance. Since 2006, all growth promoters have been banned from European agriculture by Regulation No 1831/2003 (European Parliament and Council, 2003) and therefore have not been taken into consideration in the following reflections. For cattle and swine, individual antibiotic treatment may be practical, but for poultry, antibiotics are applied orally with feed or water. For instance, antimicrobials in cattle are used for the treatment of mastitis in cows and of respiratory infections in calves. In pigs, they are mainly administered to treat gastrointestinal disorders in the weaning period or pneumonia later in life. Many of these antibiotic products are closely related to antibiotics used in human medicine, including ß-lactams, tetracyclines, sulphonamides with or without trimethoprim, macrolides, lincosamides and quinolones (Figure 1). An overview of current data on animal antibiotics world-wide, especially tylosin, tetracycline and sulphonamides, was given by Sarmah et al. (2006).

Because they are bioactive substances, acting highly effectively at low doses and excreted after a short time of residence, antibiotics are not completely eliminated in animal organisms. They are optimised with regard to their pharmacokinetics in the organisms: organic accumulation is, as in other pharmaceutics, objectionable and thus, they are excreted as parent compounds or metabolites (Kümmerer et al., 2000; Thiele-Bruhn, 2003). Excretion rates are dependant on the substance, the mode of application, the excreting species and time after administration, but it has been shown that rates vary between 40% to 90% for tetracyclines and sulphonamides (Berger et al., 1986; Haller et al., 2001; Halling-Sørensen, 2001). Sulphamethoxazole degrades to about 85%, whereas other substances are relatively inert in the body, e.g. the degradation rate for amoxicillin is between only 10% and 20% (Hirsch et al., 1999). Excretion rates of antibiotics are summarised by Jjemba (2002) and Zuccato et al. (2001). If intracorporal degradation takes place, it is often proceeded in the faeces, but if antibiotics are not metabolised, recalcitrants persist in the environment (Kümmerer et al., 2000). Additionally, antibiotic metabolites can be transformed back to their parent compound after excretion (Langhammer, 1989). For instance, some antibiotics are transformed to conjugates such as acetylated metabolites, becoming inactive and analytically camouflaged, but in manure the acetyl group can be cleaved, releasing the original active ingredient (Christian et al., 2003). For fluorchinolones and sulphonamides, the adsorption to faeces, being rich in organic matter, is strong (Marengo et al., 1997). Even by aeration of manure and increasing temperatures (Winckler and Grafe, 2001), these substances are not transformed and consecutively, distributed in the environment in an unaltered state. Possible entry paths of veterinary antibiotics are displayed in Figure 3.

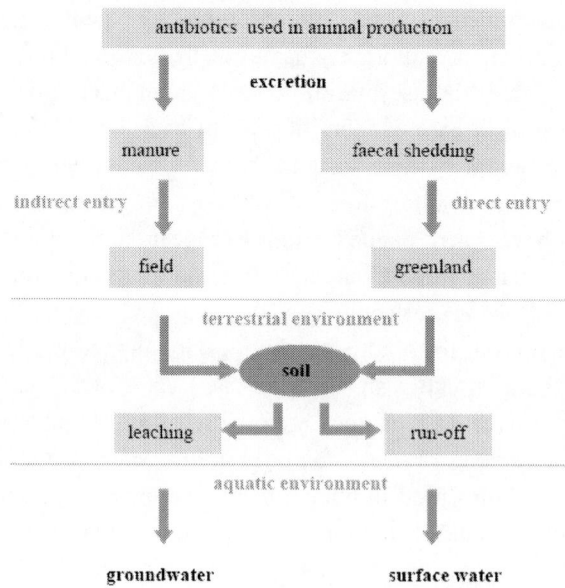

Figure 3. Veterinary antibiotics in the environment: anticipated exposure pathways (Kemper, 2008).

Current Methodological Approaches

Multianalytic methods have been developed have been developed since the late 1990s, contributing to the realisation of studies on the occurrence, transport and degradation processes of antibiotics into and in the environment. Intense work has been undertaken towards the design of analytical methods for the detection of various antibiotics, especially in wastewater and the aquatic environment (Golet et al., 2001; Hirsch et al., 1999). These methods may serve as basis for a sound risk assessment of antibiotics in the environment.

The need for extraction complicates the chemical analysis of antibiotics from different matrices. As antibiotics often consist of a non-polar core and polar functional groups, they dissociate or protonate depending on the pH of the medium (Juhel-Gaugain et al., 2000). Very polar and non-polar extractants can lead to an incomplete extraction, representing a serious analytical problem. In general, weakly acidic buffers in combination with organic solvents serve as extractants. Sample clean-up is performed via 0.45 μm filtration or solid phase extraction. A detailed review of current extraction and detection methods is given by Thiele-Bruhn (2003). To date, high-performance liquid chromatography in combination with UV and Diode-Array Detection (HPLC-UV, -DAD) or liquid chromatography with mass-spectrometry (LC-MS) or tandem mass-spectrometry (LC-MS/MS) are the most sensitive methods (Hamscher et al., 2002; Oka et al., 2000). LC-MS is especially suitable for a multitude of compounds (Niessen, 1998). A detailed description of high-performance liquid chromatography combined with electrospray ionisation tandem mass-spectrometry (LC-ESI-MS/MS) was published by Hamscher et al. (2002). High recovery rates of about 70% for oxytetracycline, chlortetracycline, and tylosin in a difficult matrix such as soil enable this method for the analysis of antibiotics in soil even in the low microgram per kilogram range. Detailed descriptions of methodologies for extraction and analysis of antibiotics in different sample material are found in Christian et al. (2003). Additionally, ELISA (Enzyme-Linked Immuno Sorbent Assay) tests, originally developed for sulphadimidine detection in milk, plasma, urine and tissue, were optimised for the analysis of environmental samples (Christian et al., 2003; Fránek et al., 1999). Thiele-Bruhn (2003) stated that the antibiotic potential of antibiotics has to be assessed by microbial assays in addition to the quantity to completely evaluate an antimicrobial substance. Limits of quantification of various antibiotics analysed with high-performance liquid chromatography combined with tandem mass-spectrometry (HPLC-MS/MS) are listed in Figure 4.

class	compounds	limit of quantification ng/l	limit of detection ng/l
ß-lactams: penicillins	amoxicillin ampicillin benzylpenicillin cloxacilin dicloxacilin flucloxacillin methicillin mezlocillin nafcillin oxacillin piperacillin phenoxymethylcill in	10	5
macrolides	azithromycin	5	1
	clarithromycin	2	0.5
	clindamycin	5	1
	erythromycin	5	2
	roxithromycin	5	2
	spiramycin	5	2
	tylosin	5	2
	vancomycin	50	30
sulphonamides	sulphadimidine sulphamethoxazol e	5	2
trimethoprim		5	2
fluorochinolones	ciprofloxacin	10	5
	ofloxacin	5	2
tetracyclines	chlortetracycline	25	10
	doxycycline	20	10
	oxytetracycline	20	10
	tetracycline	20	10

Figure 4. Limits of quantification for HPLC-MS/MS (Färber, 2001; Kemper et al., 2008).

The Fate of Antibiotics in the Environment

Depending on pharmacokinetic and pharmacodynamic parameters in the organism, antibiotics or their metabolites are excreted and spread in the environment via different pathways. Once in the environment, antibiotic efficiency depends on the physical-chemical properties, prevailing climatic conditions, soil types and a variety of other environmental factors.

Concentration limits of antibiotics in the environment are not regulated, even though the growing concern has been taken into account with the prescription of environmental risk assessment of veterinary pharmaceuticals in the U.S and Europe (EMEA, 1997; Thiele-Bruhn, 2003). Risk assessment is realised by the calculation of predicted environmental concentrations (PEC) and comparison with predicted, biological non-effective concentrations (PNEC) (Kümmerer, 2001b). In the U.S.A., the US Food and Drug Administration website provides information about the assessment on environmental risks of veterinary antibiotics (www.fda.gov/cvm/efoi/ea/ea.htm). Detailed emission and distribution models as well as environmental risk assessment for veterinary medicinal products are provided by Montforts (2003).

To start with, the fate of antibiotics in soil is described. The behaviour of antibiotics in soil has been recognised as one of the emerging issues in environmental chemistry. Antibiotics used for veterinary purposes are excreted by the animals and end up in soils via grazing livestock or manure used as agricultural fertiliser (Jørgensen and Halling-Sørensen, 2000). The loads of antibiotics shed by manuring have been estimated up to kilograms per hectare (Winckler and Grafe, 2000). Other minor agricultural entries into the environment may originate from antibiotics in the dust from the exhaust air of stable ventilation, as reported by Hamscher et al. (2003). Often, antibiotics are released into the environment only slightly transformed, or even unchanged and conjugated to polar molecules. Chemical and physical behaviour in the soil depends on the molecular structure of the pharmaceutical. An overview of the fate of antibiotic compounds in soils and the sorption coefficients in soils, sediment and slurry was also published by Thiele-Bruhn (2003). With regard to their various structural classes, antibiotics are ionised, amphiphilic or amphoteric and for this reason, adsorption to soils take place.

Due to these physical-chemical properties, such as their molecular structure, size, shape, solubility and hydrophobicity, the sorption and fixation of these substances in soils differ considerably. Many substances are polar, lowly water soluble and therefore strongly retarded in soils. For example, the transport of tetracyclines seems to be restricted to fast preferential and macropore flow or to be facilitated by co-transport with mobile colloids such as dissolved organic matter (Thiele-Bruhn, 2003). Most antibiotics are adsorbed very fast. Their antibiotic potency is mostly decreased by sorption and fixation, but that does not necessarily mean a complete elimination of the antimicrobial activity (Sengeløv et al., 2003). However, experimental studies on the antimicrobial activity of soil-bound tetracycline and tylosin have shown that even though these compounds are tightly adsorbed by clay particles, they remain active, showing antimicrobial effects that may influence the selection of antibiotic resistant bacteria in the terrestrial environment (Chander et al., 2005). A detailed overview of the sorption of veterinary pharmaceutical in soils is represented by Tolls (2001). If the application of contaminated manure on soil exceeds the degradation rate of antibiotics, an accumulation of this compound has to be expected. In general, the concentration of antibiotics in certain soil layers is termed as terracumulation (Rooklidge, 2004). These adsorbed compounds pose a reservoir of pollutants that can be mobilised in soils and further contaminate ground water by leaching or by erosion to surface waters (Pedersen et al., 2003). Figure 5 represents various antibiotic compounds detected in soils.

class	substance	concentration ng/kg	literature
macrolides	clarithromycin	-67 000	(Schüller, 1998)
	lincomycin	8 500	(Boxall et al., 2005)
sulphonamides	sulphadiazine	1 000	(Boxall et al., 2005)
	sulphadimidine	11 000	(Höper et al., 2002)
	sulphametazine	2 000	(Hamscher et al., 2005)
trimethoprim		500	(Boxall et al., 2005)
fluorochinolones	ciprofloxacin	6 000-52 000	(Schüller, 1998)
tetracyclines	tetracycline	450 000-900 000 -200 000	(Winckler & Grafe, 2000) (Hamscher et al., 2002)
	oxytetracycline	305 000	(Boxall et al., 2005)
	chlortetracycline	39 000	(Hamscher et al., 2005)

Figure 5. Antibiotics in soil (Kemper, 2008).

To date, only a few studies on mobility and transport of antibiotics in soil exist. Alder et al. (2001) reported diffuse contamination of surface water after antibiotic leaching from agricultural soils. Examinations of ground water and leachate from fields with intensive livestock production and manuring detected none or only antibiotics in small numbers (Hirsch et al., 1999; Kemper et al., 2008). Column experiments showed, depending on the soil type, the retention of the adsorbing tylosin at different depths, while olaquindox, only weakly adsorbing, leached trough the columns and oxytetracycline was not transported at all into deeper soil segments as this compound is strongly adsorbed to soil (Rabølle and Spliid, 2000). For oxytetracyclines and tylosin, distribution coefficients in manure are smaller than in soils (Loke et al., 2002). A lowering effect of manure was also detected for sulphachloropyridazine: the distribution coefficient decreases with an increasing proportion of manure in soils, mainly due to the pH effect of alkalinic manure (Boxall et al., 2002). For tetracyclines, detection at soil depths of up to 30 cm over long time periods was described by Hamscher et al. (2002). This data demonstrated that tetracyclines not only occur in significant amounts in soil after fertilisation with liquid manure, but also persist and accumulate in the environment. This strong binding to soil-organic matter is based on the ability of the tetracyclines to form complexes with double-charged cations, such as calcium, which occur in high concentrations in soil (Samuelsen et al., 1992).

The decomposition of antibiotics is driven by many factors. Photodegradation, as described for fluorchinolones, tetracyclines and sulphonamides (Sengeløv et al., 2003), does not play a major role since the influence of light is reduced when antibiotics are protected in sludge or slurry. Degradation in soil is mainly brought about by microbial activity, especially enzymatic reactions, transforming the parent compound via hydroxylation and oxidative decarboxylation (Al-Ahmad et al., 1999). Even though these reactions are reversible, antibiotics usually further degrade in manure and soil (Ingerslev and Halling-Sørensen, 2000). Biodegradation in soil increases when manure or sludge with high numbers of micro-organisms is added (Ingerslev and Halling-Sørensen, 2001).

The soil serves as a vast reservoir for micro-organisms. High numbers of bacteria, ranging from 10^6/g in agricultural soils to as high as 10^9/g in forest soils, are important in maintaining mineral immobilisation and decomposition processes (Nwosu, 2001). Antibiotics are affected in two ways: on the one hand, the microbial community can be severely disturbed by antibiotic activities; on the other hand, these environmental bacteria can acquire and provide gene-encoding resistance. Some soil micro-organisms possess a natural tolerance towards antibiotics (Esiobu et al., 2002). Especially *Pseudomonas* spp. often have an intrinsic resistance to antimicrobials (Sengeløv et al., 2003). In other bacteria, antimicrobial-specific resistance develops after the application of antibiotics. For instance, soil micro-organisms became resistant after the application of tetracycline-contaminated manure (Fründ et al., 2000). Regarding this promotion of resistance, an overview of the acquisition of genes coding for resistance in soil bacteria is presented by Seveno et al. (2002). Furthermore, in most cases, resistance is not provoked in the soil, but directly in the faeces and then spread to the soil by manuring. In Sweden and the Netherlands, the analysis of numerous faecal samples revealed a high prevalence of bacteria resistant against various antibiotics (Van den Bogaard et al., 2000). After manure fertilisation, tetracycline-resistant bacteria increased in soil as well as in ground water, but declined again after the cessation of slurry application to a level of non-slurry fertilised soil within eight months (Sengeløv et al., 2003). The ability to take up DNA from the environment occurs quite commonly among environmental isolates, as shown in a review of the role of natural transformation in the transfer of bacterial resistance (Lorenz and Wackernagel, 1994). Mobile genetic elements, transferring resistance from non-pathogenic to pathogenic bacteria, especially the important bacterial IncQ plasmid, were detected in microbial communities of environmental habitats and pig manure (Smalla et al., 2000; Smalla and Sobecky, 2002). The transfer of antibiotic resistance determinants is elucidated by Nwosu (2001).

Besides in soil, another major concern when talking about antibiotics in the environment is their fate and impact in the aquatic environment. Especially against the background of a continued exponential growth in human population, the demand for the Earth's limited supplies of freshwater has resulted in the claim for the protection of the integrity of water resources (Kolpin et al., 2002). In recent years, the occurrence and fate of antibiotics in the aquatic environment have been subjects to many investigations carried out in several countries. More than 30 antibiotic substances have been found in sewage influent and effluent samples, in surface waters and even ground and drinking water. Regarding antibiotics in animal husbandry, administered drugs, their metabolites or degradation products reach the aquatic environment by the application of manure or slurry to areas used agriculturally, or by pasture-reared animals excreting directly on the land, followed by surface run-off, driftage or leaching in deeper layers of earth. In this way, soils can act as a source of antibiotic contamination of the aquatic environment (Alder et al., 2001). Most of the antibiotics are water-soluble and therefore about 90% of one dose can be excreted in urine and up to 75% in animal faeces (Halling-Sørensen, 2001). According to Sarmah et al. (2006), occurrence of antibiotic residues in streams, lakes or other aquatic environment in the U.S. is not unlikely, when given an estimate of 100,000 million kg of faeces and urine being produced annually by the 60 million hogs raised in the U.S. and given that the use of their waste as fertiliser is a common practice. Besides this, animal-used antimicrobial compounds can also be released into the environment via aquaculture. Residuals and resistant bacteria from aquaculture operations have been reported during recent years (Olsen et al., 2001; Rice, 2001; Teuber, 1999).

The qualitative and quantitative influence of antibiotics on the resident marine bacterial community was summarised by Nygaard et al. (1992). The effects of sub-inhibitory concentrations against non-marine aquatic bacteria are mainly unknown, but the impact of various antibiotics remaining active against bacteria living in wastewater has been documented (Kümmerer, 2003). In wastewater and sewage treatment plants, resistant and multi-resistant bacteria have been detected, possibly entering the food chain directly via sewage sludge used as fertiliser or wastewater serving for irrigation (Feuerpfeil et al., 1999; Guardabassi et al., 1998; Kümmerer, 2003; Witte, 1998). Antibiotic effects on organisms living in the aquatic environment such as algae and daphnids (*Daphnia magna*) have been reported at concentrations between 5 and 100 μg/L (Holten-Lützøft et al., 1999; Wollenberger et al., 2000). Few studies have dealt with the impact of antibiotic use on populations of bacteria, especially indicator bacteria such as *enterococci*, in natural waters (Goni-Urriza et al., 2000; Wiggins et al., 1999).

Under test conditions in aquatic systems, most of the examined antibiotic compounds have been persistent, while only few have been partially biodegraded (Al-Ahmad et al., 1999; Kümmerer et al., 2000). To figure out the occurrence of antimicrobial drugs in surface waters and effluents from municipal sewage treatment plants, several studies have been conducted place in Germany (Christian et al., 2003), Switzerland (Alder et al., 2001; Golet et al., 2001), and the U.S. (Kolpin et al., 2002; Lindsey et al., 2001). A list of antibiotic substances detected in water samples, found to the ng/l-level, is shown in Figure 6.

Penicillins and tetracyclines are not usually expected to be found in the aquatic environment due to the easy hydrolysation of penicillins and the precipitation and accumulation of tetracyclines, as described above. The structure of ß-lactams such as penicillin, benzylpenicillin or cloxacillin, consisting of the ß-lactam-ring, contributes to the poor stability of this group in the environment: the ring can be opened by ß-lactamase, a widespread enzyme in bacteria, or by chemical hydrolysis. Thus, intact penicillins are usually not found in the environment (Myllyniemi et al., 2000). Neither tetracyclines nor tylosin were detected in any water sample by Hamscher et al. (2002). Further confirmation of these findings is supported by Lindsey et al. (2001), and Zhu et al. (2001). However, these substances have been detected in low levels in U.S. surface water samples (Kolpin et al., 2002) and in higher levels in overland flow water (Krapac et al., 2005). In Northwest Germany, a study was conducted sampling a series from surface waters, detecting a wide range of antibiotics in all samples (Christian et al., 2003): sulphonamides, macrolides and lincosamides were analysed frequently, whereas ß-lactams were rarely found. Tetracyclines were not detected because of their strong adsorption to organic matter. The presence of tetracycline-resistant bacterial isolates in lagoons and groundwater underlying two swine production facilities was published by Chee-Sanford et al. (2001).

class	substance	Concentration ng/l	source	literature
macrolides	lincomycin	21 100	surface water	(Boxall et al., 2005)
		-730	surface water	(Kolpin et al., 2002)
	clarithromycin	-260	surface water	(Hirsch et al., 1999)
	erythromycin	-1700	surface water	(Hirsch et al., 1999)
	roxithromycin	-560	surface water	(Hirsch et al., 1999)
	tylosin	-50	surface water	(Ashton et al., 2004; Daughton & Ternes, 1999)
Sulpho-namides	sulphadiazine	4 130	surface water	(Boxall et al., 2005)
	sulphamethazine	240	ground water	(Hamscher et al., 2005)
	sulphamethoxazole	-410	groundwater	(Sacher et al., 2001)
		-480	surface water	(Hirsch et al., 1999)
		-66	drinking water	(Mückter, 2006)
Trime-thoprim		20	surface water	(Boxall et al., 2005)
		-200	surface water	(Hirsch et al., 1999)
Fluoroc-hinolones	ciprofloxacin	-405	effluents	(Golet et al., 2001)
	norfloxacin	-120	effluents	(Golet et al., 2001)
		-120	surface water	(Kolpin et al., 2002)
Tetra-cyclines	tetracycline	400	groundwater	(Krapac et al., 2005)
	oxytetracycline	32 000	overland flow water	(Kay et al., 2005)
	chlortetracycline	-690	surface water	(Kolpin et al., 2002)

Figure 6. Antibiotics in water (Kemper, 2008).

MacKie et al. (2006) detected both tetracycline residues and tetracycline resistance genes in groundwater impacted by swine production facilities. However, antibiotic input by agricultural use is the minor origin of antimicrobials in the aquatic environment. Most of the analysed substances originated from discharge or sewage into rivers, only for a couple of samples could an influence of animal husbandry on the occurrence of antibiotics in surface waters be assumed. The major part of antibiotic input is carried out by human administration via hospital effluents or municipal wastewater, as reviewed by Kümmerer (2001a).

Analysis of Antibiotic Residues from Dairy Farms: An Example

To illustrate the reviewed current state of knowledge on antibiotics in the environment, a study is provided in the following as an example for applied methodologies and approaches. This research was funded by the Ministry of Agriculture, Environment and Rural Areas of the Federal State of Schleswig-Holstein and was published in 2008 (Kemper et al., 2008).

Introductory Remarks

In Germany as well as in other countries, regulations concerning drinking water quality demand that the amounts of chemical contaminants polluting or altering the quality of drinking water are kept as low as possible. To implement these regulations, the knowledge of the distributions of antibiotics in the environment is essential. The objective of this study was to verify whether animal husbandry can be a source of antibiotic residues which show up in the aquatic environment in Northern Germany. Furthermore, the occurrence of these residues and potential differences in conventional and organic farms were evaluated.

Studied Material

Liquid manure samples were collected during two seasons of leaching (October until February) in 2004/05 and 2005/06 every four weeks on two conventional and two organic dairy farms in Schleswig-Holstein, Germany. This sampling design was established to compare potential differences between these husbandry forms and was part of a long-term study on organic and conventional farms (Kemper, 2007). Manure was stirred mechanically in the slurry tank before sampling to guarantee a specimen as homogeneous as possible. All samples were filled into brown glass bottles and stored in the dark at 4°C until further processing within four days. After manure application on one maize field per farm, leachate samples were taken with the help of suction cups. Additionally, one grassland pasture was sampled in the same way while animals were grazing. During the test period, the sampling interval of four weeks could not be maintained totally due to weather conditions, as a minimum of two litres of leachate was needed for analysis. In 2004/05, a total of eight samples, containing five manure samples, were analysed. These examinations served as preliminary tests to establish the analysis conditions for manure samples and to adjust the sensitive laboratory methods. In 2005/06, 34 samples were examined, consisting of ten manure samples, eleven leachate samples from grassland and 13 leachate samples from maize fields.

Chemical analysis of antibiotics from different matrices, especially manure, is complicated by the need for extraction. Analytes need to be isolated from the sample matrix. In this study, sample clean-up was performed by a 1:50 dilution with following centrifugation and via solid-phase extraction. The sorbent for solid–phase extraction consisted on 200 mg of a surface-modified styrene-divinylbenzenecopolymer in 6 mL polypropylene cartridges (Strata X, Phenomenex Germany). All samples were analysed with high-performance liquid chromatography in combination with tandem mass-spectrometry (HPLC-MS/MS) as described by Christian et al. (2003). High recovery rates of about 70% for oxytetracycline, chlortetracycline, and tylosin recommend this method for the analysis of antibiotics in difficult matrices such as manure even in the low microgram per kilogram range. Samples were analysed for more than 20 substances, listed in Figure 4. Additionally, to discriminate residues' origins, detailed information on the antibiotics applied on these farms was recorded accurately with questionnaires for the whole sampling period.

Results

The treatment with antibiotics did not differ between conventional and organic farms, neither in the range of antibiotics used nor in the amount of administered treatments. In general, most treatment took place after mastitis with ß-lactam antibiotics and tetracyclines. Out of the list of examined pharmaceuticals, amoxicillin, ampicillin, benzylpenicillin, cloxacillin, sulphadimidine, chlortetracycline, doxycycline, oxytetracycline and tetracycline were administered during the examination period. Furthermore, animals were treated with enrofloxacin and cephalosporines, but these substances could not be analysed by the laboratory methods used.

Limits of quantification were not exceeded in any sample, regardless of sample origin. Neither in liquid manure nor in leachate were the analysed antibiotics detected at levels above the limits of quantification. In two manure samples from the sampling period 2004/05, traces of sulphadimidine were found, above the limit of detection (2 ng/l), but beneath the limits of quantification (5 ng/l) and therefore not further quantifiable.

Discussion

The negative results of this study can be attributed to three possible reasons.

(i) Use Patterns of Antibiotics in Dairy Farming

The amount of antibiotics administered in dairy farming is low compared to pig or poultry production. Treatment is usually conducted as individual animal therapy. Antibiotics are administered mainly per injection or locally, but not orally via feed medication. Antibiotics approved for use in dairy cattle must establish appropriate withdrawal times and methods of residue detection in milk. Therefore, the range of substances differs from those labelled for use in pig or poultry production. Antibiotics approved for the treatment of mastitis, the most common reason for antimicrobial treatment, are mainly ß-lactams, which decompose quickly in the environment. In contrast, veterinary antibiotics are used extensively in pig and poultry production as a medicine or prophylaxis. In most cases, individual application is not routine, but the treatment is performed on a group or flock basis via fodder. Different antibiotics are approved for the use in these species, reflecting the whole scope of antimicrobial substances. Hence, multiple classes of antibiotics, especially macrolide, sulphonamide and tetracycline classes have been commonly detected in liquid waste of swine (Campagnolo et al., 2002; Meyer et al., 1999) and poultry feeding operations (Meyer et al., 2003). MacKie et al. (2006) detected both tetracycline residues and tetracycline resistance genes in groundwater impacted by swine production facilities. The development of resistant bacteria is a documented effect of the use of antibiotics in swine and poultry production (Kümmerer, 2001b). A study on the presence of tetracycline-resistant bacterial isolates in lagoons and groundwater discovered to have come from two swine production facilities was published by Chee-Sanford et al. (2001), while other studies examining possible residues from cattle farms represent negative results (Kümmerer, 2001b).

(ii) Degradation during Manure Storage

No residues could be detected in the manure at the time of discharging on the field. This fact can be related on the one hand to the dilution of faeces from treated animals with that of non-treated ones. On the other hand, depending on the class of antibiotics, antimicrobial substances can be degraded very quickly in organic matter. Aerobic and anaerobic treatment of slurry is not influenced by residues (Bohm, 1996). Manure storage is a useful process to minimize the antibiotic residues as the substances applied to dairy cows are sensitive to degradation processes taking place during that period. The reduction of antibiotics can be accelerated by composting with wood chips or straw, as shown for oxytetracycline (Arikan et al., 2007). Furthermore, the structure of ß-lactams such as penicillin, benzylpenicillin or cloxacillin, consisting of the ß-lactam ring, contributes to the poor stability of this group in the environment. The ring can be opened by ß-lactamase, a widespread enzyme in bacteria, or by chemical hydrolysis. Thus, intact penicillins are not usually found in the environment (Myllyniemi et al., 2000).

(iii) Adsorption to Soil

The negative results in leachate from grasslands can also be attributed to the fact that possibly excreted antibiotics either degrade very quickly in the environment such as ß-lactam antibiotics or are highly adsorbent to soil such as tetracyclines and are therefore not present in leachate. This strong binding to soil-organic matter is based on the ability of the tetracyclines to form complexes with double-charged cations, such as calcium, which occur in high concentrations in soil (Samuelsen et al., 1992). Neither tetracyclines nor tylosin were detected in any water sample by Hamscher et al. (Hamscher et al., 2002). Further confirmation of these findings is supported by Lindsey et al. (2001) and Zhu et al. (2001). However, these substances have been detected at low levels in U.S. surface water samples (Kolpin et al., 2002) and at higher levels in overland flow water (Krapac et al., 2005). In Northwest Germany, a study was conducted sampling a series from surface water, detecting a wide range of antibiotics in all samples (Christian et al., 2003): sulphonamides, macrolides and lincosamides were analysed frequently, whereas ß-lactams were rarely found.

In general, most studies state that antibiotics in surface water and groundwater originate from discharge or sewage into rivers. Only for a couple of samples could an influence of animal husbandry on the occurrence of antibiotics in surface water be assumed. The major part of antibiotic input is carried out by human administration via hospital effluents or municipal wastewater, as reviewed by Kümmerer (2001a).

Concluding Remarks

In this study, liquid manure and leachate samples from dairy farms in Northern Germany were examined for the occurrence of antibiotic residues with HPLC-MS/MS. The study clearly shows that the transfer risk into the environment for the substances analysed for these sources is very low. The increasing resistance in bacteria and the diminishing impact of therapeutic drugs are without a doubt one major challenge for interdisciplinary research. Of course, the reduction of the emission of antibiotics into the environment, whether of human or veterinary medical origin, is a promising approach for proper risk assessment and management. Appropriate use of antimicrobials in livestock production will preserve the long-term efficacy of existing antibiotics, support animal health and welfare and limit the risk factors of transferring antibiotic resistance to animals and humans. However, as shown by this analysis, the pathway via manure originating from dairy cows can be neglected.

Conclusion

Scientific research in the area of the fate and transport of antibiotics has just stepped out of its infancy, although five decades have passed since the first use of antibiotics in feedlots (Addison, 1984). Up to the present, the lack of suitable analytical test methods has been one reason for the absence of antibiotic concentration measurements in the environment and recognised effects on terrestrial or aquatic micro-organisms. To date, most of the research has been done in Denmark, Germany and the UK. Still, the human health and environmental consequences of the presence of antibiotics and resistant bacteria in the environment remain indistinct. In general, the impact of antimicrobial drugs administered to animals in terrestrial and aquatic environments depends not only on the used amount and the type of administration, but also on animal husbandry practices, metabolism within the animal, manure handling and storage and degradation rates in it. However, knowledge about the extent of the occurrence of antibiotics, their transport and fate in the environment is lacking. Thus, the recommendation of the European Union on the prudent use of antibiotics and the claim for "co-ordination between human, veterinary and environment sectors... and the magnitude of the relationship between the occurrence of antimicrobial resistant pathogens in humans, animals and the environment should be further clarified" is factual then as now (The Council of the European Union, 2002).

Without a doubt, the main concern of the extended use of antimicrobials and their shedding into the environment is the promotion of resistance in bacteria of human and veterinary medical importance. Commensal and environmental bacteria can serve as a feasible reservoir of resistance genes for pathogenic bacteria. Antimicrobials released into the environment can enhance the formation of single, cross- and even multiple resistance in pathogens, commensal and environmental bacteria (Al-Ahmad et al., 1999; Wegener et al., 1996). The role of antimicrobials in the development and maintenance of single or multiple antibiotic-resistant bacterial populations, especially pathogenic bacteria, is still a subject for further studies. Additionally, there is a gap of reliable studies on the relationship between antibiotic residues and the occurrence of resistant bacteria. Even if a general link between antibiotic use and percentage of resistant strains is assumed (Nwosu, 2001), it is unclear at which threshold concentrations a shift towards an increase in resistant bacteria is to be expected. The transmission of these resistant bacterial strains is possible via direct contact or via the food chain and potentially lowers the pharmacotherapeutic effect of antibiotics to cure animals and humans (Richter et al., 1996). Attention has to be turned to known and new exposure pathways for the transfer of multidrug-resistant bacteria from animals to humans. In a recent study, a possible airborne transmission route of multidrug-resistant bacteria from concentrated swine feeding operation was reported (Chapin et al., 2005).

Resistance is provoked by repeated exposition of bacteria to sub-lethal dosages of antibiotics, as realised by continuing manuring with contaminated faeces on land used agriculturally (Gavalchin and Katz, 1994). The experimental long-term storage of pig slurry under conditions of agricultural practice has revealed that chlortetracycline, sulphadiazine and trimethoprim and their active metabolites, respectively, are only partly degraded (Grote et al., 2004). In June 2001, the Steering Committee of the Veterinary International Committee on Harmonization (VICH) enhanced the trigger value for antibiotic concentrations in soil from 10 to 100 µg/kg (VICH, 2000). Still, this higher trigger value is exceeded by some compounds, for instance tetracyclines, in soils regularly fertilised with manure (Hamscher et al., 2002). Therefore, the long-term dispersion of liquid manure on fields may result in serious contamination, especially when certain antibiotics, such as tetracycline, accumulate in the environment. A possible transfer of antimicrobials from nutrient to plant tissue has already been shown by studies on hydroponically grown plants (Schwake-Anduschus et al., 2003) and confirmed by recent studies (Grote et al., 2006).

Although some antibiotics are used both in humans and animals, most of the resistance problems in humans have arisen from human use. Animal agriculture contributes antibiotic residues and resistant bacteria to the environment, especially in rural areas, but human beings rather than animals appear to be the main origin of these contaminants. Mostly wastewater treatment plants are the source of the release of human antibiotics to the environment, as the removal in the treatment process is incomplete. New approaches aim at the use of antibiotic resistance analysis to identify sources of faecal pollution, deriving human or animal origin by the resistance to human or veterinary antibiotics presented in the analysed bacteria (Hagedorn et al., 1999; Kaspar et al., 1990; Pillai et al., 1997; Wiggins, 1996). As a result from all the facts concerning environmental and inter-species transmission and the spreading of antibiotics, mobile genetic elements or resistant bacteria summarised in this chapter, this conclusion is misleading. Bacteria isolated from faeces of animal or human origin, respectively, does not implicitly possess resistance to the correspondent antibiotic compound.

It is evident that antimicrobial treatment is required for an efficient production of animal products, but antibiotics should never be a substitute for good hygiene management. The

WHO's claim and recommendation for better monitoring of antibiotic use by data collection at different levels is a step towards a science-based effective intervention (World Health Organisation, 2001). In several countries, collections of pharmaceutical sales data and regulations on the extensive agricultural use of growth promoters have been instituted during the last decade, but are unlikely to be implemented in the United States, for instance, within the near future.

Finally, current research is just beginning to identify the risks antibiotics may pose to the environment. Up to now, data from environmental concentration measurements of the majority of compounds have indicated that environmentally relevant concentrations are significantly lower than the effective concentrations used on target species. The benefits of reducing antibiotic resistance can hardly be quantified for the limitations in assessing controlled comparison and the diversity in natural systems (Rooklidge, 2004). The right method to cope with this problem is still a matter of scientific discussion. Whether or not antibiotics have a deleterious effect on ecosystem health cannot be addressed by experimental studies only. As in experiments on transport, microbial degradability and metabolic pathway of antibiotics, laboratory studies often have a limited relevance to the environment due to changes in concentration, pH, moisture content, temperature and other environmental factors (Ingerslev and Halling-Sørensen, 2001). One proposed way to solve this task is the collection of data gained from environmental sampling and pathway mobility experiments regarding important veterinary drugs (Boxall et al., 2003), but relevant data have so far been insufficient to analyse many currently used antibiotics. Even though this lack of economic benefits complicates the call for comprehensive action by the research community, the scientific results presented in this chapter indicate that the extent of antibiotic contamination and the occurrence of resistant bacteria are not limited by geographic regions, inter-species barriers or economic circumstances. Thus, in addition to the prudent use of antibiotics as an applicable method to maintain effectiveness of human and veterinarian therapy, further studies on chronic subtle effects to different species and on additivity, antagonisms and other interactive effects on organisms in the environment and on the ecosystem as a whole are of future scientific concern.

Even if the occurrence, effects and fate of antibiotics have been put in the perspective of the scientific interest, still little is known about the actual risk to both humans and the environment. Significant gaps still exist in the understanding of the interaction between residues, metabolites and resistance promotion after excretion. But the consequences of increasing resistance in bacteria and the diminishing impact of therapeutic drugs reach far beyond geographic origins of antimicrobial compounds and are therefore of global concern. Without a doubt, a promising approach for proper risk assessment and management is the reduction of the emission of antibiotics into the environment, whether of human or veterinary medical origin. Appropriate use of antimicrobials in livestock production will preserve the long-term efficacy of existing antibiotics, support animal health and welfare and limit the risk factors of transferring antibiotic resistance to animals and humans. Scientific knowledge about these issues will be crucial in making public health decisions and in updating recommendations for better protection of the global community.

References

Acar, J. and Rostel, B. 2001. Antimicrobial resistance: an overview. *Revue Scientifique et Technique de L Office International Des Epizooties*, 20, 797-810.

Addison, J. B. 1984. Antibiotics in sediments and run-off waters from feedlots. *Residue Reviews*, 92, 1-24.

Al-Ahmad, A., Daschner, F. D. and Kümmerer, K. 1999. Biodegradability of cefotiam, ciprofloxacin, meropenem, penicillin G, and sulfamethoxazole and inhibition of waste water bacteria. *Archives of Environmental Contamination and Toxicology*, 37, 158-163.

Alder, A. C., McArdell, C. S., Golet, E. M., Ibric, S., Molnar, E., Nipales, N. S. and Giger, W. 2001. Occurence and fate of flouroquinolone, macrolide, and sulfanamide antibiotics during wastewater treatment and in ambient waters in Switzerland. *American Chemical Society, Washington D.C.*, Symposium Series, 791, 56-69.

Angulo, F. J., Nunnery, J. A. and Bair, H. D. 2004. Antimicrobial resistance in zoonotic enteric pathogens. *Revue Scientifique et Technique et Technique de L Office International Des Epizooties*, 23 (2), 1-11.

Arikan, O. A., Sikora, L. J., Mulbry, W., Khan, S. U. and Foster, G. D. 2007. Composting rapidly reduces levels of extractable oxytetracycline in manure from therapeutically treated beef calves. *Bioresource Technology*, 98, 169-176.

Ashton, D., Hilton, M. and Thomas, K. V. 2004. Investigating the environmental transport of human pharmaceuticals to streams in the United Kingdom. *The Science of the Total Environment*, 333, 167-84.

Bae, W., Kaya, K. N., Hancock, D. D., Call, D. R., Park, Y. H. and Besser, T. E. 2005. Prevalence and antimicrobial resistance of thermophilic Campylobacter spp. from cattle farms in Washington State. *Applied and Environmental Microbiology*, 71, 169-74.

Berger, K., Petersen, B. and Buning-Pfaue, H. 1986. Persistence of drugs occurring in liquid manure in the food chain. *Archiv für Lebensmittelhygiene*, 37, 99-102.

Bohm, R. 1996. Effects of residues of antiinfectives in animal excrements upon slurry management and upon soil. *Deutsche Tierarztliche Wochenschrift*, 103, 264-268.

Boxall, A., Blackwell, P., Cavallo, R., Kay, P. and Tolls, J. 2002. The sorption and transport of sulphonamide antibiotic in soil systems. *Toxicology Letters*, 131, 19-28.

Boxall, A. B. A., Fogg, L., Kay, P., Blackwell, P., Pemberton, E. and Croxford, A. 2003. Prioritisation of veterinary medicines in the UK environment. *Toxicology Letters*, 142, 207-218.

Boxall, A. B. A., Fogg, L. A., Baird, D. J., Lewis, C., Telfer, T. C., Kolpin, D. and Gravell, A. 2005. Targeted monitoring study for veterinary medicines in the UK environment. *Final Report to the UK Environmental Agency*.

Bundesinstitut für Risikobewertung. 2004. Resistenzeigenschaften bei Salmonella- und E. coli-Isolaten (Resistance in Salmonella- and E. coli-isolates). *Kurzfassung des Abschlussberichtes*.

Campagnolo, E. R., Johnson, K. R., Karpati, A., Rubin, C. S., Kolpin, D. W., Meyer, M. T., Esteban, J. E., Currier, R. W., Smith, K., Thu, K. M. and McGeehin, M. 2002. Antimicrobial residues in animal waste and water resources proximal to large-scale swine and poultry feeding operations. *The Science of the Total Environment*, 299, 89-95.

Chander, Y., Kumar, K., Goyal, S. M. and Gupta, S. C. 2005. Antibacterial activity of soil-bound antibiotics. *Journal of Environmental Quality*, 34, 1952-1957.

Chapin, A., Rule, A., Gibson, K., Buckley, T. and Schwab, K. 2005. Airborne multidrug-resistant bacteria isolated from a concentrated swine feeding operation. *Environmental Health Perspectives*, 113, 137-142.

Chee-Sanford, J., Aminov, R., Krapac, I., Garrigues-Jeanjean, N. and Mackie, R. 2001. Occurrence and diversity of tetracycline resistance genes in lagoons and groundwater underlying two swine production facilities. *Applied and Environmental Microbiology*, 67, 1494-1502.

Christian, T., Schneider, R., Färber, H. A., Skutlarek, D., Meyer, M. T. and Goldbach, H. E. 2003. Determination of antibiotic residues in manure, soil, and surface waters. *Acta hydrochimica et hydrobiologica*, 31, 36-44.

Daughton, C. G. and Ternes, T. A. 1999. Pharmaceuticals and personal care products in the environment: agents of subtle change? *Environmental Health Perspectives*, 107 Suppl. 6, 907-38.

Davis, M. A., Hancock, D. D., Besser, T. E., Daniels, J. B., Baker, K. N. and Call, D. R. 2007. Antimicrobial resistance in Salmonella enterica serovar Dublin isolates from beef and dairy sources. *Veterinary Microbiology*, 119, 221-30.

Davison, J. 1999. Genetic exchange between bacteria in the environment. *Plasmid*, 42, 73-91.

Dzidic, S., Suskovic, J. and Kos, B. 2008. Antibiotic resistance mechanisms in bacteria: Biochemical and genetic aspects. *Food Technology and Biotechnology*, 46, 11-21.

EMEA. 1997. Note for guidance: environmental risk assessment for veterinary medicinal products other than GMO-containing and immunological products. In: *Commitee for Veterinary and Medicinal Products*, pp. 42. London.

Esiobu, N., Armenta, L. and Ike, J. 2002. Antibiotic resistance in soil and water environments. *International Journal of Environmental Health Research*, 12, 133-144.

European Federation of Animal Health (FEDESA). 2001. Antibiotic use in farm animals does not threaten human health. Brussels, Belgium: FEDESA/FEFANA Press release, 13 July.

European Parliament and Council. 2003. Regulation (EC) No 1831/2003 of the European Parliament and of the Council of 22 September 2003 on additives for use in animal nutrition (Text with EEA relevance).

Färber, H. A. 2001. Rückstände von Antibiotika: Untersuchung von Krankenhausabwässern, kommunalem Abwasser, Oberflächenwasser und Uferfiltrate (Residues of antibiotics: examination of hospital effluents, communal sewage and filtrates).

Feuerpfeil, I., López-Pila, J., Schmidt, R., Schneider, E. and Szewzyk, R. 1999. Antibiotikaresistente Bakterien und Antibiotika in der Umwelt (Antibiotic-resistant bacteria and antibiotics in the environment). *Bundesgesundheitsblatt - Gesundheitsforschung - Gesundheitsschutz*, 42, 37-50.

Fránek, M., Kolár, V., Deng, A. and Crooks, S. 1999. Determination of sulfadimidine (sulfamethazine) residues in milk, plasma, urine and edible tissue by sensitive ELISA. *Food and Agricultural Immunology*, 11, 339-349.

Fründ, H. C., Schlösser, A. and Westendarp, H. 2000. Effects of tetracycline on the soil microflora determined with microtiter plates and respiration measurement. *Mitteilungen der Deutschen Bodenkundlichen Gesellschaft*, 93, 244-247.

Gavalchin, J. and Katz, S. E. 1994. The persistence of fecal-borne antibiotics in soil. *Journal - Association of Official Analytical Chemists*, 77, 481-485.

Golet, E. M., Alder, A. C., Hartmann, A., Ternes, T. A. and Giger, W. 2001. Trace determination of fluoroquinolone antibacterial agents in solid-phase extraction urban wastewater by and liquid chromatography with fluorescence detection. *Analytical Chemistry*, 73, 3632-3638.

Goni-Urriza, M., Capdepuy, M., Arpin, C., Raymond, N., Caumette, P. and Quentin, C. 2000. Impact of an urban effluent on antibiotic resistance of riverine Enterobacteriaceae and Aeromonas spp. *Applied and Environmental Microbiology*, 66, 125-32.

Grote, M., Schwake-Anduschus, C., Stevens, H., Michel, R., Betsche, T. and Freitag, M. 2006. Antibiotika-Aufnahme von Nutzpflanzen aus Gülle-gedüngten Böden - Ergebnisse eines Modellversuchs (Antibiotic intake of crop plants from manured soil - results of an experiment). *Journal Verbraucherschutz und Lebensmittelsicherheit*, 1, 38-50.

Grote, M., Vockel, A., Schwarze, D., Mehlich, A. and Freitag, M. 2004. Fate of antibiotics in food chain and environment originating from pigfattening. *Fresenius Environmental Bulletin*, 13, 1216-1224.

Guardabassi, L., Petersen, A., Olsen, J. E. and Dalsgaard, A. 1998. Antibiotic resistance in Acinetobacter spp. isolated from sewers receiving waste effluent from a hospital and a pharmaceutical plant. *Applied and Environmental Microbiology*, 64, 3499-502.

Hagedorn, C., Robinson, S. L., Filtz, J. R., Grubbs, S. M., Angier, T. A. and Reneau, R. B., Jr. 1999. Determining sources of fecal pollution in a rural Virginia watershed with antibiotic resistance patterns in fecal streptococci. *Applied and Environmental Microbiology*, 65, 5522-31.

Haller, M. Y., Muller, S. R., McArdell, C. S., Alder, A. C. and Suter, M. 2001. Quantification of veterinary antibiotics (sulfonamids and trimethoprim) in animal manure by liquid chromatography-mass spectrometry. *Journal of Chromatography*, A 952, 111-120.

Halling-Sørensen, B. 2001. Inhibition of aerobic growth and nitrification of bacteria in sewage sludge by antibacterial agents. *Archives of Environmental Contamination and Toxicology*, 40.

Hamscher, G., Pawelzick, H. T., Hoper, H. and Nau, H. 2005. Different behaviour of tetracyclines and sulfonamides in sandy soils after repeated fertilisation with liquid manure. *Environmental Toxicology and Chemistry*, 24, 861-868.

Hamscher, G., Pawelzick, H. T., Sczesny, S., Nau, H. and Hartung, J. 2003. Antibiotics in dust originating from a pig-fattening farm: A new source of health hazard for farmers? *Environmental Health Perspectives*, 111, 1590-1594.

Hamscher, G., Sczesny, S., Höper, H. and Nau, H. 2002. Determination of persistent tetracycline residues in soil fertilized with liquid manure by High-Performance Liquid Chromatography with Electrospray Ionization Tandem Mass Spectrometry. *Analytical Chemistry*, 74, 1509-1518.

Hensel, A. and Helmuth, R. 2005. Aktuelles zur Antibiotika-Resistenz: Das Problem aus veterinärmedizinischer Sicht (News on antibiotic resistance from a veterinarian point of view). *Fortbildung für ÖGD, 16.03.2005.*

Hirsch, R., Ternes, T., Haberer, K. and Kratz, K. L. 1999. Occurrence of antibiotics in the aquatic environment. *Science of the Total Environment*, 225, 109-118.

Holten-Lützøft, H. C., Halling-Sørensen, B. and Jörgensen, S. E. 1999. Algae toxicity of antibacterial agents applied in Danish fish farming. *Archives of Environmental Contamination and Toxicology*, 36, 1-6.

Höper, H., Kues, J., Nau, H. and Hamscher, G. 2002. Eintrag und Verbleib von Tierarzneimittelwirkstoffen in Böden (Input and fate of veterinary medicaments in soils). *Bodenschutz*, 4, 141-148.

Ingerslev, F. and Halling-Sørensen, B. 2000. Biodegradability properties of sulfonamids in acticated sludge. *Environmental Toxicology and Chemistry*, 19, 2467-2473.

Ingerslev, F. and Halling-Sørensen, B. 2001. Biodegradability of metronidazole, olaquindox, and tylosin and formation of tylosin degradation products in aerobic soil-manure-slurries. *Ecotoxicology and Environmental Safety*, 48, 311-320.

Jjemba, P. K. 2002. The potential impact of veterinary and human therapeutic agents in manure and biosolids on plants grown on arable land: a review. *Agriculture, Ecosystems and Environment*, 93, 267-278.

Jørgensen, S. E. and Halling-Sørensen, B. 2000. Drugs in the environment. *Chemosphere*, 40, 691-699.

Juhel-Gaugain, M., McEvoy, J. D. and van Ginkel, L. A. 2000. Measurements for certification of chlortetracycline reference materials within the European Union: standards, measurements and testing programme. *Fresenius' Journal of Analytical Chemistry*, 368, 656-663.

Kaspar, C. W., Burgess, J. L., Knight, I. T. and Colwell, R. R. 1990. Antibiotic resistance indexing of Escherichia coli to identify sources of fecal contamination in water. *Canadian Journal of Microbiology*, 36, 891-894.

Kay, P., Blackwell, P. A. and Boxall, A. B. A. 2005. Transport of veterinary antibiotics in overland flow following the application of slurry to arable land. *Chemosphere*, 59, 951-959.

Kemper, N. 2007. Tiergesundheit und Antibiotika-Rückstände in der Milchviehhaltung (Animal health and antibiotic residues in dairy husbandry). In: *Ergebnisse des Projekts "Compass"* (Ed. by Taube, F. and Kelm, M.). Kiel: CAU Kiel.

Kemper, N. 2008. Veterinary antibiotics in the aquatic and terrestrial environment. *Ecological Indicators*, 8, 1-13.

Kemper, N., Färber, H., Skutlarek, D. and Krieter, J. 2008. Analysis of antibiotic residues in liquid manure and leachate of dairy farms in Northern Germany. *Agricultural Water Management*, 95, 1288-1292.

Kolpin, D., Furlong, E., Meyer, M., Thurman, E., Zaugg, S., Barber, L. and Buxton, H. 2002. Pharmaceuticals, hormones, and other organic wastewater contaminants in U.S. streams, 1999-2000: a national reconnaissance. *Environmental Science and Technology*, 36, 1202-1211.

Krapac, I. G., Koike, S., Meyer, M. T., Snow, D. D., Chou, S. F. J., Mackie, R. I., Roy, W. R. and Chee-Sandford, J. C. 2005. Long-term monitoring of the occurrence of antibiotic residues and antibiotic resistance in groundwater near swine confinement facilities. *Report of the CSREES Project 2001-35102-10774*.

Kümmerer, K. 2001a. Drugs in the environment: emission of drugs, diagnostic aids and disinfectants into wastewater by hospitals in relation to other sources - a review. *Chemosphere*, 45, 957-969.

Kümmerer, K. 2001b. Pharmaceuticals in the environment: sources, fate, effects and risks. Berlin: Springer.

Kümmerer, K. 2003. Significance of antibiotics in the environment. *Journal of Antimicrobial Chemotherapy*, 52, 5-7.

Kümmerer, K., Al-Ahmad, A. and Mersch-Sundermann, V. 2000. Biodegradability of some antibiotics, elimination of the genotoxicity and affection of wastewater bacteria in a simple test. *Chemosphere*, 40, 701-710.

Langhammer, J. P. 1989. Untersuchungen zum Verbleib antimikrobiell wirksamer Arzneistoff-Rückstände in Gülle und im landwirtschaftlichen Umfeld (Examination on the fate of antimicrobials in manure and in the agricultural environment). Dissertation, Bonn: Universität.

Lee, M. H., Lee, H. J. and Ryu, P. D. 2001. Public health risks: Chemical and antibiotic residues - Review. *Asian-Australasian Journal of Animal Sciences*, 14, 402-413.

Levy, S. B. 1997. Antibiotic reistance: an ecological imbalance. In: *Antibiotic resistance: origins, evolution, selection and spread* (Ed. by Levy, S. B., Goode, J. and Chadwick, D. J.), pp. 1-9. New York: John Wiley and Sons.

Lindsey, M. E., Meyer, M. and Thurman, E. M. 2001. Analysis of trace levels of sulfonamide and tetracycline antimicrobials, in groundwater and surface water using solid-phase extraction and liquid chromatography/mass spectrometry. *Analytical Chemistry*, 73, 4640-4646.

Loke, L., Hallig-Sørensen, B. and Tjørnelund, J. 2002. Determination of the distribution coefficient (log Kd) of oxytetracycline, tylosin A, olaquindox and metronidazole in manure. *Chemosphere*, 48, 351-361.

Lorenz, M. G. and Wackernagel, W. 1994. Bacterial gene transfer by natural genetic transformation in the environment. *Microbiological Reviews*, 58, 563-602.

Luber, P., Wagner, J., Hahn, H. and Bartelt, E. 2003. Antimicrobial resistance in Campylobacter jejuni and Campylobacter coli strains isolated in 1991 and 2001-2002 from poultry and humans in Berlin, Germany. *Antimicrobial Agents and Chemotherapy*, 47, 3825-30.

MacKie, R. I., Koike, S., Krapac, I., Chee-Sanford, J., Maxwell, S. and Aminov, R. I. 2006. Tetracycline residues and tetracycline resistance genes in groundwater impacted by swine production facilities. *Animal Biotechnology*, 17, 157-176.

Marengo, J., Kok, R., OBrien, K., Velagaleti, R. and Stamm, J. 1997. Aerobic biodegredation of 14C-sarafloxacin hydrochloride in soil. *Environmental Toxicology and Chemistry*, 16, 462-471.

Martinez, J. L. 2008. Antibiotics and antibiotic resistance genes in natural environments. *Science*, 321, 365-367.

McDermott, P., Walker, R. and White, D. 2003. Antimicrobials: modes of action and mechanisms of resistance. *International Journal of Toxicology*, 22, 135-143.

Mellon, M., Benbrook, C. and Benbrook, K. L. 2001. Estimates of antimicrobial abuse in livestock. *UCS Food and Environment Program*.

Meyer, M. T., Bumgarner, J. E., Thurman, E. M., Hostetler, K. A. and Daughtridge, J. V. 1999. Occurrence of antibiotics in liquid waste at confined animal feeding operations and in surface and groundwater. In: *20th Meeting of the Society of Environmental Toxicology and Chemistry*, pp. 13-14. Philadelphia.

Meyer, M. T., Denver, J. M., Landy, R. B. and Bumgarner, J. E. 2003. Antibiotics in litter, stream sediment, and ambient water from poultry feeding operations. In: *24th Meeting of the Society for Environmental Toxicology and Chemistry*, pp. 48. Austin.

Montforts. 2003. Environmental risk assessment for veterinary medicinal products. *RIVM report 320202001/2003*, 1-88.

Morris, A. K. and Masterton, R. G. 2002. Antibiotic resistance surveillance: action for international studies. *The Journal of Antimicrobial Chemotherapy*, 49, 7-10.

Mückter, H. 2006. Antibiotika-Rückstände im Trinkwasser (Antibiotica residues in drinking water). In: *47. Arbeitstagung des Arbeitsgebiets Lebensmittelhygiene*. Garmisch-Patenkirchen.

Myllyniemi, A. L., Ranikko, R., Lindfors, E. and Niemi, A. 2000. Microbiological and chemical detection of incurred penicillin G, oxytetracycline, enrofloxacin and ciprofloxacin residues in bovine and porcine tissues. *Food Additives and Contaminants*, 17, 991-1000.

National Committee for Clinical Laboratory Standards. 2002. Performance standards for antimicrobial disk and dilution susceptibility tests for bacteria isolated from animals - Second Edition: Approved Standards M31-A2. Villanova, USA: NCCLS.

Niessen, W. M. A. 1998. Analysis of antibiotics by liquid chromatography mass spectrometry. *Journal of Chromatography*, A 812, 53-75.

Nwosu, V. C. 2001. Antibiotic resistance with particular reference to soil microorganisms. *Research in Microbiology*, 152, 421-430.

Nygaard, K., Lunestad, B. T., Hektoen, H., Berge, J. A. and Hormazabal, V. 1992. Resistance to oxytetracycline, oxolinic acid and furazolidone in bacteria from marine sediments. *Aquaculture*, 104, 21-36.

Ochmann, H., Lawrence, J. G. and Groisman, E. A. 2000. Lateral gene transfer and the nature of bacterial innovation. *Nature*, 405, 299-304.

Oka, H., Ito, Y. and Matsumoto, H. 2000. Chromatographic analysis of tetracycline antibiotics in foods. *Journal of Chromatography*, B 693, 337-344.

Olsen, S. J., DeBess, E. E., McGivern, T. E., Marano, N., Eby, T., Mauvais, S., Balan, V. K., Zirnstein, G., Cieslak, P. R. and Angulo, F. J. 2001. A nosocomial outbreak of fluoroquinolone-resistant salmonella infection. *The New England Journal of Medicine*, 344, 1572-9.

Onan, L. J. and LaPara, T. M. 2003. Tylosin-resistant bacteria cultivated from agricultural soil. *Fems Microbiology Letters*, 220, 15-20.

Pedersen, J., Yeager, M. and Suffet, I. 2003. Xenobiotic organic compounds in runoff from fields irrigated with treated wastewater. *Journal of Agricultural and Food Chemistry*, 51, 1360-1372.

Perreten, V., Schwarz, F., Cresta, L., Boeglin, M., Dasen, G. and Teuber, M. 1997. Antibiotic resistance spread in food. *Nature*, 389, 801-802.

Phillips, I., Casewell, M., Cox, T., De Groot, B., Friis, C., Jones, R., Nightingale, C., Preston, R. and Waddell, J. 2004. Does the use of antibiotics in food animals pose a risk to human health? A critical review of published data. *Journal of Antimicrobial Chemotherapy*, 53, 28-52.

Pillai, S. D., Widmer, K. W., Maciorowski, K. G. and Ricke, S. C. 1997. Antibiotic resistance profiles of Escherichia coli isolated from rural and urban environments. *Journal of Environmental Science and Health. Part A, Toxic/Hazardous Substances and Environmental Engineering*, 32 1665-1675.

Rabølle, M. and Spliid, N. 2000. Sorption and mobility of metronidazole, olaquindox, oxytetracycline and tylosin in soil. *Chemosphere*, 40, 715-722.

Rice, L. B. 2001. Emergence of vancomycin-resistant enterococci. *Emerging Infectious Diseases*, 7, 183-187.

Richter, A., Löscher, W. and Witte, W. 1996. Leistungsförderer mit antibakterieller Wirkung: Probleme aus pharmakologisch-toxikologischer und mikrobiologischer Sicht (Antimicrobial growth promoters: problems from a pharmacological and microbiological point of view). *Praktischer Tierarzt*, 7, 603-624.

Rooklidge, S. J. 2004. Environmental antimicrobial contamination from terraccumulation and diffuse pollution pathways. *The Science of the Total Environment*, 325, 1-13.

Sacher, F., Lange, F. T., Brauch, H. J. and Blankenhorn, I. 2001. Pharmaceuticals in groundwaters. Analytical methods and results of a monitoring program in Baden-Wurttemberg, Germany. *Journal of Chromatography*, 938, 199-210.

Samuelsen, O. B., Torsvik, V. and Ervik, A. 1992. Long-range changes in oxytetracycline concentration and bacterial resistance towards oxytetracycline in a fish farm sediment after medication. *The Science of the Total Environment*, 114, 25-36.

Sarmah, A. K., Meyer, M. T. and Boxall, A. B. A. 2006. A global perspective on the use, sales, exposure pathways, occurrence, fate and effects of veterinary antibiotics (VAs) in the environment. *Chemosphere*, 65, 725-759.

Schauder, S. 1989. Gefahren durch Olanquindox: Photoallergie, chronisch photosensitive Dermatitis und extrem gesteigerte Lichtempfindlichkeit beim Menschen, Hypoaldosteronismus beim Schwein (Risks of Olanquindox: photoallergy, chronic photosensitive dermatitis and extremely increased light sensibility in humans, hypoaldosteronism in pigs). *Dermatosen*, 37, 183-185.

Schüller, S. 1998. Anwendung antibiotisch wirksamer Substanzen beim Tier und Beurteilung der Umweltsicherheit entsprechender Produkte (Application of antibiotic substances in animals and evaluation of environmental safety of products). In: *3. Statuskolloquium ökotoxikologischer Forschungen in der Euregio Bodensee, 3 - 4 December 1998.*

Schwake-Anduschus, C., Nettmann, E., Betsche, T., Langenkämper, G., Freitag, M. and Grote, M. 2003. Untersuchungen zur Aufnahme von Veterinärpharmaka verschiedener Nutzpflanzen über die Wurzeln (Analyses of veterinary pharmaceuticals intake in different crop plants via the roots). In: *Tagung "Gesunde Umwelt für gesunde Pflanzen", 9.-10.10.2003.* FAL Braunschweig.

Sengeløv, G., Agersø, Y., Hallig-Sørensen, B., Baloda, S. B., Andersen, J. S. and Jensen, L. B. 2003. Bacterial antibiotic resistance levels in Danish farmland as a result of treatment with pig manure slurry. *Environment International*, 28, 587-595.

Senok, A., Yousif, A., Mazi, W., Sharaf, E., Bindayna, K., Elnima el, A. and Botta, G. 2007. Pattern of antibiotic susceptibility in Campylobacter jejuni isolates of human and poultry origin. *Japanese Journal of Infectious Diseases*, 60, 1-4.

Seveno, N. A., Kallifidas, D., Smalla, K., van Elsas, J. D., Collard, J. M., Karagouni, A. D. and Wellington, E. M. H. 2002. Occurrrence and reservoirs of antibiotic resistance genes in the environment. *Reviews in Medical Microbiology*, 13, 15-27.

Smalla, K., Heuer, H., Gotz, A., Niemeyer, D., Krogerrerecklenfort, E. and Tietze, E. 2000. Exogenous isolation of antibiotioc resistance plasmids from piggery manure slurries reveals a high prevalence and diversity of IncQ-like plasmids. *Applied and Environmental Microbiology*, 66, 4854-4862.

Smalla, K. and Sobecky, P. A. 2002. The prevalence and diversity of mobile genetic elements in bacterial communities of different environmental habitats: insights gained from different methodological approaches. *FEMS Microbiology Ecology*, 42, 165-175.

Swann Committee. 1969. Report of Joint Committee on the Use of Antibiotics in Animal Husbandry and Veterinary Medicine. London: Her Majesty's Stationary Office.

Teuber, M. 1999. Spread of antibiotic resistance with food-borne pathogens. *Cellular and Molecular Life Sciences*, 56, 755-763.

Teuber, M., Meile, L. and Schwarz, F. 1999. Acquired antibiotic resistance in lactic acid bacteria from food. *Antonie van Leeuwenhoek*, 76, 115-137.

The Council of the European Union. 2002. Council Recommendations of 15 November 2001 on the Prudent Use of Antimicrobial Agents in Human Medicine (Text with EEA relevance). Brussels, Belgium: 2002/77/EC 5 February.

Thiele-Bruhn, S. 2003. Pharmaceutical antibiotic compounds in soils - a review. *Journal of Plant Nutrition Soil Science*, 166, 145-167.

Tolls, J. 2001. Sorption of veterinary pharmaceuticals in soils: A review. *Environmental Science and Technology*, 35, 3397-3406.

Ungemach, F. 2000. Figures on quantities of antibacterials used for different purposes in the EU countries and interpretation. *Acta Veterinaria Scandinavica Supplementum*, 93, 89-97.

Union of concerned scientists. 2001. *70 Percent of all antibiotics given to healthy livestock*. Cambridge, MA, USA: Press release, 8 January.

Van den Bogaard, A. E., London, N. and Stobberingh, E. E. 2000. Antimicrobial resistance in pig faecal samples from the Netherlands (five abbatoirs) and Sweden. *Journal of Antimicrobial Chemotherapy*, 45, 663-671.

van den Bogaard, A. E. and Stobberingh, E. E. 1999. Antibiotic usage in animals - Impact on bacterial resistance and public health. *Drugs*, 58, 589-607.

VICH. 2000. Environmental impact assessments (EIAs) for veterinary medical products (VMPs): Phase I. www:\\vich.eudra.org.

Wegener, H. C. 2003. Antibiotics in animal feed and their role in resistance development. *Current Opinion in Microbiology*, 6, 439-445.

Wegener, H. C., Aarestrup, F. M., Jensen, J. B., Hammerum, A. M. and Bager, F. 1996. The association between the use of antimicrobial growth promoters and development of resistance in pathogenic bacteria towards growth promoting and therapeutic antimicrobials. *Journal of Animal Feed Science*, 7, 7-14.

White, D., Zhao, S., Simjee, S., Wagner, D. and McDermott, P. 2002. Antimicrobial resistance of foodborne pathogens. *Microbes and Infections*, 4, 405-412.

Wiggins, B. A. 1996. Discriminant analysis of antibiotic resistance patterns in fecal streptococci, a method to differentiate human and animal sources of fecal pollution in natural waters. *Applied and Environmental Microbiology*, 62, 3997-4002.

Wiggins, B. A., Andrews, R. W., Conway, R. A., Corr, C. L., Dobratz, E. J., Dougherty, D. P., Eppard, J. R., Knupp, S. R., Limjoco, M. C., Mettenburg, J. M., Rinehardt, J. M., Sonsino, J., Torrijos, R. L. and Zimmerman, M. E. 1999. Use of antibiotic resistance analysis to identify nonpoint sources of fecal pollution. *Applied and Environmental Microbiology*, 65, 3483-6.

Winckler, C. and Grafe, A. 2000. Stoffeintrag durch Tierarzneimittel und pharmakologisch wirksame Futterzusatzstoffe unter besonderer Berücksichtigung von Tetrazyklinen (Input of veterinary medicaments and food pharmaceuticals with special emphasis on tetracycline) . Berlin: UBA-Texte 44/0.

Winckler, C. and Grafe, A. 2001. Use of veterinary drugs in intensive animal production: evidence for persistence of tetracyclines in pig slurry. *Journal of Soils and Sediments*, 1, 66-70.

Witte, W. 1998. Medical consequences of antibiotic use in agriculture. *Science* 279, 996-997.

Witte, W. 2000. Selective pressure by antibiotics use in livestock. *International Journal of Antimicrobial Agents*, 19-24.

Wollenberger, L., Halling-Sørensen, B. and Kusk, K. O. 2000. Acute and chronic toxicity of veterinary antibiotics to Daphnia magna. *Chemosphere*, 40, 723-730.

World Health Organisation. 2001. Monitoring antimicrobial usage in food animals for protection of human health. (Ed. by WHO/CDS/CSR/EPH/2002.11), pp. 21. Oslo, Norway: Report of WHO consultation

World Health Organisation. 1997. The medical impact of the use of antimicrobials in food animals. Berlin, Germany: Report of a WHO meeting.

Zhu, J., Snow, D., Cassada, D. A., Monson, S. J. and Spalding, R. F. 2001. Analysis of oxytetracycline, tetracycline, and chlortetracycline in water using Solid Phase Extraction and Liquid Chromatography-Tandem Mass Spectrometry. *Journal of Chromatography*, A 928, 177-86.

Zuccato, E., Bagnati, R., Fioretti, F., Natangelo, M., Calamari, D. and Fanelli, R. 2001. Environmental loads and detection of pharmaceuticals in Italy. In: *Pharmaceuticals in the Environment-Sources, Fate, Effects and Risks* (Ed. by Kümmerer, K.), pp. 19-27. Berlin: Springer.

Index

B

D

E

F

G

I

M

S

T

U

V